Social Behavior and Skills in Children

Johnny L. Matson

Editor

Social Behavior and Skills in Children

in Children

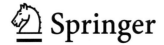

Editor
Johnny L. Matson
Department of Psychology
Louisiana State University
Baton Rouge, LA 70803
USA
johnmatson@aol.com

ISBN 978-1-4419-0233-7   e-ISBN 978-1-4419-0234-4
DOI 10.1007/978-1-4419-0234-4
Springer New York Dordrecht Heidelberg London

Library of Congress Control Number: 2009931923

Printed on acid-free paper

Springer is part of Springer Science+Business Media (www.springer.com)

Contents

Contributors

Jessica A. Boisjoli Department of Psychology, Louisiana State University, Baton Rouge, LA 70803, USA, jessicaboisjoli@gmail.com

Thompson E. Davis III Department of Psychology, Louisiana State University, Baton Rouge, LA 70803, USA, ted@lsu.edu

Timothy Dempsey Department of Psychology, Louisiana State University, Baton Rouge, LA 70803, USA, tdempsey82@hotmail.com

Dennis R. Dixon Manager, Research and Development, Center for Autism and Related Disorders, Inc., Tarzana, CA 91356, USA, d.dixon@centerforautism.com

Greg E. Everett Department of Psychology, Southern Illinois University-Edwardsville, Edwardsville, IL 62026, USA, geveret@siue.edu

Jill C. Fodstad Department of Psychology, Louisiana State University, Baton Rouge, LA 70803, USA, jcwill482@gmail.com

Patricia H. Hawley Department of Psychology, The University of Kansas, Lawrence, KS 66045-7556, phawley@ku.edu

Stephen D.A. Hupp Department of Psychology, Southern Illinois University-Edwardsville, Edwardsville, IL 62026, USA, sthupp@siue.edu

Allison Jack Department of Psychology, University of Virginia, Charlettesville, VA 22904-4404, USA, ajack@virginia.edu

Jeremy D. Jewell Department of Psychology, Southern Illinois University-Edwardsville, Edwardsville, IL 62026, USA, jejewel@siue.edu

Sara S. Jordan The University of Southern Mississippi, Hattiesburg, MS, USA, sara.jordan@usm.edu

Tra Ladner Northlake Supports and Services Center, Tucker, GA, USA, tladner@dhh.la.gov

Giulio E. Lancioni Department of Psychology, University of Bari, Bari, Italy, g.lancioni@psico.uniba.it

Monique LeBlanc Department of Psychology, Southeastern Louisiana University, Hammond, Louisiana, 70402, USA, monique.leblanc@selu.edu

Matthew D. Lerner Department of Psychology, University of Virginia, Charlettesville, VA 22904-4404, USA, mdlbe@virginia.edu

Rebecca Mandal-Blasio Louisiana Office for Citizens with Developmental Disabilities, Resource Center on Psychiatric and Behavior Supports, Hammond, LA 70401, USA, rmandal@dhh.la.gov

Johnny L. Matson Department of Psychology, Louisiana State University, Baton Rouge, LA 70803, USA, johnmatson@aol.com

Melissa Middleton Department of Psychology, University of Central Florida, Orlando, FL 32816, USA, mamiddle@gmail.com

Amori Yee Mikami Department of Psychology, University of Virginia, Charlettesville, VA 22904-4404, USA, mikami@virginia.edu

Melissa S. Munson Department of Psychology, Louisiana State University, Baton Rouge, LA 70803, USA, mmunson15@gmail.com

Adel Najdowski Manager, Research and Development, Center for Autism and Related Disorders, Inc., Tarzana, CA 91356, USA, a.najdowski@centerforautism.com

Mark F. O'Reilly University of Texas at Austin, Austin, TX, USA, markoreilly@mail.utexas.edu

Jacklyn M. Ratliff Department of Psychology, The University of Kansas, Lawrence, KS 66045-7556, jratliff@ku.edu

Kimberly Renk Department of Psychology, University of Central Florida, Orlando, FL 32816, USA, krenk@ucf.edu

Tessa T. Rivet Department of Psychology, Louisiana State University, Baton Rouge, LA 70803, USA, tessatr@gmail.com

George Schreiner Nortlake Supports and Services Center, Hammond, LA 70401, gschreiner@dhh.la.gov

Samantha Scott Department of Psychology, University of Central Florida, Orlando, FL 32816, USA, ssammie11@hotmail.com

Karen Sheridan Louisiana Office for Citizens with Developmental Disabilities, Resource Center on Psychiatric and Behavior Supports, Hammond, LA 70401, USA, ksherida@dhh.la.gov

Jeff Sigafoos Victoria University of Wellington, Wellington, NZ, USA, jeff.sigafoos@vuw.ac.nt

Nirbhay N. Singh ONE Research Institute, Midlothian, VA, USA, nirbsingh52@aol.com

Kathryn N. Stump Department of Psychology, The University of Kansas, Lawrence, KS 66045-7556, knstump@ku.edu

Jonathan Tarbox Manager, Research and Development, Center for Autism and Related Disorders, Inc., Tarzana, CA 91356, USA, j.tarbox@centerforautism.com

Erin V. Tarcza Department of Psychology, Louisiana State University, Baton Rouge, LA 70803, USA, evtarcza@gmail.com

Emily Warnes Pediatric Associates of Iowa City and Coralville, Iowa City, IA 52245, USA, emwarnes@yahoo.com

Rachel Wolfe Department of Psychology, University of Central Florida, Orlando, FL 32816, USA, rachel.wolfe.white@gmail.com

Yelena P. Wu Department of Psychology, The University of Kansas, Lawrence, KS 66045-7556, yelenawu@ku.edu

Chapter 1
History and Overview

Stephen D.A. Hupp, Monique LeBlanc, Jeremy D. Jewell, and Emily Warnes

Introduction

Generally speaking, friendships in childhood are associated with positive outcomes and being disliked is associated with negative outcomes (Parker & Asher, 1987). More specifically, social skills have been linked to academic achievement, psychological adjustment, coping skills, and employment (Miles & Stipek, 2006). Conversely, social skills deficits and maladaptive social behaviors are an integral part of the diagnostic criteria of a variety of disorders within the *Diagnostic and Statistical Manual of Mental Disorders-Fourth Edition, Text Revision* (DSM-IV-TR; American Psychiatric Association, 2000). Social problems are also used to demonstrate the impairment in social functioning that is considered for most diagnoses. Research involving social behavior has included many definitional inconsistencies; thus there have been many attempts to define and conceptualize social behavior in children and adolescents. In this chapter we will review basic definitions and conceptualizations of social behavior. This chapter will also provide a broad overview of the assessment and treatment of social problems.

Conceptualization of Social Behavior

Basic Definitions

By integrating the core concepts of several definitions of *social skills*, Merrell and Gimpel (1998) offer a comprehensive definition, suggesting that "... social skills are learned, composed of specific behaviors, include initiations and responses, maximize social reinforcement, are interactive and situation-specific, and can be specified as targets for intervention" (p. 5). This definition conceptualizes social skills as adaptive behaviors, whereas the failure to use social skills has been commonly described as *social skill deficits*. Additionally, *behavioral excesses* can have an effect on social skills deficits. That is, Gresham, Van, and Cook (2006) describe competing problem behaviors that often interfere with the social skill development. For example, some externalizing behavioral excesses (e.g., aggression) are often effective at gaining social reinforcement, and some internalizing behavioral excesses (e.g., depressive statements) can also be reinforced by social attention. Importantly, some behavioral excesses may not necessarily have a social function but also interfere with social development. Taken together, social skills and behavioral excesses (with social implications) can be characterized as types of *social behavior*. That is, social behaviors include both adaptive social skills and the other behaviors that influence social functioning.

In another important distinction, McFall (1982) emphasizes the difference between social skills and *social competence*. McFall conceptualizes social skills as specific behaviors needed to perform a

S.D.A. Hupp (✉)
Department of Psychology, Southern Illinois University Edwardsville, Edwardsville, IL 62026, USA
e-mail: sthupp@siue.edu

J.L. Matson (ed.), *Social Behavior and Skills in Children*, DOI 10.1007/978-1-4419-0234-4_1,
© Springer Science+Business Media, LLC 2009

task competently. On the other hand, *social competence* is a more general and evaluative term. In this framework, a person is judged to be socially competent when he or she exhibits adequate performance on a particular social task. McFall cautions against trait-based approaches to social competence, noting that social competence does not reside within a person and also suggesting that competence in one social situation does not signify that a child will be socially competent in all situations. Individual social skills contribute to overall social competence; however, no single behavior is sufficient for competence. Gresham and Elliott (1987) also place social skills under the broader construct of social competence, suggesting that social competence includes both social skills and other adaptive behaviors (e.g., independent functioning, physical development, self-direction, personal responsibility, and functional academic skills). Vaughn and Hogan (1990) identify four components of social competence: effective social skills, absence of maladaptive behavior, positive relations with others, and accurate social cognition. Similarly, Cavell (1990) presents a tri-component model of social competence. At the top of the hierarchy, *social adjustment* is defined as meeting important developmental goals, such as peer status and familial cohesion. *Social performance* is defined as the extent to which social responses meet socially valid criteria or the adequacy of behavior within a particular and relevant social situation. Lastly, *social skills* are the specific abilities that allow competent performance of social situations, including overt behavior, social cognitive skills, and emotional regulation.

In a further attempt to integrate several definitions of social skills and social competence, Gresham (1986) identifies three types of definitions related to social behavior: peer acceptance, behavioral, and social validity. In the *peer acceptance* definition, children are determined to be socially skilled if they are rated as popular or accepted by peers. These definitions appear throughout early work in the 1970s and 1980s (e.g., Asher, Markell, & Hymel, 1981) and are based upon sociometric assessment of peer acceptance status (Elliott & Gresham, 1987; Rose-Krasnor, 1997). This type of definition has some predictive validity, as research has linked peer rejection with negative outcomes, such as delinquent behavior (Rose-Krasnor, 1997).

On the other hand, one problem with this conceptual approach is that the particular social behaviors which lead to peer acceptance are not specified, limiting treatment utility (Bierman & Welsh, 2000; Gresham, 2002; Nangle, Erdley, Carpenter, & Newman, 2002).

The second definition involves describing social skills with *behavioral* terms. Using behavioral definitions, social skills are considered to be situation-specific behaviors that are more likely to be reinforced and less likely to be punished (Elliott & Gresham, 1987; Gresham, 1986). This type of definition is typically used in the behavior therapy and applied behavior analysis literatures (Gresham, 2002). Regarding measurement, researchers utilizing behavioral definitions of social skills most often conduct observations of behavior in specific settings. Behavioral definitions appear to have advantages over peer acceptance definitions because specific antecedents, behaviors, and consequences can be defined and targeted for treatment (Elliott & Gresham, 1987). However, Gresham (2002) indicates that behavioral definitions are also limited as there is no mechanism to ensure that the targeted social skills are socially significant or related to socially important outcomes. That is, behaviors which are selected by researchers or clinicians may not be associated with important outcomes because behaviors are often identified intuitively rather than empirically (Gresham & Elliott, 1984; Matthys, Maassen, Cuperus, & van Engeland, 2001).

The third approach includes *social validity* definitions, which address the limitations of the first two types of definitions (Gresham, 1986; 2002). With this approach, social skills are defined as specific behaviors that are predictive of important social outcomes for children in particular situations (Gresham & Elliott, 1984). Important social outcomes may include acceptance by others (e.g., peers, teachers, & parents), school adjustment, and psychological adjustment (Elliott & Gresham, 1987; Gresham, 2002). Walker, Colvin, and Ramsey (1995) add that social skills are behaviors that assist the child in coping with and adapting to increasingly demanding social environments. Social validity definitions include an evaluative component in which significant others determine whether an outcome is important. Using this type of definition, assessment of social skills includes observations of behavior, sociometric ratings, and ratings by others. Behaviors targeted for treatment are chosen due to their associative relationship with socially valuable goals. Thus, the social validity approach makes an explicit link between social skills and social competence. A possible weakness of this approach is that behaviors viewed as socially valid can be culturally biased or biased in other ways (Rose-Krasnor, 1997).

As in most areas, consideration of social validity is needed when defining, assessing, and treating social skills in children (Lane, Beebe-Frankenberger, Lambros, & Pierson, 2001). Social validity has been described as a multidimensional construct with three levels: social significance, social importance, and social acceptability (Wolf, 1978; Gresham, 1986). When considering the *social significance* dimension of validity, a clinician would ask: Is this social skill significant, related to a valued societal goal, and considered necessary by the child's significant others? Social significance often involves the subjective judgment of someone important to the child, such as parents, teachers, and other important individuals in the child's environment. In the *socially important* dimension of validity, a clinician would ask: Does the social skill predict important social outcomes, make a difference in the child's functioning in society, and have practical significance? Socially important outcomes are subjective in nature and have been traditionally assessed through sociometric ratings by peers and teachers as well as parent ratings of behavior (Gresham, 1986). In the *social acceptability* dimension of validity, a clinician would ask: Is the social skills intervention acceptable to others? That is, social acceptability generally involves the degree to which consumers like the psychological treatments that are offered (Witt & Elliott, 1986). Only accepted treatments will be used and implemented with integrity, resulting in long-term social skills changes (Lane et al., 2001; Witt & Elliott, 1986).

Social Skills Classification and Domains

One approach to classification of social skills focuses on the type of social skills deficit. Following a social learning theory (Bandura, 1977) of social

skills deficits, these deficits are conceptualized as problems in acquiring or in performing social behaviors (Gresham, 1981; Gresham & Elliott, 1989). More specifically, Gresham (1998; 2002) describes three types of social skills deficits. First, *acquisition deficits* involve the lack of particular social skills. That is, in an acquisition deficit, the child does not know how to perform the targeted social skill, regardless of the social situation. This type of deficit is often described as a "can't do" problem. Social skills interventions for acquisition deficits involve teaching the child the targeted social skill, thereby adding the skills to the child's behavioral repertoire. Second, *performance deficits* involve knowing how to perform a social skill without exhibiting it appropriately. A performance deficit is often described as a "won't do" problem. That is, the child is failing to exhibit the desired behavior in the appropriate situation despite the presence of the skill in the child's behavioral repertoire. An appropriate target for treatment would then involve prompting or reinforcing the appropriate use of the behavior. Finally, *fluency deficits* describe an acquired skill that is being used in an awkward manner. The child may have had insufficient modeling or opportunities to exhibit and practice the behavior; therefore, social skills training could involve increasing opportunities to practice the skill and build fluency. One major advantage of this classification approach is that it provides a clear pathway from assessment to treatment based on each type of deficit (Gresham & Elliott, 1989; Gresham, 2002). Additionally, this deficit model is enhanced by also considering the behavioral excesses that may be interfering with social skill development.

In another conceptualization, McFall (1982) argues for an empirically derived taxonomy based on the type of social situations. The development of a classification system which adequately captures the complexity of social skills, while also facilitating communication amongst clinicians and researchers, has been the focus of some empirical study. One early approach includes the development of the Taxonomy of Problematic Social Situations for Children (TOPS; Dodge, McClaskey, & Feldman, 1985), which is a teacher-rating scale developed and validated with a fifth grade sample. This scale identifies social skills problems in six different social situations: peer group entry, response to provocations, response to failure, response to success, social expectations, and teacher expectations. A more recent investigation of the measure in school-age Dutch children found a four-factor model including being disadvantaged, coping with competition, social expectations of peers, and teacher expectations (Matthys et al., 2001).

Caldarella and Merrell (1997) utilize a behavioral dimensions approach to construct a taxonomy of child and adolescent social skills. They describe the behavioral dimensions approach as using statistical techniques to derive clusters of highly correlated behaviors. For the study, they located 21 empirically based dimensional research studies of social skills in children and adolescents conducted from 1974 to 1994. These studies involved more than 22,000 children and adolescents, with the majority utilizing teacher ratings of children (aged 3–6 years). Caldarella and Merrell identify five dimensions of social skill. First, the *peer relations* dimension involves positive peer behaviors, such as giving compliments, offering help, and inviting others to play. Second, the *self-management skills* dimension includes behaviors such as controlling temper, following rules, and compromising. Third, *academic skills* are behaviors related to being productive in independent classroom settings, such as accomplishing tasks independently, completing individual seatwork, and listening to teacher directions. Fourth, *compliance* involves behaviors related to complying with social rules, such as appropriately using free time and sharing. Finally, the *assertion skills* dimension includes behaviors such as initiating conversations, acknowledging compliments, and making friends.

As suggested by Caldarella and Merrell (1997), this approach can be useful for design and evaluation of social skills interventions by providing a common framework for researchers and clinicians. The authors also note that understanding positive social behaviors expands the focus of researchers and clinicians away from a pathological perspective of child development to a more health-based approach. This can be related to social validity as increasing the emphasis of positive behaviors may lead to more meaningful intervention efforts. Key limitations to the Caldarella and Merrell study include overreliance on research with younger children and overreliance on teacher reports.

Assessment of Social Skills

Traditional Assessment of Social Skills

Social skills assessment has traditionally focused on identifying individual social deficiencies within a child and evaluating treatment outcomes (Sheridan & Walker, 1999). Researchers and practitioners have used a variety of methods by which to assess children's social skills. One of the most common assessment techniques includes using the evaluations of others (e.g., ratings and reports from peers, teachers, and parents). Rating scales are one way that information can be gathered from others in a child's environment (Elliott & Busse, 1991; Merrell & Gimpel, 1998; Sheridan & Walker, 1999). These scales require teachers and/or parents to rate children on a number of specified criteria. In addition to providing information about a child's individual social behaviors, many of these scales are standardized and allow for a comparison of the child's behavior to that of a same-age norm group.

Teacher nominations and rankings comprise an additional evaluative assessment of a child's social skills (Elliott & Busse, 1991; Foster, Inderbitzen & Nangle, 1993; Sheridan & Walker, 1999). Using this technique, teachers are asked to provide a list of students who demonstrate a specific behavioral characteristic to the greatest or least extent in comparison to classmates (e.g., "is the most disruptive"). This allows for a relative comparison of a child's social skills to that of other children in the classroom. Peer ratings and/or nominations (i.e., sociometrics) are conducted in much the same way with peers rating or nominating other children according to specific behavioral characteristics.

Self-report provides information about a child's subjective perceptions of his or her own social competence (Elliott & Busse, 1991; Foster et al., 1993; Merrell & Gimpel, 1998; Sheridan & Walker, 1999). This technique requires that a child report thoughts and opinions about his or her social behaviors and relationships. Children also can be asked to report how they would handle various social situations or interactions. Although self-reports can provide unique information regarding a child's perceptions of his or her social behavior, the subjective nature of this technique precludes criterion-related validity

and as such is not often used as a stand-alone procedure for assessing social competence.

Direct behavioral observation is another method
of assessing a child's social skills (Elliott & Busse,
1991; Foster et al., 1993; Merrell & Gimpel, 1998;
Sheridan & Walker, 1999). Using an observational
coding system that defines specific categories of
behavior, observers can record the behavior of a
child over a period of time. When conducted in a
naturalistic setting, behavioral observation allows
for an understanding of the frequency and range of
social behaviors in the child's repertoire. Behavioral
observation can also be a way to develop hypotheses about the function of the child's behavior in
the environment (e.g., any influential antecedent,
sequential, or consequent conditions that may
maintain or discourage particular social behaviors).

Contextual Approach to Social Skills Assessment

Each of the traditional assessment techniques provides unique information regarding a child's social
skills. Building on this traditional approach, recent
assessment techniques have also focused on contextual factors that impact social functioning (Haring,
1992; Sheridan, Hungelmann, & Maughan, 1999;
Sheridan & Walker, 1999; Warnes, Sheridan,
Geske, & Warnes, 2005). Traditional approaches
tend to provide information regarding the various
behaviors that a child does and does not exhibit.
Therefore, it is assumed that based on this information, interventions can be developed by looking at
excesses and deficits in the child's behavioral repertoire and then teaching appropriate behavioral
adjustments. However, being exclusively focused
on behavioral excesses and deficits to determine
targets for intervention has the potential to over-
look the meaningfulness of various social behaviors
within a given context. Even though new behaviors
may be taught to a child, these behaviors may not be
functional or relevant within that child's social network (Sheridan et al., 1999; Sheridan & Walker,
1999; Warnes et al., 2005).

The limitations of traditional social skills assessment have led to the emergence of a contextual
approach to understanding social competence and

assessing social behaviors. A contextual approach
requires not only consideration of the goals and
motivations of social behavior from the child's perspective but also consideration of the responses of
others in the environment that reinforce or discourage the social behavior of the child (Haring, 1992;
Sheridan & Walker, 1999; Warnes et al., 2005). This
principle can be understood by considering the various settings in which children frequently interact
such as at school and home. Each of these settings
clearly requires different behaviors for appropriate
social functioning as the expectations and normative behavior both vary across home and school
contexts. Children must be able to negotiate the
differences in expectations and demands across settings and behave in a way that adapts to the parameters of the context.

When social skills are meaningful they are more
likely to be reinforced in the child's social context,
and the process of "behavioral entrapment" may
occur whereby newly learned social skills come
under the control of naturally occurring reinforcers
(McConnell, 1987). Within this framework, newly
learned social skills must be naturally reinforced to
generalize to a child's natural environment (Fox &
McEvoy, 1993; McConnell, 1987). When others in
the environment reinforce the social skills being
used, children are more likely to continue to use
the skills on a regular basis. Because parents, teachers, and peers are relevant information sources, it
can be assumed that the social skills identified as
important by these sources may be those that will be
naturally reinforced in the environment.

Sheridan et al. (1999) describe a procedure
designed to gather contextually relevant information regarding the behavior of socially competent
children. With this procedure, teachers, peers, and
independent observers each provide a written list of
behaviors that are deemed important for children's
social competence. In gathering information from
these various sources, specific behaviors could be
identified that correspond to social competence for
a particular group of children within a given context. The identified behaviors would in essence comprise a "template" for social competence. These
authors suggest that this template eventually could
be used to help identify target behaviors for social
skills interventions by comparing the behaviors of
children with social difficulties to those behaviors

on the template. Any behaviors on the template for social competence, but not exhibited by the child, could be targets for intervention.

A similar technique of "template matching" has been suggested as a method for identifying important social skills of children (Hoier & Cone, 1987). In one study, 8- and 9 year-old children participated in a 50-item Q-sort procedure to identify specific behaviors that were critical for being a good friend (Hoier & Cone, 1987). The identified behaviors were described as comprising a "template" of a socially competent child. These "template" behaviors were validated by manipulating the behaviors in nonscripted confederates and assessing the impact of the manipulations on behavioral and sociometric measures from the original subjects involved in the Q-Sort procedure. Results indicated that the template behaviors were preferred and led to increased sociometric ratings of confederate children.

Warnes et al. (2005) expanded the research on contextualized approaches to the assessment of social skills by using a procedure similar to that outlined by Sheridan et al. (1999) to gather information from parents, teachers, and peers regarding the specific behaviors that were important for social competence in second- and fifth-grade children. Results of this study illustrate a wide range of differences and similarities among the types of behaviors reported as important for social competence by parent, teacher, and child reporters within each grade level. Many of the social behaviors identified as important in this study (e.g., empathy, humor, communication about problems) reflect dimensions of social functioning that have not always been consistently assessed through traditional standardized rating scales (Caldarella & Merrell, 1997; Warnes et al., 2005), thus strengthening support for incorporation of a contextualized approach with the traditional methods of social skills assessment.

Applications with Children

Theoretical approaches to social skills interventions can be divided into molecular and process approaches (Gumpel & Golan, 2000). In the *molecular* model, social behaviors are thought to be

responses to social discriminative stimuli and link to form a behavioral chain (Gumpel & David, 2000). Corresponding models of intervention focus upon increasing specific behaviors that would be reinforced in the natural environment. Examples of overt behaviors targeted for intervention would include eye contact, asking questions, smiling, and tone of voice. Under this framework, the original objectives of social skills training were increasing skill acquisition (Gresham, 1997) but were expanded to include promoting skill performance, eliminating competing behaviors, and generalization of treatment gains (Gresham, 2002). Modeling, coaching, behavioral rehearsal, performance feedback, and reinforcement are procedures used to accomplish these objectives (Nangle et al., 2002).

Numerous empirical studies in the 1980s utilized the molecular approach in designing and evaluating social skills training. One limitation of the molecular approach has been problems with the lack of generalization of the skills beyond the treatment setting (Gresham, 1997; Gumpel & David, 2000; Gumpel & Golan, 2000; Hansen, Nangle, & Meyer, 1998). In response, researchers and practitioners were cautioned to provide greater attention to generalization across situations, responses, and time (Gresham, 1998; Mathur & Rutherford, 1996). *Process* models also began to be developed that focused on self-mediated processes that might help increase generalization for some children. Some examples include social problem solving, self-monitoring, and self-reinforcement (Gumpel & Golan, 2000; Hansen et al., 1998). That is, corresponding interventions focus on teaching children general cognitive strategies for social situations (Gumpel & David, 2000; Hansen et al., 1998). Molecular and process models have led to a broad range of individual strategies, combinations of strategies, and entire treatment packages targeting social behavior in children.

Types of Interventions

Operant Techniques

As described by Matson and Fee (1991), some of the earliest attempts at increasing social skills used positive reinforcement strategies, such as token economies, edibles, and social reinforcement, with individuals having intellectual disabilities (Brodsky, 1967; Whitman, Mercurio, & Caponigri, 1970). Whitman, Burish, and Collins (1972) also combined reinforcers with instructions to improve conversational speech. In some of the early research on social behavior, punishment (e.g., social disapproval) was also shown to decrease maladaptive social behavior in individuals with intellectual disabilities (Schutz, Wehman, Renzaglia, & Karan, 1978). Thus, operant approaches first attempted to modify a small number of discrete behaviors with a relatively basic reinforcement approach; however, over time operant techniques became more sophisticated by attempting to modify larger related sets of behavior with important change agents, such as parents, teachers, and other children (Matson & Ollendick, 1988). While operant techniques were often effective at changing social behavior, several limitations became evident when operant techniques were used in isolation. That is, the benefits were often lost when the reinforcer was no longer available. Also, operant techniques were not effective at teaching new skills (Matson & Fee, 1991). Thus, operant techniques were quickly paired with several other strategies in order to facilitate the acquisition of new social skills in a wide range of populations.

Social Skills Training

Social skills training studies that focused on several types of problems in adults emerged in the 1970s, some of which include shyness (Twentyman & McFall, 1975), schizophrenia (Edelstein & Eisler, 1976), alcohol problems (O'Leary, O'Leary, & Donovan, 1976), explosive behavior (Matson & Stephens, 1978), and depression (Wells, Hersen, Bellack, & Himmerelhoch, 1979). During that time, similar approaches were also being used to improve the social behavior of youth evidencing intellectual disabilities (Nietupski & Williams, 1976), social isolation (Oden & Asher, 1977), and conduct problems (Spence & Marzillier, 1979).

The social skills training model of intervention assumes that the child lacks the appropriate social skills and the ensuing intervention attempts to use a variety of teaching techniques to correct this deficit (Nangle et al., 2002). Typically, social skills training procedures attempt to teach the appropriate skills by using some combination of modeling, instructions, rehearsal, feedback, and reinforcement. For example, a typical intervention focused on social greeting behavior would begin with verbal instructions regarding the behavior, modeling of the behavior by the interventionist, rehearsing the behavior with the child, providing feedback (including corrective feedback and praise) about the use of the skill. Social skills training programs are able to intervene with a number of social skills deficits. In one study, Ladd (1981) tested the effectiveness of social skills training in increasing the question-asking, leading, and supportive behaviors of third-grade children identified as having low acceptance. Students in the social skills training condition demonstrated improvements in observations of social behavior and peer acceptance compared to students in attention control and nontreatment control conditions.

Early studies also examined the effectiveness of some of the individual and combined components of social skills training. For example, with third and fourth grade students identified as being social isolated, Gresham and Nagle (1980) examined four conditions, including videotape modeling alone, coaching (i.e., instructions, rehearsal, feedback, and reinforcement) alone, a combination of abbreviated forms of both modeling and coaching, and a control condition. The dependent variables included behavioral observations of social skills such as initiating positive peer interactions. Overall results indicated that modeling alone, coaching alone, and the combined treatment were all equivalent procedures for increasing social skills.

In another study, Mize and Ladd (1990) examined the effectiveness of a social skills training program applied to preschoolers described as being low-status. The program consisted of an instructional phase using hand puppets, followed by a rehearsal phase during which the participants used the hand puppets to practice the skills taught previously. Afterward, a recall phase was implemented in which participants viewed a videotaped social interaction and were asked to apply the skills previously taught. Finally, participants were given an opportunity to practice the social skills with children who were not present during the intervention.

Four specific skills were focused on during the intervention (e.g., asking a question directed toward a peer). Results indicated significant improvements in social skill knowledge and use in the classroom for the trained participants compared to a control group, while no differences on sociometric measures was found.

It is important to note that many of the early social skills training procedures included a cognitive component as well. For example, the modeling condition of the Gresham and Nagle (1980) study included models of children "thinking over" a difficult social situation and then making a good choice by using positive self-statements. The inclusion of this component was influenced by Meichenbaum's concept of cognitive modeling (Meichenbaum, 1977). Similarly, Mize and Ladd (1990) use the term cognitive-social learning in the description of their social skills training intervention. The primary focus of these social skills training studies, however, is on the modeling and coaching of specific overt skills, while the cognitive-behavioral skills training approach (described below) has a greater focus on changing thoughts in order to influence overt behavior.

Cognitive-Behavioral Skills Training

Cognitive-behavioral skills training, a process approach, shares the same goal of positive social skills change as the traditional social skills training interventions. However, cognitive-behavioral skills training focuses more on improving cognitive social problem solving skills with the assumption that appropriate behavioral change will follow (Nangle et al., 2002). Typical cognitive skills that are targeted include generating alternative behavioral responses as well as improving social perspective-taking. Early studies demonstrated that interventions were successful at changing children's cognitions related to impulsive behavior (Winer, Hilpert, Gesten, Cowen, & Schubin, 1982), interpersonal problems (Shure & Spivack, 1982), and aggression (Vaughn, Ridley, & Bullock, 1984); however, these studies were inconsistent in demonstrating a link between cognitive changes and improved overt behavior (Nangle et al., 2002).

Follow-up studies examining the long-term effects of social problem solving have also been conducted. For example, Kazdin, Bass, Siegel, and Thomas (1989) examined the short- and long-term effectiveness of social problem solving on the antisocial behavior of children in psychiatric inpatient units. The study examined social problem solving both with and without in vivo practice and compared it to relationship therapy and a contact-only control condition. Results from the study indicate that both of the social problem solving training conditions resulted in significantly greater immediate and long-term improvements in prosocial behavior and a decline in antisocial behavior compared to the relationship therapy and contact-only control conditions. Additionally, the social problem solving condition with in vivo practice showed immediate improvement over social problem solving without such practice, but these differences disappeared at the one year follow-up. Overall, research supports cognitive-behavioral skills training; however, this type of intervention may not be appropriate for younger children or some learners with limited intellectual abilities.

Multicomponent Interventions

Cognitive-behavioral skills training targets cognitive deficits and distortions in an attempt to improve social skills, while multicomponent cognitive-behavioral skills training also addresses the mood and physiological responses related to anger or anxiety (Nangle et al., 2002). Typical components added to these intervention programs include identifying physiological cues to building anger or anxiety and implementing behavioral techniques such as relaxation training. An example of this type of training program is offered by Deffenbacher, Lynch, Oetting, and Kemper (1996) as they investigated the effects of a cognitive relaxation coping skills (CRCS) program compared to a typical social skills training program and a control group. The CRCS program included relaxation skills training, identifying and reframing cognitive biases, cognitive skills training, and rehearsal with feedback. Results indicated that both CRCS and social skills training improved functioning in a number of areas, including feelings of anger and anxiety as well as anger expression; however, the CRCS program had some additional benefits on other measures of shyness, depression, and school deviance (Deffenbacher et al., 1996).

Spence (2003) describes multimodal skills training as assuming that prosocial behavior relies on a number of behavioral, affective, and cognitive components. The multimodal skills training approach also assumes that prosocial behavior is determined by a number of environmental influences (Spence, 2003). Thus, the theoretical assumptions underlying this type of intervention integrate behavioral theory, cognitive theory, and social learning theory. Based on this, Spence (2003) describes a multimodal training program that addresses deficits or biases in each of these areas. This program includes behavioral social skills training, social perception skills training, self-instructional and self-regulation techniques, social problem solving, and the reduction of competing problematic social responses. This program strives to integrate the various behavioral, cognitive, affective, and environmental components necessary for positive social skills change, and compelling evidence for the effectiveness of this program is offered by Spence (1995).

Other Aspects of Intervention Delivery

In addition to the type of intervention targeting social skills, there are several other aspects of intervention delivery worth discussion. One aspect of intervention delivery involves the inclusion of the child's significant others during the social skills intervention. For example, teachers, parents, siblings, and peers have all been included in interventions targeting social skills. In one example, Dodd, Hupp, Jewell, and Krohn (2008) use both parents and siblings to help in an intervention for two children diagnosed with an Autism Spectrum Disorder. Teachers and parents are also used in some prevention programs (Webster-Stratton & Reid, 2003). Regarding peers, sometimes the peers are already known to the target child, and other times unknown peers have been used.

Another aspect of intervention delivery involves the intensity of treatment or the level of prevention. Weisz, Sandler, Durlak, and Anton (2005) present a comprehensive model of treatment and prevention programs for overall children's mental health with three treatment intensities (i.e., continuing care, enhanced therapy, and time-limited therapy), three levels of prevention for (i.e., universal, selected, indicated), and an additional level of health promotion that has "the goal of enhancing strengths so as to reduce the risk of later problem outcomes and/or to increase prospects for positive development" (p. 632). Thus, some programs target established social problems, some attempt to minimize the effects of risk factors, and others focus primarily on building strengths.

A third aspect of intervention delivery involves the use of technology. Technology has been part of interventions targeting social skills in even some of the earliest studies. For example, Brown and MacDougal (1972) videotaped social interactions of school-age children and reviewed the tapes with the children. Many different variations of videotape modeling continue today. More recent advances with computers and the Internet have also provided interesting opportunities for assessment (Harman, Hansen, Cochran, & Lindsey, 2005; Mikami, Huang-Pollock, Pfiffner, McBurnett, & Hangai, 2007) and intervention (Fenstermacher, Olympia, & Sheridan, 2006; Parsons, Leonard, & Mitchell, 2006).

Finally, generalization of social skills from the training situation to the natural environment has long been a consideration in the literature. Stokes and Baer (1977) describe the typically ineffective "train and hope" approach of most studies at the time. Stokes and Baer also outline several strategies for intentionally increasing the likelihood that the learned skills will generalize. For example, generalization is more likely to occur if skills are chosen that will likely contact natural reinforcers. Stokes and Baer (1977), and later Stokes and Osnes (1989), discuss several other strategies for promoting generalization. Influenced by these reviews, researchers and clinicians have been increasingly assessing for generalization and intentionally using strategies to promote generalization (Berler, Gross, & Drabman, 1982; Tofte-Tipps, Mendonca, & Peach, 1982).

Range of Populations

Social skills interventions have targeted a broad range of skills and populations. Much of the social competence literature can be categorized into studies targeting developmental problems (e.g., autism spectrum disorders, intellectual disabilities), internalizing problems (e.g., withdrawal, depression, anxiety), externalizing problems (e.g., aggression, oppositional behavior, anger), at-risk groups of children, as well as typically developing children without any identified problem.

Regarding developmental problems, Matson, Matson, and Rivet (2007) categorize five types of social skills treatments that have been used for children diagnosed with autism spectrum disorders. First, interventions focusing on *reinforcement schedules and activities* were identified as being particularly useful for young children, or those with limited ability, as there are no sophisticated conceptual skills needed for this type of intervention. Second, *modeling and reinforcement,* includes several studies that attempted to prompt discrete behaviors through modeling and provided reinforcement for the demonstration of the behavior. Third, studies using *peer-mediated interventions* attempt to use typically developing peers during the intervention in an attempt to improve generalization outside of the training setting. This approach often involves peer modeling or prompting appropriate social skills. Fourth, *scripts or social stories* interventions use written work, often brief stories (written by the therapist with help from the parent, teacher, or child) that describe appropriate social skills and possible consequences of exhibiting these skills. Nichols, Hupp, Jewell, and Zeigler (2005) provide a review of social story interventions. Finally, Matson et al. include a *miscellaneous* category to describe a range of possible interventions, such as self-management training, that did not easily fit into any of the other categories. While most of the studies focus on children diagnosed with autism, a few studies include children with Asperger's Disorder (e.g., Apple, Billingsley, & Schwartz, 2005) and Pervasive Developmental Disorder – Not Otherwise Specified (e.g., Hupp & Reitman, 2000).

Similar approaches have also been used with children with intellectual disabilities, and Sukhodolsky and Butter (2007) describe several of these approaches. First, some research has focused on improving basic interaction skills. For example, Matson, Kazdin, and Esveldt-Dawson (1980) demonstrated that social skills training was effective at improving both verbal (e.g., number of words spoken) and nonverbal (e.g., eye contact) skills in two children with moderate intellectual disabilities. Second, social skills during free play time have also been successfully targeted (e.g., Matson, Fee, Coe, & Smith, 1991). Third, peer-mediation strategies have also shown some success for children with intellectual disabilities (Hughes, Killian, & Fischer, 1996). Fourth, social problem-solving methods have recently been successfully applied (Crites & Dunn, 2004; Edeh, 2006). Finally, Sukhodsky and Butter review studies that use board games to teach social skills (e.g., Foxx & McMorrow, 1983).

Internalizing problems in children have largely been addressed with different variations of cognitive-behavioral therapy (CBT). CBT for both depression (Stark, Reynolds, & Kaslow, 1987) and social anxiety (Spence, Donovan, & Brechman-Toussaint, 2000) includes a behavioral component of teaching social skills and a cognitive component of addressing cognitive distortions about social interactions. Some interventions for depression have also used social problem-solving techniques (Jaycox, Reivich, Gillham, & Seligman, 1994). Another approach to treating depression, called interpersonal psychotherapy, focuses on improving relationships, particularly as related to role disputes, role transitions, and interpersonal deficits (Mufson et al., 2004).

There have been two primary types of interventions targeting the social behavior of children diagnosed with ADHD. First, traditional social skills training programs in clinic settings have been conducted both concurrently with behavioral parent training (Frankel, Myatt, Cantwell, & Feinberg, 1997; Tutty, Gephart, & Wurzbacher, 2003) and as independently from behavioral parent training (Antschel & Remer, 2003). Second, behavioral peer interventions in recreational settings have also been used to target social behavior in children. These interventions are typically conducted in the context of comprehensive summer treatment programs that also include academic and parenting interventions. Studies include both group designs (Pelham et al., 2000) and single-case research designs (Hupp, Reitman, Northup, O'Callaghan, & LeBlanc, M., 2002).

Similarly, treatment programs for disruptive behavior typically have the goal of replacing disruptive behavior with appropriate social skills. There have been three major types of programs with these goals. First, behavioral parent training has been applied to programs in which the parent's behavior is targeted in an attempt to ultimately affect the child's behavior. Behavioral parent training programs usually target younger children between the ages of 3 and 8 years, and examples include Parent-Child Interaction Therapy (Brinkmeyer & Eyberg, 2003), the Positive Parenting Program (Sanders, 1999), the Helping the Noncompliant Child approach (Peed, Roberts, & Forehand, 1977), and the Incredible Years program (Webster-Stratton & Reid, 2003). The Oregon Model of Parent Management Training (Patterson, Chamberlain, & Reid, 1982) is another type of behavioral parent training that applies to a broader age range. Several brands of cognitive-behavioral therapy have also been applied to older children and adolescents with disruptive behavior. Some notable programs include Anger Control Training (Lochman, Barry, & Pardini, 2003), Group Assertiveness Training (Huey & Rank, 1984), Problem-Solving Skills Training (Kazdin, 2003), and the Rational Emotive Mental Health Program (Block, 1978). Finally, a few multicomponent interventions have been used, including Multisystemic Therapy (Henggeler & Lee, 2003) and Multidimensional Treatment Foster Care (Chamberlain & Smith, 2003).

Webster-Stratton and Reid (2008) review social skills prevention programs that are aimed at enhancing social competence in "at-risk" populations, particularly children that are socioeconomically disadvantaged. First, several promising parent-focused programs are discussed and include the Positive Parenting Program (Sanders & Dadds, 1993), Coping Skills Parenting Program (Cunningham, Bremmer, & Boyle, 1995), DARE to Be You (not to be confused with Drug Abuse Resistance Education; Miller-Heyl, MacPhee, & Fritz, 1998), and the Incredible Years program (Webster-Stratton & Hancock, 1998). Notably, the Incredible Years program also includes child-focused and teacher-focused interventions. Second, promising programs that combine classroom-based child programs with parent programs include First Step to Success (Walker et al., 1998), the Montreal Longitudinal Experimental Study (Tremblay, Pagani, Masse, & Vitaro, 1995), and Linking the Interests of Families and Teachers (Reid, Eddy, Fetrow, & Stoolmiller, 1999). Finally, two additional child-focused programs include Al's Pals (Wingspan, 1999) and Promoting Alternative THinking Strategies (PATHS; Kusche & Greenberg, 1994). Although not in their review, the Second Step (Cooke et al., 2007) program also has some research support. In the conclusion to their review, Webster-Stratton and Reid (2008) suggest that that most promising approaches use interconnected programs that target both parenting and teacher behavior management skills and child-focused social competence skills.

In addition to the problems already discussed, interventions and prevention programs targeting social skills have been used with many additional populations, some of which include children with learning disabilities (Kavale & Mostert, 2004), physical disabilities (Bennett & Hay, 2007), hearing impairment (Ducharme & Holborn, 1997), visual impairment (Celeste, 2007), drug use (Ellickson, McCaffrey, Ghosh-Dastidar, & Longshore, 2003), fetal alcohol syndrome (O'Connor et al., 2006), and problems with bullying (Fox & Boulton, 2003). Thus, social skills are cross-cutting skills that are important to many facets of life for all children.

Current State of the Research

Meta-analyses of Social Skills Interventions

Several meta-analytic studies have been conducted regarding the effectiveness of interventions targeting social skills. These studies calculate overall effect sizes as well as the effect size for particular dependent measures and interventions. The influence of different participant characteristics (e.g., age, type of problem, etc.) is also commonly reported. It is worth noting that the authors of different meta-analyses often use different methods for calculating effect sizes, and the terms used to describe the effects vary but have similar meaning (e.g., "medium effect," "moderate effect," "intermediate effect"). For this chapter, we will use the terms used by the authors of each individual meta-analysis.

Schneider (1992) conducted a meta-analysis of 79 studies. To be included in the meta-analysis, the studies had to examine a planned social skills treatment that had a measure of social behavior and some type of control group. Participants in these studies included several different groups including children that were described as aggressive, withdrawn, unpopular, at-risk, or normal. The overall effect size of social skills interventions was characterized as moderate, and Schneider calculated that social skills interventions were a "success" for 70% of the participants, compared to only 30% for the participants in control groups. While only one third of the studies included follow-up measures (ranging from less than 1 to 12 months), the effect size in the follow-up period was in the medium range. The meta-analysis also compared four different types of social skills interventions, revealing that studies with modeling or coaching had higher effect sizes than studies using social-cognitive techniques (i.e., social problem solving, perspective taking, or self-statements) or multiple techniques (multimodal combinations of the other techniques). Also, social skills interventions had higher effect sizes when done individually than when done in small groups or entire classrooms.

Beelmann, Pfingsten, and Lösel (1994) reviewed 49 studies using interventions targeting social competence in children (aged 3–15 years) with a range of problems (i.e., internalizing, externalizing, intellectual), as well as at-risk groups of children and "normal" children without any identified problem. Overall, the authors report that the social competence interventions had a high effect for social-cognitive skills, an intermediate effect for social interaction skills, a small effect for social adjustment, and no effect for self-related cognitions/affects. Regarding types of interventions, both monomodal and multimodal approaches all demonstrated significant effects, and there were not significant differences in the effect sizes between these approaches. However, generally speaking, the multimodal approaches were more likely to have significant effects on more types of dependent variables than monomodal approaches. Regarding client characteristics, social competence treatments had the greatest effect for the at-risk groups of children and the lowest (but still significant) effects for the normal children, with children

with internalizing and externalizing problems in between the other two groups. Also, though leading to significant changes for all age groups, the social competence treatments had a significantly greater effect for the youngest group (i.e., 3–5 years old) than the other groups (i.e., 6–8 years old, 9–11 years old, and 12–15 years old). Unlike in the Schneider (1992) meta-analysis, this review reported that significant follow-up effects could not be confirmed for most of the treatments except for social problem solving.

In the same year as the previous meta-analysis, Erwin (1994) examined 43 studies focusing on social skills training in "ordinary" classrooms. Studies were excluded if they focused on clinical and handicapped populations, and only published studies that used an experimental design and a social status behavioral measure were included. Overall, Erwin reports that the social skills interventions had a medium effect for changing behavioral measures of social interaction at post-test. Social skills interventions had a small effect for changing sociometric status as well as cognitive problem-solving ability. Importantly, these improvements lasted during the follow-up measurements. Children described as isolated tended to show better improvements in social interaction and status than children that were not isolated. A one-way ANOVA revealed that all three of the major training approaches (i.e., modeling, coaching, and cognitive problem solving) were equally effective. A multiple regression examined some specific strategies and revealed that the most significant predictors of sociometric status were film modeling, training in problem solving, feedback, and role play, in that order. Erwin acknowledges that many of the major training approaches, as well as the specific strategies, were often used in different combinations, and thus the review provides some support for multimodal interventions.

Several additional meta-analyses have been conducted with more specific groups of children. For example, social skills interventions have been somewhat successful with children diagnosed with learning disabilities; however, the effect is fairly small (Forness & Kavale, 1996; Kavale & Mostert, 2004). Similarly, minimal effects have been found for classroom social skills interventions aimed at children with emotional or behavioral disorders (Magee Quinn, Kavale, Mathur, Rutherford, & Forness,

1999). On the other hand, a recent meta-analysis examining cognitive-behavioral therapy for anger in youth revealed a medium effect size (Sukhodolsky, Kassinove, & Gorman, 2004). In this meta-analysis, skills training and multimodal CBT approaches were more effective at improving social skills than problem-solving and affective education (i.e., education about emotions). In discussing these meta-analytic studies Foster and Bussman (2008) emphasize that the effect size heterogeneity across different studies suggests that the effectiveness of different types of social skills training programs varies considerably. It is also important to note that differences in effectiveness may be due to the population in the study.

Classification of Evidence-Based Treatments Targeting Social Skills

Beginning with the Task Force on Psychological Intervention Guidelines (American Psychological Association, 1995), the American Psychological Association has made significant progress in attempting to identify effective interventions. Since that time, the label used to describe research-supported interventions has changed from "empirically validated treatments" to "empirically supported treatments" and most recently to "evidence-based treatments"; however, the actual definition has undergone little revision (Silverman & Hinshaw, 2008). Silverman and Hinshaw (2008) offer the introductory article to the Society of Clinical Child and Adolescent Psychology's special issue on evidence-based treatments. As described in the article, a treatment can be categorized as a "well-established" evidence-based treatment if it has at least two well-conducted (e.g., randomized controlled) group design studies by at least two different research teams. Also, a treatment can be categorized as a "probably efficacious" evidence-based treatment if it has two group design studies that either do not have as strong designs as the well-established category or are conducted by the same research team. Also, multiple well-conducted single-case research designs have been another avenue for contributing to determinations about evidence-based interventions; however, most of the articles in the special issue focus primarily on group design studies.

In this special issue Rogers and Vismara (2008) review comprehensive treatments for early autism and conclude that the Lovaas model of Applied Behavior Analysis meets the well-established category, specifically for intellectual performance. That is, the reviewed studies focused primarily on intellectual performance (e.g., IQ, academic success) as the primary dependent variable (Lovaas, 1987, 1993; Sallows & Graupner, 2005; Smith, Groen, & Wynn, 2000). The Lovaas model of Applied Behavior Analysis, however, also broadly covers many other skills, many of which are social in nature. Unfortunately, the randomized control trials did not tend to focus on social skills outcomes, although the improvements in cognitive ability and language that often led to less restrictive placement likely also had many positive social benefits. In the Rogers and Vismara (2008) review, Pivotal Response Training, another behavioral approach, is also argued to meet the criteria as being a probably efficacious treatment due to several well-conducted single-case research design studies (see Delprato, 2001 for a review). Pivotal Response Training has social communication as the major focus (Koegel, Dyer, & Bell, 1987) providing further evidence that the social behavior of many children with Autism Spectrum Disorders can be improved with intervention. There are two major limitations of the Rogers and Vismara (2008) review that specifically relate to social skills. First, the review focuses on young children with autism, with less focus on older children or adolescents with Asperger's Disorder. This critique is largely a function of the treatment literature which has tended to have the same focus. Second, the review focuses on comprehensive treatments, with less discussion about other specific approaches (e.g., social stories) that have a growing evidence base.

Internalizing problems (i.e., depression and anxiety) were also reviewed in the special issue on evidence-based treatments. David-Ferdon and Kaslow (2008) review evidence-based treatments for depression. In this review they consider both specific approaches as well as broader theoretical models. They also distinguish between treatments for children and treatments for adolescents. The theoretical model of CBT is categorized as being well-established for *both* children and adolescents, with most of the studies focusing on group therapy rather than individual therapy. For children, two specific types of CBT, Self-Control Therapy and the Penn Prevention Program, were classified as probably efficacious. Self-Control Therapy (Stark, Rouse, & Livingston, 1991) is a school-based program that incorporates social skills training and assertiveness training with cognitive techniques. Similarly, the Penn Prevention Program (Jaycox et al., 1994) incorporates social problem solving with other cognitive techniques. For adolescents, the Coping with Depression program (Lewinsohn, Clarke, Hops, & Andrews, 1990) is a specific type of CBT that is classified as probably efficacious. In addition to CBT, the theoretical model of interpersonal psychotherapy (Mufson et al., 2004) is also classified as well-established and targets social relationships.

Regarding phobic and anxiety disorders, Silverman, Pina, and Viswesvaran (2008) report that no treatment is well-established; however, they focus only on specific interventions, and had they taken the approach of David-Ferdon and Kaslow (2008) to also consider broad theoretical models, CBT would have likely met the criteria for being well-established. Also, group CBT (Spence et al., 2000), which emphasizes social skills training, is also characterized as being probably efficacious for social phobia. Social Effectiveness Training (Beidel, Turner, & Morris, 2000) is also classified as probably efficacious for social phobia.

Eyberg, Nelson, and Boggs (2008) review treatments for disruptive behavior. The Oregon model of Parent Management Training (Patterson, Reid, Jones, & Conger, 1975) is classified as well-established. Parent Management Training focuses on teaching parents antecedent- and consequence-based strategies for increasing prosocial behavior while decreasing challenging behaviors in children and younger adolescents. The review also includes 10 probably efficacious treatments (as well as a few additional variations), many of which could be considered a form of behavioral parent training that is similar to Parent Management Training. For example, the Incredible Years program (Webster-Stratton & Reid, 2003) uses behavioral parent training with parents of Head Start children. Interestingly, the Incredible Years program also has a specific child-focused prevention component that teaches prosocial skills to children in Head Start. Some

other notable examples of probably efficacious treatments that are related to social behavior in children include Group Assertiveness Training (Wells & Egan, 1988) and Problem-Solving Skills Training (Kazdin, 2003), both of which target social behavior in older children.

Children diagnosed with ADHD frequently have significant peer relation problems. In fact, Pelham and Fabiano (2008) estimated that each year the average child diagnosed with ADHD has approximately half a million negative social interactions. ADHD has three well-established interventions (Pelham & Fabiano, 2008). Both behavioral parent training (Wells et al., 2000) and behavioral classroom management (Barkley et al., 2000) often focus on increasing prosocial behavior while decreasing the hyperactive, impulsive, and other challenging behavior that can interfere with peer relationships. Often these two treatments are used in combination with each other, as well as in combination with stimulant medication. Additionally, behavioral peer interventions in recreational settings (Pelham et al., 2000) are classified as well-established. Behavioral peer interventions typically teach social skills in the context of a sports setting and have usually been applied during summer programs. Pelham and Fabiano (2008) also stress that traditional social skills training (i.e., in a psychologist's office) has not been effective for children diagnosed with ADHD.

As a final note to this section, it is import to mention that recent attempts have also been made to identify *prevention* programs with a firm research base. Specifically, the Substance Abuse and Mental Health Services Association (SAMHSA) has a growing list of "model," "effective," and "promising" programs that commonly have the promotion of social skills as a component (http://www.nrepp.samhsa.gov/). Different programs have a focus in one or more of the following areas: substance use, child abuse, disruptive behavior, interpersonal skills, health, academic success, and violence.

Summary and Future Directions

Conceptual understanding and research examining social skills has flourished over the last four decades. While no single framework has been adopted by every researcher and clinician, many core conceptual issues, such as the distinction between social skills and social competence, have had a dramatic impact on the path to understanding social behavior. New assessment and intervention approaches have continued to be applied with children and adolescents, and the earlier approaches have also continued to show value for children.

In this chapter we discussed both the traditional approach and contextual approach to assessment. The traditional approach continues to yield significant benefits for case conceptualization and is complimented by the contextual approach. Although the contextual approach to the assessment of social skills can provide unique and meaningful information to the assessment process, it requires more research to examine validity and treatment utility. Similarly, several broad approaches to intervening with social skills were discussed, including operant techniques, social skills training, cognitive-behavioral skills training, and multicomponent interventions. As represented in both meta-analyses and reviews of evidence-based treatments, all of these approaches continue to have value in treating different types of social skills problems with different populations. Future research should continue to examine specific interventions targeting social skills for specific populations. It is particularly important to continue researching the treatments classified as "probably efficacious" to examine whether they will eventually meet the criteria for "well-established" or not.

Also regarding treatment, there are a number of variables that may mediate the effectiveness of social skills interventions that continue to receive little attention from researchers (Nangle et al., 2002). Some of these variables are demographic in nature, such as age, gender, and ethnicity. While much of the research on social skills interventions restricts the age range of participants in order to create a more homogeneous sample, some existing research fails to take age into account. Additionally, controversy exists as to the most and least appropriate social skills interventions for young children. For example, Nangle et al. (2002) review a number of studies finding cognitive interventions to be more successful with adolescents and relatively ineffective with young children. However, research by Doherr, Reynolds, Wetherly, and Evans (2005) found that children as young as 5 years hold the prerequisite

cognitive skills necessary for them to benefit from cognitive approaches.

Gender is another important demographic variable to consider when examining the effectiveness of social skills interventions. For example, a recent review of research on relational aggression by Crick, Ostrov, and Kawabata (2007) examines the gender differences in the expression of physical and relational aggression across the developmental life span. Although the literature on relational aggression and gender differences in aggression has been building in recent years, gender continues to be frequently overlooked as a possible mediating variable in the effectiveness of social skills training programs. Additionally, ethnicity of children and adolescents is another demographic variable that has received very little attention on this topic. For example, while African-American youth continue to be incarcerated for violent offenses at a disproportionate rate (Dryfoos, 1990), virtually no large-scale studies exist that attempt to understand whether social skills interventions vary in their effectiveness depending on participant ethnicity.

Beyond participant demographic variables, there are a number of other shortcomings and complications existing within the current literature on the effectiveness of social skills interventions. First, the heterogeneity of participants' problem behavior within and between studies threatens the reliability and generalizability of the results of those studies (Nangle et al., 2002). For example, many studies do not select participants based on formal categorical diagnoses (e.g., Conduct Disorder), but rather they are often selected from a rather vague and dimensional continuum (e.g., exhibiting antisocial behavior). The implication of this is that heterogeneity within a sample may lead to unreliable results and compromise our understanding as to how behavior severity may impact program effectiveness. Similar problems exist with regard to social cognition as fewer studies take into account participants' level of social cognition prior to an intervention program (Nangle et al., 2002). While the social information processing model holds that social cognition and processing mediates one's social behavior, a number of studies fail to measure these social information processing variables prior to intervention. The result of this omission is that while the theory proposes social information processing as a mediating variable, this mediational model is relatively untested.

A third shortcoming in the literature exists with regard to peer group influences (Nangle et al., 2002). Specifically, while participants of various social skills intervention programs may exhibit individual improvement in social skills knowledge and performance, they often continue to be rejected within their natural social setting based on a previously established social status (Gresham & Nagle, 1980). These results reflect the theoretical assumptions of the ecological model that propose that environmental 'fit' determines one's emotional and behavioral functioning. While some research exists on programs that attempt to influence the larger peer group as a component of a social skills intervention, more research on this topic is warranted. Additionally, research involving parents in social skills interventions and prevention programs has been encouraging (e.g., Webster-Stratton & Reid, 2003); however, future research should continue to examine the role of parents in social skills interventions.

References

American Psychiatric Association. (2000). *Diagnostic and statistical manual of mental disorders* (4th ed., Text Revision). Washington, DC: Author.

American Psychological Association Task Force on Psychological Intervention Guidelines. (1995). *Template for developing guidelines: Interventions for mental disorders and psychological aspects of physical disorders.* Washington, DC: American Psychological Association.

Antschel, K. M., & Remer, R. (2003). Social skills training in children with attention deficit hyperactivity disorder: A randomized-controlled clinical trial. *Journal of Clinical Child and Adolescent Psychology, 32,* 153–165.

Apple, A. L., Billingsley, F., & Schwartz, I. S. (2005). Effects of video modeling alone and with self-management on compliant-giving behavior of children with high-functioning autism spectrum disorders. *Journal of Positive Behavior Interventions, 7,* 33–46.

Asher, S. R., Markell, R. A., & Hymel, S. (1981). Identifying children at risk in peer relations: A critique of the rate-of-interaction approach to assessment. *Child Development, 52,* 1239–1245.

Bandura, A. (1977). *Social learning theory.* Oxford, England: Prentice-Hall.

Barkley, R. A., Shelton, T. L., Crosswait, C., Moorehouse, M., Fletcher, K., Barrett, S., et al. (2000). Multi-method psychoeducational intervention for preschool children with disruptive behavior: Preliminary results at post-treatment. *Journal of Child Psychology and Psychiatry and Allied Disciplines, 41,* 319–332.

Beelmann, A., Pfingsten, U., & Lösel, F. (1994). Effects of training social competence in children: A meta-analysis of recent evaluation studies. *Journal of Clinical Child Psychology, 23,* 260–271.

Beidel, D. C., Turner, S. M., & Morris, T. L. (2000). Behavioral treatment of childhood social phobia. *Journal of Consulting and Clinical Psychology, 68,* 1072–1080.

Bennett, K. S., & Hay, D. A. (2007). The role of family in the development of social skills in children with physical disabilities. *International Journal of Disability, Development and Education, 54,* 381–397.

Berler, E. S., Gross, A. M., & Drabman, R. S. (1982). Social skills training with children: Proceed with caution. *Journal of Applied Behavior Analysis, 15,* 41–53.

Bierman, K. L., & Welsh, J. A. (2000). Assessing social dysfunction: The contributions of laboratory and performance-based measures. *Journal of Clinical Child Psychology, 29,* 526–539.

Block, J. (1978). Effects of a rational-emotive mental health program on poorly achieving, disruptive high school students. *Journal of Applied Counseling Psychology, 25,* 61–65.

Brinkmeyer, M. Y., & Eyberg, S. M. (2003). Parent-child interaction therapy for oppositional children. In A. E. Kazdin & J. R. Weisz (Eds.), *Evidenced-based psychotherapies for children and adolescents* (pp. 204–223). New York: Guilford.

Brodsky, G. (1967). The relationship between verbal and non-verbal behavior change. *Behaviour Research and Therapy, 5,* 183–191.

Brown, J. A., & MacDougall, M. A. (1972). Simulated social skill training for elementary school children. *Elementary School Guidance and Counseling, 6,* 175–179.

Caldarella, P., & Merrell, K. W. (1997). Common dimensions of social skills of children and adolescents: A taxonomy of positive behaviors. *School Psychology Review, 26,* 264–278.

Cavell, T. A. (1990). Social adjustment, social performance, and social skills: A tri-component model of social competence. *Journal of Clinical Child Psychology, 19,* 111–122.

Celeste, M. (2007). Social skills intervention for a child who is blind. *Journal of Visual Impairment and Blindness, 101,* 521–533

Chamberlain, P., & Smith, D. K. (2003). Antisocial behavior in children and adolescents: The Oregon Multidimensional Treatment Foster Care Model. In A. E. Kazdin & J. R. Weisz (Eds.), *Evidenced-based psychotherapies for children and adolescents* (pp. 282–300). New York: Guilford.

Cooke, M., Beaulieu, F., Julian, L. J., Bourke, C., Newell, L., & Lapidus, G. (2007). The effects of city-wide implementation of "Second Step" on elementary school students' prosocial and aggressive behaviors. *Journal of Primary Prevention, 28,* 93–115.

Crick, N. R., Ostrov, J. M., & Kawabata, Y. (2007). Relational aggression and gender: An overview. In D. J. Flannery, A. T. Vazsonyi, & I. D. Waldman (Eds.) *The Cambridge handbook of violent behavior and aggression.* (pp. 245–259). New York, NY: Cambridge University Press.

Crites, S. A., & Dunn, C. (2004). Teaching social problem solving to individuals with mental retardation. *Education and Training in Developmental Disabilities, 39,* 301–309.

Cunningham, C. E., Bremmer, R., & Boyle, M. (1995). Large group community-based parenting programs for families of preschoolers at risk for disruptive behavior disorders: Utilization, cost effectiveness, and outcome. *Journal of Child Psychology and Psychiatry, 36,* 1141–1159.

David-Ferdon, C., & Kaslow, N. J., (2008). Evidence-based psychosocial treatments for child and adolescent depression. *Journal of Clinical Child and Adolescent Psychology, 37,* 62–104.

Deffenbacher, J. L., Lynch, R. S., Oetting, E. R., & Kemper, C. C. (1996). Anger reduction in early adolescents. *Journal of Counseling Psychology, 43,* 149–157.

Delprato, D. J. (2001). Comparisons of discrete-trial and normalized behavioral language intervention for young children with autism. *Journal of Autism and Developmental Disorders, 31,* 315–325.

Dodd, S., Hupp, S. D. A., Jewell, J., & Krohn, E. (2008). Using parents and siblings during a Social Story intervention for two children diagnosed with PDD-NOS. *Journal of Developmental and Physical Disabilities, 20,* 217–229.

Dodge, K. A., McClaskey, C. L., & Feldman, E. (1985). Situational approach to the assessment of social competence in children. *Journal of Consulting and Clinical Psychology, 53,* 344–353.

Doherr, L, Reynolds, S., Wetherly, J., & Evans, E. (2005). Young children's ability to engage in cognitive therapy tasks: Associations with age and educational experience. *Behavioural and Cognitive Psychotherapy, 33,* 201–215.

Dryfoos, J. G. (1990). *Adolescents at risk: Prevalence and prevention.* New York, NY: Oxford University Press.

Ducharme, D. E., & Holborn, S. W. (1997). Programming generalization of social skills in preschool children with hearing impairments. *Journal of Applied Behavior Analysis, 30,* 639–651.

Edeh, O. M. (2006). Cross-cultural investigation of interest-based training and social interpersonal problem solving students with mental retardation. *Education and Training in Developmental Disabilities, 41,* 163–176.

Edelstein, B. A., & Eisler, R. M. (1976). Effects of modeling and modeling with instructions and feedback on the behavioral components of social skills. *Behavior Therapy, 7,* 382–389.

Ellickson, P. L., McCaffrey, D. F., Ghosh-Dastidar, B., Longshore, D. L. (2003). New Inroads in preventing adolescent drug use: Results from a large-scale trial of project ALERT in middle schools. *American Journal of Public Health, 93,* 1830–1836.

Elliott, S. N., & Busse, R. T. (1991). Social skills assessment and intervention with children and adolescents. *School Psychology International, 12,* 63–83.

Elliott, S. N., & Gresham, F. M. (1987). Children's social skills: Assessment and classification practices. *Journal of Counseling and Development, 66,* 96–99.

Erwin, P. G. (1994). Effectiveness of social skills training with children: A meta-analytic study. *Counseling Psychology Quarterly, 7,* 305–310.

Eyberg, S. M., Nelson, M. M., & Boggs, S. R. (2008). Evidence-based psychosocial treatments for children and adolescents with disruptive behavior. *Journal of Clinical Child and Adolescent Psychology, 37,* 215–237.

Fenstermacher, K., Olympia, D., & Sheridan, S. M. (2006). Special section: Changing practice, changing schools. *School Psychology Quarterly, 21,* 197–224.

Forness, S. R., & Kavale, K. A. (1996). Treating social skill deficits in children with learning disabilities: A meta-analysis of the research. *Learning Disability Quarterly, 19,* 2–13.

Foster, S. L., & Bussman, J. R. (2008). Evidence-based approaches to social skills training with children and adolescents. In R. G. Steele, T. D. Elkin, & M. C. Roberts (Eds.), *Handbook of evidence-based therapies for children and adolescents: Bridging science and practice* (pp. 409–427). New York: Springer.

Foster, S. L., Inderbitzen, H. M., & Nangle, D. W. (1993). Assessing acceptance and social skills with peers in childhood: Current Issues. *Behavior Modification, 17,* 255–286.

Fox, C. L., & Boulton, M. J., (2003). Evaluating the effectiveness of a social skills training (SST) programme for victims of bullying. *Educational Research, 45,* 231–247.

Fox, J. J., & McEvoy, M. A. (1993). Assessing and enhancing generalization and social validity of social-skills interventions with children and adolescents. *Behavior Modification, 17,* 339–366.

Foxx, R. M., & McMorrow, M. J. (1983). *Stacking the deck: A social skills game for retarded adults.* Champaign, IL: Research Press.

Frankel, F., Myatt, R., Cantwell, D. P., & Feinberg, D. T. (1997). Parent-assisted transfer of children's social skills training: Effects on children with and without attention-deficit hyperactivity disorder. *Journal of the American Academy of Child and Adolescent Psychiatry, 36,* 1056–1064.

Gresham, F. M. (1981). Assessment of children's social skills. *Journal of School Psychology, 19,* 120–133.

Gresham, F. M. (1986). Conceptual and definitional issues in the assessment of children's social skills: Implications for classification and training. *Journal of Clinical Child Psychology, 15,* 3–15.

Gresham, F. M. (1997). Social competence and students with behavior disorders: Where we've been, where we are, and where we should go. *Education and Treatment of Children, 20,* 233–249.

Gresham, F. M. (1998). Social skills training with children: Social learning and applied behavioral analytic approaches. In T. S. Watson & F. M. Gresham (Eds.), *Handbook of child behavior therapy* (pp. 475–497). New York, NY: Plenum Press.

Gresham, F. M. (2002). Teaching social skills to high-risk children and youth: Preventive and remedial strategies. In M. R. Shinn, H. M. Walker, & G. Stoner (Eds.), *Interventions for academic and behavior problems II: Preventive and remedial approaches* (pp. 403–432). Washington, DC: National Association of School Psychologists.

Gresham, F. M., & Elliott, S. N. (1984). Assessment and classification of children's social skills: A review of methods and issues. *School Psychology Review, 13,* 292–301.

Gresham, F. M., & Elliott, S. N. (1987). The relationship between adaptive behavior and social skills: Issues in definition and assessment. *The Journal of Special Education, 21,* 167–181.

Gresham, F. M., & Elliott, S. N. (1989). Social skills deficits as a primary learning disability. *Journal of Learning Disabilities, 22,* 120–124.

Gresham, F. M., & Nagle, R. J. (1980). Social skills training with children: Responsiveness to modeling and coaching as a function of peer orientation. *Journal of Consulting and Clinical Psychology, 48,* 718–729.

Gresham, F. M., Van, M. B., & Cook, C. R. (2006). Social skills training for teaching replacement behaviors: Remediating acquisition deficits in at-risk students. *Behavioral Disorders, 31,* 363–377.

Gumpel, T. P., & David, S. (2000). Exploring the efficacy of self-regulatory training as a possible alternative to social skills training. *Behavioral Disorders, 25,* 131–141.

Gumpel, T. P., & Golan, H. (2000). Teaching game-playing social skills using a self-monitoring treatment package. *Psychology in the Schools, 37,* 253–261.

Hansen, D. J., Nangle, D. W., & Meyer, K. A. (1998). Enhancing the effectiveness of social skills interventions with adolescents. *Education & Treatment of Children, 21,* 489–513.

Haring, T. G. (1992). The context of social competence: Relations, relationships, and generalization. In S. L. Odom, S. R. McConnell, & M. A. McEvoy (Eds.), *Social competence of young children with disabilities: Issues and strategies for intervention* (pp. 307–320). Baltimore, MD: Paul H. Brookes.

Harman, J. P., Hansen, C. E., Cochran, M. E., & Lindsey, C. R. (2005). Liar, liar: Internet faking but not frequency of use affects social skills, self-esteem, social anxiety, and aggression. *CyberPsychology & Behavior, 8,* 1–6.

Henggeler, S. W., & Lee, T. (2003). Multisystemic treatment of serious clinical problems. In A. E. Kazdin & J. R. Weisz (Eds.), *Evidenced-based psychotherapies for children and adolescents* (pp. 301–322). New York: Guilford.

Hoier, T. S., & Cone, J. D. (1987). Target selection of social skills for children: The template-matching procedure. *Behavior Modification, 11,* 137–163.

Huey, W. C., & Rank, R. C. (1984). Effects of counselor and peer-led group assertive training on black-adolescent aggression. *Journal of Counseling Psychology, 31,* 95–98.

Hughes, C., Killian, D. J., & Fischer, G. M. (1996). Validation and assessment of a conversational interaction intervention. *American Journal of Mental Retardation, 100,* 493–509.

Hupp, S. D. A., & Reitman, D. (2000). Parent-assisted modification of pivotal social skills for a child diagnosed with PDD: A clinical replication. *Journal of Positive Behavior Interventions, 2,* 183–187.

Hupp, S. D. A., Reitman, D., Northup, J., O'Callaghan, P., & LeBlanc, M. (2002). The effects of delayed rewards, tokens, and stimulant medication on sportsmanlike behavior with ADHD-diagnosed children. *Behavior Modification, 26,* 148–162.

Jaycox, L., Reivich, K., Gillham, J. E., & Seligman, M. E. P. (1994). Prevention of depressive symptoms in school children. *Behavioral Research and Therapy, 32,* 801–816.

Kavale, K. A., & Mostert, M. P. (2004). Social skills interventions for individuals with learning disabilities. *Learning Disability Quarterly, 27,* 31–43.

Kazdin, A. E. (2003). Problem-solving skills training and parent management training for conduct disorder. In A. E. Kazdin & J. R. Weisz (Eds.), *Evidenced-based psychotherapies for children and adolescents* (pp. 241–262). New York: Guilford.

Kazdin, A. E., Bass, D., Siegel, T., & Thomas, C. (1989). Cognitive-behavioral therapy and relationship therapy in the treatment of children referred for antisocial behavior. *Journal of Consulting and Clinical Psychology, 57*(4), 522–535.

Koegel, R. L., Dyer, K., & Bell, L. K. (1987). The influence of child-preferred activities on autistic children's social behavior. *Journal of Applied Behavior analysis, 210,* 243–252.

Kusche, C. A., & Greenberg, M. T. (1994). *The PATHS curriculum.* Seattle, WA: Developmental Research and Programs.

Ladd, G. W. (1981). Effectiveness of a social learning method for enhancing children's social interaction and peer acceptance. *Child Development, 52,* 171–178.

Lane, K. L., Beebe-Frankenberger, M. E., Lambros, K. M., & Pierson, M. (2001). Designing effective interventions for children at-risk for antisocial behavior: An integrated model of components necessary for making valid inferences. *Psychology in the Schools, 38,* 365–379.

Lewinsohn, P. M., Clarke, G., Hops, H., & Andrews, J. (1990). Cognitive-behavioral treatment for depressed adolescents. *Behavior Therapy, 21,* 385–401.

Lochman, J. E., Barry, T. D., & Pardini, D. A. (2003). Anger control training for aggressive youth. In A. E. Kazdin & J. R. Weisz (Eds.), *Evidenced-based psychotherapies for children and adolescents* (pp. 263–281). New York: Guilford.

Lovaas, O. I. (1987). Behavioral treatment and normal educational and intellectual functioning in young autistic children. *Journal of Consulting and Clinical Psychology, 55,* 3–9.

Lovaas, O. I. (1993). The development of a treatment-research project for developmentally disabled and autistic children. *Journal of Applied Behavior Analysis, 26,* 617–630.

Magee Quinn, M., Kavale, K. A., Mathur, S. R., Rutherford, R. B. Jr., & Forness, S. R. (1999). A meta-analysis of social skill interventions for students with emotional or behavioral disorders. *Journal of Emotional and Behavioral Disorders, 7,* 54–64.

Mathur, S. R., & Rutherford, R. B. (1996). Is social skills training effective for students with emotional or behavioral disorders? Research issues and needs. *Behavioral Disorders, 22,* 21–28.

Matson, J. L., & Fee, V. E. (1991). Social skills difficulties among persons with mental retardation. In J. L. Matson & J. A. Mulick (Eds.), *Handbook of mental retardation* 2nd ed., pp. 468–478). New York: Pergamon Press.

Matson, J. L., Fee, V. E., Coe, D. A., & Smith, D. (1991). A social skills program for developmentally delayed preschoolers. *Journal of Clinical Child Psychology, 20,* 428–433.

Matson, J. L., Kazdin, A. E., & Esveldt-Dawson, K. (1980). Training interpersonal skills among mentally retarded and socially dysfunctional children. *Behaviour Research and Therapy, 18,* 419–427.

Matson, J. L., Matson, M. L., & Rivet, T. T. (2007). Social-skills treatments for children with autism spectrum disorders. *Behavior Modification, 31,* 682–707.

Matson, J. L., & Ollendick, T. H. (1988). *Enhancing Children's Social Skills: Assessment and Training.* New York: Pergamon Press.

Matson, J. L., & Stephens, R. M. (1978). Increasing appropriate behavior of explosive chronic psychiatric patients with a social-skills training package. *Behavior Modification, 2,* 61–76.

Matthys, W., Maassen, G. H., Cuperus, J. M., & van Engeland, H. (2001). The assessment of the situational specificity of children's problem behaviour in peer-peer context. *Journal of Child Psychology and Psychiatry, 42,* 413–420.

McConnell, S. R. (1987). Entrapment effects and the generalization and maintenance of social skills training for elementary school students with behavioral disorders. *Behavioral Disorders, 12,* 252–263.

McFall, R. M. (1982). A review and reformulation of the concept of social skills. *Behavioral Assessment, 4,* 1–33.

Meichenbaum, D. (1977). *Cognitive-behavior modification.* New York: Plenum Press.

Merrell, K. W., & Gimpel, G. A. (1998). *Social skills of children and adolescents: Conceptualization, assessment, treatment.* Mahwah, NJ: Lawrence Erlbaum Associates, Inc.

Mikami, A. Y., Huang-Pollock, C. L., Pfiffner, L. J., McBurnett, K., & Hangai, D. (2007). Social skills differences among attention-deficit/hyperactivity disorder types in a chat room assessment task. *Journal of Abnormal Child Psychology, 35,* 509–521.

Miles, S. B., & Stipek, D. (2006). Contemporaneous and longitudinal associations between social behavior and literacy achievement in a sample of low-income elementary school children. *Child Development, 77,* 103–117.

Miller-Heyl, J., MacPhee, D., & Fritz, J. J. (1998). DARE to be you: A family-support, early prevention program. *The Journal of Primary Prevention, 18,* 257–285.

Mize, J., & Ladd, G. W. (1990). A cognitive-social learning approach to social skill training with low-accepted preschool children. *Developmental Psychology, 26,* 388–397.

Mufson, L. H., Dorta, K. P., Wickramartne, P., Nomura, Y., Olfson, M., & Weissman, M. M. (2004). A randomized effectiveness trial of interpersonal psychotherapy for depressed adolescents. *Archives of General Psychiatry, 61,* 577–584.

Nangle, D. W., Erdley, C. A., Carpenter, E. M., & Newman, J. E. (2002). Social skills training as a treatment for aggressive children and adolescents: A developmental-clinical integration. *Aggression and Violent Behavior, 7,* 169–199.

Nichols, S. L., Hupp, S. D. A., Jewell, J. D., & Zeigler, C. S. (2005). Review of Social Story interventions for children diagnosed with autism spectrum disorders. *Journal of Evidence Based Practices for Schools, 6,* 90–120.

Nietupski, J., & Williams, W. (1976). Teaching selected telephone related social skills to severely handicapped students. *Child Study Journal, 6,* 139–153.

O'Connor, M. J., Frankel, F., Paley, B., Schonfeld, A. M., Carpenter, E., Laugeson, E. A., et al. (2006). Controlled social skills training for children with fetal alcohol spectrum disorders. *Journal of Consulting and Clinical Psychology, 74,* 639–648.

Oden, S., & Asher, S. R. (1977). Coaching children in social skills for friendship making. *Child Development, 48,* 495–506.

O'Leary, D. E., O'Leary, M. R., & Donovan, D. M. (1976). Social skill acquisition and psychosocial development of alcoholics: A review. *Addictive Behaviors, 1,* 111–120.

Parker, J. G., & Asher, S. R. (1987). Peer relations and later personal adjustment: Are low-accepted children "at risk"? *Psychological Bulletin, 102,* 357–389.

Parsons, S., Leonard, A., & Mitchell, P. (2006). Virtual environments for social skills training: Comments from two adolescents with autistic spectrum disorder. *Computers and Education, 47,* 186–206.

Patterson, G. R., Chamberlain, P., & Reid, J. B. (1982). A comparative evaluation of a parent-training program. *Behavior Therapy, 13,* 638–650.

Patterson, G. R., Reid, J. B., Jones, R. R., & Conger, R. E. (1975). *A social learning approach to family intervention: Families with aggressive children* (Vol. 1). Eugene, OR: Castalia.

Peed, S., Roberts, M., & Forehand, R. (1977). Evaluation of the effectiveness of a standardized parent training program in the altering the interaction of mothers and their noncompliant children. *Behavior Modification, 1,* 323–350.

Pelham, W. E., & Fabiano, G. A. (2008). Evidence-based psychosocial treatments for attention-deficit/hyperactivity disorder. *Journal of Clinical child and Adolescent Psychology, 37,* 184–214.

Pelham, W. E., Gnagy, E. M., Greiner, A. R., Hoza, B., Hinshaw, S. P., Swanson, J. M., et al. (2000). Behavioral vs. behavioral and pharmacological treatment in ADHD children attending a summer treatment program. *Journal of Abnormal Child Psychology, 28,* 507–525.

Reid, J. B., Eddy, J. M., Fetrow, R. A., & Stoolmiller, M. (1999). Description and immediate impacts of a preventive intervention for conduct problems. *American Journal of Community Psychology, 27,* 483–517.

Rogers, S. J., & Vismara, L. A. (2008). Evidence-based comprehensive treatments for early autism. *Journal of Clinical Child and Adolescent Psychology, 37,* 8–38.

Rose-Krasnor, L. (1997). The nature of social competence: A theoretical review. *Social Development, 6,* 111–135.

Sallows, G. O., & Graupner, T. D. (2005). Intensive behavioral treatment for children with autism: Four-year outcome and predictors. *American Journal on Mental retardation, 110,* 417–438.

Sanders, M. R. (1999). Triple p-positive parenting program: Towards an empirically validated multilevel parenting and family support strategy for the prevention of behavior and emotional problems in children. *Clinical Child and Family Psychology Review, 2,* 71–90.

Sanders, M. R., & Dadds, M. R. (1993). *Behavioral family intervention.* Needham Heights, MA: Allyn & Bacon.

Schneider, B. H. (1992). Didactic methods for enhancing children's peer relations: A quantitative review. *Clinical Psychology Review, 12*, 363–382.

Schutz, R., Wehman, P., Renzaglia, A. M., Karan, O. (1978). Efficiency of contingent social disapproval on inappropriate verbalizations of two severely retarded males. *Behavior Therapy, 9*, 657–662.

Sheridan, S. M., Hungelmann, A., & Maughan, D. P. (1999). A contextualized framework for social skills assessment, intervention and generalization. *School Psychology Review, 28*, 84–103.

Sheridan, S. M., & Walker, D. (1999). Social skills in context: Considerations for assessment, intervention, and generalization. In C. R. Reynolds & T. B. Gutkin (Eds.), *The handbook of school psychology* (3rd ed., pp. 686–708). New York: Wiley & Sons.

Shure, M. B., & Spivack, G. (1982). Interpersonal problem-solving in young children: A cognitive approach to prevention. *American Journal of Community Psychology, 10*, 341–356.

Silverman, W. K., & Hinshaw, S. P. (2008). The second special issue on evidence-based psychosocial treatments for children and adolescents: A 10-year update. *Journal of Clinical Child and Adolescent Psychology, 37*, 1–7.

Silverman, W. K., Pina, A. A., & Viswesvaran, C. (2008). Evidence-based psychosocial treatments for phobic and anxiety disorders in children and adolescents. *Journal of Clinical Child and Adolescent Psychology, 37*, 105–130.

Smith, T., Groen, A. D., & Wynn, J. W. (2000). Randomized trial of intensive early intervention for children with pervasive developmental disorder. *American Journal on Mental Retardation, 105*, 269–285.

Spence, S. H. (1995). *Social skills training: Enhancing social competence and children and adolescents.* Windsor, UK: The NFER-NELSON Publishing Company Ltd.

Spence, S. H. (2003). Social skills training with children and young people: Theory, evidence and practice. *Child and Adolescent Mental Health, 8*, 84–96.

Spence, S. H., Donovan, C., & Brechman-Toussaint, M. (1999). Social skills, social outcomes, and cognitive features of childhood social phobia. *Journal of Abnormal Psychology, 108*, 211–221.

Spence, S. H., Donovan, C., & Brechman-Toussaint, M. (2000). The treatment of childhood social phobia: The effectiveness of a social skills training-based, cognitive-behavioral intervention, with and without parental involvement. *Journal of Child Psychology and Psychiatry, 41*, 713–726.

Spence, S. H., & Marzillier, J. S. (1979). Social skills training with adolescent male offenders: Short term effects. *Behaviour Research and Therapy, 17*, 7–16.

Stark, K. D., Reynolds, W. M., & Kaslow, N. J. (1987). A comparison of the relative efficacy of self-control therapy and behavior problem-solving therapy for depression in children. *Journal of Abnormal Child Psychology, 15*, 91–113.

Stark, K. D., & Rouse, L., & Livingston, R. (1991). Treatment of depression during childhood and adolescence: Cognitive behavioral procedures for the individual and family. In P. Kendall (Ed.), *Child and adolescent therapy* (pp. 165–206). New York: Guilford.

Stokes, T. F., & Baer, D. M. (1977). An implicit technology of generalization. *Journal of Applied Behavior Analysis, 10*, 349–367.

Stokes, T. F., & Osnes, P. G. (1989). An operant pursuit of generalization. *Behavior Therapy, 20*, 337–355.

Sukhodolsky, D. G., & Butter, E. M. (2007). Social skills training for children with intellectual disabilities. In J. W. Jacobson, J. A. Mulick, & J. Rojahn (Eds.), *Handbook of intellectual and developmental disabilities* (pp. 601–618). New York: Springer.

Sukhodolsky, D. G., Kassinove, H., & Gorman, B. S. (2004). Cognitive-behavioral therapy for anger in children and adolescents: A meta-analysis. *Aggression and Violent Behavior, 9*, 247–269.

Tofte-Tipps, S., Mendonca, P., & Peach, R. V. (1982). Training and generalization of social skills. *Behavior Modification, 6*, 45–71.

Tremblay, R. E., Pagani, K. L., Masse, L. C., & Vitaro, F. (1995). A biomodal preventive intervention for disruptive kindergarten boys: Its impact through mid-adolescence. Special Section: Prediction and prevention of child and adolescent antisocial behavior. *Journal of Consulting and Clinical Psychology, 63*, 560–568.

Tutty, S., Gephart, H., & Wurzbacher, K. (2003). Enhancing behavioral and social skill functioning in children newly diagnosed with attention-deficit hyperactivity disorder in a pediatric setting. *Developmental and Behavioral Pediatrics, 24*, 51–57.

Twentyman, G. T., & McFall, R. M. (1975). Behavioral training of social skills in shy males. *Journal of Consulting and Clinical Psychology, 43*, 384–395.

Vaughn, S., & Hogan, A. (1990). Social competence and learning disabilities: A prospective study. In H. L. Swanson & B. K. Keogh (Eds.), *Learning disabilities: Theoretical and research issues.* (pp. 175–191). Hillsdale, NJ: Lawrence Erlbaum Associates, Inc.

Vaughn, S. R., Ridley, C. A., & Bullock, D. D. (1984). Interpersonal problem-solving skills training with aggressive young children. *Journal of Applied Developmental Psychology, 5*, 213–224.

Walker, H. M., Colvin, G., & Ramsey, E. (1995). *Antisocial behavior in school: Strategies and best practices.* Belmont, CA: Thomson Brooks/Cole Publishing Co.

Walker, H. M., Kavanagh, K., Stiller, B., Golly, A., Severson, H. H., & Feil, E. G. (1998). First Step to success: An early intervention approach for preventing school antisocial behavior. *Journal of Emotional and Behavioral Disorders, 6*, 66–80.

Warnes, E. D., Sheridan, S. M., Geske, J., & Warnes, W. A. (2005). A contextual approach to the assessment of social skills: Identifying meaningful behaviors for social competence. *Psychology in the Schools, 42*, 173–187.

Webster-Stratton, C., & Hancock, L. (1998). Parent training: Content, methods and processes. In E. Schaefer (Ed.), *Handbook of parent training* (2nd ed., pp. 98–152). New York: Wiley.

Webster-Stratton, C., & Reid, M. (2003). The Incredible Years parents, teachers, and children training series: A multifaceted treatment approach for young children with conduct problems. In A. E. Kazdin & J. R. Weisz

(Eds.), *Evidence-based psychotherapies for children and adolescents* (pp. 224–240). New York: Guilford.

Webster-Stratton, C., & Reid, M. (2008). Strengthening social and emotional competence in young children who are socioeconomically disadvantaged. In W. H. Brown, S. L., Odom, & S. R. McConnell (Eds.), *Social competence of young children: Risk, Disability, & Intervention* (pp. 185–203). Baltimore, MD: Paul H. Brookes Publishing Co.

Weisz, J. R., Sandler, I. N., Durlak, J. A., & Anton, B. S. (2005). Promoting and protecting youth mental health through evidence-based prevention and treatment. *American Psychologist, 60,* 628–648.

Wells, K. C., & Egan, L. (1988). Social learning and systems family therapy for childhood oppositional disorder: Comparative treatment outcome. *Comprehensive Psychiatry, 29,* 138–146.

Wells, K. C., Hersen, M., Bellack, A. S., & Himmerelhoch, J. (1979). Social skills training in unipolar nonpsychotic depression. *American Journal in Psychiatry, 136,* 1331–1332.

Wells, K. C., Pelham, W. E., Kotkin, R. A., Hoza, B., Abikoff, H. B., Abramowitz, A., et al. (2000). Psychosocial treatment strategies in the MTA study: Rationale, methods, and critical issues in the design and implementation. *Journal of Abnormal Child Psychology, 28,* 483–505.

Whitman, T. L., Burish, T., & Collins, C. (1972). Development of interpersonal language responses in two moderately retarded children. *Mental Retardation, 10,* 40–45.

Whitman, T. L., Mercurio, J. R., & Caponigri, V. (1970). Development of social responses in two severely retarded children. *Journal of Applied Behavior Analysis, 3,* 133–138.

Winer, J. L., Hilpert, P. L., Gesten, E. L., Cowen, E. L., & Schubin, W. E. (1982). The evaluation of a kindergarten social problem-solving program. *Journal of Primary Prevention, 2,* 205–216.

Wingspan, L. L. C. (1999). *Al's Pals: Kids making healthy choices.* Richmond, VA: Author.

Witt, J. C., & Elliott, S. N. (1986). Acceptability of classroom management strategies. In T. R. Kratochwill (Ed.), *Advances in school psychology* (Vol. 4, pp. 261–288). Hillsdale, NJ: Lawrence Erlbaum.

Wolf, M. M. (1978). Social validity: The case for subjective measurement or how applied behavior analysis is finding its heart. *Journal of Applied Behavior Analysis, 11,* 203–214.

Chapter 2
Theories of Social Competence from the Top-Down to the Bottom-Up: A Case for Considering Foundational Human Needs

Kathryn N. Stump, Jacklyn M. Ratliff, Yelena P. Wu, and Patricia H. Hawley

Social competence is an oft-studied, little understood construct that nonetheless remains a hallmark of positive, healthy functioning across the life span. Social competence itself, however, remains a nebulous concept in the developmental literature, particularly in the peer relations field. Dodge (1985) pointed out that there are nearly as many definitions of social competence as there are researchers in the field. Likewise, Ladd (2005) outlined the century-long academic history of research on social competence and also noted its numerous conceptualizations.

Social competence has been viewed as a multi-faceted construct involving social assertion, frequency of interaction, positive self-concept, social cognitive skills, popularity with peers, and the list goes on and on (Dodge, 1985). Whereas numerous studies outline the components, indices, and correlates of social competence, little headway has been made in generating a unified theory of social competence. In other words, much of our academic energy has been devoted to exploring a top-down approach to social competence in which we analyze and delineate the different manifestations of social competence (e.g., by identifying behaviors that we believe to be socially competent or those that are socially appealing or virtuous) and then search for common underpinnings. By instead adopting a bottom-up approach in which we examine underlying roots of competent behavior, we can form a more

cohesive picture of the construct and develop theories to predict and explain children's social behavior.

The purpose of this chapter is fourfold. First, we briefly review commonly employed approaches to social competence, especially as they relate to peer relationships and aggression. Second, we outline self-determination theory as a useful meta-theoretical lens through which we can examine children's social behavior. Third, we will introduce resource control theory (Hawley, 1999) as an evolutionary-based theory of social competence (i.e., a bottom-up approach) with which we will raise questions about the nature of social competence and provide explanations as to how a resource control theoretic perspective compares to traditional representations of social competence. Fourth, we will provide examples of how self-determination and resource control theoretic perspectives of social competence can relate to applied settings.

Top-Down Approaches to Social Competence

By "top-down approaches to social competence," we mean specific practices in which researchers first identify behaviors and components of relationship functioning that they believe to be "socially competent" and then search for commonalities among their indices. Thus, from a top-down system, the nature of social competence itself refers to the similarities of the *a priori* defined indices. The

P.H. Hawley (✉)
Department of Psychology, University of Kansas, Lawrence, KS 66045-7556, USA
e-mail: phawley@ku.edu

J.L. Matson (ed.), *Social Behavior and Skills in Children*, DOI 10.1007/978-1-4419-0234-4_2,
© Springer Science+Business Media, LLC 2009

practice of first defining outward manifestations of social competence before defining the actual construct creates difficulties in generating theories or root causes of social competence. Imagine, for example, social competence being portrayed as a tree. A top-down approach to social competence would involve gazing at the leaves of the tree (i.e., the manifestations of social competence) and attempting to aggregate them all together to find the common branch. As we will soon illustrate, the practice of analyzing "leaves" soon becomes a value-laden process in which virtuous and morally infused behaviors are deemed socially competent. Conversely, a bottom-up approach is one in which researchers focus on underlying roots of behaviors, thereby allowing multiple pathways to lead to competence (and not only those that involve behavioral profiles that conform to a top-down, value-laden approach). We will discuss bottom-up approaches to social competence in greater detail later.

Culturally Valued Attributes and Skills

In 1973, a panel of child development experts met to explore the construct of "social competence" with the intention of establishing an operational definition of the previously amorphous concept (Anderson & Messick, 1974). After discussing everything from Plato to *Oliver Twist*, the committee was unable to offer an explicit definition of social competence. Instead, they noted the dynamic nature of competence (i.e., competence in one social context may not necessarily translate into competence in another context) and proposed 29 facets of social competence, ranging from personal maintenance and cleanliness to fine motor dexterity.

While an excellent starting point, one can see how quickly the facet-creation can break down into a simple listing of attributes that are pleasant or valued in group situations, or contribute to manageability in classroom settings. Many of these qualities reflect culturally specific "values," perhaps especially values characteristic of middle class public educational contexts. It is fairly easy to derive counter-examples in which various behaviors and orientations lead to effective, adaptive functioning in harsh, deprived urban environments

or chaotic family conditions, but yet are counted as "unskilled" or disruptive in other contexts. Notably, Ogbu (1981), an acclaimed anthropologist, described the "competent bias" inherent to models that reflect a certain moral righteousness as a strategy that might not necessarily result in achieving competence in different cultures or contexts. In this way, skills-based models of social competence conform to what Kohlberg and Mayer (1972) refer to as "bag of virtues" models of social competence, an umbrella term meant to signify a cluster of ideals. Anderson and Messick (1974) also refer to these models as "Boy Scout" or "Sunday School" approaches. Social competence then comes to be defined by such ideals and as such largely reflects positive, if not romantic, standards.

Peer Regard Approaches

One way to embody culturally valued skills and attributes without actually listing the attributes is to measure one's social competence by one's social success, or the extent to which one is positively received in one's social context. To this end, acceptance by peers has long been identified as a healthy developmental and affiliative goal (Berndt & Savin-Williams, 1993; Parker & Asher, 1987). Historically, social status has been analyzed from two discrete research traditions and therefore yielded two distinct measures of status. Research from the first tradition involves directly asking children and adolescents about their social preferences (i.e., liking). Thus, the construct of *group acceptance* (or social preference) represents the variability among children in the extent to which individuals are well-liked by a wide range of their peers. Interest in social preference has been driven partly by assumptions that adaptive membership in significant peer groups is important to an individual's social (Parker & Gottman, 1989), emotional (Coleman, 1961), and identity development (Kroger, 2003; Newman & Newman, 2001; Vandell & Hembree, 1994). This link is presumed to exist partly because humans have a universal and evolutionary-based need to belong (Baumeister & Leary, 1995; see also Adler, 1924; Maslow, 1971, Sullivan, 1953) and peer groups meet this need to belong, at least after early childhood and into adolescence (Aseltine, 1995; Coleman, 1961). In addition, acceptance by a peer group also provides opportunities for interpersonal communication and social skills development, outlets for physical activity, and protection from victimization. Accordingly, longitudinal assessments reveal that early peer acceptance predicts long-term well-being (Parker & Asher, 1987). On the other hand, individuals with low group acceptance lack influence in their social environments (Parkhurst & Hopmeyer, 1998) and may be vulnerable to victimization by more powerful peers.

The second research tradition involves asking children and adolescents who they believe is popular and unpopular. This method was borne from ethnographic studies of children and adolescents in their natural school environments (Adler & Adler, 1998; Eder, 1985). When children were asked to describe their popular peers, their descriptions did not conform to the traditional social preference view of status (Eder, 1985). Instead, middle school children and adolescents described the socially elite and powerful, many of whom were actually disliked by their peers (Adler & Adler, 1998; Eder, 1985). Therefore, individuals who are perceived to be popular by the group need not be well-liked (Cillessen & Mayeux, 2004; but see Hawley, Little, & Card, 2007). This line of research centers on the construct of "perceived popularity" (Parkhurst & Hopmeyer, 1998; Prinstein & Cillessen, 2003), a measure reflecting social prominence. Rather than emphasizing actual differences among group members in the extent to which they are well-liked by the peer group at large, social prominence reflects differences among individuals in the extent to which they have a reputation in the group for being a member of the popular elite, emulated, "cool," or socially central and powerful (Cillessen & Rose, 2005; Rodkin, Farmer, Pearl, & Van Acker, 2006).

Because of the power and distinction associated with a high positioning in the peer group, most adolescents, in particular, desire membership in the subgroups with the highest power, visibility, or influence in the larger peer group (Hawley, 1999; Parkhurst & Hopmeyer, 1998). Dishion, Patterson, and Griesler (1994) refer to this process as "shopping" for status. The practice of seeking out high status peers begins long before adolescence, however. Even kindergarten age children are acutely cognizant of the existing pecking order in their social environments and report feeling more anxiety associated with status and peer relations than with school entry and academic performance (Ladd, 1990; see also Hawley & Little, 1999 for power manifestation in the preschool years).

Though social prominence may be the most salient index of status for children and adolescents (Duncan, 2004), many peer relations researchers consider social preference and acceptance to be better indices of social competence because of the emphasis on affiliation over competition or deviance (Cairns & Cairns, 1994; Rose-Krasnor, 1997). Nonetheless, "agentic goals" such as competition have long been recognized to reflect an underlying human need, presumably the satisfaction of which would itself be reflected in social competence. This is a point to which we will turn next.

Effective Goal Attainment and Balancing the Self and Other

Several developmental approaches to social competence recognize that children have differing goals, and meeting these goals in the social group gives rise to transactional challenges in the social group. Rose-Krasnor's (1997) "Social Competence Prism" hierarchically organizes several facets of social competence (social skills, sociometric status, relationships, and functional outcomes) by broadly defining competence as "effectiveness in interaction" with explicit consideration of children's motivations and goals in the social arena. Goal-oriented approaches suggest that one is effective to the degree that one successfully balances the goals of self and other (Bost, Vaughn, Washington, Cielinski, & Bradbard, 1998; Rubin & Rose-Krasnor, 1992; Weinstein, 1969). These models consider the importance of the self in that they incorporate aspects of social functioning (such as perspective taking and conflict negotiation) in judging effectiveness in interaction. In effect, according to these models, goals related to the self are important to the extent that individuals are not subordinate to the group. However, by these models, social dominance is also an inappropriate individual goal; social preference, that is, being liked by one's peer group is a valued social goal but striving to be socially elite or emulated is not. Though these models consider the role of the self, they still maintain that group cohesion and affiliation remain the primary criteria for evaluation. In other words, according to these goal-oriented approaches, subordination is undesirable, but dominance is inappropriate. To our way of thinking, simply cataloging "positive" self-oriented goals that children may have (e.g., to stop a teasing peer) contributes little more than top-down approaches that involve listing "value-laden" skills. Moreover, because of their foci on values and group cohesion, all of these perspectives rule out aggression as an appropriate or effective method of goal attainment. Aligning aggression with maladaptation may or may not be an appropriate assumption.

Aggression

Within the psychological literature (e.g., Coie & Dodge, 1998), researchers consider aggressive acts as those intended to hurt a target. For the greater part of the 20th century, aggression was considered to manifest exclusively in direct, physical forms (Coie & Dodge, 1998). Further, physically and verbally aggressive behaviors were more consistent with the goals of physical dominance and instrumentality, both typically regarded as "male goals" (Block, 1983). As a result, males were considered to be more aggressive than females (Maccoby & Jacklin, 1980). More recently, researchers have begun investigating alternative, more indirect, forms of aggression which are more inclusive to female perpetrators (Crick & Grotpeter, 1995; Galen & Underwood, 1997; Lagerspetz, Björkqvist, & Peltonen, 1988). Researchers have identified this alternative form of aggression as relational (Crick & Grotpeter, 1995) or social aggression (Galen & Underwood, 1997). Together, these forms appear to be more consistent with relational goals and social interactions than with physical dominance (Crick & Grotpeter, 1995; but see Hawley, Little, & Card, 2008). The alternative forms of aggression, though they maintain slightly dissimilar definitions, share a common behavioral thread; they each involve behaviors such as excluding, gossiping, and sabotaging relationships.

Regardless of the form that aggression takes (i.e., physical, relational), aggression is nearly unilaterally considered to be an index of social incompetence, possibly because aggression is presumably associated with peer rejection, a condition that is antithetical to acceptance (Coie & Dodge, 1998; Newcomb, Bukowski, & Pattee, 1993). Moreover, researchers have identified associations between aggression and long-term negative developmental outcomes (Brook & Newcomb, 1995; Coie & Dodge, 1983), lack of certain skills (perspective taking, empathy), and positive personality traits (e.g., agreeableness). As a result of these assumed relationships, aggression has been viewed as immoral, evil and, thus, antithetical to the "virtuous character" depicted through the top-down skills approach.

More recently, however, researchers have questioned this straightforward unilateral approach to aggression (see Bukowski, 2003; Smith, 2007; Vaughn & Santos, 2007). As a result, in addition to the different *forms* of aggression (e.g., physical or relational), researchers have begun investigating different *functions* of aggression (Little, Jones, Henrich, & Hawley, 2003). Generally speaking, reactive aggression has been conceptualized as a relatively uninhibited response to provocation whereas instrumental aggression has been described as somewhat more thoughtful, planned out, and self-serving. Both forms of aggression can manifest through these functions; in other words, both relational and physical aggression can be reactive or instrumental. Little, Jones and colleagues (2003) discovered that different functions of aggression are differentially associated with negative outcomes. For example, reactive aggression, regardless of form, was positively associated with self- and other-rated hostility and frustration intolerance, whereas instrumental aggression shared only a weak negative relationship or no relationship at all with the same outcomes. As such, Little, Jones et al. (2003) have suggested that, because instrumental aggression requires a certain degree of social skill and control, it may be more indicative of social competence than reactive aggression.

The idea that instrumental and reactive functions of aggression have differing social consequences may address a puzzle that has been evident to developmentalists throughout the

20th century. Namely, how can a behavior with ill social and personal repercussions be adaptive in an evolutionary sense? The answer may partially lie in the fact that the consequences to instrumental aggression may not be as negative to all as we are wont to believe. To help solve this paradox we turn our attention to basic and fundamental human needs as addressed by self-determination theory, with its deep roots in human motivational systems.

SDT: Theory Building from the Bottom Up

Self-determination theory (SDT; Deci & Ryan, 2000) is an organismic evolutionary-based meta-theoretical perspective of adaptive functioning (e.g., healthy development, coherent sense of self, well-being). Due to its focus on the organism and its basic needs and need fulfillment, SDT allows us to consider more explicitly the primary role of self-interest in adaptive human functioning (versus the traditional perspectives outlined above that seem to place higher premium on other-interest in terms of harmonious group functioning). As its basic premise, SDT recognizes that humans universally have three innate needs: competence, autonomy, and relatedness (Ryan, Kuhl, & Deci, 1997).[1] Different means or methods are employed to meet these needs based on context and culture. Further, the different means and methods that individuals use can be either intrinsically (from within) or extrinsically (externally controlled) motivated to varying degrees. Each will be taken in turn.

Innate Needs

Self-determination theory (e.g., Deci & Ryan, 2000) adopts the perspective of innate psychological needs from the drive and need theory traditions (e.g., Hull, 1943; Murray, 1938). Autonomy, the first of the three identified needs, refers to the degree to

which behaviors are perceived to be caused by the self versus directed by others (deCharms, 1968; Deci, 1980). Here the autonomous organism is self-directed and feels free from external force or coercion. Competence needs, derived from White's (1959) *effectance motivation*, refer to the motivation for successful and proficient interactions with the environment. The need for competence is centered on skills, action, and the ability to master the environment (Elliot, McGregor, & Thrash, 2002). Last, satisfaction of relatedness needs means one feels connected to others (Baumeister & Leary, 1995; Bowlby, 1988, Ryan, 1993).

Greater need satisfaction pursued autonomously leads to better mental health, more positive and intimate relationships, enhanced personal agency, well-being, and optimal functioning (Ryan & Deci, 2000a; Patrick, Knee, Canevello, & Lonsbary, 2007; Ryan, Deci, & Grolnick, 1995). Inadequate need fulfillment can lead to significant deficits in psychosocial functioning. For example, environments that do not promote autonomy (e.g., controlling, chaotic, punishing, or neglecting) may contribute to anxiety, alienation, inner conflict, and depression. Additionally, the nonautonomous individual is more likely to experience ill-being and, at the extreme, psychopathology such as obsessive-compulsive disorder, depression, eating disorders, and personality disorders (Ryan et al., 1995). In our conceptualization of social competence, we believe that the socially competent individual will have satisfied or met all three of these needs within the context of social interactions (see also Buhrmester, 1996).

Intrinsic vs. Extrinsic Motivation

According to SDT, individuals are differentially driven to achieve their needs or goals. To this end, goals are optimally pursued when driven by intrinsic motives (energized by personal interests and internalized values). External inducement or control can undermine pleasurable goal pursuit and concomitant positive outcomes (Frodi, Bridges, & Grolnick, 1985). More specifically, extrinsically motivated behaviors are externally directed (e.g., forced; out of the organism's direct control; Ryan & Deci, 2000a). As a result,

---

[1] SDT is not the only perspective to recognize the tension between agentic and communal needs (see also Adler, 1924; Bakan,1966; Freud, 1930/1964; Maslow, 1971).

individuals who are extrinsically motivated experience less need satisfaction, diminished well-being and personal agency, and later maladaptation (e.g., Kasser & Ryan, 2001; Sheldon & Kasser, 1998). For example, externally controlled individuals may experience difficulties integrating and internalizing behavioral social values and norms. We will return to this point later.

Conversely, psychological health and performance are fostered by behaviors that are intrinsically motivated (Deci & Ryan, 2000; Ryan & Deci, 2000a; Sheldon & Kasser, 1998). The healthiest children are those who are inherently motivated to seek out new challenges, new situations, and to energetically explore their environments. Social contextual events such as providing challenges and competence promoting feedback will facilitate intrinsic motivated behaviors and goals (Deci & Ryan, 2000; Ryan & Deci, 2000a). Promoting intrinsic motivation while also reducing external motivation may be construed as one of the greatest challenges of modern educational environments (Ryan & Brown, 2005).

SDT and Attachment Theory

Self-determination theory (SDT) may yet be relatively foreign to developmentalists and clinicians. In contrast, attachment theory is well known and often applied in these domains. Although these different theoretical traditions reside in different literatures, they share several points of contact relevant for our present purposes. Namely, Bowlby and Ainsworth construed the *secure base* as allowing the child to explore in ever-widening circles until he or she internalizes the secure base functions of the caregivers in the form of schemas and attachment working models (see Ainsworth, Blehar, Waters, & Wall, 1978; Bowlby, 1969/1980, 1988). These working models underlie confidence and autonomy. Accordingly, securely attached children become increasingly efficacious individuals who believe that (a) they are lovable and worthy of support, (b) they are self-directed, and (c) the world is a safe and predictable place where goals and material resources can be readily attained (Ainsworth et al., 1978;

Bartholomew & Horowitz, 1991; Bowlby, 1969/1980; Brennan, Clark, & Shaver, 1998). In this sense, secure attachments lay the foundation for meeting one's relatedness, autonomy, and competence needs. Indeed, La Guardia, Ryan, Couchman, and Deci (2000) investigated the relations among attachment, need satisfaction, and well-being and discovered that secure attachment satisfies all three basic needs.

As a biologically based theory, attachment theory, like SDT, is less likely to define adaptive functioning in terms of what is good for others but rather focuses primary attention on the organism actively coping with environmental inputs to maximize need satisfaction. As such, SDT and attachment theory can be construed as laying the foundations for bottom-up approaches to social competence.

A Bottom-Up Approach to Social Competence

As introduced earlier, bottom-up approaches to social competence (in contrast to top-down approaches) first consider the nature of the organism interacting in its environment. In essence, social competence refers to the ability of an individual to thrive in his or her social environment. SDT and attachment theory can both be considered bottom-up approaches because they address foundational, innate human needs as the primary drive for competence and strategies for attaining these human needs (i.e., manifestations of competence) only secondarily. Bowlby first identified the functions of behaviors and then attended to the forms of those behaviors. For example, though gazing and tantrum throwing involve dissimilar actions and appearances (i.e., forms), they share the same function – both are means to gain attention from caretakers and thus to satisfy relatedness needs. A bottom-up approach might consider both crying and gazing as effective strategies for satisfying needs. From a top-down approach, however, non-evolutionary researchers may only consider gazing to be an appropriate means of need satisfaction because it is the most pleasing method.

Both SDT and attachment theory provide useful insights into the basic foundations of human behavior and what ultimately drives it. In this sense, we feel we have the roots upon which a functional theory of social competence may be built. Until now, we have argued that the principal obstruction to developing a unified theory of social competence in the peer relations literature is that the definition of social competence is convoluted and in some senses atheoretical (competence is what is morally "good" or pleasant to others). With focus on such outward indices of "competence" such as friendship quality, popularity, social skills, and information processing, researchers risk becoming entangled in the proximate manifestations of social competence instead of exploring the foundations of competence. In contrast, a bottom-up approach strips social competence from a moral framework and instead explores competence as goal attainment, thereby considering multiple strategies as effective avenues to social competence.

Bukowski (2003), himself searching for the roots of competent behavior, explored the linguistic lineage of "*competence*" and discovered that it shares a common linguistic ancestry with "*compete.*" More specifically, Bukowski (2003) suggested "that being competent means that one is able to compete in the company of others" (p. 394). This definition of competence aligns well with White's (1959) premise that competence refers to "an organism's capacity to interact effectively with its environment" (p. 297) which underlies the understandings of competence (needs) from both SDT and Attachment theoretic perspectives. That all of these views have biological roots is not coincidental. Evolutionarily oriented approaches tend to focus on adaptation to environments both ultimately and proximally. Thus, if we were to adopt an evolutionary theoretical perspective, we may do well to consider social competence to imply effective competition in social contexts. Whereas competition is typically considered to be less than socially desirable (though it seems to be represented in a softer form in "agency needs"; Buhrmester, 1996), it lies at the heart of resource control theory, an evolutionary perspective focusing on children's competitive strategies, competitive success, and consequent developmental outcomes (both social and personal).

Resource Control Theory

Resource control theory (RCT; Hawley, 1999), like attachment theory, focuses first on individual adaptation to local circumstances, and group response as a secondary outcome of that adaptation process. *Resource control* in general refers to the extent to which individuals successfully access social, informational, or material resources. This definition includes access to and attention from high status others (social), objects denoting status (material), and valuable information regarding work, school projects, or events (informational; Hawley, 1999; Keltner, Gruenfeld, & Anderson, 2003).

Resource control strategies. According to resource control theory, there are two primary classes of strategy that can be employed to access resources. Coercive strategies are those represented well in the primate literature and include behaviors that are viewed negatively by others such as threats, aggression, and manipulation (i.e., instrumental aggression). Setting the present theory apart from other theories of social dominance (e.g., Bernstein, 1981) are prosocial strategies of resource control, or behaviors that access resources via socially acceptable means such as cooperation or reciprocation. These strategies are those that are viewed positively by the group because they are consistent with accepted norms of behavior and tend to build interpersonal bonds. In contrast, coercive strategies tend to be viewed negatively by others because they generally operate outside of accepted norms and they are assumed to break bonds with others. As we will explore later, this latter assumption may be an oversimplification and the use of coercive strategies under some conditions may actually enhance one's interpersonal reputation and interconnections within the social network.

There are several important consequences to defining resource control strategies in these ways. First, the theory implies that prosociality can well serve competition. Typically, prosociality is seen as other-oriented from most psychological perspectives. However, when evolution is invoked, discussions of prosociality often turn to the long-term benefit of interacting positively with others (such as long-term resource acquisition and predator defense). Second, if aggression is associated with effective resource control, then, by extension, coercion can be associated with competence insofar as it leads to effective interaction with the material environment. Thus, in terms of White's (1959) effectance motivation, and Deci and Ryan's (2000) competence, both strategies may facilitate the satisfaction of competence needs.[2]

Third, resource control theory employs a person-centered, typological approach, in which instead of describing the relations between variables (i.e., via correlations and regressions; a variable-centered approach) we classify individuals into "types" depending on their relative employment of the two strategies. Assessment of the "types" differs by age or developmental level. In observational studies conducted with very young children (Hawley, 2002), for example, prosocial strategies included making suggestions, issuing polite requests, and offering unsolicited help. Coercive strategies involved taking, aggression, and insults. By the time children are in late elementary school, we can administer self-report measures. Questionnaire items for prosocial strategies include "I get what I want by reciprocating," "... by being nice," or "... promising friendship." Coercive strategies include, "I get what I want by taking," "... threatening," or "... bullying." For adolescents, we can use similar items for peer nomination (e.g., "Who gets what they want by ...") and friendship inventories ("My friend gets what they want by ..."). Teacher report is useful for all ages (Hawley, 2003a, 2003b).

On the basis of the relative degree of self-report endorsement or teacher- or peer-reported employment of the strategies, subgroups of individuals can be defined depending on their standing in the distributions of prosocial and coercive strategies divided into thirds: bistrategic controllers, by definition, are in the top third of both prosocial and coercive strategies, coercive controllers are in the top third of coercive strategies only, prosocial controllers are in the top third of prosocial strategies only, and noncontrollers are in the lowest third of both strategies. Typical controllers comprise the largest remaining group. Bistrategic controllers, regardless of the reporter (e.g., teacher report,

self-report, or peer nomination), are the most successful at resource control by far, followed by prosocial and coercive controllers, with the noncontrollers being the least successful. Thus, from this perspective, bistrategic controllers are considered to be of the highest social dominance status and noncontrollers the lowest by definition.

Explorations of the personal and social outcomes of the types have yielded informative patterns that in some ways have confronted a number of cherished ideals in psychology. First, prosocial controllers routinely display appealing characteristics such as intrinsic motivations for pursuing friendships (e.g., for joy and personal fulfillment; Hawley, Little, & Pasupathi, 2002), agreeableness, and social skills. Presumably as a consequence, they are well-liked by peers and enjoy intimate, high-quality friendships (Hawley et al., 2007). In the parlance of self-determination theory, they are highly effective at meeting their relatedness needs while demonstrating competent interaction with the material world. This pattern associated with the prosocial controllers comes as no surprise as it certainly matches patterns anticipated from most perspectives. Also not surprising, coercive controllers are aggressive, hostile, unskilled, and motivated by power and popularity (rather than intimacy; Hawley, 2003b; Hawley et al., 2002). Consequently, they maintain low-quality and conflictual friendships, thus undermining the optimal satisfaction of relatedness needs (Hawley et al., 2007). Taken together, prosocial and coercive controllers accurately illustrate most social competence perspectives that maintain that good things go together, as do negative.

More instructive to us, however, are the bistrategic controllers. As mentioned, they are by far the most successful at resource control. Indeed, they place the highest value on the material world of all the groups (Hawley, Shorey, & Alderman, in press). At the same time, their behavioral profile and reception from the social group confronts commonly held assumptions in developmental psychology such as the predominant belief that aggressive individuals should be unskilled and socially repellant (Parker, Rubin, Erath, Wojslawowicz, & Buskirk, 2006). Like coercive controllers, bistrategics are aggressive, manipulative, and value power and popularity over intimacy. Yet, what sets them

---

[2] Though presumably Deci and Ryan would point out that aggression would heavily thwart relatedness needs. This point will be explored in more detail below.

starkly apart from coercive controllers is that they appear to have many of the skills of prosocial controllers; they have a relatively well-developed understanding of others, well-developed social skills, and a certain moral attunement (Hawley, 2003a, 2003b).

Where bistrategic resource controllers diverge from prosocial controllers is their self-professed high levels of overt (i.e., physical) and relational aggression (e.g., gossip). Nevertheless, our studies with preschoolers and adolescents have repeatedly shown that bistrategic controllers enjoy positive attention from others. When preschoolers nominate who they like (i.e., in sociometric procedures), bistrategic controllers garner among the most nominations (Hawley, 2003a). In adolescence, bistrategic controllers not only win "like nominations," but they also secure among the most "s/he is my best friend" nominations and are viewed as popular by others (Hawley et al., 2007; cf. Cillessen & Mayeux, 2004).

Further, the aggression of the bistrategic controller is neither subtle nor unobservable; their peers describe them as aggressive and their best friends report aggressive acts even within the relationship (Hawley et al., 2007). At the same time, bistrategic controllers appear to also enjoy reasonably high quality friendships. Bistrategic controllers and their friends report among the highest levels of fun, closeness, and companionship in their friendships relative to other resource control subtypes.[3]

Very nearly opposite in profile to the bistrategic is the noncontroller. Noncontrollers are among the least preferred social partners in the classroom (Hawley, 2003b). In middle school and high school they are at risk for rejection and victimization. The social response to these children cannot be accounted for by interpersonal aggression alone because they are among the least aggressive of all children. Overall, they lack agency (they do not interact effectively with the material world) and defer to others in play situations (Hawley & Little, 1999). They do not fully understand the perspectives and goals of others, and they lack the associated social skills necessary for

these tasks. These deficits are reflected in the quality of their friendships; noncontrollers' friendships, unlike bistrategics' friendships, are low in closeness, fun, and companionship (Hawley et al., 2007).

RCT & Aggression

What is the allure of this highly aggressive and powerful individual and why would a nonaggressive child be socially repellant? The magnetism of the bistrategic (and the opposite effect of the noncontroller) is not well explainable from predominant developmental psychopathology perspectives that hold aggression to be a clear risk factor for peer rejection and more (Coie & Dodge, 1998). In contrast to these theories, RCT predicts that the socially dominant individuals will hold social power and be socially central because of their evident mastery over the material world (i.e., competence). Social subordinance, in contrast, is thought to be associated with high risk from this perspective (social centrality hypothesis; Hawley, 1999).

Perhaps the most startling implications of RCT are those related to aggression. From this perspective, aggression can be conceptualized as an adaptive strategy because it aids in resource acquisition (Hawley, 2007; Hawley, Johnson, Mize, & McNamara, 2007). Whereas developmentalists suggest that the overall frequency of children's displayed aggressive behaviors dampens over time (Brame, Nagin, & Tremblay, 2001), we find that coercion remains a measurable strategy for resource control across the life span (Hawley, 2002; Hawley et al., 2007; Hawley et al., in press; Little, Brauner, Jones, Nock, & Hawley, 2003). Smith (2007) notes that although aggressive behavior may be "socially undesirable," we should not confuse this with "socially incompetent" or "maladaptive." Taken together, these results support Hawley's (1999) claims that aggression need not lead to negative developmental outcomes but can be associated with positive outcomes for both males and females (Hawley et al., 2008). These findings suggest that aggression alone does not determine peer acceptance. Rather, a prosocial profile, whether displayed alone or in conjunction with a coercive profile, appears to be positively related to peer acceptance.

---

[3] This is in contrast to perspectives that speculate that aggressive popular youth experience deficits at the level of the relationship (e.g., Cillessen & Mayeux, 2004; Cillessen & Rose, 2005).

RCT, Competence, Relatedness, and Autonomy

If individuals wield this power and achieve superior material success (i.e. competence) in ways that evidently draw others to them, could they also satisfy their relatedness needs? This is an important and interesting question to which we do not know the answer. At this point in our explorations, bistrategic resource controllers do not appear to sacrifice social success in the same way that coercive controllers do, perhaps because coercive controllers are unable to effectively balance their negative behaviors with positive ones. In fact, bistrategics appear to have the greatest pool of possible friends from which to choose; when individuals select their best friends, many more individuals nominate bistrategics as best friends than bistrategics reciprocate (Hawley et al., 2007). At the same time, bistrategic controllers need not defer to others; on the contrary, others generally defer to them. In this sense, then, they enjoy a good deal of autonomy. In contrast, non-controllers are the least autonomous of all children because of their chronic deferral to others; in other words, their own goals are subordinated to the goals of others.

Overall, prosocial strategies better fulfill relatedness needs than coercive strategies alone (in terms of quantity and quality of friendships). From this perspective, it should not be surprising that both prosocial and bistrategic controllers enjoy rewarding personal relationships – they share a common prosocial profile. Bistrategic controllers also display strongly coercive strategies, suggesting that coerciveness (in conjunction with prosociality) is not repellant to all peers. Also, it could be argued that bistrategic controllers are the most autonomous; as the most effective competitors (i.e., highest in social dominant status), they are free to behave outside the will of another (Hawley, 2002). All others must defer to some degree to the will of high status others, a sure sign that autonomy has been undermined. Thus, from this perspective, optimal ontogenetic adaptation is achieved through successful competition by means of prosocial strategy employment alone or prosociality balanced by coercion. However, unlike some top-down approaches to social competence, this perspective does *not* suggest that

competence is defined by the level of group contentment (i.e., relationships with bistrategics are not without cost; Hawley et al., 2007). Thus, resource control theory and self-determination theory do not fit well with the "bag of virtues," top-down approaches, but instead suggest that human behavior is incredibly complex, a central premise to evolutionary-based perspectives.

In summary, we wonder whether bistrategic resource control is consistent with our conceptualizations of social competence. Bistrategic controllers are socially central and maintain close (though conflictual) interpersonal relationships, suggesting that they are effectively balancing the needs of the self (i.e. getting ahead) with the needs of the group (i.e. getting along). Further, bistrategic resource controllers enjoy positive outcomes associated with the pursuit of relatedness, competence, and autonomy.

All of these standpoints, from both top-down and bottom-up perspectives, rely on environmental factors in terms of learning and available opportunities. Autonomy in the social domain, competence, and relatedness needs cannot be adequately achieved in neglecting and stifling environments. Successfully fostering needs satisfaction is a subject on which we focus next.

Implications for Children's Social Development and Fostering Social Competence

As discussed above, existing conceptualizations of social competence do not explicitly address the underlying biological needs that drive social behavior. Although some literature acknowledges the importance of social goals (e.g., seeking comfort or assistance; Brown, Odom, & Holcombe, 1996; Erdley & Asher, 1999), there may be additional important social goals to consider. For example, RCT suggests that competition affects children's social behavior in centrally important ways. RCT and SDT may therefore inform existing conceptualizations of social competence by addressing motivations underlying social behavior. Thus far, neither SDT nor RCT have been expressly applied to models of social competence. Nevertheless, both of these theories may have important implications for clinicians, clinical researchers, and educators. Specifically, practitioners in child development fields should be aware that children's environment (e.g., school) can foster or thwart need fulfillment and thus affect children's developing social competence.

Developing social competence in school. According to SDT (and by extension, RCT), healthy social development is predicated on children's sense of relatedness, competence, and autonomy (Ryan & Deci, 2000b). Well-being and optimal effective functioning are also predicated on the fulfillment of these needs. Recent policies focused on high stakes standardized testing may inadvertently decrease the ability to satisfy these needs in both children and teachers, creating particularly nonnutritive environments for children's optimal social development.

First, teachers who are understandably focused on helping their students succeed on standardized tests (Barksdale-Ladd & Thomas, 2000) are less likely to devote time to fostering children's autonomy, competence, and relatedness needs by, for example, deemphasizing guidance for executing appropriate social behavior and providing adequate socialization opportunities (e.g., prosocial ways of coping with conflicts; Pelletier, Seguin-Levesque, & Legault, 2002). Moreover, teachers' own sense of autonomy (how and what they teach) may be undermined, which in turn can affect their personal sense of competence and well-being. Thus, the high stakes testing movement may well have trickle down effects to teachers with negative social implications for children.

Second, policies emphasizing standardized testing often lead to standardized curricula, thus restricting socialization opportunities that are ultimately responsible for the development of social competence. For example, placing emphasis on performance standards results in rewarding didactic methods of teaching (Wood, 2004) and discouraging learning through peer collaboration (Barksdale-Ladd & Thomas, 2000). In addition, the focus on academic standards has led to the elimination of "non-academic" classes such as art, drama, and music. These non-academic classes, however, provide children with a range of enriching social development opportunities; drama classes help children develop their communication skills and improve social skills (Deasy, 2002) and art and music encourage children to express themselves in different ways than "academic" activities. Using art or music as a prosocial method of expressing oneself may improve children's relationships with other people by fostering perspective-taking and interpretative skills, essential skills for participating in healthy social interactions (Chandler, 1973). Furthermore, recess and gym, both essential outlets for children's physical and emotional energy and contexts for unstructured play where children can practice social skills, have been eliminated from some schools because they detract from performance standards.

Last, policies focused on testing may undermine children's perceptions of their own competence, particularly in the academic domain (Barksdale-Ladd & Thomas, 2000; Ryan & Brown, 2005), and poor performance may lead to further social difficulties (Roeser, Eccles, & Sameroff, 2000).

By turning our attention to high stakes testing, we wish only to point out the dangers of ignoring children's innate needs. Programs and interventions can have unintentional detrimental effects when the whole child is not considered. For example, what implications does RCT have for therapeutic interventions? If coercive behavior is not always harmful to the social well-being of the child (as in the case of bistrategic resource controllers), should we target the behavior of a bistrategic controller for intervention? Indeed, do these children even catch the attention of school personnel like the coercive controllers most assuredly do? These are difficult questions to answer, and we are not advocating implementing specific treatments or interventions but merely discussing the difficulty and complexity associated with taking the social goals of the child into consideration. We are in good company in voicing our apprehension regarding interventions; educators in the early 20th century have worried that policies centering on reducing aggressive behavior regardless of circumstances lead to the suppression of executive skills, particularly in girls (Wooley, 1925). These deep questions regarding the nature of social competence and the importance of individuals' social goals are often ignored in the developmental literature.

Conclusion

Most peer relations researchers are prosocial purists, describing "bag of virtues" models in which individuals help, self-sacrifice, and cooperate their way to competence. According to RCT, though individuals can in fact help and cooperate their way to resource control, being a highly successful competitor means one is able to balance "getting along" with "getting ahead" (Hogan, 1982); in other words, many successful competitors, even if aggressive, can remain socially dominant while also maintaining intimate social relationships. These descriptions may conjure an unsettling resemblance to the unscrupulous Machiavellian, but even Machiavelli (1513/2003) described the necessity of rewarding citizens with celebrations and of maintaining favor with the people: "[I]t is necessary for a prince to have the friendship of the people; otherwise he has no remedy in times of adversity" (p. 43). Whereas prosocial behaviors such as throwing festivals are not necessarily devoid of manipulative objectives (i.e., they are not *altruistic*), they are not purely coercive or tyrannical either. Prosociality is indeed an effective strategy of resource control, but so too are coercion and aggression. Prosocial and coercive behaviors exhibit different outward manifestations (e.g., doing favors vs. taking by force) but share the same ultimate function (gaining resources). By stripping prosociality and coercion from a moral framework in which prosociality should always be encouraged and coercion always discouraged, we can now consider each tactic to be a viable method to gain resources and satisfy foundational human needs. Researchers and practitioners perhaps should not only evaluate the resulting outcomes in the group context but also the extent to which each strategy is successfully implemented on its own and in combination.

References

Adler, A. (1924). *The practice and theory of individual psychology*. Oxford, England: Harcourt, Brace.

Adler, P. A., & Adler, P. (1998). *Peer power: Preadolescent culture and identity*. New Brunswick, NJ: Rutgers University Press.

Ainsworth, M. S., Blehar, M. C., Waters, E., & Wall, S. (1978). *Patterns of attachment: A psychological study of the strange situation*. Oxford, England: Lawrence Erlbaum.

Anderson, S., & Messick, S. (1974). Social competency in young children. *Developmental Psychology, 10*, 282–293.

Aseltine, R. H. (1995). A reconsideration of parental and peer influences on adolescent deviance. *Journal of Health and Social Behavior, 36*(2), 103–121.

Bakan, D. (1966). *The duality of human existence*. Boston: Beacon Press.

Barksdale-Ladd, M. A., & Thomas, K. F. (2000). What's at stake in high-stakes testing: Teachers and parents speak out. *Journal of Teacher Education, 51*, 384–397.

Bartholomew, K., & Horowitz, L. M. (1991). Attachment styles among young adults: A test of a four-category model. *Journal of Personality and Social Psychology, 61*(2), 226–244.

Baumeister, R., & Leary, M. R. (1995). The need to belong: Desire for interpersonal attachments as a fundamental human motivation. *Psychological Bulletin, 117*, 497–529.

Berndt, T. J., & Savin-Williams, R. C. (1993). Peer relations and friendships. In P. H. Tolan, & B. J. Cohler (Eds.), *Handbook of clinical research and practice with adolescents* (pp. 203–219). Oxford, England: John Wiley & Sons.

Bernstein, I. S. (1981). Dominance: The baby and the bathwater. *Behavioral and Brain Sciences, 4*(3), 419–457.

Block, J. H. (1983). Differential premises arising from differential socialization of the sexes: Some conjectures. *Child Development, 54*(6), 1335–1354.

Bost, K. K., Vaughn, B. E., Washington, W. N., Cielinski, K. L., & Bradbard, M. R. (1998). Social competence, social support, and attachment: Demarcation of construct domains, measurement, and paths of influence for preschool children attending head start. *Child Development, 69*(1), 192–218.

Bowlby, J. (1969/1980). *Attachment and loss*. New York, NY: Basic Books.

Bowlby, J. (1988). *A secure base: Parent-child attachment and healthy human development*. New York: Basic Books.

Brame, B., Nagin, D. S., & Tremblay, R. E. (2001). Developmental trajectories of physical aggression from school entry to late adolescence. *Journal of Child Psychology and Psychiatry, 42*(4), 503–512.

Brennan, K. A., Clark, C. L., & Shaver, P. R. (1998). Self-report measurement of adult attachment: An integrative overview. In J. A. Simpson, & W. S. Rholes (Eds.), *Attachment theory and close relationships*. (pp. 46–76). New York, NY: Guilford Press.

Brook, J. S., & Newcomb, M. D. (1995). Childhood aggression and unconventionality: Impact on later academic achievement, drug use, and workforce involvement. *Journal of Genetic Psychology, 156*(4), 393–410.

Brown, W. H., Odom, S. L., & Holcombe, A. (1996). Observational assessment of young children's social behavior with peers. *Early Childhood Research Quarterly, 11*, 19–40.

Buhrmester, D. (1996). Need fulfillment, interpersonal competence, and the developmental contexts of early adolescent friendship. In W. M. Bukowski, A. F. Newcomb, & W. W. Hartup (Eds.), *The company they keep: Friendship in childhood and adolescence*. (pp. 158–185). New York, NY, US: Cambridge University Press.

Bukowski, W. M. (2003). What does it mean to say that aggressive children are competent or incompetent? *Merrill-Palmer Quarterly. Special Issue: Aggression and Adaptive Functioning: The Bright Side to Bad Behavior, 49*(3), 390–400.

Cairns, R. B., & Cairns, B. D. (1994). *Lifelines and risks: Pathways of youth in our time.* New York, NY, US: Cambridge University Press.

Chandler, M. J. (1973). Egocentrism and antisocial behavior: The assessment and training of social perspective-taking skills. *Developmental Psychology, 9*, 326–332.

Cillessen, A. H. N., & Mayeux, L. (2004). From censure to reinforcement: Developmental changes in the association between aggression and social status. *Child Development, 75*(1), 147–163.

Cillessen, A. H. N., & Rose, A. J. (2005). Understanding popularity in the peer system. *Current Directions in Psychological Science, 14*(2), 102–105.

Coie, J. D., & Dodge, K. A. (1983). Continuities and changes in children's social status: A five-year longitudinal study. *Merrill-Palmer Quarterly, 29*(3), 261–282.

Coie, J. D., & Dodge, K. A. (1998). Aggression and antisocial behavior. In W. Damon & N. Eisenberg (Eds.), *Handbook of child psychology, social, emotional, and personality development.* (5th ed., Vol. 3, pp. 779–862). Hoboken, NJ: John Wiley & Sons Inc.

Coleman, J. S. (1961). *The adolescent society: The social life of the teenager and its impact on education.* Oxford, England: Free Press of Glencoe.

Crick, N. R., & Grotpeter, J. K. (1995). Relational aggression, gender, and social-psychological adjustment. *Child Development, 66*(3), 710–722.

Deasy, R. J. (Ed.). (2002). *Critical links: Learning in the arts and student academic and social development* (Arts Education Partnership, Washington, DC). Washington, DC: Department of Education.

deCharms, R. (1968). *Personal causation.* New York: Academic Press.

Deci, E. L. (1980). *The psychology of self-determination.* Lexington, MA: Lexington Books.

Deci, E. L., & Ryan, R. M. (2000). The "what" and "why" of goal pursuits: Human needs and the self-determination of behavior. *Psychological Inquiry, 11*, 227–268.

Dishion, T. J., Patterson, G. R., & Griesler, P. C. (1994). Peer adaptations in the development of antisocial behavior: A confluence model. In L. R. Huesmann (Ed.), *Aggressive behavior: Current perspectives* (pp. 61–95). New York, NY, US: Plenum Press.

Dodge, K. A. (1985). Facets of social interaction and the assessment of social competence in children. In B. Schneider, K. H. Rubin, & J. Ledingham (Eds.), *Children's peer relations: Issues in assessment and intervention* (pp. 3–22). New York: Springer-Verlag.

Duncan, N. (2004). It's important to be nice, but it's nicer to be important: Girls, popularity and sexual competition. *Sex Education. Special Issue: Sex/Sexuality and Relationships Education Conference, 4*(2), 137–152.

Eder, D. (1985). The cycle of popularity: Interpersonal relations among female adolescents. *Sociology of Education, 58*(3), 154–165.

Elliot, A. J., McGregor, H. A., & Thrash, T. M. (2002). The need for competence. In E. Deci & R. Ryan (Eds.), *Handbook of self-determination theory* (pp. 361–387). Rochester, NY: University of Rochester Press.

Erdley, C. A., & Asher, S. R. (1999). A social goals perspective on children's social competence. *Journal of Emotional and Behavioral Disorders, 7*, 156–167.

Freud, S. (1930/1964). *Civilization and its discontents.* New York: W. W. Norton.

Frodi, A., Bridges, L., & Grolnick, W. S. (1985). Correlates of mastery related behavior: A short-term longitudinal study of infants in their second year. *Child Development, 56*, 1291–1298.

Galen, B. R., & Underwood, M. K. (1997). A developmental investigation of social aggression among children. *Developmental Psychology, 33*(4), 589–600.

Hawley, P. H. (1999). The ontogenesis of social dominance: A strategy-based evolutionary perspective. *Developmental Review, 19*(1), 97–132.

Hawley, P. H. (2002). Social dominance and prosocial and coercive strategies of resource control in preschoolers. *International Journal of Behavioral Development, 26*, 167–176.

Hawley, P. H. (2003a). Strategies of control, aggression, and morality in preschoolers: An evolutionary perspective. *Journal of Experimental Child Psychology, 85*, 213–235.

Hawley, P. H. (2003b). Prosocial and coercive configurations of resource control in early adolescence: A case for the well-adapted Machiavellian. *Merrill-Palmer Quarterly. Special Issue: Aggression and Adaptive Functioning: The Bright Side to Bad Behavior, 49*(3), 279–309.

Hawley, P. H. (2007). Social dominance in childhood and adolescence: Why social competence and aggression may go hand in hand. In P. H. Hawley, T. D. Little, & P. C. Rodkin (Eds.), *Aggression and adaptation: The bright side to bad behavior* (pp. 1–29). Mahwah, NJ: Lawrence Erlbaum Associates, Inc.

Hawley, P. H., Johnson, S. E., Mize, J. A., & McNamara, K. A. (2007). Physical attractiveness in preschoolers: Relationships with power, status, aggression and social skills. *Journal of School Psychology, 45*(5), 499–521.

Hawley, P. H., & Little, T. D. (1999). On winning some and losing some: A social relations approach to social dominance in toddlers. *Merrill-Palmer Quarterly, 45*(2), 185–214.

Hawley, P. H., Little, T. D., & Card, N. A. (2007). The allure of a mean friend: Relationship quality and processes of aggressive adolescents with prosocial skills. *International Journal of Behavioral Development, 31*(2), 170–180.

Hawley, P. H., Little, T. D., & Card, N. A. (2008). The myth of the alpha male: A new look at dominance-related beliefs and behaviors among adolescent males and females. *International Journal of Behavioral Development, 32*(1), 76–88.

Hawley, P. H., Little, T. D., & Pasupathi, M. (2002). Winning friends and influencing peers: Strategies of peer influence in late childhood. *International Journal of Behavioral Development, 26*(5), 466–474.

Hawley, P. H., Shorey, H. S., & Alderman, P. M. Attachment correlates of resource control strategies: Possible origins of social dominance and interpersonal power differentials. Journal of Social and Personal Relationships. *The origins of social dominance and power: Perspectives from resource control and attachment theories.* Manuscript submitted for publication.

Hogan, R. (1982). A socioanalytic theory of personality. *Nebraska Symposium on Motivation, 30*, 5–89.

Hull, C. L. (1943). *Principles of behavior: An introduction to behavior theory.* New York: Appleton-Century-Crofts.

Kasser, T., & Ryan, R. M. (2001). Be careful what you wish for: Optimal functioning and the relative attainment of intrinsic and extrinsic goals. In P. Schmuck & K. Sheldon (Eds.), *Life goals and well-being.* Gottingen: Hogrefe.

Keltner, D., Gruenfeld, D. H., & Anderson, C. (2003). Power, approach, and inhibition. *Psychological Review, 110*, 265–284.

Kohlberg, L., & Mayer, R. (1972). Development as the aim of education. *Harvard Educational Review, 42*, 449–496.

Kroger, J. (2003). Identity development during adolescence. In G. R. Adams & M. D. Berzonsky (Eds.), *Blackwell handbook of adolescence* (pp. 205–226). Malden, MA: Blackwell Publishing.

La Guardia, J. G., Ryan, R. M., Couchman, C. E., & Deci, E. L. (2000). Within-person variation in security of attachment: A self-determination theory perspective on attachment, need fulfillment, and well-being. *Journal of Personality and Social Psychology, 79*, 367–384.

Ladd, G. W. (1990). Having friends, keeping friends, making friends, and being liked by peers in the classroom: Predictors of children's early school adjustment? *Child Development, 61*(4), 1081–1100.

Ladd, G. W. (2005). *Children's peer relations and social competence: A century of progress.* New Haven, CT: Yale University Press.

Lagerspetz, K. M., Björkqvist, K., & Peltonen, T. (1988). Is indirect aggression typical of females? Gender differences in aggressiveness in 11- to 12-year-old children. *Aggressive Behavior, 14*(6), 403–414.

Little, T. D., Brauner, J., Jones, S. M., Nock, M. K., & Hawley, P. H. (2003). Rethinking aggression: A typological examination of the functions of aggression. *Merrill-Palmer Quarterly. Special Issue: Aggression and Adaptive Functioning: The Bright Side to Bad Behavior, 49*(3), 343–369.

Little, T. D., Jones, S. M., Henrich, C. C., & Hawley, P. H. (2003). Disentangling the "whys" from the "whats" of aggressive behaviour. *International Journal of Behavioral Development, 27*(2), 122–133.

Maccoby, E. E., & Jacklin, C. N. (1980). Sex differences in aggression: A rejoinder and reprise. *Child Development, 51*(4), 964–980.

Machiavelli, N. (1513/2003). *The prince and other writings.* New York: Barnes and Noble Classics.

Maslow, A. H. (1971). *The farther reaches of human nature.* Oxford, England: Viking.

Murray, H. A. (1938). *Explorations in personality.* New York: Oxford University Press.

Newcomb, A. F., Bukowski, W. M., & Pattee, L. (1993). Children's peer relations: A meta-analytic review of popular, rejected, neglected, controversial, and average sociometric status. *Psychological Bulletin, 113*(1), 99–128.

Newman, B. M., & Newman, P. R. (2001). Group identity and alienation: Giving the we its due. *Journal of Youth and Adolescence, 30*, 515–538.

Ogbu, J. U. (1981). Origins of human competence: A cultural-ecological perspective. *Child Development, 52*, 413–429.

Parker, J. G., & Asher, S. R. (1987). Peer relations and later personal adjustment: Arelow-accepted children at risk? *Psychological Bulletin, 102*(3), 357–389.

Parker, J. G., & Gottman, J. M. (1989). Social and emotional development in a relational context: Friendship interaction from early childhood to adolescence. In T. J. Berndt & G. W. Ladd (Eds.), *Peer relationships in child development* (pp. 95–131). Oxford, England: John Wiley & Sons.

Parker, J. G., Rubin, K. H., Erath, S. A., Wojslawowicz, J. C., & Buskirk, A. A. (2006).Peer relationships, child development, and adjustment: A developmental psychopathology perspective. In D. Cicchetti & D. J. Cohen (Eds.), *Developmental psychopathology: Theory and methods* (2nd ed., Vol. 1, pp. 419–493). Hoboken, NJ: John Wiley & Sons Inc.

Parkhurst, J. T., & Hopmeyer, A. (1998). Sociometric popularity and peer-perceived popularity: Two distinct dimensions of peer status. *Journal of Early Adolescence, 18*(2), 125–144.

Patrick, H., Knee, C. R., Canevello, A., & Lonsbary, C. (2007). The role of need fulfillment in relationship functioning and well-being: A self-determination theory perspective. *Journal of Personality and Social Psychology, 92*(3), 434–457.

Pelletier, L. G., Seguin-Levesque, C., & Legault, L. (2002). Pressure from above and pressure from below as determinants of teachers' motivation and teaching behaviors. *Journal of Educational Psychology, 94*, 186–196.

Prinstein, M. J., & Cillessen, A. H. N. (2003). Forms and functions of adolescent peer aggression associated with high levels of peer status. *Merrill-Palmer Quarterly. Special Issue: Aggression and Adaptive Functioning: The Bright Side to Bad Behavior, 49*(3), 310–342.

Rodkin, P. C., Farmer, T. W., Pearl, R., & Van Acker, R. (2006). They're cool: Social status and peer group supports for aggressive boys and girls. *Social Development, 15*(2), 175–204.

Roeser, R. W., Eccles, J. S., & Sameroff, A. J. (2000). School as a context of early adolescents' academic and social-emotional development: A summary of research findings. *The Elementary School Journal, 100*, 443–472.

Rose-Krasnor, L. (1997). The nature of social competence: A theoretical review. *Social Development, 6*, 111–135.

Rubin, K. H., & Rose-Krasnor, L. (1992). Interpersonal problem solving and social competence in children. In V. B. Van Hasselt & M. Hersen (Eds.), *Handbook of social development: A lifespan perspective* (pp. 283–323). New York, NY: Plenum Press.

Ryan, R. M. (1993). Agency and organization: Intrinsic motivation, autonomy and the self in psychological development. In J. Jacobs (Ed.), *Nebraska symposium on motivation: Developmental perspectives on motivation* (Vol. 40, pp. 1–56). Lincoln, NE: University of Nebraska Press. Rochester Press.

Ryan, R. M., & Brown, K. W. (2005). Legislating competence: High-stakes testing policies and their relations with psychological theories and research. In A. J. Elliot & C. S.

Dweck (Eds.), *Handbook of competence and motivation* (pp. 354–372). New York: The Guilford Press.

Ryan, R. M., & Deci, E. L. (2000a). Intrinsic and extrinsic motivations: Classic definitions and new directions. *Contemporary Educational Psychology, 25*, 54–67.

Ryan, R. M., & Deci, E. L. (2000b). Self-determination theory and the facilitation of intrinsic motivation, social development, and well-being. *American Psychologist, 55*, 68–78.

Ryan, R. M., Deci, E. L., & Grolnick, W. S. (1995). Autonomy, relatedness, and the self: Their relation to development and psychopathology. In D. Cicchetti & D. J. Cohen (Eds.), *Developmental psychopathology: Theory and methods* (Vol. 1, pp. 618–655). New York: Wiley.

Ryan, R. M., Kuhl, J., & Deci, E. L. (1997). Nature and autonomy: An organizational view on the social and neurobiological aspects of self-regulation in behavior and development. *Development and Psychopathology, 9*, 701–728.

Sheldon, K. M., & Kasser, T. (1998). Pursuing personal goals: Skills enable progress, but not all progress is beneficial. *Personality and Social Psychology Bulletin, 24*, 1319–1331.

Smith, P. K. (2007). Why has aggression been thought of as maladaptive? In P. H. Hawley, T. D. Little, & P. C. Rodkin (Eds.), *Aggression and adaptation: The bright side to bad behavior* (pp. 65–83). Mahwah, NJ: Lawrence Erlbaum Associates, Inc.

Sullivan, H. S. (1953). *The interpersonal theory of psychiatry*. Oxford, England: Norton & Co.

Vandell, D. L., & Hembree, S. E. (1994). Peer social status and friendship: Independent contributors to children's social and academic adjustment. *Merrill-Palmer Quarterly, 40*(4), 461–477.

Vaughn, B. E., & Santos, A. J. (2007). An evolutionary/ecological account of aggressive behavior and trait aggression in human children and adolescents. In P. H. Hawley, T. D. Little, & P. C. Rodkin (Eds.), *Aggression and adaptation: The bright side to bad behavior* (pp. 31–63). Mahwah, NJ: Lawrence Erlbaum Associates, Inc.

Weinstein, M. S. (1969). Achievement motivation and risk preference. *Journal of Personality and Social Psychology, 13*(2), 153–172.

White, R. W. (1959). Motivation reconsidered: The concept of competence. *Psychological Review, 66*, 297–333.

Wood, G. (2004). A view from the field: NCLB's effects on classrooms and schools. In D. Meier & G. Wood (Eds.), *Many children left behind: How the No Child Left Behind act is damaging our children and our schools* (pp. 33–50). Boston: Beacon Press.

Wooley, H. T. (1925). Agnes: A dominant personality in the making. *Pedagogical Seminary, 32*, 569–598.

Chapter 3
Etiology and Relationships to Developmental Disabilities and Psychopathology

Jeremy D. Jewell, Sara S. Jordan, Stephen D.A. Hupp, and Gregory E. Everett

Introduction

This chapter reviews a variety of developmental disabilities and psychological disorders that children experience, first describing the relevant symptoms of these disorders and second attempting to understand how social skills are related to the disorder. One theme throughout this chapter is the question of whether social skills deficits can be understood etiologically or whether these deficits are rather a behavioral consequence of a disorder. Specifically, social skills deficits are often either a diagnostic criterion of a particular disorder or a direct consequence of the disorder itself (or both). As such, the social skills deficits co-occur with the disorder. However, in some cases there is evidence to suggest that a prior social skills deficit precedes the manifestation of the disorder and therefore is part of the etiology of the disorder. This is similar to the perennial chicken and the egg question but reframed as, which came first, the disorder or the social skills deficit?

A second theme throughout this chapter is that of *reciprocity*. Regardless of the directional relationship between social skills deficits and disorders, these deficits usually assist in the maintenance of the disorder. Therefore, with many disorders a lack of competence in the social domain is related to greater severity of the disorder, higher risk of comorbid disorders, and poorer prognosis. For example, an adolescent who enters a depressive episode with a larger social network, frequent involvement in activities, and a greater repertoire of social competencies prior to the depressive episode will more likely experience a more mild depressive episode that is relatively short in length and is less likely to be chronic. In this case, the individual's social skills prior to the onset of the depressive episode serve as a protective factor against the disorder.

Understanding the social skills deficits as they relate to particular disorders is critical in the planning of prevention and intervention programs as well. While some have concluded that social skills training is not by itself sufficient to treat various disorders, social skills training is often a component of various multi-method prevention and intervention programs (Spence, 2003). Understanding which specific social skills are in need of addressing often depends on the specific disorder that one is attempting to treat or prevent. This chapter will also review research that describes some surprising and counterintuitive results suggesting that some social skills that were assumed to be related to a disorder are relatively unrelated, while some positive social skills may actually help maintain some disorders as well.

Developmental Disabilities

Intellectual Disability

Symptoms of Intellectual Disability

Characterized by subaverage intellectual functioning, deficits in adaptive behavior, and onset before

J.D. Jewell (✉)
Department of Psychology, Southern Illinois University
Edwardsville, Edwardsville, IL 62026, USA
e-mail: jejewel@siue.edu

J.L. Matson (ed.), *Social Behavior and Skills in Children*, DOI 10.1007/978-1-4419-0234-4_3,
© Springer Science+Business Media, LLC 2009

age 18, intellectual disability is estimated to affect 7.8 people per thousand of the noninstitutionalized population of the United States (Larson et al., 2001). Although often used interchangeably, the terms "intellectual disability" and "mental retardation" indicate slight definitional variations between that of the American Association on Intellectual and Developmental Disabilities (AAIDD; formerly the American Association on Mental Retardation) and the *Diagnostic and Statistical Manual of Mental Disorders, Fourth Edition – Text Revision* (DSM-IV-TR) of the American Psychiatric Association (APA, 2000). Although both include all three criteria listed above, the AAIDD definition emphasizes a functional approach to classification based on the amount of support needed to promote the well-being of those with the disability (Luckasson et al., 2002) while the DSM-IV-TR emphasizes degree of impairment (APA, 2000). As trends in the field indicate a shift toward "intellectual disability" and away from "mental retardation" (Schalock et al., 2007), we shall use the former throughout the course of the current chapter.

Of the required criteria for an intellectual disability diagnosis, deficits in adaptive functioning are most important for distinguishing the condition from both other developmental disabilities (e.g., autism) and other disorders of decreased cognitive performance (e.g., specific learning disabilities). Regarding adaptive behavior, persons with an intellectual disability may evidence deficits in conceptual (e.g., language or academic), practical (e.g., daily living and self-care), and/or social (e.g., interpersonal) skills (see Luckasson et al., 2002 for a comprehensive discussion of all forms and manifestations of adaptive behavioral deficits). As the focus of the current chapter is the relation between various disabilities and forms of psychopathology on the social skills of children, only adaptive skill difficulties related to the social domain will be discussed further.

Relationship Between Symptomatology and Social Skills

Social skills difficulties of those with an intellectual disability are associated with a number of related variables. A wide body of research has delineated several characteristics of those with intellectual disabilities with which social skills problems are correlated, including, but not limited to (a) degree of intellectual impairment (Bielecki & Swender, 2004), (b) presence of comorbid problem behaviors including self-injury and stereotypy (Matson, Minshawi, Gonzalez, & Mayville, 2006), and (c) presence of psychopathological symptoms (Matson, Smiroldo, & Bamburg, 1998). For example, research has consistently shown that as the degree of intellectual impairment increases, social skills decrease; meaning those with a "severe" or "profound" intellectual disability consistently demonstrate less developed social skills than those with "mild" or "moderate" classifications. In addition, the developmental level of the impaired individual directly influences the topography of displayed social skills, as the manners in which social skills are displayed vary across childhood development (Guralnick & Neville, 1997; Witt, Elliott, Daly, Gresham, & Kramer, 1998).

In addition to their association with differing subject-related variables, social skills of children with intellectual impairment vary widely according to observed behavioral manifestation. According to Dodge (1986) the display of social skills by children includes the correct interpretation of the social situation and associated problems, the selection of a strategy with which to deal with the problem, and the implementation of the selected strategy; each of which may be problematic for children with intellectual disabilities. Although difficulties with the first two steps, collectively referred to as social problem solving (Jacobs, Turner, Faust, & Stewart, 2002), indicate children with intellectual disabilities are less accurate in their interpretation of social situations and may posit solutions more hostile than their same-aged, nondisabled peers (Gomez & Hazeldine, 1996; Jacobs et al., 2002), broad-based generalizations cannot yet be made due to the lack of comprehensive research in this area. Conversely, conclusions regarding the specific types of social skills difficulty displayed by children with intellectual disabilities are more widely documented and indicate a host of problems, including (a) social skills deficits (Vaughn et al., 2003; Wallander & Hubert, 1987), (b) social skills excesses (Bielecki & Swender, 2004), (c) decreased social status among peers (Berkson, 1993), (d) poor ratings by teachers (Taylor, Asher, & Williams, 1987), and (e) increased social isolation (Pearl et al., 1998).

In sum, children with intellectual disabilities are categorized as such based in part on adaptive behavior difficulties (of which social skills are a component), which may vary according to the presence of several associated subject variables and are manifested in a number of different ways. Thus one can view social skills deficits as a symptom of the disorder, while social skills themselves are also affected by other symptoms of the disorder such as impaired cognitive processing.

Autism Spectrum Disorders

Symptoms of Autism Spectrum Disorders

Including autistic disorder, Asperger's disorder, and Pervasive Developmental Disorder-Not Otherwise Specified (PDD-NOS), children with autism spectrum disorders (ASD) comprise a group with widely varying social, cognitive, and language abilities. Although definitive prevalence estimates of ASD do not currently exist because of issues, including broadening diagnostic criteria, better understanding of the disorders, and methodological differences across prevalence studies, recent estimates indicate a rate of approximately 6.0 per 1000 for all spectrum disorders (Charman, 2002). Common across ASD are the necessary diagnostic criteria of impaired social reciprocity and restricted or repetitive patterns of behaviors, interests, or activities (APA, 2000). In addition, autistic disorder requires the display of impaired development in both nonverbal and verbal communication skills. Asperger's disorder is distinguished from autism by relatively normal communication, with the additional qualification that Asperger's disorder cannot be diagnosed in the presence of an intellectual disability (Macintosh & Dissanayake, 2006). A diagnosis of PDD-NOS is made when social functioning, stereotypy, or communication impairments fail to reach the threshold for autism or Asperger's, include atypical symptomatology, or first occur after age 3 (APA, 2000). It is this high degree of overlap that has led many to question the

validity of separate diagnostic categories versus a single disorder encompassing varying degrees of symptomatology (Macintosh & Dissanayake, 2004; Schopler, Mesibov, & Kunce, 1998). Regardless of classification as separate disorders or a singular construct of varying levels of severity, significant impairment in social functioning is a hallmark of all ASD.

Relationship Between Symptomatology and Social Skills

Children with ASD display a wide variety of social skills difficulties that may be discussed broadly in terms of problems with both reciprocal social interaction and emotional expression and recognition (Volkmar, Carter, Grossma, & Klin, 1997). Such deficits have been found to occur across those with ASD regardless of language or cognitive abilities (Carter, Davis, Klin, & Volkmar, 2005) and do not decrease as development progresses but rather may become more prominent throughout childhood and adolescence due to increased awareness regarding personal social difficulties (White, Keonig, & Scahill, 2007). Commonly identified social difficulties observed across children with ASD include problems with turn-taking that may negatively influence a variety of interactions including play and conversation, inability to both initiate and maintain social interactions, engagement in one-sided interactions, a lack of awareness of other's feelings, odd verbal behaviors and gestures such as atypical voice pitch and inflection, impaired expression of own emotions, and decreased understanding of nonliteral language (Kasari, Chamberlain, & Bauminger, 2001; Macintosh & Dissanayake, 2004; White et al., 2007).

Although apparent across all children with ASD, researchers have attempted to delineate more specifically the social difficulties of children with differing levels of impairment, including differences between those with high-functioning autism (HFA; autism without intellectual impairment) and those with intellectual impairment or Asperger's disorder. For example, Bauminger (2002) found that in addition to difficulties with reciprocal peer interaction, children with HFA commonly display problems with social cognition including difficulties with emotional recognition of self and others, a tendency to give more attention to peripheral, as opposed to, central details in social situations, and lack of knowledge of appropriate social behaviors in common social tasks. In addition, children with HFA are better able to engage in more complex social relationships and display more complex emotions than those with some degree of cognitive impairment (Kasari et al., 2001). Regarding the social behaviors of children with HFA versus Asperger's disorder, Macintosh and Dissanayake (2004) report that although both groups evidence social impairment when compared to typically developing peers, a diagnosis of Asperger's may indicate more advanced social skills in areas including greeting others, interest sharing, parental affection, and peer interest. Although such findings indicate likely differences between children with HFA and other spectrum disorders, firm conclusions are lacking due to the limited research on this topic.

A great deal of research indicates that most psychological disorders significantly impact the social skills of children, several of which are outlined in other sections of the current chapter. Although the symptoms of all disorders currently covered either directly or indirectly influence childhood social functioning, the previous presentation outlines the only two disorders for which social deficits are required diagnostic criteria. That is, in order for children to be diagnosed with either an intellectual disability or ASD they must evidence significant social functioning difficulty (APA, 2000). In this manner, both intellectual disability and all variations of ASD are described by the DSM-IV-TR (APA, 2000) as childhood disorders *of* social behavior. However, the research reviewed also describes how other related symptoms of these disorders may directly or indirectly negatively impact social skills as well. For example, children with autism exhibit problems with communication as well as social skills deficits. Undoubtedly, the level of communication impairment present will influence the level of social impairment in these children, yet less is currently known about this relationship.

Mood and Anxiety Disorders

Mood Disorders

Symptoms

The term mood disorder describes a variety of psychiatric disorders, including Major Depressive Disorder, Dysthymia, and Bipolar I and II Disorders (APA, 2000). Most mood disorders are defined by the presence of either a depressive episode, manic episode, or both. In some cases, criteria are not reached for a full depressive episode, such as in the case of dysthymia, or a full manic episode (known as a hypomanic episode) as in the case of Bipolar II Disorder (APA, 2000). However, all mood disorders include a disturbance of mood that is either depressive or manic in nature, or both. Typical symptoms of a depressive episode include depressed mood, anhedonia, a significant change in appetite or weight, insomnia or hypersomnia, psychomotor agitation or retardation, fatigue, feelings of worthlessness, poor concentration and indecisiveness, and suicidal ideation. Typical symptoms of a manic episode include grandiosity, diminished need for sleep, pressured speech, racing thoughts, distractibility, and increased pleasure-seeking behaviors such as compulsive gambling or hypersexuality (APA, 2000).

While the previous discussion of ASD reviewed disorders that first occur in childhood, mood disorders are often first diagnosed in adulthood though they can occur in childhood or adolescence as well. The prevalence rate of Major Depressive Disorder (MDD) in children is rather low at an estimated 2%, though this rate rises to between 4–8% in adolescence (Birmaher, Ryan, & Williamson, 1996). This review indicates that the incidence of MDD is similar in males and females in childhood but is twice as prevalent in females compared to males during adolescence. Additionally, another 5–10% of children and adolescents suffer significant symptoms of depression yet do not qualify for a diagnosis of MDD (Fergusson, Horwood, Ridder, & Beautrais, 2005).

Relationship Between Symptomatology and Social Skills

As one can see from a brief perusal of these criteria, symptoms of either a depressive or manic episode would certainly have serious consequences for one's social functioning. Symptoms of a depressive episode, such as fatigue and poor concentration, can reflect a significant decline in physical and mental energy that occurs during this episode, thus negatively affecting one's ability to relate to others. Similarly, symptoms of a manic episode such as pressured speech and distractibility can also impede one's social functioning. Regarding social skills impacted during a depressive episode, Tse and Bond (2004) describe three social skills components that are effected by depressive symptomatology. The first social skills component that may be effected is perceptual. There are two facets to the perceptual component of social skills, which are the selection process that guides people to attend to particular social stimuli (or not) as well as the tendency for people with depression to hold negative cognitive biases. The second social skills component effected by a depressive episode is cognitive in nature. The cognitive component comprises several facets, including the decreased ability to accurately judge emotion in others, mistakenly perceiving aggression in the behavior of others, and a general restriction of social response options available to the person experiencing a depressive episode. The third component of social skills effected during a depressive episode is the performance component. This component is primarily described by the anhedonia that one experiences during a depressive episode. There are two facets to anhedonia as relating to social situations. First, the depressed person is often unwilling to participate in socially rewarding behaviors (going out with friends) and, secondly, is viewed by others as withdrawn and perhaps uninterested in social participation.

Relevant research by D'Zurilla, Chang, Nottingham, and Faccini (1998) examined the effects of social problem-solving skills, hopelessness, and depression on suicidal risk in a series of three studies with three different adult samples; college students, admitted psychiatric patients, and suicidal psychiatric patients. All three studies found significant relationships between poor social problem-solving skills and suicidal risks, hopelessness, and depression. These results suggest that there is a similar link between social skills and depressive symptomatology and is consistently found across a continuum of participants ranging from the nondisordered to the moderately and severely disordered (D'Zurilla et al., 1998).

Many studies have documented correlations between social skills and symptoms of either a manic or depressive episode (Goldstein, Miklowitz, & Mullen, 2006; Stednitz & Epkins, 2006). However, understanding the potentially reciprocal relationship between social skills and a disorder's symptomatology is more complex. As discussed in the beginning of this chapter, the symptoms of a particular disorder can be viewed as a simple behavioral consequence that co-occurs with the disorder or can also be viewed as one of the causes of the disorder itself. For example, does a person exhibit anhedonia as a consequence of their dysthymic mood or does the behavior related to anhedonia (e.g., not "going out" with one's friends) lead that person to experience a dysthymic mood? It is possible that both statements are true in that these symptoms are both a reflection of the disorder and a contributing factor to the initiation and maintenance of the disorder. The cognitive model as described by Aaron Beck (1963) and Judith Beck (1995) exemplifies the reciprocal relationship between depressive cognitions and behaviors, including social behavior. Specifically, during a depressive episode, there are a number of typical cognitive distortions (Beck, 1995) such as "I am a failure" or "No one cares about me", which would lead to consequences for one's social behavior. For example, someone experiencing this type of thinking would be more likely to withdraw when in social situations and not take full advantage of other social situations such as not returning a call from a friend. This model also explains how a mood disorder can effect one's perception of a social situation, consequently affecting their social functioning as well. For example, someone experiencing a depressive episode may be more likely to believe that if a friend does not return their phone call within the day, then that friend no longer cares for them. That belief can then lead to a continued impairment in social functioning whereby the individual is caught in a cycle of misperception, distorted cognitions, and dysfunctional social behavior, similar to the social skills deficits described by Tse and Bond (2004). Therefore, the cognitive model is another useful paradigm that can help explain the reciprocal relationship between mood disorders and social functioning by describing the effect of typical depressive cognitions on consequent social behaviors.

Tse and Bond (2004) also provide an excellent review of some of the literature to date that attempts to understand this reciprocal relationship. These authors argue that a predominant amount of the literature in this area provides evidence that social skills deficits occur concurrently with depressed mood. In other words, social skills deficits manifest themselves during a state of depressed mood rather than preceding and potentially causing the depressed mood. The authors argue that social skills deficits are transient and occur *with* rather than *prior to* a depressive episode. For example, Tse and Bond (2004) cite research by Bouhuys, Bloem, and Groothuis (1995) in which researchers induced a depressed mood in nondisordered participants. These participants then displayed more negative attributions regarding neutral social situations once this depressed mood was induced (Bouhuys et al., 1995 as cited in Tse & Bond, 2004)

However, the argument that social skills deficits only occur during a state of depressed mood is contradicted by the results of a study by Cole, Martin, Powers, and Truglio (1996). The authors of this study measured academic and social competence and symptoms of depression in third and sixth graders at the beginning of the study as well as six months later. The authors used structural equation modeling to determine the predictive relationship between these variables from time 1 to time 2. Results indicated that for both age groups, depression at time 1 had very little effect on social competence at time 2 (while controlling for social competence at time 1). However, for sixth graders, lower social competence at time 1 significantly predicted higher ratings of depression at time 2 (while controlling for depression at time 1). This result was not significant for third graders, however. The authors argue that social competence does, in fact, precede and predict the development of depressive symptoms, at least in their sixth grade sample. They posit that this relationship may not hold true for younger children, however, as family and parent relationships are more influential in the lives of younger children.

Other researchers have examined the possible risk and protective factors that are involved in the relationship between social skills and depressive symptomatology. For example, McFarlane, Bellissimo, and Norman (1995) examined the relationship between social self-efficacy, peer support, and family support predicting depression. Participants consisted of tenth grade students who were surveyed twice over a 6-month time period. The results indicated that in general, social support from family predicted fewer symptoms of depression. Social self-efficacy was also negatively predictive of symptoms of depression, and social self-efficacy was positively related to peer and family support (McFarlane et al., 1995). Overall, these findings reflect the variety of risk and protective factors that may both directly and indirectly predict social skills and symptoms of depression.

While there is a relatively large literature on social skills and symptoms of depression, there is less research on the relationship between social skills and symptoms of mania or bipolar disorder. However, one such study by Goldstein et al. (2006) compared the social skills knowledge and performance of adolescents with bipolar disorder with a nondisordered group. Results of this study indicated that both groups had comparable levels of social skills *knowledge* as measured by the Interpersonal Negotiation Strategy Interview (INS; Selman, Beardslee, Schultz, Krupa, & Podorefsky, 1986). However, the self and parent-rated social skills *performance* of bipolar youth was significantly impaired compared to nondisordered youth. The conclusions of this study are extended in a study by Lewinsohn, Klein, and Seeley (2000) that found psychosocial impairment to be greater in young adults with bipolar disorder compared to a healthy control group.

Overall, research to date has revealed a relationship between social skills and symptoms of depressive and manic episodes. There is still some controversy that exists as to whether these social skills deficits precede and potentially influence the initiation of a depressive episode, or whether these social skills deficits are simply symptomological of the depressive episode. A resolution of this controversy will only be found with the implementation of studies that are longitudinal in nature and that take advantage of causal models of analysis. Other issues that warrant future research include determining how the relationship between social skills and depressive symptomatology might be different given varying gender and age effects.

Anxiety Disorders

Symptoms

There are several anxiety disorders that children and adolescents may suffer from with a long list of diagnostic criteria for each. However, as this chapter is focused less on the diagnosis of any particular anxiety disorder, the following section will often consider the generalities of anxiety instead. Thus, anxiety can be considered a normal response to potentially dangerous stimuli. Lang (1968) presented anxiety as a multidimensional construct involving a physiological response (e.g., increased heart rate), behavioral response (e.g., running away), and cognitive response (e.g., fearful thoughts). More recently, a fourth component, emotional response (e.g., the subjective feeling of anxiety), has also been explored (Hannesdottir & Ollendick, 2007; Southam-Gerow & Kendall, 2002). Anxiety can be considered a disorder rather than a normal response when it significantly interferes with the quality of a child's life and when the anxiety experienced is disproportionate to the situation.

Relationship Between Symptomatology and Social Skills

All of the anxiety disorders in the DSM-IV-TR (APA, 2000) have some relationship to social skills; however, this relationship is most evident with social phobia. To be diagnosed with social phobia a child must have a significant fear of embarrassment or humiliation in either a social (e.g., during recess) or performance (e.g., giving a speech) situation. Typically, children with social phobia have

feelings of panic that may be expressed through crying, tantrums, etc., and they attempt to avoid the anxiety-provoking situation. School refusal is common with this disorder as well. For children, the symptoms must last at least six months and cause significant impairment (APA, 2000). Two closely related disorders to social phobia include separation anxiety disorder and selective mutism, both of which are usually diagnosed first in childhood. Children diagnosed with separation anxiety disorder often withdraw from others when separated from a caregiver, and children diagnosed with selective mutism refuse to speak in certain situations. Behaviors associated with both disorders obviously interrupt some social opportunities for these children.

While many of the anxiety disorders do not always relate specifically to social situations, they often do have some resulting social impairments. For example, children with generalized anxiety disorder have a difficult time controlling a range of worries that often include worries about social competence. Additionally, specific phobia may, at times, include fear of specific groups of people (Madonna, 1990), and some children with post-traumatic stress disorder may avoid people that elicit memories of a traumatic event. Finally, people with obsessive-compulsive disorder sometimes refuse to shake someone's hand for fear of contamination, and evidence other compulsive behaviors (e.g., counting, ordering, etc.) that lead to the child being ostracized. One common thread between all of the anxiety disorders (also including panic disorder and agoraphobia) is that the person's avoidance of anxiety-provoking stimuli often leads to experiencing fewer social events.

The direction of the relationship between social behavior and anxiety disorders is difficult to untangle with three primary possibilities. First, impairments in social behavior may lead to an anxiety disorder. For example, a child with poor social skills may start becoming clinically anxious in social situations. Second, an existing anxiety disorder may lead to avoidance of social situations, thus interfering with the development of social behavior. Third, some other variable (e.g., genetics, certain environments) may lead to both clinical anxiety and impairments in social behavior at the same time.

Most etiological theories of anxiety include both a genetic and environmental contribution (Elizabeth, King, & Ollendick, 2004). Twin and adoption studies support a genetic contribution to anxiety in children. In fact, the 5-HTT allele has specifically been identified as a contributor to shyness, although some studies have yielded mixed results on the exact nature of the relationship (Gregory & Eley, 2007). Interestingly, genetics research with adults has indicated that heritability is stronger for some anxiety disorders than others (Kendler, Neale, Kessler, Heath, & Eaves, 1992). Gregory and Eley (2007) also suggest that genetic influence may vary depending on one's period of development.

The same studies that support a genetic contribution to anxiety also support a major environmental contribution because the expression of anxiety is often different for identical twins, especially when they are raised apart (Gregory & Eley, 2007). Some research has also demonstrated an interesting gene-environment interaction. For example, Fox et al. (2005) reported that the genetic contribution to behavioral inhibition was stronger for families in which the mother reported less social support than in families with more social support.

There are several theories regarding how the environment can influence anxiety. In an early study, Watson and Watson (1921) demonstrated how the fear response (e.g., crying) could be learned through classical conditioning. In their research they repeatedly paired a stimulus that elicited fear in an infant (i.e., loud sound) with a stimulus that did not elicit fear (i.e., a white rat), and after a few pairings the infant also demonstrated the fear response to the white rat. In addition to the direct pathway of classical conditioning, Rachman's (1977) theory added two indirect pathways. That is, Rachman suggested anxiety can also be developed without direct experience by observing other people's fears (i.e., vicarious learning) and learning what to fear from the language of others (i.e., information transmission). Finally, operant conditioning has also been suggested to influence anxiety. For example, in an early conceptualization, Mowrer (1939) posited that fearful behaviors can be reinforced when they serve to decrease anxiety.

Research has supported the influence of vicarious learning, information transmission, and operant conditioning on the social anxiety of children

(c.f., Fisak & Grills-Taquechel, 2007). In an example of vicarious learning, one study manipulated mothers' responses to strangers and examined the effect on their children (de Rosnay, Cooper, Tsigara, & Murray, 2006). Participants in the study were 24 infants (12–14 months old) and their mothers. Infants observed their mothers interact with two strangers. With one stranger, the mother was instructed to act in a comfortable manner, and with the other stranger the mother was instructed to act in an anxious way. When mothers purposely demonstrated anxious behavior in response to the stranger their infants were also observed to demonstrate more anxious behavior with that stranger. Again, this study reflects how social behavior can be observed in others and later modeled by oneself. These results may offer some support to the idea that the observation and imitation of anxious behavior may precede the existence of the anxiety disorder itself.

Regarding information transmission, researchers have manipulated the type of information that is provided by peers (Field, Hamilton, Knowles, & Plews, 2003). In this study, a peer read one of three stories (positive, negative, or neutral) about a public speaking experience to research participants ages 10–13. Interestingly, positive information about public speaking elicited significantly more anxiety about public speaking for children. The authors suggested that when the participants learned about another child who did well on a speech, the participants then compared themselves to that child and assumed they would do worse. It is also interesting to note that similar information provided by teachers (instead of peers) did not have a significant impact on the anxiety of the participants.

Research has also examined parents' reinforcement of anxious behaviors. In a retrospective study, college students were surveyed regarding their current panic symptoms and their parents' reinforcement of symptoms in childhood (Watt, Stewart, & Cox, 1998). College students with current symptoms of panic retrospectively reported more parent encouragement of panic symptoms during their childhood. The questionnaire examining parent encouragement focused on both negative reinforcement (e.g., letting the child stay home from school) and positive reinforcement (e.g., being allowed to do special activities) following panic symptoms.

This study also revealed that the learning experiences of the participants were not only limited to the reinforcement of panic symptoms but also to other somatic symptoms as well. That is, the researchers suggested parents were reinforcing "sick-role behavior" in general. These conclusions drawn from this study may also indicate the possibility that children with anxiety disorders may elicit particular social behaviors in others, such as sympathy and caretaking behaviors.

Additional research has examined the cognitive style of children. In one study by Barrett, Rapee, Dadds, and Ryan (1996), over 200 children aged 7–14 years were classified in one of three groups. Children in the anxious group were referred for an anxiety treatment program. The study also included a nonclinic control group, as well as a second control group that met the diagnostic criteria for oppositional defiant disorder. All of the children were interviewed individually about their interpretations of hypothetical ambiguous scenarios. For example, one scenario described a situation in which a child wants to join another group of students but notices that they are laughing. The participants are then prompted to decide whether the group of students is either (a) telling secrets about the child, (b) wanting the child to join them, (c) getting ready to push the child, or (d) smile at the child. Parents of all of the children in the study were also interviewed separately from their children regarding their interpretation of the scenarios. Results of the Barrett et al. study (1996) indicated that children in the anxious group and oppositional group interpreted the scenarios as more threatening than children in the nonclinic control group. Thus, children with anxiety experience impairment in their perception of social situations. Importantly, mothers and fathers of children in the anxious and oppositional groups also interpreted the scenarios as more threatening. Parents and children in the study also later discussed two of the ambiguous scenarios, and were required to come up with a solution. After the family discussion, children in the anxious group came up with more avoidant solutions than children from the other groups. In fact, the solutions of children in the anxious group were significantly more avoidant after they discussed the scenario with their parents than before discussing the scenarios with their parents. This study suggests that parents may model, prompt, and reinforce socially anxious cognitions and behaviors as well.

DiBartolo and Helt (2007) also review another area of research examining the influence of parental warmth and control on childhood anxiety. The results for parental warmth were mixed with less than half of the reviewed studies finding that parents of anxious children were less warm to their children. However, the results for parental control were clearer with all of the studies in the review suggesting that parents of anxious children exhibited more control (e.g., sometimes described as overprotection) than parents of comparison children. Chorpita and Barlow (1998) suggest that when parents are overly controlling, children develop a style of learned helplessness and anxiety. Rubin and Mills (1991) suggest that levels of parental control may be partly influenced by the child's temperament. That is, an inhibited temperament may prompt protective parental behaviors. In turn, the parental control begins to interfere with the child's ability to explore the social environment; thus, the child has less opportunity to develop appropriate social behavior. Thus, while Chorpita and Barlow (1998) may argue that parents influence the development of an anxiety disorder in their children, Rubin and Mills (1991) posit that the innate temperament of the child elicits their parents' protective behaviors.

As discussed, many different variables have been hypothesized (and supported by research) to influence childhood anxiety and related social behavior. These theories include classical conditioning, operant conditioning, vicarious learning, information transmission, cognitive style, and parent control. Most theories account for an interaction between genetics and environment. Understanding the relationship between social behavior and anxiety disorders is made more complicated by the possibility that different causative pathways exist for different anxiety disorders of individual children.

Externalizing Behavior Disorders

Externalizing behavior disorders are widely recognized as the most common psychiatric problem in childhood. Externalizing behavior disorders include attention-deficit/hyperactivity disorder (ADHD), and the disruptive behavior disorders, oppositional defiant disorder (ODD) and conduct disorder (CD). Collectively, the disruptive behavior associated with these disorders, accounts for the majority of childhood clinic referrals (Brinkmeyer & Eyberg, 2003), and if left untreated are associated with significant academic, occupational, and social impairment.

Attention-Deficit/Hyperactivity Disorder (ADHD)

Symptoms

According to the DSM-IV-TR, ADHD is an externalizing behavior disorder affecting 3–7% of children in the United States (APA, 2000). A 2003 report from the Centers for Disease Control and Prevention (CDC) drawn from the National Child Health Survey suggests that 4.4 million children between the ages of 4 and 17 in the United States have ADHD (CDC, 2005). ADHD is characterized by a persistent pattern of inattention and hyperactivity/impulsivity that causes impairment in daily functioning. Symptoms must be present for at least 6 months and be both excessive and developmentally inappropriate. Inattentive symptoms include making careless mistakes, difficulty maintaining attention, failing to listen, failing to follow through with assignments or responsibilities, organizational problems, avoiding or disliking tasks that require sustained attention, losing necessary materials, being easily distracted, and being forgetful. Hyperactive symptoms include frequent fidgeting, being out of seat, running or climbing in inappropriate situations, difficulty playing quietly, and excessive talking. Impulsive symptoms include prematurely blurting out answers, difficulty waiting, and frequently interrupting others' activities. In addition, the DSM-IV-TR (APA, 2000) requires that these symptoms have an onset prior to age 7, be present in more than one setting (e.g., home, school, community), and not be better explained by another psychiatric condition such as autism or a mood disorder. Children are diagnosed with one of

three subtypes: Predominantly Inattentive (at least 6 of 9 inattentive symptoms), Predominantly Hyperactive/Impulsive (at least 6 of 9 hyperactive and/or impulsive symptoms), or Combined Type (at least 6 of 9 from both sets of symptoms).

Relation Between Symptomatology and Social Skills

Although not a defining feature of the disorder, children with ADHD often experience a range of impairments in social interactions, commonly resulting in peer and adult conflict, peer rejection, and social isolation (De Boo & Prins, 2007; Dumas, 1998). The nature and cause of these impairments have been debated (Guevremont & Dumas, 1994; Nixon, 2001). Explanatory factors that have been proposed include the core symptoms of ADHD, subtype, comorbidity with disruptive behavior disorders, social communication impairments, and social cognitive functioning. Social functioning of children with ADHD is critical because peer rejection is predictive of meaningful long-term outcomes, including negative social status and psychopathology (Greene, Biederman, Faraone, Sienna, & Garcia-Jetton, 1997). Given the high rates of peer relationship difficulties among children with ADHD (Dumas, 1998), the implications for long-term social consequences is great.

Children with ADHD often exhibit a range of social impairments, beyond the core symptoms of inattention, hyperactivity, and impulsivity (Frick & Lahey, 1991). It is estimated that 40–70% of children with ADHD exhibit negative and aggressive behavior (Barkley, 2003). Verbal and physical aggression, problems with group entry, and disruptive behavior are associated with peer rejection (Guevremont & Dumas, 1994; Landau & Moore, 1991). Consequently, about 50% of children with ADHD experience peer rejection (Dumas, 1998; Milich & Landau, 1982). Erhardt and Hinshaw (1994) found that children who are more hyperactive, noncompliant, or aggressive tend to both receive more negative peer ratings on sociometric measures and experience higher rates of peer rejection. Peer rejection also happened quite quickly, even after one day of interacting with a child with ADHD (Erhardt & Hinshaw, 1994).

Whalen and Henker (1992, 1998) identified five aspects of social functioning that are characteristic of children with ADHD. First, children with ADHD tend to respond to social interactions in a disruptive and impulsive manner. Second, their style of approach tends to be intense, dysregulated, and lacking awareness with respect to subtle social cues. Third, children with ADHD appear to have adequate social information processing and knowledge of social acts but difficulty putting that knowledge into practice. Some researchers have characterized this as a performance or motivational deficit rather than a lack of knowledge or awareness (Whalen, Henker, & Granger, 1990). Fourth, these children are at greater risk for negative peer interactions, which translates into both active rejection by peers, difficulty developing and maintaining friendships, and consequently, lower social status. This appears to stem, at least partly, from hyperactivity. Finally, there appears to be a reciprocal effect between ADHD symptoms and the social behaviors of others as the expression of ADHD symptoms negatively impacts both peer play and parenting practices.

The cause of the social impairments associated with ADHD has been a source of considerable discussion. Researchers generally agree that some degree of social impairment can be attributed to core symptoms of ADHD (Nijmeijer et al., 2008). Hyperactivity and inattention have been shown to negatively influence peer relationships independent of aggression that may co-occur with ADHD (Pope, Bierman, & Mumma, 1991). Furthermore, inattention and impulsivity disrupt social processes and typical peer relations, resulting in peer rejection (Dumas, 1998).

Yet, despite the high rates of social problems among children with ADHD, social impairment is not universal (Nijmeijer et al., 2008). Thus, ADHD subtype and comorbidity have been examined for differential relations with social impairment. Lahey et al. (1998) examined differences in functional impairment across ADHD subtypes in children aged 3–7. Social problems, including disruptive

behavior and poor self-control, were more evident among children with Combined and Hyperactive types. Children with the Combined type were also more likely to be rated by peers as "actively disliked" than comparison peers. Similarly, Carlson, Lehy, Frame, Walker, and Hynd (1987) found that children with the combined type symptom profile were at greater risk for peer rejection than those with the Inattentive type. With respect to comorbidity, across clinic and community samples of children with ADHD, as many as 30–67% also have ODD, and 20–50% develop comorbid CD (Barkley, 2003; Spencer, 2006). The available evidence suggests that comorbidity with disruptive behavior disorders is associated with greater social impairments, including aggression, more negative peer relationships, and more parent–child relational difficulties. Thus, some researchers have questioned whether ADHD with and without ODD/CD are distinct disorders (Nijmeijer et al., 2008).

Social communication deficits, such as difficulty attending to social cues and responding appropriately in social interactions, has also been suggested as an area of weakness for children with ADHD (Dumas, 1998; Nixon, 2001). The role of social cognitive factors in social impairments has been less clear. Earlier studies implicated social-information processing skills deficits and suggested that social problem solving and social knowledge were impaired among children with ADHD (Dodge & Coie, 1987; Guevremont & Dumas, 1994). More recent evidence has contradicted these findings, suggesting that children with ADHD have adequate knowledge of social behavior, but that they fail to apply that knowledge in social contexts (Barkley, 1997; Whalen et al., 1990; Whalen & Henker, 1998).

Social impairment among children with ADHD can have long-term and far-reaching consequences. It has been well established that children with ADHD are at a greater risk of delinquency, criminal behavior, conduct disorder, and antisocial personality disorder. However, co-occurring social impairments may exacerbate these long-term negative outcomes. In a study comparing children with ADHD with and without social dysfunction, Greene et al. (1997) found that ADHD with social dysfunction was associated with higher rates of mood disorders, anxiety disorders, ODD, CD, and various forms of substance abuse. Even after controlling baseline levels of psychopathology, aggressive behavior, and attention problems, ADHD with social dysfunction predicted later conduct disorder and substance abuse. Thus, better understanding of the causes of social difficulties associated with ADHD is necessary.

There is a large body of literature supporting the efficacy of various psychosocial interventions in the reduction of ADHD symptomatology. While stimulants have consistently been shown to have rapid and sizeable effects on the core symptoms of ADHD, 10–30% of children do not respond well to stimulant medications or are unable to tolerate side effects (U.S. Department of Health and Human Services, 1999). Thus, psychosocial interventions and multimodal approaches have also been considered an important component of comprehensive ADHD treatment. Efficacious psychosocial interventions have consisted primarily of behavioral approaches, including parent training, classroom management, and peer interventions (Pelham & Fabiano, 2008; Pelham, Wheeler, & Chronis, 1998). Successful peer interventions have focused on improving peer relations, largely in the context of multimodal summer treatment programs (e.g., Pelham & Hoza, 1996). These behavioral interventions have focused on brief social skills training followed by coaching during organized recreational activities in the context of a contingency management system (Pelham & Fabiano, 2008).

Studies of traditional social skills training (SST) as an intervention for ADHD have generally received mixed or limited support, and thus, SST has not been considered efficacious (see Pelham et al., 1998; Pelham & Fabiano, 2008). Recent studies have shown greater effects both in behavioral improvement and generalization across settings for SST when combined with parent training, relative to social skills training or parent training alone (Chronis, Jones and Raggi, 2006). The results of these treatment studies potentially speak to the relationship between social skills problems and ADHD symptomatology. Specifically, it may be that typical attentional and executive functioning process deficits found with ADHD may limit the effectiveness of SST alone. On the other hand, changes in family environment and the addition of operant conditioning procedures employed by parents or others may enhance the benefits of SST (Chronis et al., 2006; Pelham & Fabiano, 2008; Pelham et al., 1998).

Disruptive Behavior Disorders

Symptoms

The disruptive behavior disorders include ODD and CD. ODD is a persistent pattern of hostile, defiant, and negative behavior that is frequently associated with noncompliance (APA, 2000). The DSM-IV-TR requires four or more symptoms lasting more than 6 months including losing temper, arguing with adults, defiance or noncompliance with rules or requests, purposefully annoying others, blaming others for mistakes, being "easily annoyed," "angry and resentful," or "spiteful or vindictive" (APA, 2000). Like ADHD, this pattern of symptoms must be associated with impaired social, occupational, or academic functioning and must not be better explained by a psychotic or mood disorder. Unlike ADHD, ODD may be diagnosed if the behavior only occurs in one setting, although children with ODD often have difficulties in multiple contexts. ODD affects 2–15% of children (Loeber, Burke, Lahey, Winters, & Zera, 2000) and is a common precursor to CD. If CD is present, the CD diagnosis supersedes an ODD diagnosis.

Untreated, about one-fourth of children with ODD go on to develop CD (Hinshaw & Lee, 2003), although some children, particularly adolescents, may develop CD in the absence of a significant history of ODD (APA, 2000). CD is a persistent pattern of deviant behavior involving serious violation of social norms. To qualify for a diagnosis of CD, a child must exhibit at least 3 symptoms for the prior 6 months, with at least 1 symptom lasting at least a year. Symptoms fall into one of four categories, including aggression, property destruction, deceitfulness/theft, and serious rule violations. Aggression may include behaviors such as bullying or threatening others, fighting with or without a weapon, cruelty to people or animals, armed robbery, or forced sexual activity. Property destruction involves intent to damage others' goods or property, including by fire setting. Deceitfulness or theft refers to breaking and entering, frequent lying, and stealing (e.g., shoplifting). Serious rule violations include staying out too late before age 13, running away, and truancy. Furthermore, this deviant pattern of behavior causes significant social, occupational, or academic impairment. The severity can be rated from mild to severe, and the onset can be specified as either childhood onset (some symptoms prior to age 10) or adolescent onset (after age 10).

Relationship Between Symptomatology and Social Skills

The aggressive and antisocial behaviors characteristic of disruptive behavior disorders are fundamentally different from the inattentive, hyperactivity, and impulsive actions characteristic of ADHD (Hinshaw & Lee, 2003). Unlike ADHD, children with ODD and CD typically experience tremendous social difficulties interacting with parents, teachers, and, especially peers, as a matter of course. Aggression and delinquent or antisocial behaviors are associated with significant social sequelae, including hostile and coercive parent-child interactions, peer conflict, and ultimately, peer rejection and social isolation or affiliation with deviant peers. In turn, ODD and CD are associated with long-term negative outcomes including delinquency, substance abuse, school dropout, depression, and criminal behavior. A substantial portion (25–40%) of individuals with CD goes on to develop antisocial personality disorder (Hinshaw & Lee, 2003). Thus, disruptive behavior disorders are associated with significant societal costs as well.

Behaviors associated with interpersonal relational difficulties include verbal (i.e., yelling, criticizing, threatening) and physical aggression (i.e., hitting, fighting). Hinshaw and Lee (2003) distinguish between subtypes of aggression. *Proactive* aggression is similar to *instrumental* aggression in that it is goal oriented or purposeful. Threatening or bullying are considered proactive because they achieve certain desired outcomes and are more characteristic of ODD/CD. By contrast, *reactive* aggression refers to aggressive acts that may be more impulsive and less intentional, typically in response to an external stimulus. Hitting in response to being hit is considered reactive. Subtypes of aggression are important because they are differentially predicted by models of social cognition.

A great deal of attention has focused on the relation between age of onset of aggressive and antisocial behavior and subsequent long-term stability of antisocial behavior. Researchers have identified a subgroup of "early starter" offenders who are at increased risk for developing CD and subsequent APD (Moffitt, 1993). Moffitt's (1993) Transactional Analysis Model suggests that conduct problems develop through distinct pathways. The Life-Course type (also known as the Early Starter path) has onset in preschool or early childhood and may include ADHD. It is characterized by very early development of aggression, conduct problems, and substance use. This pathway is associated with chronic, severe antisocial behavior, and greater risk of psychopathy and criminality in adulthood. The Limited-duration type (also known as the Adolescent onset or Late Starter path) has onset in adolescence and is associated with mild or moderate conduct problems. This pathway has been characterized as an exaggeration of age-appropriate rebellion. The majority of youth with this subtype desist from antisocial and criminal actions as they move into adulthood, although less is known about protective factors and why these youth desist (Loeber & Stouthamer-Loeber, 1998). Characteristics including early onset of and greater severity of conduct problems, aggression, ADHD, lower IQ, parental history of antisocial or criminal behavior, dysfunctional family environment and socioeconomic disadvantage have been identified as risk factors for more chronic conduct problems (Frick & Loney, 1999).

The etiology of persistent aggressive and antisocial behavior is complex, multifaceted, and transactional (Hinshaw & Lee, 2003). Genetic factors appear to play a role, accounting for about 50% of the variance (Mason & Frick, 1994), although twin studies suggest greater heritability for adults than children. Frick (1998a; b) has argued that this is evidence of the heterogeneity of conduct problems among children and that different subgroups may have different etiologies. A number of biological correlates have been associated with antisocial behavior, including autonomic underreactivity and psychophysiological arousal (Hinshaw & Lee, 2003.). Familial factors associated with antisocial behavior include parental depression, antisocial behavior, and substance abuse (Loeber & Farrington, 2000), as well as structural factors like single parenthood, larger family size, and younger maternal age (Hinshaw & Lee, 2003). Disrupted parenting practices, as indicated in Patterson's (1982) Coercive Family Process model (discussed further below), have also been implicated as factors contributing to aggression and antisocial behavior. Peer rejection in childhood and involvement with deviant peer groups in later middle childhood and adolescence are also important predictors of later antisocial behavior and delinquency (Coie & Dodge, 1998; Patterson, DeBaryshe & Ramsey, 1989). Finally, neighborhood and socioeconomic contextual factors like poverty have consistently related to ASB (specifically early onset), but are largely mediated by parenting variables (Capaldi & Patterson, 1994).

A number of integrative models have been developed to explain the development of aggressive and antisocial behavior seen in children with ODD/CD. The most elaborate social cognitive model is Crick and Dodge's (1994) social information processing model, which is a six-stage model suggesting impairment in social cognitive processes. The stages of information processing include encoding and interpretation of social cues, clarification of social goals, response construction, response decision, behavioral enactment, and evaluation/response. This model is the basis for the hostile attribution bias, which suggests that biases in the cognitive processing of ambiguous social information explain aggressive behavior. In other words, these children tend to perceive hostile intent in ambiguous situations. This may be an adequate explanation for reactive aggression, and thus, may explain some of the aggression seen in children with impulse-control problems like ADHD, but fails to adequately explain the instrumental aggression that is more characteristic of chronic antisocial behavior (Frick, 1998a). Empirical investigations of this model do support distorted information processing at various stages of the model among aggressive youth, including failure to attend to relevant social cues, attributing hostile intent in ambiguous situations, identification of fewer assertive solutions, and

an expectation that aggressive responses will produce reward (Crick & Dodge, 1994). However, lower than expected effect sizes suggest that this model does not fully explain antisocial behavior (Coie & Dodge, 1998).

Patterson's Coercive Family Process model (1982; Patterson et al., 1989; Patterson, Reid, & Dishion, 1992) is supported by more than 30 years of observational research, and as such, is one of the most comprehensive accounts of the development of antisocial behavior and delinquency. This model is based on social-learning theory and suggests that delinquency and conduct problems are learned. The model places a primary focus on parenting skills deficits, with hostile and coercive parent-child interactions and poor monitoring and supervision promoting development of early childhood conduct problems. These conduct problems lead to peer rejection and academic failure by middle school, which together promote involvement with deviant peers and delinquency by adolescence. Furthermore, Patterson's work suggests that a number of contextual factors including low income and education, neighbourhood, and ethnicity; parental antisocial behavior; and family stressors such as unemployment and marital conflict all work together to disrupt parenting practices resulting in antisocial behavior (Patterson et al., 1989). Despite its solid empirical foundation, critics of the model suggest it is limited by its failure to address development of more serious delinquent behavior (Loeber & Stouthamer-Loeber, 1998).

Well established and probably efficacious treatments for ODD and CD (see Eyberg, Nelson, & Boggs, 2008 for a complete review) have included various forms of parent training (McMahon & Forehand, 2003; Brinkmeyer & Eyberg, 2003; Webster-Stratton & Hammond, 1997), problem solving skills training (Kazdin, 1997), and anger control training (Lochman, Barry, & Pardini, 2003). Parent training approaches, including parent management training (Patterson, Chamberlain, & Reid, 1982), behavioral parent training (McMahon & Forehand, 2003), parent management training (Kazdin, 1997), parent-child interaction therapy (Brinkmeyer & Eyberg, 2003), and the *Incredible Years* videotape modeling (Webster-Stratton & Hammond, 1997), have been among the most effective interventions for reducing conduct problems of young children. These programs are founded on the assumption that a change in the family environment, parent modeling of appropriate social skills, and operant conditioning procedures employed by parents will overcome social skills problems in their children. Problem-solving skills training approaches rely on cognitive-behavioral techniques to alter responses in social situations. This is typically used during middle childhood and adolescence and has been shown to be probably efficacious both with and without parent training (Kazdin, 2003). The problem-solving skills training programs assume a deficit in social cognition primarily and address these deficits at the cognitive level. Anger Control Training (Lochman et al., 2003) maps directly onto Crick and Dodge's (1994) social information processing model and has also shown promise in preventing later conduct problems among aggressive, at-risk youth in later middle childhood.

Other Disorders Impacting Social Skills

Childhood social skills deficits are associated with a number of other clinical problems including psychosis, personality disorders, and substance abuse. Although these clinical concerns often do not arise until adolescence, in many cases, a clear history of social impairments may have been evident for years.

Social impairment is a significant early marker for psychosis. Psychosis is a prominent feature of psychotic depression in children, bipolar disorder, and schizophrenia and related disorders (e.g., schizoaffective disorder) (Volkmar, 1996). Children experiencing psychosis in the context of a primary mood disorder may experience social withdrawal or other impairment, but it is generally restricted to the active phase of the disorder and is not a salient feature between episodes. By contrast, children developing schizophrenia usually experience more chronic premorbid shyness and social withdrawal (Ropcke & Eggers, 2005). Childhood onset schizophrenia (COS) is exceedingly rare, with the more common presentation occurring in late adolescence and early adulthood (Volkmar, 1996). Yet childhood onset is insidious rather than acute and associated with a more severe and debilitating course (Asarnow, Tompson, & Goldstein, 1994; Eggers &

Bunk, 1997; Ropcke & Eggers, 2005). There is now substantial evidence that premorbid social functioning is often impaired among individuals who develop schizophrenia (Lewine, Watt, Prentky, & Fryer, 1980) and that social withdrawal and isolation may be prodromal signs of the disorder (Gonthier & Lyon, 2004). Poor social functioning at initial psychotic episode also predicts worse prognosis (Addington & Addington, 2006), while social competence and social support have been conceptualized as potential protective factors against development of COS (Asarnow & Asarnow, 2003).

Although social skills training has been successfully applied to the treatment of adult schizophrenia (Kurtz & Mueser, 2008), there is an absence of controlled studies examining social skills training and other psychosocial interventions in psychotic children (Asarnow & Asarnow, 2003). Based on the adult literature, social skills training and other behavioral treatment approaches targeting problem-solving skills and communication should be further evaluated.

Impaired social skills are also a prominent feature in certain personality disorders (PD). PDs are not diagnosed in childhood, but traits are often present by adolescence. According to the DSM-IV, schizoid PD is characterized by social detachment and disinterest in interpersonal relationships. Individuals with schizoid PD often lack friends, prefer being alone, and appear indifferent to social reinforcement. As a result, they often fail to attend to normal social cues and pragmatics of social discourse. Schizotypal PD is associated with similar social detachment and diminished interest and capacity for interpersonal relationships but includes odd thought patterns, magical thinking, perceptual disturbances, and eccentricities not seen in schizoid PD. Schizoid PD may precede schizophrenia and both schizoid and schizotypal PD can be associated with transient psychotic symptoms and are common among relatives of individuals with schizophrenia (APA, 2000).

Social behavior is also a prominent aspect of Antisocial PD and Avoidant PD. Antisocial PD is the adult extension of conduct disorder, marked by disregard for social normal and violation of others' rights. This may include aggression, violence, and criminal behavior. A portion of antisocial individuals display psychopathy, which is a particularly deviant variant. Psychopathic individuals may actually be quite socially skilled and charming and are able to manipulate and successfully "con" others in order to fit their self-serving agendas. Yet they are quite callous and lack feelings of guilt, empathy, and remorse (APA, 2000). By contrast, Avoidant PD is characterized by pervasive social inhibition and fear of negative evaluation, including criticism and negative evaluation. Avoidant PD is associated with shyness and anxiety, and commonly results in social isolation and both social and work-related impairment (APA, 2000).

The relationship between social skills and substance abuse is perhaps more complex. Studies have shown that poor social skills put individuals at increased risk for substance abuse and that substance abuse is associated with greater social impairment (Becker & Curry, 2007). The social stress model of substance abuse reviewed by Rhodes and Jason (1990) describes the three social components that may serve as protective factors to substance use, which are social networks, social competence, and resources. Conversely, specific risk factors include inconsistent caregivers, peer modeling of substance use, and lack of alternatives to substance use. Data gathered by Rhodes and Jason attempted to test this model empirically in an adolescent sample using structural equation modeling. The results indicated that while several measures of family problems as well as low levels of assertiveness predicted higher substance use, a number of hypothesized paths were not significant. For example, perceived stress, socioeconomic status, and school environment did not predict substance use.

The role of social skills in predicting substance use is complex as well. A longitudinal study by Pandina, Labouvie, Johnson, and White (1991) gathered data from a sample of substance using adolescents followed at the ages of 12, 15, and 18. Surprisingly, higher competence in making friends and becoming more socially oriented led to higher rates of substance use from age 12 to 15. However, rates of use between ages 15 and 18 declined when participants became more socially oriented. This study also found that having an older sibling and a substance abusing sibling predicted higher substance use. These results only begin to shed light on the complex relationship between social skills and substance use. For example, it may not be important whether a child can make friends, but perhaps it is more important as to whether those friends are substance abusing themselves. These results also point to a possible time interaction effect, whereby initial drug use is related to increased social skills, but then continued drug use leads to a decline in social skills (Pandina et al., 1991).

Conclusion & Future Research

The following review of the literature on social skills as they relate to developmental disabilities and psychopathology reveals several major points, as well as current gaps in the literature and opportunities for future research. First, with relation to social skills, there appear to be two types of disorders. The first type of disorder holds social skills deficits as a diagnostic criterion. An example of this would be social problems as being required for any diagnosis of an ASD. The second type of disorder does not require a social skills deficit as part of its diagnostic criteria, though social skills are almost always negatively impacted by the disorders that have been reviewed.

Another important point that has emerged from the literature is the complex and reciprocal relationship between social skills and the disorder itself. Specifically, it is still debatable for many disorders as to whether an existing social skills deficit first promotes the initiation of the disorder or whether the social skills deficits only exist during the disorder. An example of this would be whether an existing social skills deficits influences the development of an anxiety disorder in a prodromal fashion or whether the social skills deficits only occurs while the person is in an affective state of anxiety. Evidence on both sides of this argument exists, and future research on the topic is needed for many of the disorders that have been reviewed. A definitive answer to this question for each of the disorders reviewed is critical to the development of effective prevention and intervention programs. For example, knowing whether a specific social skills deficit may be strongly predictive of a particular anxiety disorder would certainly influence the content of a prevention program focused on that disorder as well as assist in the selection of youth that might benefit the most from the prevention program.

Thus, there is a critical need for more research that examines that reciprocal relationship between psychopathology and social skills. Research that is longitudinal in nature is especially important, as this type of data would allow for causal models of analysis such as structural equation modeling. While the beginnings of this research exist, some studies point to other variables that may be of interest. For example, a number of studies have revealed that relationships between psychopathology and social skills deficits may appear, disappear, or change direction depending on the developmental period of the participant (Cole et al., 1996; Pandina et al., 1991). Additionally, little research exists that attempts to understand how gender may affect the relationship between social skills and psychopathology. While some disorders may find few gender differences (e.g., intellectual disability), there are several disorders that are either more prevalent in females (e.g., MDD) or males (e.g., ADHD) in which the relationship between social skills and symptomatology are quite different depending on the gender of the participant. Similarly, there is virtually no research examining how social skills deficits may be attenuated or strengthened based on the ethnicity or cultural background of the child with any particular disorder.

The need for future research on this topic is critical when one considers that the treatment of many of the reviewed disorders often includes a social skills component. For example, if one component of a substance abuse program includes social skills training, it is important to know that substance abusing youth may not have difficulty initiating friendships, but rather they often choose friends who are substance abusing themselves. This knowledge would certainly have an impact on the content of this substance abuse program or even related prevention programming. Similarly, prevention and intervention programs related to depression and suicide often have social skills components that are related to help-seeking, building social support networks, etc. (Stark et al., 2008). However, only recently are these programs considering how male and female youth develop social skills differently and how these deficits may affect the initiation and maintenance of a particular disorder differently.

Therefore, future research on intervention and prevention programming must answer three related questions. First, for which disorders do significant gender differences exist? Second, how can these gender differences be described? And finally, how do these gender differences impact the content of the intervention or prevention program. Finally, there is virtually no research on whether social skills deficits (and related prevention and intervention program effectiveness) may differ based on the youth's ethnicity. Given cultural differences in various normative social skills, research such as this is critical (Sasao, & Sue,1993).

References

Addington, J., & Addington, D. (2006). Poor social and interpersonal functioning prior to diagnosis predicts poor outcome for people with first episode psychosis. *Evidence-Based Mental Health, 9*, 5–9.

American Psychiatric Association (2000). *Diagnostic and statistical manual of mental disorders* (4th ed., Text Revision). Washington, DC: Author.

Asarnow, J. R., & Asarnow, R. F. (2003). Childhood-onset schizophrenia. In E. J. Mash & R. A. Barkley (Eds.), *Child psychopathology* (2nd ed., pp. 455–485). New York: Guilford.

Asarnow, J. R., Tompson, M. C., & Goldstein, M. J. (1994). Childhood-onset schizophrenia: A followup study. *Schizophrenia Bulletin, 20*, 599–617.

Barkley, R. A. (1997). Behavioral inhibition, sustained attention, and executive functions: Constructing a unifying theory of ADHD. *Psychological Bulletin, 121*, 65–94.

Barkley, R. A. (2003). Attention-deficit/hyperactivity disorder. In E. J. Mash & R. A. Barkley (Eds.), *Child psychopathology* (2nd ed., pp. 75–143). New York: Guilford.

Barrett, P. M., Rapee, R. M., Dadds, M. M., & Ryan, S. M. (1996). Family enhancement of cognitive style in anxious and aggressive children. *Journal of Abnormal Child Psychology, 24*, 187–203.

Bauminger, N. (2002). The facilitation of social-emotional understanding and social interaction in high-functioning children with autism: Intervention outcomes. *Journal of Autism and Developmental Disorders, 32*, 283–298.

Beck, A. (1963). Thinking and depression: 1, Idiosyncratic content and cognitive distortions. *Archives of General Psychiatry, 9*, 324–333.

Beck, J. S. (1995). *Cognitive therapy: Basics and beyond.* New York, NY: Guilford Press.

Becker, S. J., & Curry, J. F. (2007). Interactive effect of substance abuse and depression on adolescent social competence. *Journal of Clinical Child and Adolescent Psychology, 36*, 469–475.

Berkson, G. (1993). *Children with handicaps: A review of behavioral research*. Hillsdale, NJ: Erlbaum.

Bielecki, J., & Swender, S. L. (2004). The assessment of social functioning in individuals with mental retardation. *Behavior Modification, 28*, 694–708.

Birmaher B., Ryan N. D., Williamson D. E. et al. (1996). Childhood and adolescent depression: a review of the past ten years. Part I. *Journal of the American Academy of Child and Adolescent Psychiatry, 35*, 1427–1439.

Bouhuys, A. L., Bloem, G. M., & Groothuis, T. G. G. (1995). Induction of depressed and elated mood by music influences the perception of facial emotional expressions in health subjects. *Journal of Affective Disorders, 33*, 215–226.

Brinkmeyer, M. Y., & Eyberg, S. M. (2003). Parent-child interaction therapy for oppositional children. In A. E. Kazdin & J. R. Weisz (Eds.), *Evidence-based psychotherapies for children and adolescents* (pp. 204–223). New York: Guilford.

Capaldi, D. M., & Patterson, G. R. (1994). Interrelated influences of contextual factors on antisocial behavior in childhood and adolescence for males. In D. C. Fowles, P. Sutker, & S. H. Goodman (Eds.), *Progress in experimental personality and psychopathology research* (pp. 165–198). New York: Springer.

Carlson, C. L., Lehy, B. B., Frame, C. L., Walker, J., & Hynd, G. W. (1987). Sociometric status of clinic-referred children with ADD with and without hyperactivity. *Journal of Abnormal Child Psychology, 15*, 537–547.

Carter, A. S., Davis, N. O., Klin, A., & Volkmar, F. R. (2005). Social development in autism. In F. R. Volkmar, R. Paul, A. Klin, & D. Cohen (Eds.), *Handbook of autism and pervasive developmental disorders: Diagnosis, development, neurobiology, and behavior* (Vol. 1). Hoboken, NJ: John Wiley & Sons.

Centers for Disease Control and Prevention. (2005). Mental health in the United States: Prevalence of diagnosis and medication treatment for attention-deficit/hyperactivity disorder – United States, 2003. *Morbidity and Mortality Weekly Report, 54*(34), 842–847.

Charman, T. (2002). The prevalence of autism spectrum disorders: Recent evidence and future challenges. *European Child & Adolescent Psychiatry, 11*, 249–256.

Chorpita, B. F., & Barlow, D. H. (1998). The development of anxiety: The role of control in the early environment. *Psychological Bulletin, 124*, 3–12.

Chronis, A. M., Jones, H. A., & Raggi, V. L. (2006). Evidence-based psychosocial treatments for children and adolescents with attention-deficit/hyperactivity disorder. *Clinical Psychology Review, 26*, 486–502.

Coie, J. D., & Dodge, K. A. (1998). Aggression and antisocial behavior. In W. Damon (Series Ed.) & N. Eisenberg (Vol. Ed.), *Handbook of child psychology: Social, emotional, and personality development* (5th ed., Vol. 3, pp. 779–862). New York: Wiley.

Cole, D. A., Martin, J. M., Powers, B., & Truglio, R. (1996). Modeling causal relations between academic and social competence and depression: A multitrait-multimethod longitudinal study of children. *Journal of Abnormal Psychology, 105*, 258–270.

Crick, N. R., & Dodge, K. A. (1994). A review and reformulation of social information-processing mechanisms in children's social adjustment. *Psychological Bulletin, 115*, 74–101.

De Boo, G. M., & Prins, P. J. M. (2007). Social incompetence in children with ADHD: Possible moderators and mediators in social-skills training. *Clinical Psychology Review, 27*, 78–97.

de Rosnay, M., Cooper, P. J., Tsigara, N., & Murray, L. (2006). Transmission of social anxiety from mother to infant: An experimental study using a social referencing paradigm. *Behaviour Research and Therapy, 44*, 1165–1175.

DiBartolo, P. M., & Helt, M. (2007). Theoretical models of affectionate versus affectionless control in anxious families: A critical examination based on observations of parent-child interactions. *Clinical Child and Family Psychology, 10*, 253–274.

Dodge, K. A. (1986). A social information processing model of social competence in children. In M. Perlmutter (Ed.), *The Minnesota symposium on child psychology* (Vol. 18, pp. 77–125). Hillsdale, NJ: Erlbaum.

Dodge, K. A., & Coie, J. D. (1987). Social information processing factors in reactive and proactive aggression in children's peer groups. *Journal of Personality and Social Psychology, 6*, 1146–1158.

Dumas, M. C. (1998). The risk of social interaction problems among adolescents with ADHD. *Education and Treatment of Children, 21*, 447–461.

D'Zurilla, T. J., Chang, E. C., Nottingham, E. J., & Faccini, L. (1998). Social problem-solving deficits and hopelessness, depression, and suicidal risk in college students and psychiatric inpatients. *Journal of Clinical Psychology, 54*, 1091–1107.

Eggers, C., & Bunk, D. (1997). The long-term course of childhood-onset schizophrenia: A 42-year followup. *Schizophrenia Bulletin, 23*, 105–117.

Elizabeth, J., King, N., & Ollendick, T. H. (2004). Etiology of social anxiety disorder in youth. *Behaviour Change, 21*, 162–172.

Erhardt, D., & Hinshaw, S. P. (1994). Initial sociometric impressions of attention-deficit hyperactivity disorder and comparison boys: Predictions from social behaviors and from nonbehavioral variables. *Journal of Consulting and Clinical Psychology, 62*, 833–842.

Eyberg, S. M., Nelson, M. M., & Boggs, S. R. (2008). Evidence-based psychosocial treatments for children and adolescents with disruptive behavior. *Journal of Clinical Child & Adolescent Psychology, 37*, 215–237.

Fergusson, D. M., Horwood, L. J., Ridder, E. M., & Beautrais, A. L. (2005). Subthreshold depression in adolescence and mental health outcomes in adulthood. *Archives of General Psychiatry, 62*, 66–72.

Field, A. P., Hamilton, S. J., Knowles, K. A., & Plews, E. L. (2003). Fear information and social phobic beliefs in children: A prospective paradigm and preliminary results. *Behaviour Research and Therapy, 41*, 113–123.

Fisak, B., & Grills-Taquechel, A. E. (2007). Parental modeling, reinforcement, and information transfer: Risk factors in the development of child anxiety? *Clinical child and Family Practice, 10*, 213–231.

Fox, N. A., Nichols, K. E., Henderson, H. A., Rubin, K., Schmidt, L., Hamer, D., et al. (2005). Evidence for a gene-environment interaction in predicting behavioral inhibition in middle childhood. *Psychological Science, 16*, 921–926.

Frick, P. J. (1998a). Conduct disorders. In T. H. Ollendick & M. Hersen (Eds.), *Handbook of child psychopathology* (3rd ed., pp. 213–237). New York: Guilford.

Frick, P. J. (1998b). *Conduct disorders and severe antisocial behavior.* New York: Plenum.

Frick, P. J., & Lahey, B. B. (1991). The nature and characteristics of attention-deficit/hyperactivity disorder. *School Psychology Review, 20*, 163–173.

Frick, P. J., & Loney, B. R. (1999). Outcomes of children and adolescents with oppositional defiant disorder and conduct disorder. In H. C. Quay & A. E. Hogan (Eds.), *Handbook of disruptive behavior disorders* (pp. 507–524). Dordrecht, Netherlands: Kluwer Academic Publishers.

Goldstein, T. R., Miklowitz, D. J., & Mullen, K. L. (2006). Social skills knowledge and performance among adolescents with bipolar disorder. *Bipolar Disorders, 8*, 350–361.

Gomez, R., & Hazeldine, P. (1996). Social information processing in mild mentally retarded children. *Research in Developmental Disabilities, 17*, 217–227.

Gonthier, M., & Lyon, M. A. (2004). Childhood-onset schizophrenia: An overview. *Psychology in the Schools, 41*, 803–811.

Greene, R. W., Biederman, J., Faraone, S. V., Sienna, M., & Garcia-Jetton, J. (1997). Adolescent outcome of boys with attention-deficit/hyperactivity disorder and social disability: Results for a 4-year longitudinal follow-up study. *Journal of Consulting and Clinical Psychology, 65*, 758–767.

Gregory, A. M., & Eley, T. C. (2007). Genetic influences on anxiety in children: what we've learned and where we're heading. *Clinical Child and Family Psychology, 10*, 199–212.

Guevremont, D. C., & Dumas, M. C. (1994). Peer relationship problems and disruptive behavior disorders. *Journal of Emotional & Behavioral Disorders, 2*, 164–173.

Guralnick, M. J., & Neville, B. (1997). Designing early intervention programs to promote children's social competence. In M. J. Guralnick (Ed.), *The effectiveness of early intervention* (pp. 579–610). Baltimore: Brookes.

Hannesdottir, D. K., & Ollendick, T. H. (2007). The role of emotion regulation in the treatment of child anxiety disorders. *Clinical Child and Family Psychology Review, 10*, 275–293.

Hinshaw, S. P., & Lee, S. S. (2003). Conduct and oppositional defiant disorders. In E. J. Mash & R. A. Barkley (Eds.), *Child Psychopathology* (2nd ed., pp. 144–198). New York: Guilford.

Jacobs, L., Turner, L. A., Faust, M., & Stewart, M. (2002). Social problem solving of children with and without mental retardation. *Journal of Developmental and Physical Disabilities, 14*, 37–50.

Kasari, C., Chamberlain, B., & Bauminger, N. (2001). Social emotions and social relationships in autism: Can children with autism compensate? In J. Burack, T. Charman, N. Yirmiya, & P. Zelazo (Eds.), *Development and autism: Perspectives from theory and research.* Hillsdale, NJ: Erlbaum Press.

Kazdin, A. E. (1997). Parent management training: Evidence, outcomes, and issues. *Journal of the American Academy of Child and Adolescent Psychiatry, 36*, 1349–1356.

Kazdin, A. E. (2003). Problem-solving skills training and parent management training for conduct disorder. In A. E. Kazdin & J. R. Weisz (Eds.), *Evidence-based psychotherapies for children and adolescents* (pp. 241–262). New York: Guilford.

Kendler, K. S., Neale, M. C., Kessler, R. C., Heath, A. C., & Eaves, L. J. (1992). The genetic epidemiology of phobias in women: The interrelationship of agoraphobia, social phobia, situational phobia, and simple phobia. *Archives of General Psychiatry, 49*, 273–281.

Kurtz, M. M., & Mueser, K. T. (2008). A meta-analysis of controlled research on social skills training for schizophrenia. *Journal of Consulting and Clinical Psychology, 76*, 491–504.

Lahey, B. B., Pelham, W. E., Stein, M. A., Loney, J., Greenhill, L., Hynd, G. W., et al. (1998). Validity of DSM-IV attention-deficit/hyperactivity disorder for younger children. *Journal of the American Academy of Child and Adolescent Psychiatry, 37*, 695–702.

Landau, S., & Moore, L. A. (1991). Social skills deficits in children with ADHD. *School Psychology Review, 20*, 235–251.

Lang, P. (1968). Fear reduction and fear behavior: Problems in treating a construct. In J. M. Shlien (Ed.), *Research in psychotherapy* (pp. 90–102). Washington, DC: American Psychological Association.

Larson, S. A., Lakin, K. C., Anderson, L., Kwak, N., Lee, J. H., & Anderson, D. (2001). Prevalence of mental retardation and developmental disabilities: Estimates from the 1994/1995 national health interview survey disability supplements. *American Journal on Mental Retardation, 106*, 231–252.

Lewine, L. R., Watt, N. F., Prentky, R. A., & Fryer, J. H. (1980). Childhood social competence in functionally disordered psychiatric patients and in normals. *Journal of Abnormal Psychology, 89*, 132–138.

Lewinsohn, P. M., Klein, D. N., & Seeley, J. R. (2000). Bipolar disorder during adolescence and young adulthood in a community sample. *Bipolar Disorders, 2*, 281–293.

Lochman, J., Barry, T. D., & Pardini, D. A. (2003). Anger control training for aggressive youth. In A. E. Kazdin & J. R. Weisz (Eds.), *Evidence-based psychotherapies for children and adolescents* (pp. 263–281). New York: Guilford.

Loeber, R., Burke, J. D., Lahey, B. B., Winters, A., & Zera, M. (2000). Oppositional defiant and conduct disorder: A review of the past 10 years, Part I. *Journal of the American Academy of Child & Adolescent Psychiatry, 39*, 1468–1484.

Loeber, R., & Farrington, D. P. (2000). Young children who commit crime: Epidemiology, developmental origins, risk factors, early intervention and policy implications. *Development and Psychopathology, 12*, 737–762.

Loeber, R., & Stouthamer-Loeber, M. (1998). Development of juvenile aggression and violence: Some common misconceptions and controversies. *American Psychologist, 53*, 242–259.

Luckasson, R., Borthwick-Duffy, S., Buntinx, W. H. E., Coulter, D. L., Craig, E. M., Reeve, A., et al. (2002). *Mental retardation: Definition, classification, and systems of supports* (10th ed.). Washington, DC: American Association on Mental Retardation.

Macintosh, K., & Dissanayake, C. (2004). Annotation: The similarities and differences between Autistic disorder and Asperger's disorder: A review of the empirical evidence. *Journal of Child Psychology and Psychiatry, 45*, 421–434.

Macintosh, K., & Dissanayake, C. (2006). Social skills and problem behaviours in school aged children with high-functioning autism and Asperger's disorder. *Journal of Autism and Developmental Disorders, 36*, 1065–1076.

Madonna, J. M. (1990). An integrated approach to the treatment of a specific phobia in a nine-year-old boy. *Phobia Practice and Research Journal, 3*, 95–106.

Mason, D. A., & Frick, P. J. (1994). The heritability of antisocial behavior: A meta-analysis of twin and adoption studies. *Journal of Psychopathology and Behavioral Assessment, 16*, 301–323.

Matson, J. L., Minshawi, N. E., Gonzalez, M. L., & Mayville, S. B. (2006). The relationship of comorbid problem behaviors to social skills in persons with profound mental retardation. *Behavior Modification, 30*, 496–506.

Matson, J. L., Smiroldo, B. B., & Bamburg, J. W. (1998). The relationship of social skills to psychopathology for individuals with severe or profound mental retardation. *Journal of Intellectual and Developmental Disability, 23*, 137–145.

McFarlane, A. H., Bellissimo, A., & Norman, G. R. (1995). The role of family and peers in social self-efficacy: Links to depression in adolescence. *American Journal of Orthopsychiatry, 65*, 402–410.

McMahon, R. J., & Forehand, R. L. (2003). *Helping the noncompliant child: Family-based treatment for oppositional behavior* (2nd ed.). New York: Guilford.

Milich, R., & Landau, S. (1982). Socialization and peer relations in hyperactive children. In K. D. Gadow & I. Bialer (Eds.), *Advances in learning and behavioural disabilities: A research annual* (pp. 283–339). Greenwich, CT: JAI Press.

Moffitt, T. E. (1993). Adolescence-limited and life-course persistent antisocial behavior: A developmental taxonomy. *Psychological Review, 100*, 674–701

Mowrer, O. H. (1939). A stimulus-response analysis of anxiety and its role as a reinforcing agent. *Psychological Review, 46*, 553–565.

Nijmeijer, J. S., Minderaa, R. B., Buitelaar, J. K., Mulligan, A., Hartman, C. A., & Hoekstra, P. J. (2008). Attention-deficit/hyperactivity disorder and social dysfunctioning. *Clinical Psychology Review, 28*, 692–708.

Nixon, E. (2001). The social competence of children with attention deficit hyperactivity disorder: A review of the literature. *Child Psychology & Psychiatry Review, 6*, 172–180.

Pandina, R. J., Labouvie, E. W., Johnson, V., & White, H. R. (1991). The relationship between alcohol and marijuana use and competence in adolescence. *Journal of Health & Social Policy, 1*, 89–108.

Patterson, G. R. (1982). *Coercive family process*. Eugene, OR: Castalia.

Patterson, G. R., Chamberlain, P., & Reid, J. B. (1982). A comparative evaluation of a parent-training program. *Behavior Therapy, 13*, 638–650.

Patterson, G. R., DeBaryshe, B. D., & Ramsey, E. (1989). A developmental perspective on antisocial behavior. *American Psychologist, 44*, 329–335.

Patterson, G. R., Reid, J. B., & Dishion, T. J. (1992). *Antisocial boys*. Eugene, OR: Castalia.

Pearl, R., Farmer, T. W., Van Acker, R., Rodkin, P., Bost, K. K., Coe, M., et al. (1998). The social integration of students with mild disabilities in general education classrooms: Peer group membership and peer-assessed social behaviour. *The Elementary School Journal, 99*, 167–186.

Pelham, W. E., & Fabiano, G. A. (2008). Evidence-based psychosocial treatment for attention-deficit/hyperactivity disorder. *Journal of Clinical Child & Adolescent Psychology, 37*, 184–214.

Pelham, W. E., & Hoza, B. (1996). Intensive treatment: A summer treatment program for children with ADHD. In E. Hibbs & P. Jensen (Eds.), *Psychosocial treatments for child and adolescent disorders: Empirically based strategies for clinical practice* (pp. 311–340). New York: APA Press.

Pelham, W. E., Wheeler, T., & Chronis, A. (1998). Empirically supported psychosocial treatments for attention deficit hyperactivity disorder. *Journal of Clinical Child Psychology, 27*, 190–205.

Pope, A. W., Bierman, K. L., & Mumma, G. H. (1991). Relations between hyperactivity and aggressive behavior and peer relations at three elementary grade levels. *Journal of Abnormal Child Psychology, 17*, 253–267.

Rachman, S. (1977). The conditioning theory of fear-acquisition: A critical examination. *Behavior Research and Therapy, 15*, 375–387.

Rhodes, J. E., & Jason, L. A. (1990). A social stress model of substance abuse. *Journal of Consulting and Clinical Psychology, 58*, 395–401.

Ropcke, B., & Eggers, C. (2005). Early-onset schizophrenia: A 15-year follow-up. *European Child and Adolescent Psychiatry, 14*, 341–350.

Rubin, K. H., & Mills, R. S. L. (1991). Conceptualizing developmental pathways to internalizing disorders in childhood. *Canadian Journal of Behavioural Science, 23*, 300–317.

Sasao, T., & Sue, S. (1993). Toward a culturally anchored ecological framework of research in ethnic-cultural communities. *American Journal of Community Psychology, 21*, 705–727.

Schalock, R. L., Luckasson, R. A., Shogren, K. A., Borthwick-Duffy, S., Bradley, V., Buntix, W. H. E., et al. (2007). The renaming of mental retardation: Understanding the change to the term intellectual disability. *Intellectual and Developmental Disabilities, 45*, 116–124.

Schopler, E., Mesibov, G. B., & Kunce, L. J. (Eds.). (1998). *Asperger syndrome or high-functioning autism?* New York: Plenum Press.

Selman, R. L., Beardslee, W., Schultz, L. H., Krupa, M., & Podorefsky, D. (1986). Assessing adolescent interpersonal negotiation strategies: Toward the integration of structural and functional models. *Developmental Psychology, 22*, 450–459.

Southam-Gerow, M. A., & Kendall, P. C. (2002). Emotion regulation and understanding: Implications for child psychopathology and therapy. *Clinical Psychology Review, 22*, 189–222.

Spence, S. H. (2003). Social skills training with children and young people: Theory, evidence, and practice. *Child and Adolescent Mental Health, 8*, 84–96.

Spencer, T. J. (2006). ADHD and Comorbidity in childhood. *Journal of Clinical Psychiatry, 67*(Suppl 8), 27–31.

Stark, K. D., Hargrave, J., Hersh, B., Greenberg, M., Herren, J., & Fisher, M. (2008). Treatment of childhood depression: The ACTION Treatment Program. In J. R. Abela & B. L. Hankin (Eds.), *Handbook of depression in children and adolescents* (pp. 224–229). New York, NY, US: Guilford Press.

Stednitz, J. N., & Epkins, C. C. (2006). Girls' and mothers' social anxiety, social skills, and loneliness: Associations after accounting for depressive symptoms. *Journal of Clinical Child and Adolescent Psychology, 35*, , 148–154.

Taylor, A. R., Asher, S. R., & Williams, G. A. (1987). The social adaptation of mainstreamed mildly retarded children. *Child Development, 58*, 1321–1334.

Tse, W. S., & Bond, A. J. (2004). The impact of depression on social skills: A review. *The Journal of Nervous and Mental Disease, 192*, 260–268.

US Department of Health and Human Services (1999). *Mental health: A report of the surgeon general*. Rockville, MD: US Department of Health and Human Services, Substance Abuse and Mental Health Services Administration Center for Mental Health Services, National Institutes of Health, National Institutes of Mental Health.

Vaughn, S., Kim, A., Morris Sloan, C. V., Hughes, M. T., Elbaum, B., & Sridhar, D. (2003). Social skills intervention for young children with disabilities: A synthesis of group design studies. *Remedial and Special Education, 24*, 2–15.

Volkmar, F. R. (1996). Childhood and adolescent psychosis: A review of the past 10 years. *Journal of the American Academy of Child & Adolescent Psychiatry, 35*, 843–851.

Volkmar, F. R., Carter, A., Grossma, J., & Klin, A. (1997). Social development in autism. In D. J. Cohen & F. R. Volkmar (Eds.), *Handbook of autism and developmental disorders* (pp. 173–194). New York: Wiley.

Wallander, J. L., & Hubert, N. C. (1987). Peer social dysfunction in children with developmental disabilities: Empirical basis and a conceptual model. *Clinical Psychology Review, 7*, 205–221.

Watson, J. B., & Watson, R. R. (1921). Studies in infant psychology. *Scientific Monthly, 13*, 493–515.

Watt, M. C., Stewart, S. H., & Cox, B. J. (1998). A retrospective study of the learning history origins of anxiety sensitivity. *Behaviour Research and Therapy, 36*, 505–525.

Webster-Stratton, C., & Hammond, M. (1997). Treating children with early-onset conduct problems: A comparison of child and parent training interventions. *Journal of Consulting and Clinical Psychology, 65*, 93–109.

Whalen, C. K., & Henker, B. (1992). The social profile of attention-deficit hyperactivity disorder: Five fundamental facets. *Child and Adolescent Psychiatric Clinics of North America, 1*, 395–410.

Whalen, C. K., & Henker, B. (1998). Attention-deficit/ hyperactivity disorders. In T. H. Ollendick & M. Hersen (Eds.), *Handbook of child psychopathology* (3rd ed., pp. 181–211). New York: Guilford.

Whalen, C. K., Henker, B., & Granger, D. A. (1990). Social judgment processes in hyperactive boys: Effects of methylphenidate and comparisons with normal peers. *Journal of Abnormal Child Psychology, 18*, 297–316.

White, S. W., Keonig, K., & Scahill, L. (2007). Social skills development in children with autism spectrum disorders: A review of the intervention research. *Journal of Autism and Developmental Disorders, 37*, 1858–1868.

Witt, J. C., Elliott, S. N., Daly III, E. J., Gresham, F. M., & Kramer, J. J. (1998). *Assessment of at-risk and special needs children* (2nd ed.). Boston: McGraw Hill.

Chapter 4
General Methods of Assessment

Jessica A. Boisjoli and Johnny L. Matson

Introduction

People encounter social interactions throughout the course of a day at their home, job, school, grocery store, and anywhere people are present. What contributes to the accord or conflict during these interactions are social skills. Adequate and poor social skills can be easily identified, even by the lay observer, yet defining what social skills are and what behaviors constitute a person being skilled or unskilled is more difficult. Numerous definitions of social skills exist; many of which are used in the assessment and treatment literature (Merrell & Gimpel, 1998). Social skills definitions can be consolidated into three broad categories: a behavioral model, peer acceptance model, and social validity model (Gresham & Elliott, 1984).

The behavioral approach to defining social skills is the most commonly presented in the literature. This is not a surprise given that the most widely used interventions for social skills are behavioral in nature (Matson & Wilkins, 2007). Many of the currently accepted behavioral definitions have a common underlying theme; that is, both verbal and nonverbal behaviors are learned and that these behaviors result in either reinforcement or punishment during social interactions. Depending on the discipline or theoretical orientation of the clinician or researcher, the definition of social skills may differ. However, all can

agree that a person who is socially skilled is able to maneuver through life with the ability to avoid conflicts and can easily remedy conflicts through communication, should they arise (Matson & Ollendick, 1988). Conversely, a person lacking in the social skills domain may encounter more interpersonal difficulties in comparison to the socially skilled individual.

The peer acceptance definitions propose that a person who is accepted by his/her peers is socially skilled. That is, the individual engages in behaviors that are approved of by his/her peers. The social validity definitions describe a person who is socially skilled as being able to use certain behaviors that result in socially important outcomes. These latter two definitions of social skills touch upon the construct of social competence. Social competence is different from social skills in that social competence is social behavior that is effective in producing, maintaining, and enhancing effective interactions with others (Foster & Ritchey, 1979). In comparison, social skills are components or discrete behaviors of the broader construct of social competence. Social competence can be described as how well persons use the social skills they have in their repertoire. Social competence in children is generally assessed through sociometrics such as peer nomination and other peer-report measures.

While a person can be described as either socially skilled or socially unskilled, there is also a gray area where many children lie. These children may evince some pro-social skills, yet they also exhibit some social skill excesses and deficits that need remediation. The purpose of assessing social skills is to identify strengths and weaknesses to target for treatment intervention as well as monitor treatment progress. It is well

J.A. Boisjoli (✉)
Department of Psychology, Louisiana State University,
Baton Rouge, LA 70803, USA
e-mail: jessicaboisjoli@gmail.com

J.L. Matson (ed.), *Social Behavior and Skills in Children*, DOI 10.1007/978-1-4419-0234-4_4,
© Springer Science+Business Media, LLC 2009

documented in the literature of child psychology that social skills deficits are related to many unfavorable outcomes with children. Children with poor social skills are more likely to experience substance abuse (Greene et al., 1999), depression (Sato, Ishikawa, Arai, & Sakano, 2005), antisocial behavior (Dodge et al., 2003), and delinquency and criminality in adulthood (Roff & Wirt, 1984). Furthermore, deficits in social skills are defining characteristics for some developmental disabilities. Social skills are a core deficit in the diagnosis of intellectual disabilities as defined by the American Association of Intellectual and Developmental Disabilities (Grossman, 1973) and Pervasive Developmental Disorders according to the *Diagnostic and Statistical Manual of Mental Disorders-4th edition-Text Revision* (American Psychiatric Association, 2000). Conversely, adequate social skills predict academic achievement (Wentzel, 1993), popularity, and better adjustment later in life. The implications of social skills difficulties necessitate accurate assessment.

While there are numerous definitions of social skills and measures to assess these behaviors, a taxonomy of social skills has not been established (Merrell & Gimpel, 1998). There is no universally agreed upon set of behaviors that are known as social skills. Most measures do assess interpersonal behaviors; however, item content varies from measure to measure. In an attempt to develop a taxonomy of social skills, Caldarella and Merrell (1997) conducted a meta-analysis of research studies involving the assessment of social skills in children from 1974 to 1994 using 21 well-established social skills measures. The analysis yielded a taxonomy of 5 social skill dimensions. The dimensions represented in this synthesis were peer relations, self-management, academic, compliance, and assertion. Analyzing psychometrically sound assessment measures provided a step toward the identification of behavioral dimensions that compose the concept of social skills.

History of Assessment

The earliest assessment and treatment of social skills involved assertiveness training for shy men nearly 40 years ago (McFall & Marston, 1970). Following the success of these early studies on identifying behavioral targets and implementing

effective treatment, the study of social skills was soon applied to other groups, including children. Early studies on the assessment of social skills involved children and adults with more severe forms of psychopathology. Researchers employed role-play assessments to identify specific treatment targets for these special populations.

Due to the connection of interpersonal difficulties and undesirable outcomes, the study of assessment and treatment of social skills became a popular area of clinical interest (Matson & Ollendick, 1988). The assessment of social skills have been applied to various populations such as those with schizophrenia, anxiety, intellectual disabilities, autism, sensory impairments, depression, learning disabilities, emotional disturbance, as well as typically developing children (Agaliotis & Kalyva, 2008; Garland & Fitzgerald, 1998; Matson, 1990; Matson, Macklin, & Helsel, 1985; Matson, Rotatori, & Helsel, 1983; Matson & Wilkins, 2007; Raymond & Matson, 1989; Rojahn & Warren, 1997). More recently, the assessment of social skills has expanded to individuals with medical conditions, including epilepsy, spina bifida, and chronic illness (Lemanek, Jones, & Lieberman, 2000; Matson, Luke, & Mayville, 2004; Meijer, Sinnema, Bijstra, Mellenbergh, & Wolters, 2000; Tse, Hamiwka, Sherman, & Wirrell, 2007). By accurately assessing the social skills of these special populations, effective treatments can be implemented.

From the contributions made by role-play assessments, other techniques have been developed to assess children's social skills. More recently, researchers and clinicians have used direct behavioral observation and developed informant-based rating scales, self-report measures, and sociometrics to assess the social skills of children.

Assessment Methods

Role-Play

Role-play is a behavioral observation method of social skills assessment. This method of measuring social skills was one of the first in the field of psychology. With role-play assessments, the individual is given a sample situation and then directed to respond to the situation. Objective measures such as eye contact, voice volume, number of words spoken, and facial expression are recorded and rated on both accuracy and performance (Matson & Ollendick, 1988). Typically, the clinician or researcher presents the person with a vignette or scenario and directs him/her to react as they would if the situation were actually occurring. This method of social skills assessment can be conducted in most settings.

An early study by McFall and Marston (1970) focused on shy men. Operationally defined target behaviors were identified for the participants. Next the participants were asked to respond to particular vignettes and the target behaviors were rated. The McFall and Marston study provided the men with feedback on their performance and appropriate social behaviors were modeled. With role-play assessments, there is considerable overlap between assessment and treatment, emphasizing the utility of this assessment technique and contributing to its popularity during this time (Matson & Wilkins, 2009). Given the nature of the role-play assessment, they have since been applied to other populations, including children.

Role-play assessments were not standardized assessments for children until the introduction of the *Behavioral Assertiveness Test for Children* (BAT-C) (Bornstein, Bellack, & Hersen, 1977). The BAT-C was designed for children experiencing difficulty with assertiveness. The child is presented with nine scenes. Four scenes involve an opposite sex role model and five scenes involve a same sex role model. The children are presented with each of the scenes on three separate occasions. Scene settings are school related, and the situations are those that the authors felt are common to children. For example, scenes may involve such topics as the child having his seat taken by another child, having his loaned pencil broken, or being skipped on his turn. The objective measures for this assessment include ratio of eye contact to the duration of speech, volume of speech, making a request to change behavior, and overall assertiveness. Inter-rater reliability is high and validity studies have also been conducted. Thus, a significant relationship between BAT-C scores and sociometric ratings exists (Hobbs, Walle, & Hammersly, 1984). The BAT-C has also been used to compare group differences such as between gender and race (Hobbs et al., 1984).

Another role-play assessment developed to measure social skills, in addition to assertiveness, is the *Social Skills Test for Children* (SST-C) (Williamson, Moody, Granberry, Lethermon, & Blouin, 1983). The SST-C is designed to be used with children of elementary school age. The 30 role-play scenes are read to the child by a narrator, with another person present to prompt the child for responses. Five broad categories of scenes comprise the SST-C. Four of the categories present pro-social skills: accepting help, accepting praise, giving help, and giving praise. The last scene addresses assertiveness. Each broad category consists of six scenes. The child is rated on speech content, gestures, intonation, duration of speech, ratio of eye contact to speech duration, head position, posture, fluency, latency of response, and an overall rating of skill. Validity studies have been conducted using sociometric ratings, teacher ratings, and self ratings. None of the specific behaviors of the SST-C and the other measures of social skills (i.e., criterions) were highly correlated. These findings were similar to previous studies, finding low correlations between role-play assessments and other measures of social skills. However, when analyses were employed looking at the relationship between sets of variables, correlational relationships between the role-play scenes and other clusters of social skills were found to be significant. For example, short response latency, high overall skill, and non-erect head were moderately associated with positive ratings by peers and high ratings by teachers. While more significant associations were reported after using this particular analysis, the majority of associations were moderate at best (Williamson et al., 1983).

The role-play method of social skills assessment has a long history in the field of assessment and treatment of social skills. However, this method has since fallen out of favor due to poor validity (Matson, Esveldt-Dawson, & Kazdin, 1983). Bellack and his associates conducted studies that while there was some relationship between role-play assessments and structured interviews, overall validity of this method was questionable (Bellack, 1979). Due to the uncertain validity of this assessment method, its use should be cautioned (Hersen & Bellack, 1981; Matson & Senatore, 1981) and not be the sole measure of a child's social skills (Matson & Ollendick, 1988).

Direct Behavior Observation

Direct behavioral observation of target behaviors is hallmark to the field of behaviorism. Direct behavioral observation is used to assist in the identification of antecedents and consequences of a particular behavior, as well as gain information on the frequency, intensity, and duration of the behavior. The target behaviors, which may be either positive and/or negative social skills, are operationally defined. The child is observed and the occurrence of the target behavior is recorded. Because this is a direct behavioral observation, only observable behavior can be targeted; as opposed to mental states. Furthermore, the observation may occur in the natural environment or in a contrived environment. Methods of conducting an observational assessment may also use a comparison child. That is, during the observation of the target child, another child is employed as a comparison of behavior.

One standardized behavioral observation method to assess a child's social functioning is the PLAY (Farmer-Dougan & Kaszuba, 1999). For this play-based assessment, preschool aged children are observed during free-play and circle time in their classroom. Each child is rated according to their sophistication of play and interactions with others. The authors of this study found that ratings of children's behavior during circle time were predictive of scores on a social skills rating measure and the socialization portion of a developmental inventory. However, children's behavior during free-play was not predictive of ratings on social skills measures. Implications from the results of this study include selecting appropriate times and activities for the observation of children's social skills. Furthermore, because the child's ratings of social skills were not correlated with free-play, a time when social behavior would be expected, but were correlated with circle-time, indicates that the clinician should only measure a particular type of social skill specific to certain contexts.

Just as with any behavioral observation method of assessment, the same factors that affect ratings are also applied to behavioral observation of social skills. In particular, reactivity to being observed may affect the person's behavior. Another complicating factor with the behavioral observation method is that many behaviors that are targeted for assessment may be of low frequency and difficult to observe (Bellack, 1979). Furthermore, certain targeted behaviors may only be displayed in certain environments and not in others. Due to problems with low rate behaviors and context issues, multiple observations may be required. Observers need to be well-trained on behavioral observation methods and, for some situations, need to be available for multiple observations. This last point (multiple observations), in particular, makes the use of the behavioral observation for most settings such as homes, schools, and outpatient clinics difficult. Nonetheless, behavioral observation is an important component of thorough assessments and has great implications for intervention strategies. One approach that would incorporate behavioral observations in the assessment process, while being sensitive to time and financial constraints, is the use of behavioral observations following the identification of a child who may be experiencing social difficulties. Identifying children in need of a more thorough assessment can be accomplished through the use of broadband screening measures or social skills rating scales. These measures can be administered to a larger number of children and, thus, are more efficient than behavioral observations.

Rating Scales

Rating scales are an increasingly popular method of assessing constructs in the mental health and education fields. Rating scales and behavioral checklists consist of a list of items that are representative of the construct to be measured. Typically for social skills rating scales, each item is rated according to how common a particular behavior occurs for the target child (e.g. "0" = never, "1" = sometimes, "2" = often, and "3" = always). On average, rating scales consist of 25–75 items and take approximately 10–30 minutes to complete (Matson & Wilkins, 2009). For most rating scales, the child's score is compared to a normative group of similar age and gender. Informants for childhood social skill rating scales are usually parents or teachers—a person who knows the child well and is able to report on their social behaviors. Scales used to assess social skills generally assess both adaptive and maladaptive social skills, therefore providing useful information for treatment planning.

An advantage to using rating scales is that less frequent behaviors may be rated. For example, behaviors such as advocating for one's own rights may not occur multiple times per day, making this skill difficult to collect data on through the use of just behavioral observation. The information provided from a rating scale is an overall measure of the child's social skills, rather than just a time sample of exhibited social behaviors. Furthermore, rating scales are an efficient tool for use in settings where time and resources may be limited, such as schools and outpatient clinics.

Numerous measures exist which assess social skills as a component of the overall measure. The well-known measures are *Behavioral Assessment System for Children* (Second Edition) (Reynolds & Kamphaus, 1992), *Vineland Adaptive Behavior Scale* (VABS; Sparrow, Balla, & Cicchetti, 1984), and the *Child Behavior Checklist* (Achenbach, 1980). These broadband measures screen other constructs in addition to social skills, such as adaptive behavior and emotional difficulties. While these measures are good screeners for social skill deficits, the review presented in this chapter will be limited to measures that comprehensively assess social skills only.

A recent review by Matson and Wilkins (2009) reported that there are 48 different norm referenced measures of social skills for children. While there are numerous scales, few have been extensively researched. Two of the most commonly studied measures of social skills of children is the *Matson Evaluation of Social Skills in Youngsters* (MESSY), and the *Social Skills Rating System* (SRSS) (Matson & Wilkins, 2009). Research on the MESSY has primarily focused on older children and special populations, while the SSRS has had more of a focus on younger children (Matson & Wilkins, 2009). A review of some of the more popular measures of children's social skills follows, with a more detailed review provided for the MESSY and the SSRS. This review is not intended to be all-inclusive.

MESSY

The MESSY (Matson et al., 1983) is one of the most well-known measures of social skills in children and has been extensively researched over the past 25 years. The 64-item informant-based measure uses a 5-point Likert-type rating scale. Each item is based on observable behaviors that are representative of social skills of children. The MESSY takes approximately 10–25 minutes to administer, and the teacher report form may be used with any adult who knows the child well (Matson, 1990). There are two factors for the measure: assertiveness/impulsiveness and appropriate social skills. The MESSY is a useful tool that can be used for the identification of children experiencing social skills deficits, assessment of social skills for Individualized Education Plans, treatment monitoring, evaluation of social skills of children with various handicapping conditions, developing educational programs with social skills curricula, and for scientific research purposes (Matson, 1990). The manual states that user qualifications are personnel with at least a master's degree in a mental health-related field (e.g. social work, psychology) or a certified teacher. The original norms for the measure consisted of 744 children, not identified as having any handicapping conditions (Matson, Helsel, Bellack, & Senatore, 1983). Good reliability and validity have been reported in multiple studies of the MESSY (Kazdin, Matson, & Esveldt-Dawson, 1984; Matson et al., 1983; Wierzbicki & McCabe, 1988). Normative samples of children with handicapping conditions, such as hearing and visual impairments, have also been published for the MESSY (Matson et al., 1983; Matson, Heinze, Helsel, Kapperman, & Rotatori, 1986; Matson et al., 1985).

International recognition on the utility of the MESSY has been established as it has been translated into numerous languages including German, Japanese, Spanish, Chinese, Dutch, Hindi, and Turkish with psychometric properties reported for many of these languages (Bacanli & Erdogan, 2003; Kee-Lee, 1997; Méndez, Hidalgo, & Inglés, 2002; Sharma, Sigafoos, & Carroll, 2000; van Manen, Prins, & Emmelkamp, 1999). In addition to the MESSY's usefulness with typically developing children and cross-culturally, the measure has also been used to study social skill characteristics of children with chronic illness (Meijer et al., 2000), hearing impairment (Matson et al., 1985; Raymond & Matson, 1989), depression (Garland & Fitzgerald, 1998), visual impairment (Matson, 1986), and autism (Matson, Stabinsky Compton, & Sevin,

1991). The MESSY is a well-established, useful tool for the identification of social skill functioning with most children, including those who are typically developing, and those with disabilities and psychopathology.

Social Skills Rating System (SSRS)

The SSRS (Gresham & Elliott, 1990) is another well-known and extensively researched assessment of children's social skills. The SSRS consists of three separate rating forms: parent and teacher informant and self-report. There are three different versions of the SSRS for different ages: preschool, elementary, and secondary age groups. The third-party informant versions of the SSRS will be reviewed in this section. The self-report version of the SSRS will be reviewed in a subsequent section. The items of the SSRS are rated on a 3-point Likert-type scale. The parent and teacher versions consist of a social skills scale and problem behaviors scale. The teacher version also includes an academic competence component. The social skills scale consists of five factors: cooperation, assertion, responsibility, empathy, and self-control. The problem behaviors scale includes three factors: externalizing, internalizing, and hyperactivity. Depending on the version of the scale (i.e. informant and age), the number of items on the measure ranges from 34 to 57 items. Each of the different versions of the SSRS can be administered in approximately 15–25 minutes. According to the manual, user qualifications for administration of the measure are any personnel in the mental health field; however, scoring and interpretation should only be conducted by psychologists trained in assessment. The standardization sample included more than 4,000 children in grades 3–10. Standardization sample sizes for the other age groups were considerably smaller.

Reliability and validity analyses of the SSRS have been conducted with each of the versions during the original standardization studies. The reliability estimate for the pre-school version of the SSRS is good (Gresham & Elliott, 1990; Rich, Shepherd, & Nangle, 2008). The original factor analysis of the pre-school version revealed three factors for the social skills domain: self-control, assertion, and cooperation. The problem behaviors scale included

two factors: internalizing and externalizing. However, recent analysis of the pre-school, teacher report version of the SSRS failed to replicate the social skills factors but did replicate the problem behaviors factors in a sample of low-income children (Fantuzzo, Manz, & McDermott, 1998). Results by Fantuzzo and colleagues have been replicated in another study of children enrolled in Head Start (Rich et al., 2008). Analyses using the parent report of the pre-school version did not replicate the original factor structure and also found no relationship between the parent and teacher forms (Manz, Fantuzzo, & McDermott, 1999). However, it should be noted that the sample used for the original analyses of the pre-school version of SSRS was small and was referred to as a trial sample.

For the elementary version of the SSRS, the original four-factor solution is labeled cooperation, assertion, responsibility, and self-control (Gresham & Elliott, 1990). Reliability analyses revealed adequate to excellent internal consistency and excellent test-retest reliability according to the manual (Gresham & Elliott, 1990). However the original factor model of the SSRS elementary version, parent report failed to replicate in other studies, including studies with African American participants (Manz et al., 1999) and a mainly Caucasian, midwestern sample (Whiteside, McCarthy, & Miller, 2007). The adolescent version of the SSRS has been used in a Norwegian sample revealing adequate reliability and replicating the factor structure by Gresham and Elliott (1990).

Like the MESSY, the SSRS has been studied internationally and has been translated into the following languages: Spanish (Jurado, Cumba-Aviles, Collazo, & Matos, 2006), Iranian (Shahim, 2004), Dutch (Van der Oord et al., 2005) and Japanese (Van Horn, Tamase, & Hagiwara, 2001). The SSRS has also been used with special populations such as those with Attention Deficit/Hyperactivity Disorder (Van der Oord et al., 2005), neurofibrosis (Barton & North, 2004), and spina bifida (Lemanek et al., 2000). The SSRS has been used to study social skills of different racial groups, in addition to Caucasian, including Native-American (Powless & Elliott, 1993) and African American (Manz et al., 1999). While the SSRS is a widely used measure of social skills in children, critics suggest that the manual is less than adequate in sufficiently providing the psychometric properties of the measure and information on test construction methods for the consumer to adequately assess the measure (Whiteside et al., 2007).

Home and Community-Based Social Behavior (HCBSB)

The HCBSB (Merrell & Caldarella, 2002) is a 64-item, 5-point Likert-type rating scale for children between the ages of 5 and 18. The aim of the measure is to assess social competence and antisocial behavior. The authors state that the social competence domain is representative of social skills consistent with well-adjusted children (Merrell & Caldarella, 2002). The measure is composed of 4 subscales: peer relations, self-management/compliance, defiant/disruptive, and antisocial/aggressive. Reliability analyses for inter-rater and test-retest coefficients were good to excellent. Convergent and discriminant validity has been supported through correlations with other known measures of children's social skills.

School Social Behavior Scales (SSBS)

The SSBS (Merrell, 1993) is the companion instrument of the HCBSC for school settings. The SSBS has undergone a recent revision and is now the SSBS, Second Edition (SSBS-2) (Merrell, 2002). The SSBS-2 is intended for children between the ages of 5 and 18 with teachers serving as informants. Each item is rated on a 5-point Likert-type scale. The measure consists of 64 items, with 32 items each on the two subscales: social competence and anti-social problem behavior. The items reflect behaviors that involve peer-related and teacher-related social adjustment, which the authors state is necessary for social success in school. Factor analytic studies were conducted on both of the subscales of the SSBS. The social competence subscale yielded a three-factor solution representing the following constructs: interpersonal skills, self-management skills, and academic skills. The antisocial behavior scale also yielded a three-factor solution. The factors represent constructs consistent with hostile-irritable, antisocial-aggressive, and disruptive-demanding behaviors. Reliability analyses revealed

excellent internal consistency, and test-retest and inter-rater reliability were both adequate-to-good for both subscales of the measure. Validity studies have been conducted using the *Waksman Social Skills Rating Scale*, the *Connors Teacher Rating Scales*, and inter-correlations among the subscales of the SSBS (Merrell, 2002).

Waksman Social Skills Rating Scale (WSSRS)

The WSSRS (Waksman, 1985) is a 21-item rating scale of social skills in children from elementary age through high school age. Each item is rated on a 4-point Likert-type scale by teachers. The items of the measure represent negative social skills; no pro-social skills are included. Items were generated for this measure by a review of common components of social skills training programs. A factor analysis of the original sample yielded two factors: aggressive and passive. Reliability analyses were conducted and internal consistency was strong, test-retest reliability for both of the domains was adequate, and inter-rater reliability for the aggressive domain was adequate. However, inter-rater reliability for the passive domain was poor (Waksman, 1985). The author of the original study for the WSSRS also reported validity studies with the WSSRS compared to a measure of problem behaviors, *The Portland Problem Behavior Checklist – Revised*. These analyses revealed adequate correlations between the two measures.

Age-Specific Rating Scales

Social Skills Inventory

The Social Skills Inventory (Riggio, 1986) is a 105-item measure of social skills which has mainly been used with undergraduate populations. This self-report measure not only inquires about skills the individuals perceive themselves as exhibiting, it also inquires about how they think they are perceived by other people. The items are rated on a 9-point Likert-type scale. The measure is broken down into seven social skill dimensions including emotional expressivity, emotional sensitivity, emotional control, social expressivity, social sensitivity, social control, and social manipulation. Each of the dimensions was confirmed through factor analysis. Initial reliability studies reported adequate internal consistency and good-to-excellent test-retest reliability. Convergent and discriminant validity has been reported with other measures of nonverbal social skills (Riggio, 1986).

Teenage Inventory of Social Skills (TISS)

The TISS (Inderbitzen & Foster, 1992) is a self-report measure of social skills with adolescents. The authors of the TISS state that the purpose for the development of the measure is to recognize individuals who have social skills problems and to identify specific behaviors to target for intervention. The measure consists of 40 items which load onto either a positive or negative social skills scale. Test-retest correlations for the positive and negative scales were good, and internal consistency was acceptable. Furthermore, convergent validity was supported through analyses correlating the TISS with self-monitoring, other measures of social skills, and peer ratings of the TISS (Inderbitzen & Foster, 1992).

Preschool and Kindergarten Behavior Scales (PKBS)

The PKBS (Merrell, 1994) is an informant-based rating scale of social skills for children between the ages of 3 and 6 years. Parents, caretakers, and teachers may serve as informants. Items of the PKBS are specific to early childhood development. The PKBS comprises two scales: social skills and problem behavior. The 76 items of the measure are rated on a 4-point Likert-type scale according to frequency of occurrence. According to the manual, internal consistency and inter-rater reliability between teachers and classroom aids is good (Merrell, 1994). Validity studies have been conducted with adequate correlations between the PKBS and other social skills rating measures (Gresham & Elliott, 1990) and also for convergent and divergent validity (Canivez & Rains, 2002).

Behavioral rating scales have major benefits including standardization, efficiency, and relatively little training required for administration. However, there are some weaknesses to using this method for behavioral assessment. Rating scales do not allow for the assessment of environmental variables that may affect the behavior, that is, antecedent and consequences of an action or performance or skill deficits. Because with rating scales only discrete behaviors are measured, there is a need for follow-up evaluation. As is the case of any assessment, multi-method assessments are always warranted. Furthermore, researchers and clinicians need to be consistently aware of biases effecting ratings, such as halo effects.

Sociometrics

In addition to gathering information on a child's social skills from a parent/teacher or behavioral observation, peers are also a valuable source of information on a child's social functioning. Rating of a peer's social skills is often referred to as sociometrics. Peer ratings of social status have been used for many years in classrooms to identify children in need of remediation (Moreno, 1953). The advantage of this assessment method is that evaluation of social skills is done within the context of a group. That is, an outside observer is not employed to make ratings, rather someone within the social dynamic, who may be aware of behaviors that adults are not, make the ratings (Merrell & Gimpel, 1998).

Sociometric assessments can be in the form of peer nomination or peer ratings (Mpofu, Carney, Lambert, & Hersen, 2006). Peer nomination measures, such as the *Peer Nomination Inventory* (Wiggins & Winder, 1961), instruct the child to provide the name of a peer who best fits with a particular question (e.g. "Who is the most liked person in the class?"). For older children, the peer writes the name of the child who best fits the question. Adaptations for younger peers include the use of pictures of children mounted on a piece of paper and the child is instructed to point to the picture of the child that best fits a particular question/statement. This assessment method may inquire about both positive and negative attributes of peers. The number of nominations a child receives is tallied. Interpretations are then made regarding the number of nominations a child receives for each item.

A published peer nomination measure is the *Revised Class Play* (Masten, Morison, & Pellegrini, 1985). This measure is an updated version of the original *Class Play* (Lambert & Bower, 1961) in that positive aspects of social functioning were added and items that represented polar opposites of other items were also included. The *Revised Class Play* consists of 15 positive and 15 negative roles. Children are instructed to assign classmates to roles of a hypothetical play that would be most appropriate for that child. Initial reliability analyses for the *Revised Class Play* were good-to-excellent for internal consistency, inter-rater, and test-retest analyses (Masten et al., 1985). Preliminary studies on validity were good when comparing scores of the *Revised Class Play* to other measures of social skills (Masten et al., 1985).

Another method of acquiring sociometric information of children is through the use of peer ratings. This assessment method is typically done via rating forms where the peer is asked to rate other children on certain attributes or behaviors. This method is similar to rating scales used with parents or teachers. Each child is rated on each item typically using Likert-type scoring. For younger children, like the peer nomination method, pictures of each child can be used. For example, the clinician could use three boxes with one labeled "children I like a lot," the next labeled "children I like a little," and the third labeled "children I don't like at all." The peer is instructed to place the pictures of the children in the appropriate box (Balda, Punia, & Singh, 2005). The number of ratings the child receives is tallied and interpretations are made from the items endorsed. Peer ratings may be a reliable method of assessing social status of children (Balda et al., 2005).

While sociometric methods appear to be a reliable method of assessing a child's social functioning within the peer group, the information provided by the measures may have limited utility for treatment planning purposes. The assessors generally obtain information on the popularity of the children, not explicit deficiencies. Specifically for the peer nomination format, some children may not be nominated at all, thereby offering no information on that child's social functioning. Furthermore, information on specific behaviors that may lead to the child's social status is not provided. Perhaps the use of sociometric ratings along with other informant-based rating measures of social skills, such as the MESSY, could provide information on the status of the child in the peer group along with observable behaviors that can be targeted for treatment.

Self-Report

Parent and teacher rating scales of children's social skills are generally limited to observable behaviors. With self-report rating scales, the child is able to report on their cognitions and perceptions of their own social skills (Danielson & Phelps, 2003). Self-report measures are similar to third-party informant-based rating scales with regard to format. The measures are generally relatively short with a force-choice response format. Self-report measures may be a beneficial method of identifying a child's perception of their own social functioning; however, this method's utility is limited to those children who are able to identify the strengths and weaknesses of their own social behavior. Particularly with children of elementary age, parent report, as opposed to self-report, may be a more reliable method of determining a child's social functioning (Byrne & Bazana, 1996). This consideration would also apply to special groups that may have limited cognitive functioning. A review of self-report measures follows.

The SSRS Self-Report (Gresham & Elliott, 1990) is similar in format to the other versions of the SSRS. The Self-Report forms are intended for children of elementary and secondary age. Subscales of the measure include empathy, cooperation, self-control, and assertion. Original studies, using the standardization sample, reported that internal consistency was adequate for the total score but was not acceptable for the each of the factors. In addition, test-retest and inter-rater reliability were low. Reliability analyses by Diperna and Volpe (2005) were consistent with the original analyses with the total score exhibiting acceptable internal consistency and the factors failing to meet an acceptable level. Test-retest at 6 months was low; however, this may be due to instability of some of the constructs over extended periods of time.

List of Social Situation Problems (LSSP)

The LSSP (Spence, 1980) is a self-report measure of social situations that may be difficult for children. The purpose of the measure is to identify behaviors to address in treatment. The measure comprises 60 social problem situations. The child responds with either a "yes" or a "no" with regard to their perception of the situation being problematic for them. Reliability analyses have been conducted with excellent test-retest correlations (Spence & Marzillier, 1981) and good internal consistency (Spence & Liddle, 1990). Factor analytic studies revealed eight factors representing anxiety with assertiveness, strangers, conflict situations, parents, hetero-social relationships, and issues relating to temper control, social discomfort, and lack of friends (Spence & Liddle, 1990). One concern with the LSSP, evidenced through the factor analytic study, is that in addition to measuring a child's perceived social skill, it appears that the instrument may also be measuring other constructs, such as anxiety (Danielson & Phelps, 2003).

A recent measure has been developed to address some of the shortcomings of other self-report measures of social skills in children such as length, wording, and assessing constructs in addition to social skill. This relatively new measure is the *Children's Self-report Social Skills Scale* (CS^4) (Danielson & Phelps, 2003). The CS^4 is a brief 21-item measure, rated on a 5-point Likert-type scale. Items were carefully selected so as to avoid items that were redundant, addressed affect rather than behavior, and addressed constructs other than social skills. Sixteen of the items measure pro-social skills and five of the items address poor social skills. Reliability analyses have been conducted with test-retest correlations being adequate-to-good and internal consistency was excellent (Danielson & Phelps, 2003). Further analyses are warranted.

Child Characteristics

In addition to identifying which social behaviors are present and which are absent, other considerations should be addressed during the assessment of social skills with children. When assessing a child's social skills it is important to consider whether a behavior, or absence of a behavior, is due to performance or skill deficits. It is just one aspect of a thorough assessment to identify the behaviors that need intervention; however, it is also necessary to identify *why* the behavior is

occurring, or not occurring, to aid in treatment planning. When the child has not learned the necessary behaviors that are effective in social situations, this is considered a skill deficit. Alternatively, the child has the necessary skills in its repertoire to effectively engage in social situations; however, the child fails to display the behavior (Erdlen, Rickrode, Christner, Stewart, & Freeman, 2007). The reason for not displaying a behavior can have various reasons, including using the skill at the wrong time or motivational issues (Matson & Ollendick, 1988). Information on skill and performance deficits will guide more effective intervention. For example, interventions for skill or acquisition-related social deficiencies may include teaching the child the skill through behavioral procedures, such as modeling. For performance deficits, a reinforcement program may be implemented to increase motivation.

In addition to identifying whether behaviors are due to performance or skill deficits, the child's behavior must also be evaluated with individual characteristics considered. Such characteristics include the child's gender, socioeconomic status, race/ethnicity, and culture (Bain & Pelletier, 1999; Bierman & Montminy, 1993; Chen & French, 2008; Crombie, 1988). Just as with any area of assessment in psychology, clinicians should have a thorough understanding of the population being served and how individual characteristics differ according to groups. For example, assertiveness and sociability may be encouraged in one culture, while these characteristics are discouraged in more group-oriented cultures (Chen & French, 2008). Furthermore, the developmental level of the child should also be considered with regard to social skills (Bierman & Montminy, 1993). Developmental differences in social skills are observed in children of different ages and should be considered during the assessment process.

Social Validity

The concept of social validity was introduced by Montrose Wolf in 1979. The rigor of collecting data on observable behavior, as opposed to mental states, is often associated with applied behavior analysis. However, the concept of the social importance of assessments and interventions began to fall in the hands of the editors of behavioral journals, such as *Journal of Applied Behavior Analysis,* in the late 1960s and early

1970s (Wolf, 1978). Ratings of other people's perceptions on the importance of the assessments and interventions were incorporated into the studies. The new focus on assessment and intervention with regard to its significance to society, the socially appropriateness of the treatments procedures, and the importance of the effects on society, is referred to as social validity (Wolf, 1978).

Social validity is a concept that is an important topic in the study of social skills in children. However, despite the importance of social validity in research, few studies using social skills as treatment targets report the social validity of their studies (Matson, Matson, & Rivet, 2007). Kazdin and Matson (1981) state that for social validity the focus of the intervention needs to be acceptable, and the behavioral change needs to be important. These components of social validity can be studied with social skills of children through the use of subjective measurement and/or social comparison. A study by Charlop and Milstein (1989) used video modeling to teach children with autism more appropriate conversational skills. To assess the social validity of the treatment targets, parents of typically developing children observed video tapes of the participants prior to intervention and subsequent to intervention. The parents were then asked to rate items that reflected social importance for each of the conversations. Example items include "The child shows an interest in the conversation" and "My child would like to talk with this child."

Social comparison involves using a norm group as a comparison for an individual's behavior. A recent study of a child with a learning disability and withdrawn behavior by Christensen and colleagues (2007) was published using social comparison. Twenty-one students of the same age as the target child were selected and observed. Their behavior was utilized as a standard for comparison to the target child. Following treatment, the child's behavior was compared to the behavior of the comparison group on performance and frequency of specific behaviors.

Current Trends and Future Directions

Enormous interest in the area of social skills of children has developed over the past 40 years. Matson and Wilkins (2009) suggest that there has been a large increase in the number of published studies on the topic, particularly in the last 10 years. This attention to children's social functioning may be largely credited to the connection between mental health problems and social functioning.

The definition of what are social skills has not been agreed upon by clinicians and researchers. Many scales exist that address interpersonal situations of children, yet, these scales vary in context, format, item wording, and informant. Furthermore, while still measuring the same broad category of social skills, these assessment methods may, in addition, measure different aspects of socialization. For example, peer nominations and behavioral observations may address different social behaviors than rating scales (Farmer-Dougan & Kaszuba, 1999; Gresham, 1981). Some of the measures provide information on a peer's perspective, while others inquire about the child's own perspective of their social skills. The different methods of assessing children's social skills all have their own strengths and weaknesses.

Many of the current studies of social skills and children use only a small number assessment measures, in particular the MESSY and the SSRS (Matson & Wilkins, 2009). Because of the different information provided by the different scales, there is a need for a variety of social skills measures. Furthermore, these different assessment methods, in general, need continuing study of their psychometric properties, and, more specifically, in their application with different types of populations.

Despite the numerous scales to assess social skills in children, few treatment studies use assessment measures to identify treatment targets or to monitor treatment progress (Matson et al., 2007). Studies using standardized measures need to be the rule not the exception. Additionally, social validity should be addressed in all assessment and treatment studies of social skills with children. Further development of assessment targets that are both operationally defined and socially valid is an area that warrants additional study.

The next step for research and clinical practice of social skills with children is a focus on the identification of specific behaviors that are more likely to lead to social adjustment. Similarly, these next steps should also focus on those behaviors that may lead to maladjustment, including psychopathology. The identification and prioritization of behaviors that will have the most impact on the child's functioning is an area of great importance (Bosch & Fuqua, 2001).

Consistent with studying social skills of different groups is the need for connecting research with clinical practice. There are measures available to assess children's social skills but consistently using psychometrically sound measures in practice is not the norm. Using these measures to identify differences in groups and which behaviors are consistent across groups may assist with the identification of common pathways to mental health concerns (Matson & Wilkins, 2009).

Conclusions

Role-play assessments were one of the first techniques to assess social skills in many populations, including shy men, individuals with severe psychopathology, and unassertive children. Since the introduction of the role-play, direct behavioral observation, informant-based rating scales, self-report rating scales, and sociometrics have been introduced to assess this construct. Each of these methods has strengths and weaknesses that should be considered in the context of the assessment. Rating-scales are an efficient method to gain information on the presence or absence of essential skills to social functioning, while direct behavioral observation provides information on environmental variables that affect behavior. The child's developmental level, culture, and setting should also be considered when selecting appropriate assessment methods. Just as with any assessment in the education or psychology fields, the assessment of social skills should be conducted through the use of multiple assessment methods and from a variety of sources (Merrell, 1999).

The assessment of social skills of children is, undoubtedly, of great importance. Accurate assessment leads to effective intervention, as well as knowledge on the implications of poor social functioning, group differences, and, hopefully one day, information on common pathways to psychopathology (Matson & Wilkins, 2009). Researchers are encouraged to continue the study of social skills in children to aid in the better understanding of social dysfunction and its implications within

groups, particularly those with special needs, and across cultures, and internationally.

References

Achenbach, T. M. (1980). *Child behavior checklist*. Burlington, VT: Child Behavior Checklist.

Agaliotis, I., & Kalyva, E. (2008). Nonverbal social interaction skills with learning disabilities. *Research in Developmental Disabilities, 29*, 1-10.

American Psychiatric Association. (2000). *Diagnostic and statistical manual of mental disorders-text revision* (4th ed.). Washington, DC: Author.

Bacanli, H., & Erdogan, F. (2003). Adaptation of the Matson evaluation of social skills with youngsters (MESSY) to Turkish. *Kuram ve Uygulamada Egitim Bilimleri, 3*(2), 368–379.

Bain, S. K., & Pelletier, K. A. (1999). Social and behavioral differences among a predominantly African American preschool sample. *Psychology in the Schools, 36*(3), 249–259.

Balda, S., Punia, S., & Singh, C. (2005). Assessment of peer relations: A comparison of peer nomination and rating scale. *Journal of Human Ecology, 18*(4), 271–273.

Barton, B., & North, K. (2004). Social skills of children with neurofibromatosis type 1. *Developmental Medicine & Child Neurology, 46*(8), 553–563.

Bellack, A. S. (1979). A critical appraisal of strategies for assessing social skill *Behavioral Assessment, 1*, 157–176.

Bierman, K. L., & Montminy, H. P. (1993). Developmental issues in social-skills assessment and intervention with children and adolescents. *Behavior Modification, 17*(3), 229–254.

Bornstein, M. R., Bellack, A. S., & Hersen, M. (1977). Social-skills training for unassertive children: A multiple-baseline analysis. *Journal of Applied Behavior Analysis, 10*(2), 183–195.

Bosch, S., & Fuqua, R. W. (2001). Behavioral cusps: A model for selecting target behaviors. *Journal of Applied Behavior Analysis, 34*(1), 123–125.

Byrne, B. M., & Bazana, P. G. (1996). Investigating the measurement of social and academic competencies for early/late preadolescents and adolescents: A multitrait-multimethod analysis. *Applied Measurement in Education, 9*(2), 113–132.

Caldarella, P., & Merrell, K. W. (1997). Common dimensions of social skills of children and adolescents: A taxonomy of positive behaviors. *School Psychology Review, 26*(2), 264–278.

Canivez, G. L., & Rains, J. D. (2002). Construct validity of the adjustments scales for children and adolescents and the preschool and kindergarten behavior scales: Convergent and divergent evidence. *Psychology in the Schools, 39*(6), 621–633.

Charlop, M. H., & Milstein, J. P. (1989). Teaching autistic children conversational speech using video modeling. *Journal of Applied Behavior Analysis, 22*(3), 275–285.

Chen, X., & French, D. C. (2008). Children's social competence in cultural context. *Annual Review of Psychology, 59*, 591–616.

Christensen, L., Young, K. R., & Marchant, M. (2007). Behavioral intervention planning: Increasing appropriate behavior of a socially withdrawn student. *Education & Treatment of Children, 30*(4), 81–103.

Crombie, G. (1988). Gender differences: Implications for social skills assessment and training. *Journal of Clinical Child Psychology, 17*(2), 116–120.

Danielson, C. K., & Phelps, C. R. (2003). The assessment of children's social skills through self-report: A potential screening instrument for classroom use. *Measurement & Evaluation in Counseling & Development, 35*(4), 218.

Diperna, J. C., & Volpe, R. J. (2005). Self-report on the social skills rating system: Analysis of reliability and validity for an elementary sample. *Psychology in the Schools, 42*(4), 345–354.

Dodge, K. A., Lansford, J. E., Burks, V. S., Bates, J. E., Pettit, G. S., Fontaine, R., et al. (2003). Peer rejection and social information-processing factors in the development of aggressive behavior problems in children. *Child Development, 74*(2), 374–393.

Erdlen, R. J., Jr., Rickrode, M. R., Christner, R. W., Stewart, J. L., & Freeman, A. (2007). Social skills groups with youth: A cognitive-behavioral perspective. *Handbook of cognitive-behavior group therapy with children and adolescents: Specific settings and presenting problems* (pp. 485–506). New York, NY: Routledge/Taylor & Francis Group.

Fantuzzo, J., Manz, P. H., & McDermott, P. (1998). Preschool version of the social skills rating system: An empirical analysis of its use with low-income children. *Journal of School Psychology, 36*(2), 199–214.

Farmer-Dougan, V., & Kaszuba, T. (1999). Reliability and validity of play-based observations: Relationship between the PLAY behaviour observation system and standardised measures of cognitive and social skills. *Educational Psychology, 19*(4), 429–440.

Foster, S., L., & Ritchey, W., L. (1979). Issues in the assessment of social competence. *Journal of Applied Behavior Analysis, 12*, 625–638.

Garland, M., & Fitzgerald, M. (1998). Social skills correlates of depressed mood in normal young adolescents. *Irish Journal of Psychological Medicine, 15*(1), 19–21.

Greene, R. W., Biederman, J., Faraone, S. V., Wilens, T. E., Mick, E., & Blier, H. K. (1999). Further validation of social impairment as a predictor of substance use disorders: Findings from a sample of siblings of boys with and without ADHD. *Journal of Clinical Child Psychology, 28*(3), 349–354.

Gresham, F. M. (1981). Validity of social skills measures for assessing social competence in low-status children: A multivariate investigation. *Developmental Psychology, 17*, 390–398.

Gresham, F. M., & Elliott, S. N. (1984). Assessment and classification of children's social skills: A review of methods and issues. *School Psychology Review, 13*(3), 292–301.

Gresham, F. M., & Elliott, S. N. (1990). *Social skills rating system*. Circle Pines, MN: American Guidance Services.

Grossman, H. J. (1973). *Manual on terminology and classification in mental retardation*. Washington, DC: American Association on Mental Deficiency.

Hersen, M., & Bellack, A. S. (1981). *Assessment of social skills*. New York: Wiley.

Hobbs, S. A., Walle, D. L., & Hammersly, G. A. (1984). Assessing children's social skills: Validation of the behavioral assertiveness test for children (BAT-C). *Journal of Behavioral Assessment, 6*(1), 29–35.

Inderbitzen, H. M., & Foster, S. L. (1992). The teenage inventory of social skills: Development, reliability, and validity. *Psychological Assessment, 4*(4), 451–459.

Jurado, M., Cumba-Aviles, E., Collazo, L. C., & Matos, M. (2006). Reliability and validity of a spanish version of the social skills rating system – Teacher form. *Journal of Psychoeducational Assessment, 24*(3), 195–209.

Kazdin, A. E., & Matson, J. L. (1981). Social validation in mental retardation. *Applied Research in Mental Retardation, 2*(1), 39–53.

Kazdin, A. E., Matson, J. L., & Esveldt-Dawson, K. (1984). The relationship of role-play assessment of children's social skills to multiple measures of social competence. *Behaviour Research and Therapy, 22*, 129–139.

Kee-Lee, C. (1997). The Matson evaluation of social skills with youngsters: Reliability and validity of a Chinese translation. *Personality and Individual Differences, 22*(1), 123–125.

Lambert, N. M., & Bower, E. M. (1961). *A process for in-school screening of children with emotional handicaps*. Atlanta: Office of Special Tests, Educational Testing Service.

Lemanek, K. L., Jones, M. L., & Lieberman, B. (2000). Mothers of children with spina bifida: Adaptational and stress processing. *Children's Health Care, 29*(1), 19–35.

Manz, P. H., Fantuzzo, J., & McDermott, P. A. (1999). The parent version of the preschool social skills rating scale: An analysis of its use with low-income, ethnic minority children. *The School Psychology Review, 28*, 493–504.

Masten, A. S., Morison, P., & Pellegrini, D. S. (1985). A revised class play method of peer assessment. *Developmental Psychology, 21*(3), 523–533.

Matson, J. L. (1986). Assessing social behaviors in the visually handicapped: The Matson evaluation of social skills with youngsters (MESSY). *Journal of Clinical Child Psychology, 15*(1), 78–87.

Matson, J. L. (1990). *Matson evaluation of social skills in youngsters*. Worthington, Ohio: International Diagnostic Systems, Inc.

Matson, J. L., Esveldt-Dawson, K., & Kazdin, A. E. (1983). Validation of methods for assessing social skills in children. *Journal of Clinical Child Psychology, 12*, 174–180.

Matson, J. L., Heinze, A., Helsel, W. J., Kapperman, G., & Rotatori, A. F. (1986). Assessing social behaviors in the visually handicapped: The Matson evaluation of social skills with youngsters (MESSY). *Journal of Clinical Child Psychology, 15*, 78–87.

Matson, J. L., Helsel, W. J., Bellack, A. S., & Senatore, V. (1983). Development of a rating scale to assess social skill deficits in mentally retarded adults. *Applied Research in Mental Retardation, 4*(4), 399–407.

Matson, J. L., Luke, M. A., & Mayville, S. B. (2004). The effects of antiepileptic medications on the social skills of individuals with mental retardation. *Research in Developmental Disabilities, 25*(2), 219–228.

Matson, J. L., Macklin, G. F., & Helsel, W. J. (1985). Psychometric properties of the Matson evaluation of social skills with youngsters (MESSY) with emotional problems and self concept in deaf children. *Journal of Behavior Therapy and Experimental Psychiatry*, *16*(2), 117–123.

Matson, J. L., Matson, M. L., & Rivet, T. T. (2007). Social-skills treatments for children with autism spectrum disorders: An overview. *Behavior Modification*, *31*(5), 682–707.

Matson, J. L., & Ollendick, T. H. (1988). *Enhancing children's social skills: Assessment and training* (1st ed.). New York: Pergamon Press.

Matson, J. L., Rotatori, A. F., & Helsel, W. J. (1983). Development of a rating scale to measure social skills in children: The Matson evaluation of social skills with youngsters (MESSY). *Behavior Research and Therapy*, *21*, 335–340.

Matson, J. L., & Senatore, V. (1981). A comparison of traditional psychotherapy and social skills training for improving interpersonal functioning of mentally retarded adults. *Behavior Therapy*, *12*, 369–382.

Matson, J. L., Stabinsky Compton, L., & Sevin, J. A. (1991). Comparison and item analysis of the MESSY for autistic and normal children. *Research in Developmental Disabilities*, *12*(4), 361–369.

Matson, J. L., & Wilkins, J. (2007). A critical review of assessment targets and methods for social skills excesses and deficits for children with autism spectrum disorders. *Research in Autism Spectrum Disorders*, *1*(1), 28–37.

Matson, J. L., & Wilkins, J. (2009). Psychometric testing methods for children's social skills. *Research in Developmental Disabilities*, *30*, 249–274.

McFall, R. M., & Marston, A. R. (1970). An experimental investigation of behavior rehearsal in assertive training. *Journal of Abnormal Psychology*, *76*, 295–303.

Meijer, S. A., Sinnema, G., Bijstra, J. O., Mellenbergh, G. J., & Wolters, W. H. G. (2000). Peer interaction in adolescents with a chronic illness. *Personality and Individual Differences*, *29*(5), 799–813.

Méndez, F. X., Hidalgo, M. D., & Inglés, C. J. (2002). The Matson evaluation of social skills with youngsters: Psychometric properties of the Spanish translation in the adolescent population. *European Journal of Psychological Assessment*, *18*(1), 30–42.

Merrell, K. W. (1993). Using behavior rating scales to assess social skills and antisocial behavior in school settings. *School Psychology Review*, *22*(1), 115.

Merrell, K. W. (1994). *Preschool and kindergarten behavior scales: Test manual*. Brandon, VT: Clinical Psychology Publishing Company, Inc.

Merrell, K. W. (1999). *Behavioral, social, and emotional assessment of children and adolescents*. Mahwah, NJ, US: Lawrence Erlbaum Associates Publishers.

Merrell, K. W. (2002). *School social behavior scales* (2nd ed.). Eugene, OR: Assessment-Intervention Resources.

Merrell, K. W., & Caldarella, P. (2002). *Home & community social behavior scales (HCSBS)*. Eugene, OR: Assessment-Intervention Resources.

Merrell, K. W., & Gimpel, G. A. (1998). *Social skills of children and adolescents: Conceptualization, assessment, treatment*. Mahwah, NJ, US: Lawrence Erlbaum Associates Publishers.

Moreno, J. L. (1953). *Who shall survive?* New York: Beacon House.

Mpofu, E., Carney, J., Lambert, M. C., & Hersen, M. (2006). Peer sociometric assessment. *Clinician's handbook of child behavioral assessment* (pp. 233–263). San Diego, CA: Elsevier Academic Press.

Powless, D. L., & Elliott, S. N. (1993). Assessment of social skills of Native American preschoolers: Teachers' and parents' rartings. *Journal of School Psychology*, *31*, 293–307.

Raymond, K. L., & Matson, J. L. (1989). Social skills in the hearing impaired. *Journal of Clinical Child Psychology*, *18*(3), 247–258.

Reynolds, C. R., & Kamphaus, R. W. (1992). *Behavior assessment system for children (BASC-2)* (2nd ed.). Circle Pines, MN: American Guidance Service.

Rich, E. C., Shepherd, E. J., & Nangle, D. W. (2008). Validation of the SSRS-T, preschool level as a measure of positive social behavior and conduct problems. *Education & Treatment of Children*, *31*(2), 183–202.

Riggio, R. E. (1986). Assessment of basic social skills. *Journal of Personality and Social Psychology*, *51*(3), 649 660.

Roff, J. D., & Wirt, R. D. (1984). Childhood aggression and social adjustment as antecedents of delinquency. *Journal of Abnormal Child Psychology*, *12*(1), 111–126.

Rojahn, J., & Warren, V. J. (1997). Emotion recognition as a function of social competence and depressed mood in individuals with intellectual disability. *Journal of Intellectual Disability Research*, *41*(6), 469–475.

Sato, H., Ishikawa, S. -I., Arai, K., & Sakano, Y. (2005). The relationship between childhood depression and teacher's ratings of social skills in elementary school. *Japanese Journal of Counseling Science*, *38*(3), 226–234.

Shahim, S. (2004). Reliability of the social skills rating system for preschool children in Iran. *Psychological Reports*, *95*(3), 1264–1266.

Sharma, S., Sigafoos, J., & Carroll, A. (2000). Social skills assessment of Indian children with visual impairments. *Journal of Visual Impairment & Blindness*, *94*(3), 172–176.

Sparrow, S., Balla, D., & Cicchetti, D. V. (1984). *The vineland adaptive behavior scales (survey form)* Circle Pines, MN: American Guidance Service.

Spence, S. H. (1980). *Social skills training with children and adolescents: A Cousellor's manual*. Windsor: NFER Publishing Co.

Spence, S. H., & Liddle, B. (1990). Self-report measures of social competence for children: An evaluation of the Matson evaluation of social skills for youngsters and the list of social situation problems. *Behavioral Assessment*, *12*(3), 317–336.

Spence, S. H., & Marzillier, J. S. (1981). Social skills training with adolescent male offenders – II. Short-term, long-term and generalized effects. *Behaviour Research and Therapy*, *19*(4), 349–368.

Tse, E., Hamiwka, L., Sherman, E. M. S., & Wirrell, E. (2007). Social skills problems in children with epilepsy: Prevalence, nature and predictors. *Epilepsy & Behavior*, *11*(4), 499–505.

Van der Oord, S., Van der Meulen, E. M., Prins, P. J. M., Oosterlaan, J., Buitelaar, J. K., & Emmelkamp, P. M. G. (2005). A psychometric evaluation of the social skills rating system in children with attention deficit hyperactivity disorder. *Behaviour Research and Therapy*, *43*(6), 733–746.

Van Horn, K. R., Tamase, K., & Hagiwara, K. (2001). Teachers' expectations of high school students' social skills in Japan. *Psychologia: An International Journal of Psychology in the Orient*, *44*(4), 250–258.

van Manen, T., Prins, P., & Emmelkamp, P. (1999). Een sociaal-cognitief interventieprogramma voor gedragsgestoorde kinderen, een vooronderzoek. *Gedragstherapie*, *32*(1), 33–55.

Waksman, S. A. (1985). The development and psychometric properties of a rating scale for children's social skills. *Journal of Psychoeducational Assessment*, *3*(2), 111–121.

Wentzel, K. R. (1993). Does being good make the grade? Social behavior and academic competence in middle school. *Journal of Educational Psychology*, *85*(2), 357–364.

Whiteside, S. P., McCarthy, D. M., & Miller, J. D. (2007). An examination of the factor structure of the social skills rating system parent elementary form. *Assessment*, *14*(3), 246–254.

Wierzbicki, M., & McCabe, M. (1988). Social skills and subsequent depressive symptomotology in children. *Journal of Clinical Child Psychology*, *17*, 203–208.

Wiggins, J. S., & Winder, C. L. (1961). The peer nomination inventory: an empirically derived sociometric measure of adjustment in preadolescent boys. *Psychological Reports*, *9*, 643–677.

Williamson, D. A., Moody, S. C., Granberry, S. W., Lethermon, V. R., & Blouin, D. C. (1983). Criterion-related validity of a role-play social skills test for children. *Behavior Therapy*, *14*(4), 466–481.

Wolf, M. M. (1978). Social validity: The case for subjective measurement or how applied behavior analysis is finding its heart. *Journal of Applied Behavior Analysis*, *11*(2), 203–214.

Chapter 5
General Methods of Treatment

Timothy Dempsey and Johnny L. Matson

Social Skills Treatment Overview

Problems related to social skills deficits and excesses in children are evinced in a myriad of psychopathology. Maneuvering through social interactions is one of the most complex tasks that all human beings do. Social skills involve many psychological systems, such as perception, language, and problem solving. These systems develop throughout childhood and result from biological and environmental influences. Social situations can be problematic when these systems do not function adequately. For example, a child with a language deficit may have difficulty making sense of verbal social cues and communicating desires and opinions. Impulsive children can often make quick decisions that could result in conflicts with others. This chapter will discuss classic literature regarding the nature of evidence-based interventions, who provides the intervention (e.g., parents, siblings, teachers), how best to promote generalization and maintain treatment efficacy over time. Other critical aspects of social skills treatment, as well as strengths, weaknesses, meta-analytic outcome results, and future directions for treatment, will also be reviewed.

The ability to interact successfully with one's peers and significant adults is an important aspect of a child's development. Most prominent developmental theorists have noted the relationship between social competence in childhood and psychological adjustment in adulthood. Erikson (1963) views adequately socialized children as successfully moving through a series of psychosocial stages that begin with trust in others (infancy) and eventuate in adulthood with a socially approved sense of self. Piaget (1962) and Kohlberg (1969) have delineated cognitive developmental theories of social and moral development in which socially competent children move from an egocentric to an altruistic style of social functioning. Like Erikson, Piaget and Kohlberg conceptualize social competence evolving in a series of interrelated stages which closely parallel chronological and/or mental age.

Social competence is an important developmental achievement for a variety of reasons. First, children who are poorly accepted by their peers have shown a high incidence of school maladjustment (Gronlund & Anderson, 1963), dropping out of school (Ullman, 1957), delinquency (Roff, Sells, & Golden, 1972), and adult mental health difficulties (Cowen, Pederson, Babigian, Izzo, & Trost, 1973; Kohn & Clausen, 1955; Roff, 1970). Second, children with social difficulties tend to be poorly accepted, overtly rejected, or ignored by peers (Asher & Hymel, 1981; Asher, Oden, & Gottman, 1977; Asher & Renshaw, 1981; Weintraub, Prim, & Neale, 1978). Moreover, these children typically exhibit lower levels of academic performance than their more socially competent peers (Cartledge & Milbum, 1978). Finally, children with social difficulties typically display higher rates of negative interaction and lower rates of positive interaction toward peers and adults (Bryan, 1978; Bryan,

T. Dempsey (✉)
Department of Psychology, Louisiana State University,
Baton Rouge, LA 70803, USA
e-mail: tdempsey82@hotmail.com

J.L. Matson (ed.), *Social Behavior and Skills in Children*, DOI 10.1007/978-1-4419-0234-4_5,
© Springer Science+Business Media, LLC 2009

Wheeler, Felcan, & Henek, 1976; Gresham & Nagle, 1980; Hartup, Glazer, & Charlesworth, 1967).

It is readily apparent that socially unskilled children have a high probability of experiencing severe negative outcomes in the course of development, ranging from short-term consequences (e.g., negative peer interactions) to long-term outcomes (e.g., adult mental health difficulties). The previously discussed theories of Erikson, Piaget, and Kohlberg are perhaps useful for a general conceptualization of social and moral development in children; however, they do not identify what specific social skills children need in order to be socially competent. While no unified theory of social skills exists to date, social learning theory (Bandura, 1969, 1973, 1977a) perhaps comes closest to providing a usable theory for the task of teaching social skills.

Current Guiding Theory of Social Skills Interventions

Much of the movement toward cognitive-behavioral approaches originated from Bandura's work in the area of social learning theory, particularly his research in modeling (see Bandura, 1969, 1973, 1977a). In modeling, behavior is acquired through the mediating influences of symbolic coding, cognitive organization, symbolic rehearsal, and motor rehearsal of information. Motivation to perform behaviors acquired through modeling is determined by various external reinforcement contingencies, vicarious reinforcement processes, and/or self-generated reinforcement contingencies (Bandura, 1977a, 1977b).

A critical distinction is made in social learning theory between acquisition and performance of behavior. This distinction illuminates the role of cognitive processes in cognitive-behavioral approaches for teaching social behavior to children. According to Bandura (1977a), the cognitive processes of attention and retention are responsible for response acquisition or learning. Performance of behavior is determined by motor-reproduction capabilities (e.g., physical skills, availability of response components, etc.) and motivational processes (e.g., external vicarious, and self-reinforcement contingencies). The

major difference between Bandura's conceptualization of environmental influences (e.g., reinforcement) upon behavioral performance and that of more operantly oriented theorists is that Bandura views reinforcement functioning more as antecedent rather than consequent control. That is, in social learning theory a person's anticipation of reinforcing consequences (antecedent control) has a greater impact upon behavioral performance than the consequences of any particular response (consequent control). In fact, Bandura prefers the term regulation over reinforcement, because it better describes the role of cognitive processes (e.g., awareness, information, etc.) in strengthening and maintaining behavior.

In sum, social learning theory emphasizes the role of both cognitive and environmental influences in determining behavior. Environmental influences are considered to be mediated by cognitive processes (e.g., perception, attribution, etc.). As such, the direction of influence between the organism and the environment is bidirectional as they mutually and reciprocally influence each other (Bandura, 1977a, 1977b; Craighead, 1982; Kazdin, 1982). The various approaches to teaching social behaviors reviewed here focus upon the role of cognitive processes in the acquisition of behavior. Outcomes of these cognitive-behavioral techniques are viewed in terms of actual behavior change or performance. While it is assumed that cognitive processes are primarily responsible for learning social behavior (acquisition), the efficacy of these procedures in teaching social skills must be evaluated in terms of the actual performance of these behaviors. The studies reviewed in this chapter are evaluated on the basis of several methodological issues which are presented in the following section.

Methodological Issues in Social Skills Research

Empirical studies which have used cognitive-behavioral procedures to teach social skills to children constitute the basis for the remainder of this chapter. As with any research conducted, it is necessary to know the limitations presented in the literature. Some of these methodological issues are as follows: (a) age of subjects, (b) training procedures, (c) outcome measures, (d) research design, (e) evidence for generalization, and (f) social validation. Each issue will be discussed separately.

Age

Of the reviewed studies, 12 studies were conducted with preschoolers, 15 studies with elementary-age children, and 4 studies with adolescents. These differences become more meaningful when viewed in relation to the type of technique used to teach social behavior. For example, all 9 studies utilizing symbolic modeling employed preschool-age samples. In contrast, of the 6 studies using a coaching procedure, only one (Zahavi & Asher, 1978) used preschoolers as subjects. Elementary-age children were used most often in coaching studies as well as in those studies using a combination of techniques and self-control training. Perhaps the most striking feature of the age issue is the lack of studies conducted with adolescents. Only four studies (Blackwood, 1970; Kaufman & O'Leary, 1972; Minkin, Braukmann, Minkin, Timbers and Timbers, 1976; Santogrossi, O'Leary, Romanczyk, & Kaufman, 1973) used adolescents in social skills training studies. Given the salience of the peer group during adolescence and the problems associated therewith, this lack of research is puzzling. To date, we know little about the efficacy of social skills training procedures with adolescent populations. Future research should investigate not only specific training procedures for adolescents but also focus upon the most appropriate skills to teach. Obviously, there are developmental differences in important social skills. For example, teaching sharing and cooperation is probably appropriate for preschoolers and elementary-age children but perhaps less important for adolescents. Appropriate social behaviors for adolescents might be in the area of heterosexual relationships, negotiating with parents about curfew restrictions, or dealing with peer pressure. Goldstein, Sprafkin, Gershaw, and Klein (1980) have identified at least 50 social skills that are relevant for adolescents, with training procedures for each skill. Unfortunately, these skills are based primarily upon face validity rather than

empirical relationships to important social outcomes, such as peer acceptance, job acquisition, academic achievement, or decreases in status offenses (e.g., truancy, probation violations, or running away from home).

The potential for developmental changes in social competence has been ignored by most investigators conducting social skills training (Foster & Ritchey, 1979). As a result, there is simply not enough empirical data to identify the most important social skills for each developmental level (e.g., for early and middle childhood, and adolescence).

The studies in this review are organized around four general types of training procedures: (a) symbolic modeling, (b) coaching, (c) combinations of techniques, and (d) self-control training.

Symbolic Modeling

Nine studies in this review used symbolic modeling to remediate social skill deficits. As previously mentioned, all of these studies used preschool samples. Symbolic modeling denotes the acquisition of behavior through film or verbal symbols as opposed to exposure to live models of behavior (Thelen, Fry, Fehrenbach, & Frautschi, 1979).

The pioneering study using filmed modeling to remediate social skill deficits was conducted by O'Connor (1969), who selected preschool children exhibiting low rates of social interaction and randomly assigned them to treatment and attention-control groups. The treatment group was shown a 23-minute film depicting age- and sex-appropriate models becoming increasingly involved in social interaction with other children and being reinforced for doing so. The film was narrated to draw attention to the social interaction behaviors. Attention-control subjects viewed a 20-minute Marineland dolphin video. Children in the treatment group significantly increased their rates of social interaction at posttest, whereas control children showed no interaction increases. Similar treatment effects from symbolic modeling videos have been observed by O'Connor (1972) and independent investigators (Evers-Pasquale, 1978; Evers-Pasquale & Sherman, 1975; Evers & Schwarz, 1973; Keller & Carlson, 1974). Two of these studies (Evers-Pasquale, 1978, and Evers-Pasquale & Sherman, 1975) found that children who were peer-oriented (i.e., preferred to interact with children their own age) showed greater responsiveness to the modeling videos than nonpeer-oriented children (i.e., who preferred to play alone or with adults). Although both peer-oriented and nonpeer-oriented children showed significant increases in social interaction relative to control groups, these findings suggest that modeling interventions may be more effective for children who, because of their learning histories, prefer same-age playmates. This finding, however, has not been replicated with older children (Gresham & Nagle, 1980).

One important component of modeling videos is the use of narration which enhances attention to critical behaviors exhibited by models and promotes verbal labeling of such behaviors. Jakibchub and Smeriglio (1976) used a novel approach to investigate the effects of video narration on rates of social interaction. In their study, identical modeling films were developed which differed only in the person in which the videos were narrated. That is, one video was narrated in the third person (e.g., "She is talking and playing with others") and the other video was narrated in the first person (e.g., "I am talking and playing with others"). First-person narration significantly increased the social interaction rates of withdrawn preschoolers over those children in the third-person narration group. The third-person narration condition did not produce increases in social interaction which represents a failure to replicate the previously described modeling studies. It could be hypothesized that first-person narration led to increase in perceived model-observer similarity which, in turn, led to increased attention to the modeling video. Bandura (1969, 1977a) suggests that the more closely children perceive themselves as being like a model, the greater the modeling effects. The findings of Jakibchub and Smeriglio (1976) study has yet to be replicated to see whether the first- and third-person narrations produce similar effects.

Two studies have failed to demonstrate significant modeling effects using filmed modeling (Geller & Scheirer, 1978; Gottman, 1977b). Both studies were conducted with disadvantaged withdrawn preschoolers enrolled in Head Start programs. Geller and Scheirer (1978) used three 10-minute videotapes depicting models engaging in cooperative play and

social interaction, whereas Gottman (1977b) used the previously described O'Connor (1969) film. Neither study demonstrated increases in rates of social interaction; however, these findings should be interpreted cautiously. One significant difference in these studies from previous modeling research concerns the nature of the target population and the models used in the videos. Both studies used white, middle-class models which may have created a great deal of model-observer dissimilarity, thus weakening the modeling effects. The target children in these studies (mostly lower-class blacks) could have perceived the models as being vastly different from themselves and consequently did not attend to or retain the modeled behaviors. Future research using modeling videos with disadvantaged populations should attempt to achieve model-observer similarity to investigate the effects of culturally or racially similar models on the acquisition of social skills in disadvantaged or culturally different populations.

Coaching

Coaching is a behavior-change technique which depends primarily upon the child's understanding of language and verbal concepts. Coaching typically includes three components: (a) presentation of rules and standards for behavior, (b) behavior rehearsal, and (c) response feedback and discussion. In coaching, social skills are taught through direct instruction, whereby ideas concerning appropriate social behavior are conveyed verbally and specific examples of how to translate these ideas into behavioral sequences are communicated (Asher & Renshaw, 1981).

Oden and Asher (1977) conducted one of the first well-designed coaching studies in which adult coaches taught four social skills. These skills were participation (i.e., getting involved in play situations), cooperation (i.e., taking turns, sharing) communication (listening to others, talking to others), and validation support (i.e., being friendly, fun, and nice). The coaching procedure for each skill involved three steps: (a) presentation of rules or standards for behavior (e.g., "Participation is important, because it lets you make new friends and have fun"); (b) behavior rehearsal (e.g., "I want you to play this game in which you have to participate with others"); and (c) feedback and discussion (e.g., "That was good participating. Maybe next time you could look at the person you're playing with more often"). Coaching was effective in increasing children's peer acceptance, and the gains were maintained at one-year follow-up.

In a related study, Gottman, Gonso, and Schuler (1976) used coaching to teach friendship skills to 2 third-grade females with social difficulties. Friendship skills included the following sequence: (a) greeting, (b) asking for and giving information, (c) extending an offer of inclusion, and (d) effective leave-taking. These skills were found in a previous study to discriminate well-accepted from poorly accepted children (Gottman, Gonso, & Rasmussen, 1975). Referential communication skills, in which children were taught to take the listener's perspective, were also taught. Coaching increased the frequency of experimental subjects' nominations on a sociometric measure and the target children increased their social interactions with other children. Similar findings were reported in two studies by Ladd (1979, 1981), using a coaching procedure with groups of third-grade children.

One study failed to demonstrate the superiority of coaching over other training conditions. Hymel and Asher (1977) assigned third- through fifth-grade unpopular children (i.e., low sociometric status) to one of three conditions: (a) peer-pairing in which children played games with peer partners for six sessions; (b) general coaching, identical to the Oden and Asher (1977) procedure; and (c) individualized coaching in which coaching was based upon the child's specific social skill deficits (e.g., whether child was neglected or rejected, interaction difficulties with peers, teachers, or both, etc.). There were no significant differences between the three conditions in the degree to which children changed sociometric status, as all increased in peer acceptance. Without the benefit of an untreated control group, it is difficult to interpret these findings as indicating the equal effectiveness of all treatments or regression toward the mean.

One coaching study used coaching to decrease aggressive behavior in a preschool population. Zahavi and Asher (1978) selected the eight most aggressive children, via a time-sampling procedure using behavioral observations of aggressive behavior in the classroom. Coaching involved three

concepts: (a) aggression hurts another person and makes them unhappy; (b) aggression does not solve problems; and (c) positive ways to solve conflicts are sharing, taking turns, and playing together. Each concept was taught by asking the child questions regarding aggressive behavior and providing prompts and clarification to the child's verbalization of these concepts. The entire coaching procedure lasted 10 minutes for each child. Compared to a control group, children receiving the coaching procedure decreased rates of aggressive behavior which was maintained at a 2-week follow-up.

Techniques Used in Combination

Six studies are reviewed in which various combinations of social learning techniques were used to teach social skills. These include combinations of modeling, coaching, and behavior rehearsal (Gresham & Nagle, 1980; LaGreta & Santogrossi, 1980); instructions, modeling, behavior rehearsal, and social praise (Bomstein, Bellack, & Hersen, 1977; Cooke & Apolloni, 1976; Minkin et al., 1976); and modeling, behavior rehearsal, scripts, and class discussion (Michelson & Wood, 1980). While effective in teaching social skills, one of the major difficulties in this group of studies is the dearth of research evaluating the specific components of these techniques that are responsible for therapeutic change.

Two studies used a combination of modeling, coaching, and behavior rehearsal to teach social skills to poorly accepted elementary-age children. In the first of these studies, LaGreta and Santogrossi (1980) used the above treatment combination to teach social skills to third- to fifth-grade children. The treatment consisted of target children viewing videos of peer models demonstrating the above social skills. Subsequent to viewing the videos, target children discussed how they might use the modeled skills in their daily activities with two group leaders. Target children were then coached in the use of the skills and were provided opportunities to behaviorally rehearse the skill in role-playing situations. Finally, children were given homework assignments to promote generalization of trained social skills across settings (i.e., to typical interactions with peers in school and community settings).

Compared to attention-placebo and waiting-list control groups, the social skills training group demonstrated greater verbal knowledge of appropriate social skills, greater improvement in social skills on a role-playing assessment measure, and increased frequency of social interaction rates on a generalization assessment.

LaGreta and Santogrossi (1980) failed to find significant differences between the three groups on peer acceptance ratings or in frequencies of positive social interaction. The failure to replicate the findings of Oden and Asher (1977) using peer-rating scales was unexpected, since a similar population and similar training procedures were used.

In an analogous study, Gresham and Nagle (1980) compared modeling, coaching, and an abbreviated combination of modeling and coaching (MAMC) to teach social skills to third- and fourth-grade children. Modeling consisted of children viewing videos of targeted social skills (e.g., participation, cooperation, communication, friendship making, etc.) for six sessions over a 3-week period.

Coaching was identical to the Oden and Asher (1977) procedure training the same social skills as in the modeling condition. The MAMC group received an abbreviated sequence of modeling and coaching. Contrary to the LaGreta and Santogrossi (1980) findings, Gresham and Nagle (1980) found significant increases on a play with sociometric rating scale for all treatment groups, as well as significant increases in rates of positive peer interaction in classroom settings. Gresham and Nagle (1980) also found that groups that received a coaching component (Coaching and MAMC groups) showed greater decreases in rates of negative peer interaction. This supports the earlier work of Zahavi and Asher (1978) who used a coaching procedure to decrease aggressive interaction in preschoolers.

Three studies have used combinations of instructions, modeling, behavior rehearsal, and social praise to teach social skills to skill-deficient children and adolescents. Bomstein et al. (1977) used the above combination to teach assertive behavior to four 8- to 11-year-old children. This combination of techniques increased target children's ratio of eye contact to speech duration, loudness of speech, number of requests for behavior change, and ratings of overall assertiveness. These changes generalized

to untrained role-play situations with adults and were maintained at 2- and 4-week follow-up. The degree to which these assertive behaviors generalized to interactions with other children in the natural environment was not assessed. Similar findings were reported by Cooke and Apolloni (1976) using the above treatment combination to teach smiling, sharing, positive physical contacting, and verbal complimenting.

In a study with predelinquent adolescents, Minkin et al. (1976) used the treatment combination to increase rates of questioning, positive conversational feedback, and time spent talking. An interesting feature of the Minkin et al. (1976) study was that these conversational behaviors were *socially validated* by 15 adult judges who rated videos of subjects' conversations as being more appropriate after training. Social validation is an important component of treatment evaluation, since it provides an indication of the quality and significance of trained social skills by consumers or judges of the child's behavior in naturalistic environments (see Wolf, 1978, for a discussion).

Michelson and Wood (1980) taught assertiveness to two groups of elementary school children using a combination of modeling, behavior rehearsal, scripts, and class discussion. This study differs from the rest of the reviewed studies in two ways: (a) selected subjects were not evidencing any particular problems in the area of social skills and were treated as an intact group and (b) primary outcome measures consisted of paper-and-pencil assertiveness measures (*Children's Assertive Behavior Scale* and *Rathus Assertiveness Scale Revised for Children*) rather than observational and/or sociometric measures. Using social skills training groups' differing amounts of contact (8 hours vs. 16 hours), Michelson and Wood found the treatment package to be effective in teaching assertiveness skills as measured by the paper-and-pencil measures of assertiveness. No significant differences were found as a function of training duration. Given the sample selection procedures in this study, the only statement one can make regarding training effectiveness is that the treatment package was effective in changing children's (who apparently had no social skill deficits) responses on self-report measures. It is unknown whether this treatment combination would be effective with groups of unassertive children using observational measures of assertiveness.

Self-Control Training

Behavior therapists have become interested in teaching children methods of changing their own behavior (O'Leary & Dubey, 1979). Meichenbaum (1977) asserts that the major focus of cognitive-behavioral techniques such as self-instruction is to teach children to develop verbal control over their overt behavior. As such, Meichenbaum (1977) recommends that training and practice in using language as a regulator of impulsive responding can be an effective social skills training strategy.

Another line of research that emphasizes children's control of their own social behavior has been the investigation of self-evaluation and self-reinforcement techniques (see O'Leary & Dubey, 1979, and Rosenbaum & Drabman, 1979, for review). In these studies, children are taught to self-monitor, self-record, and/or to self-reinforce behavior.

In this section, studies that have used self-instructions and self-evaluation/self-reinforcement to train social skills will be reviewed. For in-depth discussions of cognitive-behavioral theory and interventions, see reviews by Hobbs, Moguin, Tryoler, and Lahey (1980) and Kendall and Hollon (1979). Verbal mediation has been shown to be an effective social skills training strategy to exert stimulus control over disruptive or aggressive social behavior (Blackwood, 1970; Bomstein & Quevillon, 1976; Camp, Blom, Hebert, & van Doominck, 1977; Robin, Schneider, & Dolnick, 1976).

Three studies used variations of Meichenbaum and Goodman's (1971) cognitive self-guidance treatment program with impulsive children. Camp et al. (1977) modeled cognitive strategies and trained aggressive children to develop answers to four basic questions: "What is my problem? What is my plan? Am I using my plan? How did I do?" Modeling was gradually faded, and children subsequently asked these questions and planned strategies at a covert level. Cognitive self-guidance led to improved social behavior as measured by teacher's ratings of prosocial behavior. No significant differences between experimental and control groups

were demonstrated on teacher ratings of aggressive behavior. Bomstein and Quevillon (1976) reduced off-task and disruptive behavior of three preschoolers using similar procedures.

Blackwood (1970) taught verbal mediation skills to eighth- and ninth-grade children using essays which identified the misbehavior, explaining why it was inappropriate, indicated what the child should have been doing instead, and gave reasons for the desired behavior. Children were required to copy, paraphrase, and orally recite the verbal-mediation essays contingent upon disruptive classroom behavior.

Compared to controls, the verbal mediation group significantly reduced overall levels of observed disruptive behavior. The Blackwood (1970) study differs from the Camp et al. (1977) and Bomstein and Quevillon (1976) studies in that verbal mediation was used more as a punisher contingent upon inappropriate social behavior rather than a purely instructional strategy. Robin et al. (1976) combined a type of self-instructional training with relaxation to decrease children's level of aggressive behavior. Self-instruction consisted of teaching children to think of alternative solutions to problem situations and role-playing these strategies. Relaxation training consisted of teaching children to pull their arms and legs to their bodies, put their heads down on their desk, and to relax. These procedures led to reduced rates of aggressive behavior in two classrooms of aggressive children.

Five studies are reviewed which have trained children to self-evaluate and/or self-reinforce social behavior (Bolstad & Johnson, 1972; Drabman, Spitalnik, & O'Leary, 1973; Kaufman & O'Leary, 1972; Santogrossi et al., 1973; Turkewitz, O'Leary, & Ironsmith, 1975). Two studies have attempted to reduce the socially disruptive behavior of emotionally disturbed adolescents in a hospital school. Kaufman and O'Leary (1972) used self-evaluation (subjects' ratings of behavior) of classroom behavior subsequent to interventions under token reward-and-response cost conditions. Self-evaluation of social behavior maintained low levels of classroom disruptiveness equivalent to that achieved under the reward-and-cost procedures. Santogrossi et al. (1973) found negative results using self-evaluation of behavior. Self-evaluation (subjects rated their own behavior on a 0–2 scale) did not reduce disruptive behavior significantly below baseline levels. Only when teachers determined reinforcement, based upon their evaluation of the children's behavior, did disruptive behavior decrease. The differential results from these two studies may be partially attributable to the methodologies used in each. That is, in the Kaufman and O'Leary (1972) study, the subjects had been in a teacher-administered token program for 25 days before they were allowed to self-evaluate behavior. In the Santogrossi et al. (1973) study, subjects were in a teacher-administered token program for only 9 days before the self-evaluation phase. The longer exposure to the token system in the Kaufman and O'Leary (1972) study could have resulted in the subject learning how to more accurately evaluate their own behavior. Also, the self-evaluation phase in the Kaufman and O'Leary (1972) study was preceded by both token reward and response-cost phases, whereas this was not the case in the Santogrossi et al. (1973) study.

It is difficult to draw any conclusions regarding the effectiveness of self-evaluation of behavior in emotionally disturbed adolescents, since the two studies reviewed used somewhat different methodologies. It could be that self-evaluation is more effective when it is preceded by both reinforcement and punishment phases than when it is preceded by a reinforcement phase alone. Three studies have used self-evaluation of behavior to control the disruptive social behavior of children in remedial or regular classrooms. Drabman et al. (1973) taught self-evaluative behavior to eight disruptive nine- and ten-year-old boys in an after-school remedial reading class. Disruptive behavior was initially controlled by a teacher-administered token system in which points were given for appropriate social behavior (on-task, sitting in seat, being quiet, not disturbing others, etc.). Subsequent to the teacher-administered phase, subjects were reinforced for accurately matching the teacher's evaluations of the behavior. Matching was faded over a period of time so that reinforcement was entirely self-determined. Self-evaluation was as effective as the teacher-administered phase in controlling disruptive social behavior. Moreover, low levels of disruptiveness were maintained when all checking of self-evaluation was eliminated, and these low rates of disruptive behavior generalized to periods when no token or back-up reinforcement was available (generalization across stimulus conditions). Similar results were obtained by Bolstad and Johnson (1972) who found self-evaluation and self-reinforcement to be slightly more effective in controlling disruptive behavior than external regulation, such as teacher-determined reinforcement.

Turkewitz et al. (1975) taught self-evaluative behavior to eight disruptive children in an after-school reading tutorial program. Their methodology and results were similar to the Drabman et al. (1973) study. Turkewitz et al. (1975), however, did not find generalization of appropriate social behavior to the target subjects' regular classroom, although generalization to non-token intervals (intervals in which reinforcement was not available) and maintenance for 1 week after program termination were observed. It appears that self-evaluation used alone does not effect significant changes in behavior, at least for children with a history of behavioral difficulties. Only when self-evaluation is used in conjunction with, and is preceded by, teacher-administered token reinforcement does it effectively control disruptive social behavior. However, it appears that self-evaluation is as effective as externally administered token programs when preceded by teacher-administered reward phases (Bolstad & Johnson, 1972). Self-evaluation may be useful for maintaining effects when other interventions are withdrawn (e.g., token reinforcement) and seems to facilitate maintenance of treatment gains in the absence of token reinforcement (O'Leary & Dubey, 1979). Generalization has been demonstrated across stimulus conditions (token vs. non-token phases), but generalization across settings (i.e., from special classes to regular classes) has not been adequately documented.

Outcome Measures

The type of outcome measure used in the social skills literature is primarily associated with the type of training procedure used. For example, eight of the nine studies utilizing symbolic modeling employed global rates of social interaction as the sole outcome measure. The use of global rates of social interaction with socially withdrawn children has intuitive appeal; however, global social interaction rates have not been shown to predict peer acceptance (Deutsch, 1974; Gottman, 1977a, b; Jennings, 1975). Gottman (1977b) demonstrated that the quality of social interaction (positive or negative) rather than overall rate predicts social acceptance in children. This has been a rather consistent finding in the developmental literature, and it is somewhat surprising that the symbolic modeling research seems to have overlooked these findings (Hartup et al., 1967; Marshall & McCandless, 1957; McCandless & Marshall, 1957; Moore, 1967; Moore & Updegraff, 1964).

The self-control literature appears guilty of the same error, in that the outcome measures are almost exclusively global rates of aggressive/disruptive behavior. The lone exception is the study by Combs and Lahey (1981), who used a more fine-grained analysis of social behavior (e.g., rate of eye contact, verbal initiations, etc.). It should be pointed out that the Combs and Lahey (1981) study focused upon socially withdrawn children, whereas the other nine self-control studies used aggressive/disruptive subjects. In the 19 studies using either symbolic modeling or self-control procedures, none used sociometric status as an outcome measure. Although the majority of studies demonstrated rather consistent increases in global interaction rates or decreases in aggressive/disruptive behaviors, there is no indication that this results in greater peer acceptance or less peer rejection.

The 12 studies using coaching or a combination of techniques tended to employ multiple outcome measures, especially focusing upon the relationship between the quality of social interactions and sociometric status. Various skills training procedures have shown differential effects upon outcome measures. Gresham and Nagle (1980) demonstrated changes in both social interaction quality and peer acceptance using both symbolic modeling and coaching procedures. These findings have been replicated by Ladd (1979, 1981) using coaching procedures almost identical to those used by Gresham and Nagle (1980). On the other hand, LaGreta and Santogrossi (1980) failed to show changes in social interaction quality or sociometric status using group training procedures. Three

studies in this literature employed analogue role-play measures of social skills (Bornstein et al., 1977; LaGreca & Santogrossi, 1980; Minkin et al., 1976). All showed consistent increases in social skills after training on the role-play measures. A major difficulty with these data is that increases in performance on role-play measures is not predictive of either behavior in naturalistic settings or peer acceptance (Bellack, 1979; Bellack, Hersen, & Lampmorski, 1979; Bellack, Hersen, & Turner, 1978; Berler, Gross, & Drabman, 1982; Van Hasselt, Hersen, & Bellack, 1981).

Research Design

Of the reviewed studies, 23 studies used some type of group experimental design. All of the symbolic modeling and coaching studies used group experimental designs. In the studies using a combination of techniques, all but two (Bomstein et al., 1977; Cooke & Apolloni, 1976) used group experimental designs.

Of the 23 group design studies, over half (12 studies) utilized an attention control group. The addition of attention-control groups strengthens the findings of these studies because of the control over possible placebo effects. Only 5 studies in the group design literature compared the relative effects of multiple treatments (Evers & Schwarz, 1973; Evers-Pasquale & Sherman, 1975; Gresham & Nagle, 1980; Jakibchub & Smeriglio, 1976; O'Connor, 1972). Only 2 of these studies (Gresham & Nagle, 1980; Jakibchub & Smeriglio, 1976) compared cognitive-behavioral techniques. Gresham and Nagle (1980) compared symbolic modeling and coaching while Jakibchub and Smeriglio (1976) contrasted first- and third-persons narrations in a modeling film. The remaining three studies compared a symbolic modeling treatment with operant reinforcement procedures in facilitating social interaction rates.

Only 8 studies in this review used single-case experimental designs, with 5 studies using multiple baseline designs, 3 studies employing reversal designs, and one study utilizing a multielement design. Single case experimental designs, particularly the multiple baseline and reversal designs, provide strong demonstration of experimental control over dependent variables and thus possess good internal validity (Hersen & Barlow, 1976). The external validity of these designs is less convincing due to problems in generalizability from small sample sizes, differences in training procedures or conditions, and lack of convincing evidence for maintenance of treatment effects (Hersen & Barlow, 1976). Moreover, it is difficult to tease out the relative contributions of individual treatment components in studies using various treatment combinations (e.g., instructions + modeling + feedback + social reinforcement, etc.).

Generalization

One of the biggest problems in the social skills literature is the failure to either assess or demonstrate generalization effects. Generalization includes four major descriptive classes: (a) across settings, (b) across time, (c) across behaviors, and (d) across subjects (Stokes & Baer, 1977). Setting generalization refers to behavior changes in settings separate from the specific environment in which training occurred.

Only two studies demonstrated setting generalization (Bomstein et al., 1977; Cooke & Apolloni, 1976). In the Bomstein et al. (1977) study, trained social skills occurred in an analogue setting different from the training setting. The Cooke and Apolloni (1976) study was the only study in this review which demonstrated generalization across naturalistic settings. This paucity of evidence for setting generalization is discouraging, since social skills that do not occur cross-situationally have little functional or adaptive value.

Time generalization or maintenance refers to the continuation of behavior change in the treatment setting following the withdrawal of a training program. Seventeen studies demonstrated time generalization with follow-up periods ranging from 5 days (Bolstad & Johnson, 1972) to one year (Oden & Asher, 1977). The modal follow-up period for maintenance has been on the order of 2 weeks. Although the evidence for time generalization is encouraging, demonstrating continuation of behavior change for 2–3 weeks is not convincing evidence of the durability of effects produced by social skills training. The

one exception to this is the Oden and Asher (1977) study which maintained gains in sociometric status for the treatment group for one year following the cessation of treatment.

Behavior generalization refers to a change in behaviors not specifically targeted in treatment. The criterion for judging whether a behavior is same or different is whether the behavior can be defined independently of the target behavior. None of the studies reviewed demonstrated behavior generalization. This probably represents the fact that only relatively few behaviors were assessed in social skills training studies. It is conceivable that nontarget behaviors in these studies changed as a result of treatments.

Subject generalization refers to a change in the behavior of nontarget children after a training procedure has produced a change in the behavior of target children. Some authors refer to this as "spillover effects" (Strain, Shores, & Kerr, 1976), while the most frequent explanation is in terms of observational learning (Bandura, 1977a). Only one study demonstrated subject generalization with Cooke and Apolloni (1976) finding that nontarget children increased social interaction rates subsequent to training procedures for target children.

The evidence for generalization in the social skills training literature is not very overwhelming with only 18 studies demonstrating any kind of generalization. Nine of the studies simply did not assess generalization, while 4 studies assessed, but failed to demonstrate, generalization effects. There is little evidence to support the notion that social skills interventions based on social learning theory lead to a greater degree of generalization than less cognitively oriented (i.e., operant) strategies. This finding is in contradiction to reviews by O'Leary and Dubey (1979) and Rosenbaum and Drabman (1979), which suggest that interventions incorporating a cognitive component should produce greater generalization effects than more operantly based procedures.

Social Validity

The idea of social validity has intuitive appeal in the area of social skills training with children since the ultimate goal of such training is to facilitate important and valued social outcomes for children. Wolf (1978) suggests that behavior change is socially validated on three levels. First, the social significance of the goals is evaluated. That is, are the goals of behavior change of magnitude that society considers important? Second, are the means through which behavior changes are brought about socially appropriate in terms of time and ethical considerations? Third, are the outcomes of a given social skills training program considered socially important? In other words, do the quantity and quality of behavior change make a difference in terms of the individual's functioning in society? In terms of evaluating the outcome of social skills training, the social importance criterion becomes paramount.

What types of measures can be used as indices of a socially important outcome? In the area of social skills training, those measures upon which social systems (e.g., schools, courts, mental health agencies, etc.) and significant others (e.g., parents, teachers, etc.) tend to refer children can be considered socially valid. These may include such things as measures of peer acceptance, academic achievement, teacher or parent judgments of social competence, and/or certain forms of archival data (e.g., school attendance and suspension records, recidivism rates, etc.) (Gresham, 1981; Lahey & Strauss, 1982). The fact that social systems and significant others refer children to other professionals on the basis of one or more of the above measures makes them socially valid (i.e., they reflect someone's evaluation of the child's functioning in society).

The purpose of social validation is to ensure not only statistically significant but also socially important outcomes of social skills training programs. About 20% of the reviewed studies offered any evidence for social validity. Five of these studies used measures of peer acceptance to socially validate the effects of training programs (Gottman et al., 1976; Gresham & Nagle, 1980; Ladd, 1979, 1981; Oden & Asher, 1977). These studies offer some evidence to suggest that increases in certain social skills leads to a socially important outcome (i.e., increases in peer acceptance).

Two studies did not use peer acceptance as social validation measures. Kaufman and O'Leary (1972) noted increases in reading achievement that

paralleled decreases in rates of disruptive classroom social behavior. Minkin et al. (1976) showed that adult judges naive to the purpose of the investigation rated adolescent females as more socially skilled in conversation after social skills training.

Meta-analysis of Outcome Studies

Meta-analysis has been applied to social skills treatment research as a quantitative means of reviewing outcomes. A total of six meta-analyses of the social skills treatment literature have been conducted using students with or at risk for high-incidence disabilities (Beelman, Pfingsten and Losel, 1994; Coleman, Wheeler, & Webber, 1993; Denham & Almeida, 1987; Forness & Kavale, 1999; Mathur, Kavale, Quinn, Forness and Rutherford, 1998; Schneider, 1992). In a comprehensive meta-analytic investigation, Mathur et al. analyzed 35 group and 64 single-case design studies with students having emotional and behavioral disorders. On average, these students received 2.5 hours per week of social skills treatment for 12 weeks (M = 30 hours total). Overall, this research synthesis of 328 effect sizes showed that social skills treatment had an average effect size of .20 meaning that approximately 58% of children improved compared to controls not receiving social skills treatment. There were no differences between effect sizes based on the quality of research, length of social skills treatment, the method of measuring social skills, or the construct used to measure social skills. Using the percentages of nonoverlapping data points in the 64 single-case design studies, based on a summary of 463 graphs, Mathur et al. showed a moderate effect size of 62%. Based on these data, Mathur et al. concluded that social skills treatment has limited value in intervention programs for students with emotional and behavioral disorders.

Forness and Kavale (1999) conducted a meta-analysis of social skills treatment for children with specific learning disabilities. They analyzed 53 studies involving 2,113 students (average age = 11.5 years). Averaged across the 53 studies, students received an average of 3 hours per week of social skills treatment over 10 weeks. Based on the analysis of the 328 effect sizes, the mean effect size was .21

(range $= -0.674$ to 1.19). This effect size is almost identical to the one reported by Mathur et al. (1998). No differences were observed in effect sizes as a function of students' age or length of social skills treatment. Forness and Kavale concluded that social skills treatment with students having specific learning disabilities has limited empirical support at the present time.

Substantially stronger effect sizes were reported in meta-analyses conducted by Schneider (1992) and Beelman et al. (1994). Schneider reviewed 79 studies and found an overall average effect size of .87 at posttest and .75 at follow-up. Effect sizes of this magnitude mean that the average outcome for students receiving social skills treatment exceeded 78–81% of students not receiving social skills treatment. Schneider also found that social skills treatment was more effective with children described as "withdrawn" ($d = 1.90$) and least effective for children described as "aggressive" or "unpopular" ($d = 0.80$). In terms of outcome measures, social skills treatment produced the largest effect on social interaction ($d = 0.93$) and lower effect sizes on aggression ($d = 0.41$) and peer acceptance ($d = 0.45$).

Beelman et al. (1994) reported smaller effect sizes that Schneider (1992) in their analysis of 49 studies conducted with children between 3 and 15 years of age. This meta-analysis showed an average effect size of .47, meaning that the average score of the social skills treatment group was higher than the average score of about 69% of the control group. Higher effect sizes were reported for social-cognitive skills ($d = 0.77$) than for social interaction skills ($d = 0.34$), and higher effect sizes were reported for performance on social cognitive tests ($d = 0.83$) than for naturalistically observed behavior ($d = 0.49$).

Like previous reviews of the social problem-solving literature, these authors showed that social problem-solving treatments produce higher scores on measures of social problems solving but have little effect on social behavior of children in naturalistic settings, measures of peer acceptance/ rejection, or behavior ratings of social behavior. Denham and Almeida (1987) noted similar findings in their meta-analysis showing that social problem-solving interventions produced strong effects on social problem-solving measures

($d = 0.78$) but weak effects on behavior ratings ($d = 0.26$). Coleman et al. (1993) made similar interpretations by arguing that the data do not support the basic assumption that training in social skills mediates social behavior and generalizes to other behaviors or settings. Beelman et al. (1994) made a similar point by stating that social skills treatment does not produce durable treatment outcomes and perhaps should involve more ecological training procedures that do not just acknowledge children's social environments but actively include them in the intervention.

Intervention Providers

Parents and Family

The techniques and methods of child-specific intervention were developed primarily by clinical psychologists in inpatient and outpatient settings. Through studies such as the Kazdin et al. (1984) experiment, techniques initially developed for chronic schizophrenic and depressed adults were modified for use with children who evince a developmental disability (Bellack et al., 1984; Hersen, Eisler, & Miller, 1973). Since that time, special educators have made clever and useful modifications to these strategies to make them more applicable to parents and teachers. Strain and associates have been particularly active in this area. They have been instrumental in doing research to identify targets for social skills curriculums to use in school settings for children with Autism Spectrum Disorders (ASD) (Strain, 1983). They used naturally developing preschoolers to help train the peer social interactions of socially withdrawn, handicapped preschoolers (Strain, 1977; Strain, Shores, & Timm, 1977). Caregivers are encouraged to provide positive interactions between preschoolers with ASD (Strain & Danko, 1995). Positive imitations, appropriate play, and other cooperative social behaviors have emerged as key in improving how handicapped children are viewed. Exploring peers, curriculums, and using caregiver/parent participation has been an excellent way to enhance the likelihood that children with ASD can learn to perform these skills in real-world environments, while decreasing the major costs associated with such training.

Peer-mediated interventions often involve typically developing peers. These children act as therapists in this type of treatment technique. A typical child and a child with ASD are paired during an activity such as recess. However, just pairing the two children does not ensure meaningful interactions (Pierce & Schreibman, 1995). Thus, supports to typical peers (e.g., training as a therapist) are recommended to sustain the use of new interaction strategies (Saintano, Goldstein, & Strain, 1992). However, as we have noted, the typical child may not wish to give up its free time or it may wish to be paired with a child with ASD for only a brief time period. These desires and wishes must be adhered to in a sensitive fashion to ensure the rights of both children. Also, these programs are unlikely to be feasible with very young children. Children of this age are unlikely to be able to accurately perform the requisite treatment strategies accurately.

Similarly, families with several small children must be careful not to become so involved with the child with ASD that the other children receive very minimal parenting. Also, parents may live in areas that are at great distances from service centers, making daily commutes impractical. Another issue is that parents may simply not be willing to invest the amount of effort and time needed to carry out such a program, even if they can manage the time commitment. Additionally, many children may have milder symptoms of ASD and do not require such intensive care. Therefore, these children might benefit more from attending regular day programs and elementary schools. For these and many other reasons, outpatient care with some additional supports in the school and, perhaps, the home environment are much more likely to be the norm. These programs are available through many universities and medical schools.

Koegel, Koegel and Brookman (2003) provide an overview of how to coordinate services in an outpatient program using parent participation. Koegel et al. discuss the role of the clinician, parent, and school. One of the most important goals is insuring that the children and their parents and teachers can carry out the desired behaviors in real-life settings. The authors, through the University of California Santa Barbara (UCSB), run an Autism Research and Training Clinic. They note that the goal of their program is to provide comprehensive treatment in key areas to promote independence and self-education. Parents coordinate daily activities, and the treatment is provided in regular school settings. This latter point can be very important in promoting generalization.

Koegel et al. (2003) emphasized that for children with ASD, motivation and child initiations are particularly important. Given the many needs these children have, treatment can be overwhelming. Thus, the notion of prioritizing skills in a hierarchy from most to least important is quite useful. For some people, it will be possible to have similar priorities across children. The idea of grouping children with similar skills and deficits, such as children with ASD, can result in more efficient service delivery. Nonetheless, everyone is unique in their challenges and needs. Thus, some fine-tuning specific to each child is also needed.

More recent research suggests that parental involvement may lead to better outcomes (Kolko, Loar and Sturnick, 1990). However, until recently, parents have infrequently been used in social skills interventions (Budd, 1986). Frankel, Myatt, and Cantell (1995) have attempted to address this deficiency by designing a group-based social skills intervention that mobilizes parents in the development and maintenance of their children's prosocial behaviors. Overall, this intervention has shown good outcomes for preadolescent boys with difficulty making and keeping close friends, including those diagnosed with oppositional defiant disorder and/or attention deficit/hyperactivity disorder. In particular, findings suggested that the social skills intervention using parent involvement significantly increased parent and teacher ratings of social skills, as well as decreased ratings of aggression compared to similar children on a waiting list for treatment (Frankel, Myatt, Cantwell, & Feinberg, 1997).

Although Frankel et al. (1997) have demonstrated good outcomes for this intervention, findings are limited to a research setting where investigators use strict procedures to ensure treatment fidelity and adherence to the manual, such as extensive training and independent observers, procedures that are difficult to implement in a typical outpatient practice. Moreover, children typically seen in clinical practice are generally excluded from efficacy studies, including those who have comorbid diagnoses and those with developmental delays. As such, it is unclear whether the effectiveness of this intervention at posttreatment can be demonstrated in a less structured clinical setting where treatment fidelity and adherence are less strict and the inclusion criteria are more widely defined.

Peer-Mediated Interventions

This set of procedures involves employing other children in a classroom, or other naturalistic environment as a co-trainer or co-participant with the child who has ASD. The literature typically gives considerable weight to the positive aspects of such interventions, which we will do as well. However, it is important to note that these "other children" must willingly participate and should be allowed to continue to participate in such activities by their own choosing. We have seen numerous examples where children have been coerced into involvement and to stay involved in such programs when, in fact, they would prefer not to do so. Ethical concerns exist here that must be addressed whenever children are being asked or required to participate in peer-mediated interventions. Professionals or parents, should be equally concerned about the rights and well-being of all children involved and must be careful not to push one's value system upon others.

With the concern noted above addressed, there are many potential positive elements associated with the peer-mediated approach. Peer-mediated interventions have been reported to be effective for enhancing interactions of children with ASD and their peers (Goldstein & Ferrell, 1987), increasing social interaction rates (Lee & Odom, 1996), and to show that older elementary age children can implement learning-based procedures to increase the social interactions of their young siblings (Coe, Matson, Cragie, & Gossen, 1991). Peer-mediated interventions have a number of potential benefits for all the children involved in the training. One such benefit is that intervention providers are strengthening their own skills through repetition, while at the same time the children are able to see the benefits of these skills first hand when practiced by others.

The area of social skills has a technology shift that borrows a good deal from training methods used for other domains of behavior studied in children with ASD. Other areas tend to rely largely on traditional operant conditioning methods. These procedures incorporate a range of methods that could be described as social learning or cognitive behavior therapy. Techniques such as modeling, social reinforcement, and self-monitoring are commonly described. Typically, these procedures have not been described as often in the packaged programs discussed previously as operant methods. However, the potential these methods have for promoting skill acquisition and maintenance in real- life situations would seem to suggest that they deserve further attention in the future, perhaps with other skill areas, such as aberrant behavior and communication.

Teachers

A number of procedures have been identified as effective treatment methods for social skills deficits. The myriad of procedures, however, can be classified under four major headings: (a) operant conditioning, (b) modeling, (c) coaching, and (d) social-cognitive procedures. Operant conditioning interventions consist primarily of providing social or material reinforcement of targeted prosocial behaviors in naturalistic or analogue settings. Modeling interventions involve the training of desired social behaviors through videotaped or live demonstrations of the skills to be acquired. Coaching procedures consist of direct verbal instruction, accompanied by discussion of the desired social behaviors. Finally, social-cognitive interventions focus on any of several cognitive processes that have been associated with social competence and problem solving. In practice, behavioral rehearsal is often incorporated into treatment, and most effective social skills interventions are combined procedures rather than a single technique.

Promoting Generalization and Maintaining Treatment Efficacy

To be truly effective, behaviors taught in social skills training programs should generalize across time (i.e., maintenance), settings, individuals, and behaviors. Berler et al. (1982) recommended that social skills interventions not be considered valid unless generalization to the natural environment can be demonstrated. Application of social skills outside the training setting does not occur naturally; rather, generalization must be programmed actively into the training program (Weissberg, 1985). Stokes and Baer (1977) and Michelson et al. (1983) discussed several procedures, referred to as generalization facilitators, that enhance generalization beyond the specific aspects of an intervention. Examples of generalization facilitators are as follows: (a) teaching behaviors that are likely to be maintained by naturally occurring contingencies, (b) training across stimuli (e.g., persons, setting) common to the natural environment, (c) fading response contingencies to approximate naturally occurring consequences, (d) reinforcing application of skills across settings and to new and appropriate situations, and (e) including peers in training. By incorporating as many of these facilitators as possible into social skills interventions, and by offering "booster" sessions at regular intervals, maintenance and generalization of skills are enhanced.

Despite decades of research, one of the most persistent weaknesses in the social skills literature is its failure to demonstrate sufficient generalization and maintenance of instructed social skills. Two main reasons for this are commonly cited: (1) failure to adequately program for generalization and maintenance, and (2) the use of treatments in contrived and restricted setting to teach social behavior (Carey & Stoner, 1994; DuPaul & Eckert, 1994; Gresham, 1997; Haring, 1992; Scott & Nelson, 1998).

Social skills are often taught in self-contained, small group settings of four to six children and one or two adults. Haring (1992) has argued that a task-analytic approach to social skills treatment be employed that emphasizes acquisition and performance of discrete responses in contrived situations. Other researchers contend that a contextual approach would be more beneficial.

A contextual approach would occur in naturalistic settings using informal intervention procedures based on incidental learning (i.e., "teachable moments"). Incidental learning takes advantage of naturally occurring behavioral events to teach or enhance the performance of desired social behaviors. Most social skill instruction in homes, schools, and community settings is informal or incidental. Thousands of behavioral incidents occur in these settings, thereby creating numerous contextually relevant opportunities for teaching social behavior (Gresham, 1997).

Current Issues and Future Directions

The amount of treatments available for social skills deficits in children has increased over the past few decades. Studies of both clinical and community samples have furthered our understanding of the nature and course of social skills development. The continual study of new treatment methods will remain central to remediating social skill deficits in children. Classical studies conducted with children demonstrate the effectiveness of social skills training using operant behavioral and social modeling procedures. While this research is important, there is a noticeable lack of studies that show long-term gains and generalization of skills. Treatment modalities should be created that build in generalization and maintenance procedures across a variety of settings. In turn, these new therapies would need empirical support prior to widespread implementation.

References

Asher, S. R., & Hymel, S. Children's social competence in peer relations: Sociometric and behavioral assessment. In J. D. Wine & M. D. Smye (Eds.), *Social competence*. New York: Guilford Press, 1981.

Asher, S. R., Oden, S. L., & Gottman, _I. M. Children's friendships in school settings. In L. G. Katz (Ed.) (1977). *Current topics in early childhood education* (Vol. I). Norwood. NJ: Ablex.

Asher, S. R., & Renshaw, P. D. (1981). Children without friends: Social knowledge and social skill training. In S. R. Asher & J. M. Gottman (Eds.), *The development of children's friendships*. New York: Cambridge University Press.

Bandura, A. *Aggression: A social learning analysis*. Englewood Cliffs, NJ: Prentice-Hall, 1973.

Bandura, A. *Principles of behavior modification*. New York: Hoh, Rinehart, & Winston, 1969.

Bandura, A. *Social learning theory*. Englewood Cliffs, NJ: Prentice-Hall, 1977. (a)

Bandura, A. (1977b). Self-efficacy: Toward a unifying theory of behavior change. *Psychological Review, 84,* 191–215.

Beelman, A., Pfingsten, U., & Losel, F. (1994). Effects of training social competence in children: A meta-analysis of recent evaluation studies. *Journal of Clinical Child Psychology, 23,* 260–271.

Bellack, A. S. (1979). A critical appraisal for strategies for assessing social skills. Behavioral Assessment, *1,* 157–176.

Bellack, A. S., Hersen, M., & Lampmorski, D. (1979). Role play tests for assessing social skills: Are they valid? Are they useful? *Journal of Consulting and Clinical Psychology, 47,* 335–342.

Bellack, A. S., Hersen, M., & Turner, S. M. (1978). Role play tests for assessing social skills: Are they valid? *Behavior Therapy. 9,* 448–461.

Bellack, A. S., Turner, S. M., Hersen, M., & Luber, R. F. (1984). An examination of the efficacy of social skills training for chronic schizophrenic patients. *Hospital and Community Psychiatry, 35,* 1023–1028.

Berler, E. S., Gross, A. M., & Drabman, R. S. (1982). Social skills training with children: Proceed with caution. *Journal of Applied Behavior Analysis, 15,* 41–53.

Blackwood, R.O. (1970). The operant conditioning of verbally mediated self-control in the classroom. *Journal of School Psychology, 8,* 251–258.

Bolstad, O. D., & Johnson, S. M. (1972). Self-regulation in the modification of disruptive classroom behavior. *Journal of Applied Behavior Analysis, 5,* 443–454.

Bomstein, M. R., Bellack, A. S., & Hersen, M. (1977). Social skills training for unassertive children: A multiple baseline analysis. Journal of *Applied Behavior Analysis, 10,* 183–195.

Bomstein, P. H., & Quevillon, R. P. (1976). The effects of a self-instructional package with overactive preschool boys. *Journal of Applied Behavior Analysis, 9,* 179–188.

Bryan, T. S. (1978). Social relationships and verbal interactions of learning disabled children. *Journal of Learning Disabilities, 11,* 107–115.

Bryan, T. S., Wheeler, R., Felcan, I., & Henek, T. (1976). Come on dummy: An observational study of children's communications. *Journal of Learning Disabilities, 9,* 53–61.

Budd, K. S. (1986). Parents as mediators in the social skills training of children. In L. L'Abate & M. A. Milan (Eds.), *Handbook of social skills training and research* (pp. 245–262). New York: Wiley.

Camp, B. W., Blom, G. E., Hebert, F., & van Doominck, W. J. (1977). Think aloud: A program for developing self-control in young aggressive boys. *Journal of Abnormal Child Psychology, 5,* 157–169.

Carey, S., & Stoner, G. (1994). Contextual considerations in social skills instruction. *School Psychology Quarterly, 9,* 137–141.

Cartledge, G., & Milbum, J. F. (1978). The case for teaching social skills in the classroom: A review. *Review of Educational Research, 48,* 133–156.

Coe, D. A., Matson, J. L., Craigie, C. J., & Gossen, M. A. (1991). Sibling training of play skills to autistic children. *Child and Family Behavior Therapy, 13,* 13–40.

Coleman, M., Wheeler, L., & Webber, J. (1993). Research on interpersonal problem-solving training: A review. *Remedial and Special Education, 14,* 25–37.

Combs, M. L., & Lahey, B. B. (1981). A cognitive social skills training program: Evaluation with young children. *Behavior Modification, 5,* 39–60.

Cooke, T. P., & Apolloni, T. (1976). Developing positive social-emotional behaviors: A study of training and generalization effects. *Journal of Applied Behavior Analysis, 9,* 65–78.

Cowen, E. L., Pederson, A., Babigian, H., Izzo, L. D., & Trost, M. A. (1973). Long-term follow-up of early detected vulnerable children. *Journal of Consulting and Clinical Psychology, 41,* 438–446.

Craighead, W. E. (1982). A brief clinical history of cognitive-behavior therapy with children. *School Psychology Review, 2,* 5–13.

Denham, S., & Almeida, M. (1987). Children's social problem solving skills, behavioral adjustment, and interventions: A meta-analysis evaluating theory and practice. *Journal of Applied Developmental Psychology, 8,* 391–409.

Deutsch, F. (1974). Observational and sociometric measures of peer popularity and their relationship to egocentric communication in female preschoolers. *Developmental Psychology, 10,* 745–755.

Drabman, R. S., Spitalnik, R., & O'Leary, K. D. (1973). Teaching self-control to disruptive children. *Journal of Abnormal Psychology, 82,* 10–16.

DuPaul, G., & Eckert, T. (1994). The effects of social skills curricula: Now you see them, now you don't. *School Psychology Quarterly, 9,* 113–132.

Erikson, E. H. *Childhood and society.* New York: Norton, 1963.

Evers-Pasquale, W. L. (1978). The Peer Perference Test as a measure of reward value: Item analysis, crossvalidation, concurrent validation, and replication. *Journal of Abnormal Child Psychology, 6,* 175–188.

Evers-Pasquale, W. & Sherman, M. (1975). The reward value of peers: A variable influencing the efficacy of filmed modeling in modifying social isolation in preschoolers. *Journal of Abnormal Child Psychology, 3,* 179–189.

Evers, W. L., & Schwarz, J. C. (1973). Modifying social withdrawal in preschoolers: The effects of filmed modeling and teacher praise. *Journal of Abnormal Child Psychology, 1,* 248–256.

Forness, S., & Kavale, K. (1999). Teaching social skills in children with learning disabilities: A meta-analysis of the research. *Learning Disabilities Quarterly, 19,* 2–13.

Foster, S. L., & Ritchey, W. L. (1979). Issues in the assessment of social competence in children. *Journal of Applied Behavior Analysis, 12,* 625–638.

Frankel, F., Myatt, R., & Cantell, D.P. (1995). Training outpatient boys to conform with social ecology pf popular peers: Effects on parent and teacher ratings. *Journal of Clinical Child Psychology, 24,* 300–310.

Frankel, F., Myatt, R., Cantwell, D. P., & Feinberg, D. T. (1997a). Use of the child behavior checklist and DSM-III-R diagnosis in predicting outcome of children's social skills training. *Journal of Behavioral Therapy and Experimental Psychiatry, 28,* 149–161.

Geller, M. I., & Scheirer, C. J. (1978). The effect of filmed modeling on cooperative play in disadvantaged preschoolers. *Journal of Abnormal Child Psychology, 6,* 71–87.

Goldstein, H., & Ferrell, D. R. (1987). Augmenting communicative interaction between handicapped and nonhandicapped preschool children. *Journal of Speech and Hearing Disorders, 52,* 200–211.

Goldstein, A. P., Sprafkin, R. P., Gershaw, N. J., & Klein, P. (1980). *Skill-streaming the adolescent: A structured learning approach to teaching prosocial skills.* Champaign, IL: Research Press.

Gottman, J. M. (1977a). Toward a definition of social isolation in children. *Child Development, 1977, 48,* 513–517.

Gottman, J. M. (1977b) The effects of a modeling film on social isolation in preschool children: A methodological investigation. *Journal of Abnormal Child Psychology, 5,* 69–78.

Gottman, J., Gonso, J., & Rasmussen, B. (1975). Social interaction, social competence, and friendship in children. *Child Development, 46,* 709–718.

Gottman, J., Gonso. J., & Schuler. P. (1976). Teaching social skills to isolated children. *Journal of Abnormal Child Psychology, 4,* 179–197.

Gresham, F.M. (1997). Treatment integrity in single-subject research. In R. Franklin, D. Allison, & B. Gorman (Eds.), *Design and Analysis of Single Case Research.* Hillsdale, NJ: Erlbaum.

Gresham, F.M., & Nagle, R.J. (1980). Social skills training in children: Responsiveness to modeling and coaching as a function of peer orientation. *Journal of Consulting and Clinical Psychology, 48,* 718–729.

Gresham, F. M., (1981). Assessment of children's social skills. *Journal of School Psychology, 19,* 120–134.

Gronlund, H., & Anderson, L. (1963). Personality characteristics of socially accepted, socially neglected, and socially rejected junior high school pupils. In J. Seidman (Ed.), *Educating for mental health.* New York: Crowell.

Haring, N. (1992). The context of social competence: Relations, relationships, and Generalization. In S. Odom, S. McConnell, & M. McEnvoy (Eds.), *Social competence of young children with disabilities: Issues and strategies for intervention.* Baltimore: Paul H. Brookes.

Hartup, W. W., Glazer, J. A., & Charlesworth, R. (1967). Peer reinforcement and sociometric status. *Child Development, 38,* 1017–1024.

Hersen, M., Eisler, R. M., & Miller, P. M. (1973). Development of assertive responses: Clinical measurement and research considerations. *Behaviour Research and Therapy, 11,* 505–521.

Hersen, M., & Barlow, D. H. (1976). Single case experimental *designs: Strategies for studying behavior change.* New York: Pergamon Press.

Hobbs, S. A., Moguin, L. E. Tryoler, M., & Lahey, B. B. (1980). Cognitive behavior therapy with children: Has clinical utility been demonstrated? *Psychological Bulletin, 87,* 147–165.

Hymel, S. and Asher, S. R. (1977). Assessment and training of isolated children's social skills. In: *Paper presented at the biennial meeting of the Society for Research in Child Development* (1977, March).

Jakibchub, Z., & Smeriglio, V. L. (1976). The influence of symbolic modeling on the social behavior of preschool children with low levels of social responsiveness. *Child Development, 47,* 838–841.

Jennings, K. D. (1975). People versus object orientation, social behavior, and intellectual abilities in children. *Developmental Psychology, 11,* 511–519.

Kaufman, K. F., & O'Leary, K. D. (1972). Reward, cost, and self-evaluation procedures for disruptive adolescents in a psychiatric hospital school. *Journal of Applied Behavior Analysis, 5,* 293–309.

Kazdin, A. E. (1982). Current developments and research issues in cognitive-behavioral interventions: A commentary. *School Psychology Review, 11,* 75–82.

Kazdin, A. E., Matson, J. L., & Esveldt-Dawson, K. (1984). The relationship of role-play assessment of children's social skills to multiple measures of social competence. *Behaviour Research and Therapy, 22,* 129–140.

Keller, M. F., & Carlson, P. M. (1974). The use of symbolic modeling to promote social skills in preschool children with low levels of social responsiveness. *Child Development, 45,* 912–919.

Kendall, P. C., & Hollon, S. D. (Eds.). (1979). *Cognitive-behavioral interventions: Theory research, and procedures.* New York: Academic Press.

Koegel, R. L., Koegel, L. K., & Brookman, L. I. (2003). Empirically supported pivotal response interventions for children with autism. In A. E. Kazdin & J. R. Weisz (Eds.), *Evidence-based psychotherapies for children and adolescents* (pp. 341–357). New York: Guilford Press.

Kohn, M., & Clausen, J. (1955). Social isolation and schizophrenia. *American Sociological Review. 20,* 265–213.

Kohlberg, L. (1969). Stage and sequence: The cognitive-developmental approach to socialization. In D. A. Gosline (Ed.), *Handbook of socialization theory and research.* Chicago, IL: Rand McNally.

Kolko, D. J., Loar, L. L., & Sturnick, D. (1990). Inpatient social cognitive skills training groups with conduct disordered and attention deficit disordered children. *Journal of Child Psychology & Psychiatry and Allied Disciplines, 31,* 737–748.

Ladd, G. W. (1979). *A social learning approach to training social skills with low-accepted children.* Unpublished doctoral dissertation, University of Rochester, Rochester, NY.

Ladd, G.W. (1981). Effectiveness of a social learning method for enhancing children's social interactions and peer acceptance. *Child Development, 52,* 171–178.

LaGreca, A.M., & Santogrossi, D.A. (1980). Social skills training with elementary school students: A behavioral group approach. *Journal of Consulting and Clinical Psychology, 48,* 220–227.

Lahey, B. B., & Strauss, C. C. (1982). Some considerations in evaluating the clinical utility of cognitive behavior therapy with children. *School Psychology Review, 11,* 67–74.

Lee, S., & Odom, S. L. (1996). The relationship between stereotypic behavior and peer social interactions for children with severe disabilities. *Journal of the Association for Persons with Severe Handicaps, 21,* 88–95.

Marshall, H. R., & McCandless, B. R. (1957). A study in prediction of social behavior in preschool children. *Child Development, 28,* 149–159.

Mathur, S., Kavale, K., Quinn, M., Forness, S., & Rutherford, R. (1998). Social skills intervention with students with emotional and behavioral problems: A quantitative synthesis of single subject research. *Behavioral Disorders, 23*, 193–201.

McCandless, B. R., 81 Marshall, H. R. (1957). A picture sociometric technique for preschool children and itsrelation to teacher judgments of friendship. *Child Development, 28*, 139–168.

Meichenbaum, D. H. (1977). *Cognitive-behavior modification: An integrative approach.* New York: Plenum Press.

Meichenbaum, D. H. & Goodman, J. (1971). Training impulsive children to talk to themselves: A means of developing self-control. *Journal of Abnormal Psychology, 77,* 115–126.

Michelson, L., Mannarino, A.P., Marchione, K.E., Stern, M., Figeroa, J., & Beck, S. (1983). A comparative outcome study of behavioral social skills training, interpersonal problem-solving, and non-directive control treatments with child psychiatric outpatients. *Behavior Research and Therapy, 21*, 545–556.

Michelson, L., & Wood, R. (1980). A group assertive training program for elementary schoolchildren. *Child Behavior Therapy, 2*, 1–9.

Minkin, N., Braukmann, C. J., Minkin, B. L., Timbers, C. D., Timbers, F. J. Fixen, D. L., et al. (1976). The social validation and training of conversation skills. *Journal of Applied Behavior Analysis, 9*, 127–140.

Moore, S. C. (1967). Correlates of peer acceptance in nursery school children. In W. W. Hartup & N. L. Smathergill (Eds.), *The young child.* Washington, DC: National Association for the Education of Young Children.

Moore, S., & Updegraff, R. (1964). Sociometric status of preschool children related to age, sex, nurturance-giving, and dependency, *Child Development, 35*, 519–524.

O'Connor, R. D. (1969). Modification of social withdrawal through symbolic modeling. *Journal of Applied Behavior Analysis, 2*, 15–22.

O'Connor, R. D. (1972). Relative effects of modeling, shaping, and the combined procedures for modification of social withdrawal. *Journal of Abnormal Psychology, 79*, 327–334.

Oden, S., & Asher, S.R. (1977). Coaching children in social skills for friendship making. *Child Development, 56*, 495–506.

O'Leary, S.G., & Dubey. O.R. (1979). Applications of self-control procedures by children: A review. *Journal of Applied Behavior Analysis, 12*, 449–465.

Piaget, J. (1962). *The moral judgment of the child.* New York: Collier.

Pierce, K., & Schreibman, L. (1995). Increasing complex play in children with autism via peer-implemented Pivotal Response Training. *Journal of Applied Behavior Analysis, 28*, 285–295.

Robin, A., Schneider, M. & Dolnick, M. (1976). The turtle technique: An extended case study of self-control in the classroom. *Psychology in the Schools, 13*, 449–453.

Roff, M. F., Sells, S. B., & Golden, M. M. (1972). *Social adjustment and personality in children.* Minneapolis, MN: University of Minnesota Press.

Roff, M. F. (1970). Some life history factors in relation to various types of adult maladjustment. In M. F. Roff & D. F. Ricks (Eds.), *Life history research in psychopathology Vol. 1.* Minneapolis, MN: University of Minnesota Press.

Rosenbaum, M. S., & Drabman, R. S. (1979). Self-control training in the classroom: A review and critique. *Journal of Applied Behavior Analysis, 12*, 467–485.

Saintano, D., Goldstein, H., & Strain, P. (1992). Effects of self-evaluation on pre-school children's use of social interaction strategies with their classmates with autism. *Journal of Applied Behavioral Analysis, 25*, 127–141.

Santogrossi, D. A., O'Leary, K.D., Romanczyk, R.G., & Kaufman, K.F. (1973). Self-evaluation by adolescents in a psychiatric hospital school token programs. *Journal of Applied Behavior Analysis, 6*, 277–287.

Schneider, B. (1992). Didactic models for enhancing children's peer relations: A quantitative review. *Clinical Psychology Review, 12*, 363–382.

Scott, T. & Nelson, C.M. (1998). Confusion and failure in facilitating generalized social responding in the school setting: Sometimes $2 + 2 = 5$. *Behavioral Disorders, 23*, 264–275.

Stokes, T. F., & Baer, D. M. (1977). An implicit technology of generalization. *Journal of Applied Behavior Analysis, 10*, 349–368.

Strain, P. S. (1977). Effects of peer social initiations on withdrawn preschool children: Some training and generalization effects. *Journal of Abnormal Child Psychology, 5*, 445–455.

Strain, P. S. (1983). Identification of social skills curriculum targets for severely handicapped children in mainstream preschools. *Applied Research in Mental Retardation, 4*, 369–382.

Strain, P. S., & Danko, C. D. (1995). Caregivers' encouragement of positive interactions between preschoolers with autism and their siblings. *Journal of Emotional and Behavioral Disorders, 3*, 2–12.

Strain, P. S., Shores, R. E., & Kerr, M. M. (1976). Experimental analysis of spillover effects on social interaction of behaviorally handicapped preschooler children. *Journal of Applied Behavior Analysis, 21*, 34–40.

Strain, P. S., Shores, R. E., & Timm, M. A. (1977). Effects of peer initiations on social behavior of withdrawn preschoolers. *Journal of Applied Behavior Analysis, 10*, 289–298.

Thelen, M. H., Fry, R. A., Fehrenbach, P. A., & Frautschi, N. M. (1979). Therapeutic videotape and film modeling: A review. *Psychological Bulletin, 86*, 701–720.

Turkewitz, H., O'Leary, K. D., & Ironsmith, M. (1975). Producing generalization of appropriate behavior through self-control. *Journal of Consulting and Clinical Psychology, 43*, 577–583.

Ullman, C. A. (1957). Teachers, peers, and tests as predictors of adjustment. *Journal of Educational Psychology, 48*, 257–267.

Van Hasselt, V. B., Hersen, M., & Bellack, A. S. (1981). The validity of role play tests for assessing social skills in children. *Behavior Therapy, 12*, 202–216.

Weintraub, S., Prim, R. J., & Neale, J. M. (1978). Peer evaluations of the competence of children vulnerable to psychopathology. *Journal of Abnormal Child Psychology, 6*, 461–473.

Weissberg, R. P. (1985). Designing effective social problem-solving programs for the Classroom. In B. H. Schneider, K. H. Rubin & J.E. Ledingham (Eds.), *Children's peer relations: Issues in assessment and intervention* (pp. 225–242). New York, NY: Springer-Verlag.

Wolf, M. M. (1978). Social validity: The case for subjective measurement or how applied behavior analysis is finding its heart. *Journal of Applied Behavior Analysis, 11*, 203–214.

Zahavi, S. L., & Asher, S. R. (1978). The effect of verbal instructions on preschool children's aggressive behavior. *Journal of School Psychology, 16*, 146–153.

Chapter 6
Challenging Behaviors

Rebecca Mandal-Blasio, Karen Sheridan, George Schreiner, and Tra Ladner

It is widely accepted that challenging behaviors are the result of social skills deficits. Acquisition, performance, or fluency deficits related to cognitive and emotional difficulties, as well as environmental issues, may be the root of the challenging behaviors. Additionally, challenging behaviors related to social skills deficits have been found in many groups, including children diagnosed with Intellectual Disabilities (ID), Attention Deficit Hyperactivity Disorder (ADHD), Learning Disabilities (LD), and other psychiatric diagnoses. Boys, both with and without ID, exhibit more challenging behaviors than girls and these behaviors are often associated with social skills deficits (Campbell, Spieker, Burchinal, Poe, & the NICHD Early Child Care Research Network, 2006; de Ruiter, Dekker, Verhurst, & Koot, 2007; Douma, Dekker, de Ruiter, Tick, & Koot, 2007; Emerson et al., 2001). Challenging behaviors that have been found to be related to social skills deficits, in the literature, are aggression (Campbell et al., 2006; Emerson et al., 2001; Keltikangas-Järvinen, 2001), property destruction (Douma et al., 2007; Emerson et al., 2001), self-injury (Emerson et al., 2001; Matson, Minshawi, Gonzales, & Mayville, 2006), and stereotypies (Matson, Smiroldo, & Bamburg, 1998).

Researchers have consistently shown that children who demonstrate social skills deficits and/or challenging behavior experience related short- and long-term negative effects. It has been demonstrated that multiple behavioral challenges increased the probability of social skills deficits (Matson et al., 2006). In regard to short-term effects, children may encounter poor family, peer, and teacher interactions, peer rejection, and less social acceptance (Chang, 2003; Spence, 2003; Vaughn, Zaragoza, Hogan, & Walker, 1993). Furthermore, individuals displaying such deficits have been associated with risk of personal injury, injury of caregivers, the need for physical interventions, and possibility of being assigned to lower functioning/ability programming activities (Emerson et al., 2001). If the short-term effects do not receive immediate intervention, negative long-term effects may develop, including psychological, academic, and adaptive functioning difficulties (Coie, Terry, Lenox, & Lochman, 1995; Mansell, Macdonald, & Beadle-Brown, 2002), psychopathology (de Ruiter et al., 2007; Spence, 2003), unemployment, and criminality (Chung & Steinberg, 2006). Due to the fact that current research is correlational, it has not been determined whether multiple behavioral challenges or symptoms of psychopathology interfere with the acquisition of social skills or whether individuals who have fewer appropriate social skills resort to inappropriate social behavior (Matson et al., 2006). Thus, the importance of assessment of the challenging behaviors and treatment interventions related to social skills should be of immediate attention to mental health professionals.

Comorbidity and Social Skills Deficits

Children diagnosed with ID, Autism Spectrum Disorders (ASD), ADHD, and LD have been found to have fewer social skills and more challenging

R. Mandal-Blasio (✉)
Louisiana Office for Citizens with Developmental Disabilities, Resource Center on Psychiatric and Behavior Supports, Hammond, LA 70401, USA
e-mail: rebecca.mandal@la.gov

J.L. Matson (ed.), *Social Behavior and Skills in Children*, DOI 10.1007/978-1-4419-0234-4_6,
© Springer Science+Business Media, LLC 2009

behaviors compared to children without these diagnoses. For example, researchers have found that children diagnosed with ID are three to seven times more likely to exhibit behavioral and emotional problems than children without ID (Dekker, Koot, van der Ende, & Verhurst, 2002; Dykens, 2000; Emerson, 2003; Emerson et al., 2001). Specifically, de Ruiter et al. (2007) noted that children between the ages of 6–18 years with ID exhibited higher levels of challenging behaviors and are at greater risk for psychopathology than children without ID. Interestingly, both groups of children followed the same developmental course of psychopathology; however, aggressive behavior is the exception. Children with ID showed a greater decrease in aggressive behavior over time than children without ID. A more detailed description of aggressive behavior will be discussed later in this chapter.

Individuals with ASD have impairments in social functioning per diagnostic criteria (American Psychiatric Association, 2000). Social impairments such as difficulties in initiating/ joining in social activities and accurately identifying others' perceptions, suppressing inappropriate verbalizations or expression of feelings, and dominating conversations with topics of personal interest often may prohibit social connectedness with others and promote challenging behaviors (Bellini, Peters, Benner, & Hopf, 2007) As a result of social skills deficits, it has been found that children with ASD are prone to anxiety, depression, and isolation if treatment is not sought early in the child's development (Bellini, 2006; Bellini et al., 2007). Additionally, children with ASD have been found to have challenging emotional reactions and/or behaviors such as aggression and self-injury which may be the result of medical or environmental factors (Myers & Plauche-Johnson, 2007).

There is also much empirical support that children diagnosed with LD have fewer social skills and higher levels of behavior problems (Toro, Weissberg, Guare, & Liebenstein, 1990; Vaughn et al., 1993). These groups of children have more interpersonal difficulties (Marglit, 1989) and are rated by their parents as having more social skills deficits when compared to their siblings (Dyson, 2003). This finding may be due to the contributing factor that children with LD have difficulties producing solutions to problem-solving situations and tend to have less frustration tolerance to those situations.

Interestingly, parental stress (Dyson, 2003), family, economic, and interpersonal difficulties (Toro et al., 1990) have been linked to social competence and behavior problems of children with LD.

Similarly, there is considerable support in the literature for ADHD as a risk factor for social skills deficits and challenging behaviors. In fact, Fussell, Macias, and Saylor (2005) found that children diagnosed with ADHD have more social skills deficits and behavior problems in comparison to children diagnosed with only learning disabilities/learning problems. Children who are clinically diagnosed or experience hyperactivity, impulsivity, and inattention symptoms tend to exhibit challenging behaviors that are maintained throughout adulthood. This situation often leads to antisocial activities and psychiatric diagnosis such as conduct disorders (Barkley, Fischer, Smallish, & Fletcher, 2004). Some of these results may be better explained by examining research on ADHD subtypes.

Children diagnosed with ADHD-Combined type are found to make more hostile statements and exhibit more aggressive behavior which contribute to peer rejection (Mikami, Huang-Pollock, Pfiffner, McBurnett & Hangai, 2007; Landau, Milich, & Diener, 1998). Children diagnosed with ADHD-Inattentive Type were found to be more passive or socially withdrawn and were more accepted by peers than children diagnosed with ADHD-Combined Type (Mikami et al., 2007). Given the dissimilarity in the challenging behaviors and social deficits associated with each of the ADHD subtypes, it is important for clinicians to note these differences when assessing and treating this population of children since cognitive distortions or deficits may be related to social skills acquisition or performance deficits.

The Relationship Between Social Skills Deficits and Challenging Behavior

Problem behaviors are usually categorized as either internalizing (e.g., social withdrawal, depression, or anxiety) or externalizing (e.g., hyperactivity, aggression, or self-injurious behavior, stereotypies). For example, a child with a history of social anxiety may never acquire a skill such as joining in a play group or may fail to perform a skill such as sharing because of avoidance of social situations. In contrast, a child with aggression may never acquire the skill of sharing because other children avoid him, or he may fail to perform the skill of joining in a play group because bullying behavior has been reinforced by peers. Considering this, it is clear that challenging behaviors, both internal and external, often hinder either the acquisition or the performance of interpersonal skills (Gresham & Elliott, 1990).

Social skill acquisition, performance, or fluency deficits often play a role in the development of challenging behaviors. Sometimes interfering or competing problem behaviors also preclude the child from utilizing the correct social skill. Gresham and Elliott (1990) designed the social skills classification model that is discussed at length below regarding the three types of social skills deficits. It is important to assess which type of social skill deficit a child may have when identifying target skills to train and selecting intervention approaches.

Acquisition Deficits

Acquisition deficits are defined when a child does not have a certain skill within his social repertoire needed to obtain a needed or desired object or outcome (Gresham & Elliott, 1990; Gresham, Sugai, & Horner, 2001a; Spence 2003). For example, a child may not have the skill to ask for help when he becomes frustrated with an academic task; thus, he throws his book across the classroom. As a result, the child is sent to the office. In this exchange, the child's challenging behavior is reinforced since his ultimate goal of not completing the task was successful; thus the challenging behavior is likely to occur again. If the child had the skills to communicate frustration and need for assistance, then the appropriate social behavior could have been reinforced.

Performance Deficits

A performance deficit is associated with the child possessing the necessary social skills for appropriate interactions but not exercising the

skills in certain social situations (Gresham, 1997). This state of affairs may be the result of cognitive distortions, affective difficulties, or lack of motivation to perform the appropriate social skill (Spence, 2003). Each of these factors will be discussed next.

In regard to cognitive distortions, children who experience depressive symptoms sometimes have cognitive distortions about social situations. Vickerstaff, Heriot, Wong, Lopes, and Dossetor (2007) found that children with high functioning autism spectrum disorders, and who had low self-perceived social competence, reported higher levels of depressive symptomology. Children diagnosed with depression also demonstrated interpersonal difficulties with peers and parents (Garber, Weiss, & Shanley, 1993; Puig-Antich et al., 1993). They attribute negative life events to internal/stable causes and have a helpless attribution style (Asarnow & Bates, 1988; Garber et al., 1993). Hence, children who are depressed are likely to see their social situations in a pessimistic light. They also attribute their interpersonal deficits as within themselves and unchanging, rather than developing from external and transient factors. Because of this hopeless attribution style, children with depression lack the motivation to perform appropriate social skills because of the fear of negative outcomes, thus perpetuating social skills performance deficits.

Affective state may also contribute to performance deficits. Anxiety or anger may prohibit the person from using the suitable skill and consequently preventing appropriate interactions. Children with LD have been found to be at an increased risk for being rated as anxious or withdrawn when compared to children without LD (Stone & Le Greca, 1984). Also, adolescents diagnosed with high functioning ASD have been found to exhibit clinically significant anxiety levels and social skills deficits when compared to their peers without disabilities (Bellini, 2003, 2006). Because high levels of affective states sometimes prohibit children from choosing or utilizing social skills in an appropriate manner, challenging behaviors may develop. Avoidance of those types of situations, unfavorable effects on the child's self-efficacy, and lower outcome expectancies are often the result of anxiety-provoking situations (Hannesdottir & Ollendick, 2007; Ollendick & Schimdt, 1987).

Fluency Deficits

Fluency deficits consist of the desire to use social skill in the appropriate manner, but skill performance is not adequate. The child does not need remediation of the actual skill or more practice of the "unrefined" social skill. Fluency deficits occur from "a lack of exposure to sufficient or skilled models of social behavior, insufficient rehearsal or practice of a skill, and low rates or inconsistent delivery of reinforcement of skilled performances" (p. 334, Gresham et al., 2001a). For example, a child with ADHD has learned when it is appropriate to interrupt another's conversation as well as the steps to do so. However, when confronted with the actual situation the child is not successful on all steps.

Interfering or Competing Behavior

Gresham and Elliott (1990) broadened their social skills classification model to include two dimensions of social behavior: social skills and competing behaviors. (Gresham et al., 2001a; Spence, 2003). The competing behavior may be more effective, efficient, or provide more reinforcement than using the appropriate social skill, while the interfering behavior may obstruct the appropriate social skill from being displayed. Because performance of the appropriate social skills has not received consistent reinforcement in the past, the challenging behavior is performed because of the maintaining reinforcing consequences gained. Considering this, a comprehensive assessment that consists of evaluating social skills deficits and a functional behavior assessment of the challenging behavior should be the first strategic step in the process of designing interventions.

A final note on social skill deficits. One should not preclude a child from having acquisition deficits even if that child possesses affective or cognitive challenges (Spence, 2003). Oftentimes these factors are interrelated and may prohibit or delay a child from learning the skills to use, ending in challenging behavior. As a clinician, one should examine the possibility of all the deficits listed in this section by conducting a thorough assessment of the child's social skills deficits and challenging behaviors. This chapter will focus on three challenging behaviors often associated with social skills deficits: aggression, self-injury, and stereotypies.

Aggression

Sources estimate that between 2 and 7 percent of school children have significant, long-term emotional and behavioral problems that involve aggression and impair academic and social functioning (Kauffman, 2004). Patterson, Reid, and Dishion (1992) noted the role of parental factors on the development of aggressive behavior such as the following: harsh or irritable discipline, poor parental problem solving, vague commands, and poor parental monitoring and supervision of child's behavior. Other risk factors found in the research that have been linked to aggression include neighborhood and school problems and low socioeconomic status (SES). These variables have been shown to be significant even when family characteristics are taken into account (Kupersmidt, Griesler, DeRosier, Patterson, & Davis, 1995).

In 2006, Campbell et al conducted a longitudinal study investigating social outcomes and behavior problems in children between birth and 9 years of age. Maternal ratings were used to calculate probability scores used to assign children to 5 different aggression trajectory levels: Very low aggression, low-stable aggression, moderate-decreasing aggression, moderate-stable aggression, and high-stable aggression. Children on the high-stable aggression trajectory had the most severe adjustment problems (i.e., poorer social skills, more self-reported peer problems and externalizing problems). Children on the moderate-stable aggression trajectory had more inattention and reduced self-regulation skills. Further, children who had moderate levels of aggression earlier in development, and where these behaviors decreased by school age, appeared to have secure adjustment. Children that maintained low levels of aggression over time (stable) had more social and behavioral problems. Thus, it can be gleaned that the stability of aggressive behavior over time and the level of the aggression during childhood have some impact on a child's social adjustment.

Some cognitive factors have been used to explain the social deficits of many children who display aggressive behavior. Aggression may arise from misperception or errors in processing of environmental events (Berkowitz & Frodi, 1977). For example, cognitive errors in processing the child's appraisals of a social situation, anticipation of reactions of their peers, and self-statements in reaction to certain situations may all be factors contributing to childhood aggression. Others have found that children identified as aggressive showed a predisposition to assign hostile intent to others, particularly in response to social situations in which cues of actual intent were ambiguous (Dodge, 1985) or in aggression – provocative situations (Keltikangas-Järvinen, 2001).

Cognitive mediators, based on the social-cognitive development model, have also been examined in the area of aggression and children with social skills deficits. Adolescents who engaged in high levels of aggression were likely to utilize fewer problems-solving skills and support aggression as a means to solve problems. They also perceived that there would be fewer consequences that would result because of their aggressive behavior. Conversely, adolescents who had lower levels of aggression had more problem-solving skills and were less likely to use aggression as a problem-solving mechanism (Slaby & Guerra, 1988).

Peer Status

There have been conflicting results in the research concerning the relationship between aggression and peer status. Some studies report that aggression is a primary reason for low peer status (Dodge, 1983). For example, children diagnosed with ADHD often are rejected by peers due to aggression and disruptive behavior (Mikami et al., 2007). However, other investigations have failed to confirm this finding. In fact, some studies noted that children who are viewed by peers as being aggressive and dominant were perceived as popular (Parkhurst & Hopmeyer, 1998). Moderating variables, such as gender, aggression type, social structure of the environment (norms and values of the peer context), and teachers' attitudes or beliefs have been identified in order to explain these contrasting views (Chang, 2003).

Aggression in childhood and peer rejection independently predicts delinquent behavior and conduct problems during the adolescent years (Lochman & Wayland, 1994). Children who are aggressive and socially rejected by their peers are more likely to display severe behavior problems than children who are either aggressive only or rejected only (Miller-Johnson, Cole, Maumary-Gremaud, Lochman, & Terry, 1999). Vitaro, Brendgen, Pagani, Tremblay, and McDuff (1999) noted that the relationship between childhood conduct problems and adolescent delinquency is at least in part mediated by deviant peer group affiliation. Salamivalli, Huttunen, and Lagerspetz (1997) pointed out that aggressive children often associate with peers who assist or reinforce their aggressive behavior. Youth with antisocial behavior usually form relationships with peers who reciprocate (e.g., other aggressive peers) or complement (e.g., followers, victims) their behavior (Cairns, Cairns, Neckerman, Gest, & Gariépy, 1988; Pellegrini, 1998). Similarly, Synder, Horsch, and Childs (1997) found that the amount of time that preschoolers spent with aggressive peers was predictive of their level of aggression. Children who are rejected by their peers and who associate with other antisocial peers are likely to need social skills interventions that are different from those who are socially isolated. Children who associate with other aggressive peers will most likely be less motivated to give up the challenging behaviors that are valued and reinforced by their peers (Erdley & Asher, 1999; Farmer & Hollowell, 1994). Therefore, social skills interventions would need to target reframing interactions with peers in order to reduce challenging behavior.

However, peer strategies are not without their set of problems. For example, aggressive children who maintain relationships with other aggressive youth are more likely to be responsive to reinforcement from their own group than from less valued peers in artificially constructed groups or dyads. In addition, issues may arise from social interactions of aggressive children and their peers. Aggressive children may try to bully or dominate their peers, may model aggression to peers, or may become followers and support aggression of others. Considering this, it is important to monitor peer interventions in order to prevent possible conflict and escalation of challenging behaviors (Maag & Webber, 1995).

Self-Injury

While children who display aggression often have deficits in social skills, a similar relationship has been documented in research concerning the relationship between self-injurious behavior and social skills (Duncan, Matson, Bamburg, Cherry, & Buckley, 1999).

One study divided participants with profound learning disabilities into four groups – those who engaged in aggression, self-injury, aggression and self injury, and controls. Results found that individuals with profound learning disabilities who exhibited any challenging behaviors had a limited set of social skills compared to controls. In addition, Duncan et al. (1999) found these individuals were consistently assigned into the aggressive and self-injurious behavior groups based on profiles derived from subscale scores of the Matson Evaluation of Social Skills for Individuals with Severe Retardation (MESSIER; Matson, 1995a).

Stereotypies

Stereotypies, repetitive behaviors, have also been correlated with social skills deficits particularly in children with developmental disabilities. Matson et al. (2006) found that people who exhibited both self-injurious behavior and stereotypies displayed more negative nonverbal social skills (e. g., preferring to be alone, seeking isolation, etc.) than those who exhibited self-injurious behavior alone or no problem behaviors as measured by the Diagnostic Assessment for the Severely Handicapped Revised (DASH-II; Matson, 1995b). In addition, those individuals that exhibited stereotypies alone also showed significantly fewer general positive social skills than the group with no problem behaviors. Similarly, Matson et al. (1998) found those diagnosed with stereotypic movement disorder (with or without self-injurious behavior) and an intellectual disability showed less general positive and

positive nonverbal behavior compared to controls with an intellectual disability without this diagnosis.

Considering past research, many children who evidence social skills deficits also demonstrate challenging behaviors, particularly aggression, self-injury, and stereotypes, which contribute to these deficits. In order to select the most appropriate intervention for these children it is important to identify the maintaining functions of these challenging behaviors. Conducting a functional behavior assessment (FBA) is imperative in determining these factors. Results of such an assessment will inform clinicians which target social skills need to be trained as replacement behaviors; moreover, such an assessment may determine which reinforcers may be used to treat performance deficits.

Functional Assessment of Challenging Behaviors

Functional Behavior Assessments (FBA) have led to advances in assessment and treatment for children with challenging behaviors (Carr, 1994; Matson, Mayville, & Lott, 2002). The FBA allows the clinician to systematically gather information about antecedents, behaviors, and consequences so that the maintaining behaviors can be determined. Once the function (or reason) of the behavior is understood, interventions can be designed to reduce problem behaviors and to facilitate the acquisition of adaptive (replacement) behaviors (Witt, Daly, & Noelle, 2000). The function or purpose of a behavior generally falls into one of the five following categories. An individual may engage in a maladaptive behavior to (a) seek/gain attention, (b) gain access to tangible reinforcers, (c) avoid aversive tasks, (d) avoid other individuals, or (e) self-stimulation (Carr, 1994). For example, treatment for a 6-year-old child diagnosed with Moderate Mental Retardation who bangs his head to gain attention (social reinforcement) may involve teaching the adolescent alternate ways of getting attention. In contrast, the same adolescent who bangs his head in order to avoid schoolwork may receive different schoolwork that is more commensurate with his abilities. A thorough assessment is needed to design and implement effective interventions. No consensus on a single method of completing a functional behavioral analysis has emerged. The FBA may be based on indirect assessments (interviews, questionnaires, rating scales), descriptive assessments (A-B-C sheets, direct observation with no variable-environment manipulations), or experimental/traditional functional assessment (analog conditions in which variables are systematically manipulated) (Herzinger & Campbell, 2006).

Indirect Methods

Behavior rating scales/checklists, functional assessment interviews, and reviews of historical records are some of the most widely used indirect assessment methods. They are referred to as indirect because they involve the assessment of behavior that is removed in time and place from the actual occurrence of that behavior (Cone, 1978). These methods may be considered less rigorous than the experimental functional assessment. They nevertheless provide clinicians with valuable information and have been found to highly correlate with the findings of experimental functional assessments (Durand & Crimmins, 1992). The Questions About Behavioral Function (QABF; Matson & Vollmer, 1995), the Motivation Analysis Rating Scale (MARS; Wieseler, Hanzel, Chamberlain, & Thompson, 1985) and the Motivation Assessment Scale (MAS; Durand & Crimmins, 1992) represent three recognized behavior rating scales of assessing the function of behavior.

Interviews are another indirect method used in conducting a functional behavior assessment. In the handbook for conducting a functional assessment O'Neill, Horner, Albin, Sprague, Storey, and Newton (1999) provide a tool for conducting a structured interview called the *Functional Assessment Interview*. They teach that information should be obtained in the context in which the challenging behavior occurs. This approach emphasizes the specific context of behavior. Information should be obtained not only from the person displaying the behavior, but, depending on the circumstances in which the behavior occurs, interviews may occur with numerous people who know the person well in order to gain a thorough assessment. Information should be collected on what specifically the behavior looks like, how frequently it occurs, how long it lasts, and how intensely it is displayed. Identifying patterns in the occurrence of the behavior is important for prediction.

A systematic review of school records can be useful in identifying important information for a functional behavior analysis. The School Archival Records Search (SARS) can be a valuable tool for systematically quantifying and analyzing information contained in school records (Walker, Block-Pedego, Todis, & Severson, 1991). This method may be particularly important for low frequency behaviors that are not easily observed directly.

Direct (Descriptive) Methods

The direct (or descriptive) observation of maladaptive behaviors in naturalistic settings is one of the hallmarks of the FBA (Gresham, Watson, & Skinner, 2001b). Most direct observation methods stress the assessment of objective features of behavior. Features such as frequency, temporality, intensity, and permanent products (Gresham, 1985) allow the clinician to record the events immediately before and following the maladaptive behavior. This Antecedent-Behavior-Consequence analysis is used to form hypotheses about what may be maintaining the problematic target behavior. A student may throw paper (maladaptive behavior) on the floor every time his teacher talks to another student (antecedent) – the teacher may then react with a verbal reprimand (consequence). One possible hypothesis in this situation could be that the purpose (or function) of the student's behavior is to gain his teacher's attention. Depending on the nature of the target behavior, the clinician chose to employ an event-based recording strategy (for discrete behaviors with a definite beginning and a definite end) or an interval-recording strategy (for continuous behaviors). In time-based recording measures, the duration (and not its frequency) of the maladaptive behavior is of interest (Gresham et al., 2001b).

Experimental/Traditional Functional Assessment

The experimental functional assessment relies on a systematic variation in environmental conditions in order to isolate the function of the maladaptive behavior. The therapist may modify the physical or social environment in an attempt to alter the frequency of the maladaptive behavior (Herzinger & Campbell, 2006). This will allow the clinician to determine why the maladaptive behavior occurs.

The first standardized method for conducting a functional assessment was designed by Iwata, Dorsey, Slifer, Bauman, and Richman (1994). In their study, all participants showed some degree of a developmental delay, and each person had a documented history of engaging in self-injurious behavior. The researchers created four different treatment conditions believed to be analogous to "real-life" conditions: social disapproval, academic demand, unstructured play, and alone. In order to determine the function of the self-injurious behavior, each participant was randomly exposed to all four conditions.

In the first condition, the child was asked to play with toys. Every time the individual engaged in self-injury, (s)he was told, "Stop that," followed by brief physical contact of a non-punitive nature (hands on shoulder). This first condition was conceptualized as being similar to parents disapproving of their child's behavior while at the same time being more involved with their child at/or around the time of self-injury. Frankel and Simmons (1976) found that in natural environments, self-injury often results in parents given undue attention to their child at the *wrong* time. Consequently, parents or caretakers were often inadvertently reinforcing maladaptive behaviors.

In second condition, the child was directed to complete tasks such as putting a wooden puzzle together. This condition was viewed as replicating any situation during which a caretaker places a demand on a child. Every time the child self-injured, the child was allowed to discontinue working on his/her assigned task. Here, the researchers hypothesized that the self-injurious behavior is maintained as a result of an aversive task being successfully avoided (Carr, 1977; Carr, Newsome, & Binkoff, 1976).

In the third condition, the child was given ample access to toys. The child was given no instructions on what to do but received social praise following appropriate behavior (absence of self-injurious behavior). Self-injurious behavior, on the other hand, was ignored. This condition mirrored an enriched environment (Horner, 1980), in which the

parent deliberately praises adaptive behavior and ignores the maladaptive behavior.

The fourth condition was designed to approximate environments in which the child is basically left alone without access to toys or social contact (impoverished environment). Here, the self-injurious behavior may occur as an attempt to self-produce reinforcement of a sensory nature in the absence of a stimulating environment (Rincover, 1978). As the researcher/clinician compares rates of self-injurious behavior across these conditions, a conclusion as to why the behavior occurs can be drawn. If, for example, the child's rate of self-injury is highest when asked to complete a task, the researcher or clinician can reasonably conclude that the child self-injures in order to avoid aversive tasks.

One of the findings of Campbell's (2003) meta-analysis of 117 studies is that performing a pretreatment FBA increases treatment effectiveness. Similarly, Kahn, Iwata, and Lewin (2002) compared treatments based on FBAs to arbitrarily chosen ones and concluded that treatment based on FBAs are more effective. In 1997, these assessments were mandated by federal law as part of the amendments to the Individuals with Disabilities Education Act (IDEA) (Horner & Carr, 1997).

FBA is vital when selecting interventions for problem behavior. If one neglects this step in the process, several problems may present themselves. For example, the intervention selected may increase a problem behavior through inadvertent positive reinforcement. Also, the treatment may be functionally irrelevant to the problem behavior. Lastly, the treatment strategy may not provide alternative reinforcement for more appropriate behavior (Vollmer & Northup, 1996).

Training of Social Skills as Replacement Behaviors

Once a function is identified for the problem behavior, treatment should be based on one of two strategies: (1) weakening the maintaining reinforcement of the maladaptive response and (2) strengthening reinforcement for appropriate behavior that replaces the function of the maladaptive behavior (Mace, 1994). However, training social skills to children with problem behaviors, such as aggression, as replacement behaviors for these competing inappropriate behaviors may not only increase social skills and status but also reduce the dysfunctional response.

Results of functional behavior assessments should be closely examined to identify maintaining functions of challenging behaviors. This information should be helpful when selecting which treatment components to include when designing social skills interventions. For example, when problem behavior is identified as a form of communication, Carr and Durand (1985) suggest that clinicians may develop and implement more successful strategies to teach communication skills, in particular requests for some type of response from others. One technique that has been shown to be particularly effective in situations in which challenging behavior serves a communication function is functional communication training (FCT). FCT has often been used in studies with individuals with developmental disabilities to decrease challenging behavior and increase pro-social behaviors (Casey & Merical, 2006). For example, one study found that when FCT was used to train an 11-year-old boy with autism how to communicate, "I need a break", the self-injurious behavior was eliminated. Gains were maintained at 5, 12, and 24-month follow-ups (Casey & Merical, 2006). Similarly, using this intervention, Bird, Dores, Moniz, and Robinson (1989) reduced severe self-injury in two men with profound mental retardation.

When implementing FCT, there are a few variables to consider that are essential to the success of this intervention. These variables include the following: training the participant in a replacement behavior that is equivalent to the problem behavior, not just a socially appropriate act (Carr & Durand, 1985), replacement behavior must be more efficient (result in reinforcement more easily) than the challenging behavior (Horner, Sprague, O'Brien, & Heathfield, 1990), and treatment package should also include such techniques as extinction and redirection (Wacker et al., 1990).

Choice making may be another component that may be effectively utilized when developing social skills training protocols. Researchers have demonstrated that choice reduces behavioral challenges and increases learning through avoidance of aversive situations and access to larger rewards (Reid & Parson, 1991). When people have choices regarding their treatment they are more likely to be satisfied, thereby more likely to participate. Bannerman, Sheldon, Sherman, and Harchik (1990) suggest teaching preferred functional skills and using preferred methods of reinforcement. Making choices (whether real or perceived) promotes a personal sense of value that is likely to result in motivation; therefore, choice making may be useful to include in treatment packages which focus on social skills performance deficits.

Social skills training in conjunction with behavioral interventions are frequently used to prevent and treat many emotional and behavioral problems (Spence, 2003). Many different methods of instruction have been used to train social skills in the past. The following review will include information regarding the effectiveness of behavioral social skills training, cognitive interventions, and multimodal interventions in increasing social skills and reducing problem behaviors.

Behavioral Social Skills Training

Behavioral social skills packages often use techniques such as verbal instructions, modeling, behavioral rehearsal, role-play, and feedback/reinforcement. Studies have found mixed success for behavioral social skills interventions. A study conducted by Gresham, Bao Van, and Cook (2006) used behavioral social skills training (60 hours over 20 weeks) and differential reinforcement of other behavior (DRO) with a group of children chosen based on their social skill acquisition deficits. Large decreases in competing problem behaviors and improvements in social skills were noted. Maintenance effects were found in a 2-month follow-up for some target behaviors. Bulkeley and Cramer (1990) conducted a social skills training with nine subjects utilizing role-playing, positive reinforcement, and homework assignments for generalization. Participants were found to show improvements on teacher-rated and self-rated social skills questionnaire. However, there were no significant differences in peer nominations pre to post intervention. Other studies have found that behavioral interventions for social skills have shown short-term effectiveness for specific social skill responses (Gresham, 1985; McIntosh, Vaughn, & Zaragoza, 1991; Spence, 2003).

Schneider (1992) conducted a meta-analysis of didactic techniques used to improve peer relations of children. A moderate treatment effect for the interventions reviewed was noted. Withdrawn participants showed better outcomes from interventions than participants demonstrating aggression or participants lacking a diagnosis related to atypical behavior. However, a small effect size was found for aggressive populations though children with aggression may be less responsive than other populations. Modeling and coaching did demonstrate higher effect sizes than social-cognitive techniques or multi-component interventions; nonetheless, results of a multiple regression failed to show training technique as significant predictor of treatment outcome.

In another meta-analysis, Magee Quinn, Kavale, Mathur, Rutherford, and Forness (1999) examined social skills interventions for students with emotional or behavioral disorders. Results found that students showed only modest gains equaling about 8 percentile ranks on outcome measures. Additional analyses in this study found that variables such as duration of intervention and research quality did not significantly influence these results. However, interventions were found to be slightly more effective in improving prosocial skills. Disruptive behavior and aggression were the behaviors most resistant to change by social skills training.

Some meta-analyses have documented the positive effect of self-control training with externalizing behavior, such as aggression (Baer & Nietzel, 1991; Beelmann, Pfingsten, & Lösel, 1994). However, behavioral training has been more effective with socially withdrawn children. These children with externalizing behavior may not respond as well to multimodal interventions due to their emphasis on cognitive components (Beelmann et al., 1994). In addition, other researchers have (Hollinger, 1987) found that the combination of modeling, coaching, and reinforcement procedures (all behavioral components) were found to be the most effective techniques used in social skills training.

Social Stories

Social stories are another intervention that has shown success in training social skills. Social stories were originated by Carol Gray (Gray & Garand, 1993). Social stories are used to provide children with information about appropriate responses to various social situations that may be problematic for them. There have been several studies that found improvements in selected social skills following implementation of social stories for children with autism. In one study, three participants with autism increased appropriate social interactions during a free play period. Two of the three participants demonstrated improvements from baseline to intervention (7–39%; 13–28%). The participant who did not improve had a lower IQ than the other two children. In addition, this participant's peers were sometimes nonresponsive to his social initiations which may have served to inhibit appropriate social behavior (Scattone, Tingstrom, & Wilczynski, 2006). Similarly, Swaggert and Gagnon (1995) used social stories to teach three children with autism appropriate social behavior. The first participant increased appropriate social interactions from 7% at baseline to 74% after the social story intervention. An additional response cost-social story intervention was developed to treat the target behavior of aggression. Improvements in aggression were noted following implementation. The second participant's aggressive behavior was decreased from 30 to 6% and sharing behavior increased from 0 to 22%. The third participant's parallel play increased from 80 to 90% of sessions and sharing behavior improved from 0 to 35% over sessions.

Barry and Burlew (2004) conducted a study that used social stories to increase the choice and play skills of two children with autism. Both participants needed less prompting in choice making during intervention phases. In addition, one participant made substantial increases in the duration of intervals engaged in play with peers. Reynhout and Carter (2007) implemented a social story in order to decrease repetitive tapping of an eight-year-old boy with autism. During the final phase of the study, the boy's tapping behavior decreased as his comprehension of the social story increased.

Some advantages of using social stories as an intervention include simplicity, convenience, and low cost. However, social stories may not be an appropriate choice when participants are lower functioning (Scattone et al., 2006). Social stories may be best utilized as an adjunct to such interventions such as differential reinforcement schedules and other behavioral techniques particularly for children with both social deficits and challenging behaviors.

Cognitive-Based Programs

Some studies have identified cognitive factors that are involved in children's challenging behavior. For example, Keltikangas-Järvinen (2001) reported that aggressive students applied aggressive strategies systematically over different social situations in all steps of problem solving; however, sociable students consistently used more constructive and prosocial strategies. Some treatment protocols are utilizing popular behavioral methods and adding a cognitive component to further enhance social skills training. For example, Verduyn, Lord, and Forrest (1990) studied effects of an intervention which combined didactic instruction with behavioral rehearsal, problem solving, and homework assignments. The treatment group significantly improved in social activity based on parental report of social behavior. Effects were maintained at 6-month follow-up. A significant improvement in self-esteem was noted for the younger age group. However, overall, the efficacy of cognitive-behavioral treatment components (e.g., social problem solving & self-instruction) was much weaker than for other intervention components (Ager & Cole, 1991; Gresham, 1985).

Some programs rely solely on cognitive methods of training social skills. Vaughn, Ridley, and Bullock (1984) found that aggressive children who received interpersonal problem-solving training program showed significant gains in skills, following the intervention and at 3- month follow-up, compared to controls. At posttest and follow-up, the experimental group in this study showed an increase in the number of alternative solutions generated for an interpersonal problem with a peer and were more likely to produce relevant responses during the problem-solving task compared to their counterparts.

Studies utilizing samples of aggressive children and adolescents have noted that cognitively based interventions may improve behavior in a number of settings, including the home, school, and community. Results have been maintained up to 1 year following treatment (Kazdin, Esveldt- Dawson, French, & Unis, 1987; Lochman, Phillips, & Barry, 2003). Other researchers have found only weak effects of cognitive treatments on child aggression (Weissberg, Cowen, Lotyczewski, & Gesten, 1983). In order to clarify these findings, further investigation is needed on the effects of cognitive treatments with children and adolescents who demonstrate aggression and other challenging behaviors.

Multimodal Interventions

Some interventions have utilized multiple treatment components when designing social skills training protocols. Spence (2003) noted that social skills training was found to have an insignificant impact on psychopathology or global markers of social competence; however, social skills training is an acceptable component in multimodal methods of treatment of various emotional, behavioral, and developmental disorders. One multimodal intervention is the Social Skills Group Intervention (S. S. GRIN) which was described in a study by DeRosier (2004). This intervention includes social learning and cognitive-behavioral techniques. This package combines didactic instruction and active practice of skills using techniques such as modeling, role-playing, and hands-on activities. Children with peer problems who received this treatment showed increases in self-esteem, social self-efficacy, and decreased social anxiety over time compared to controls. Aggressive children who participated in the treatment reported decreased bullying behavior and antisocial affiliations over the school year compared to controls. The program was also found to benefit boys and girls equally.

A multimodal program called Aggression Replacement Training (ART) has been designed to reduce aggression in participants by utilizing social skills training, anger control techniques, and moral reasoning skills (Reddy & Goldstein, 2001). The first phase of the program uses Skills Streaming, which utilizes behavioral components such as modeling, role-play, praise, and feedback to instruct participants on prosocial skills. The second phase includes Anger Control Training (ACT) which includes instruction regarding triggers of anger, cues of arousal, strategies to reduce anger, reminders or self-statements to decrease anger, and self-evaluation. The third phase includes Moral Education Training which is characterized by training skills used in the resolution of cognitive conflict (Reddy & Goldstein, 2001). There have been a few studies testing the effects of this intervention. For example, ART was studied with a group of children with various degrees of behavioral problems in Norway. The treatment group evinced improved social skills and decreased challenging behavior at posttest (Gundersen & Svartdal, 2006). One study using a sample of juveniles incarcerated at a detention center assigned participants to a group receiving either 10 weeks of ART, or brief instructions control group, and/or no treatment. ART participants, compared to other groups, significantly acquired and transferred 4 of 10 Skill Streaming skills. Also, ART participants demonstrated less and lower intensity acting out behaviors than participants in either control group. Of those participating in ART that were later released from the detention center, these youth were rated significantly higher in community functioning in the domains of home, family, peer, and legal compared to their counterparts not receiving this treatment program (Goldstein & Glick, 1987). A similar study was conducted with adolescents at a maximum security youth center. As with the previous study, participants in the ART group transferred more streaming skills (e.g., 5 out of 10) than the other groups. The ART group in this study also showed improvements in moral reasoning compared to the other groups. In addition, a community-based study used a sample of adolescents who had been released from juvenile detention. The three groups in which participants were assigned included an ART group provided to adolescents and their parents, ART group with adolescents alone, and no treatment control. Results noted participants in both ART groups differed significantly in interpersonal skill competence and reported feeling less angry than the control group Goldstein, Glick, Irwin, Pask, & Rubama, (1989).

It should be noted that younger children may respond better to monomodal programs compared to multimodal programs. Since monomodal programs are more simplistic they place more emphasis on a certain skill set which may accelerate the development and learning of those specific skills. The integration of cognitive components of training often included in multimodal treatment packages may be more beneficial to older children (Beelmann et al., 1994). For example, Durlak, Fuhrman, and Lampman (1991) conducted a meta-analysis that children with maladaptive behavior treated with cognitive-behavioral therapy showed effect sizes twice as high when used with 11–13-year-olds compared with younger children.

Replacement Behavior Training

In examining the social skills training literature, problems often cited include poor generalization and maintenance of skills, modest effect sizes, and lack of data regarding social validity of target behavior selection. Considering these shortcomings in past literature, Maag (2005) recommended that replacement behavior training (RBT) may assist in addressing some of these issues. RBT is based on the concept of functional analysis of behavior. The goal of this intervention is to identify social behaviors that serve the same function as a problem behavior. For example, if a functional behavioral assessment was conducted with a child who demonstrated aggression, and the function of this behavior was determined to be social attention from peers and teacher; the RBT approach would select a social skill, such as shaking hands that would address the same function. In addition, Gresham and Elliott (1991) suggested that differential reinforcement schedules of other behaviors (DRO) should be implemented to increase the incidence of the new social skills and decrease the incidence of the competing problem behavior. It is important to collect baseline data on both problem behaviors and replacement behaviors, in this case social skills, in order to monitor progress on the intervention chosen. If problem behavior is not treated by teaching replacement behaviors, studies have found that youths are not likely to achieve growth in environments outside of the controlled classroom setting (Maag & Kemp, 2003; Neel & Cessna, 1993). This lack of generalization has been noted repeatedly in studies of traditional social skills training studies (Maag, 2005).

One major challenge in implementing replacement behavior training is in identifying what skill will function best for the child. This task begins with identifying a response class defined as a group of behaviors that share the same topography, consequences of reinforcement and punishment, or share the same function. Replacement behaviors that are characterized by the same topography as the problem behavior are more likely to be adopted and utilized (Maag & Kemp, 2003). In addition, a list of possible replacement behaviors is often generated by the following methods: observing high-status peers to determine what behaviors they use to obtain positive outcomes, the target participants are asked what they would like to try, and adults who are most familiar with the child are interviewed to identify appropriate behaviors they have seen the participant demonstrate to obtain positive outcomes. The final list is created from all of these sources, and the participant ranks the behaviors according to desirability. Next, the participant is assessed to determine what skill deficits he/she possesses so that an appropriate intervention can be selected to address these deficits. Lastly, a reinforcement system is implemented to motivate the participant to utilize the replacement behaviors selected. Eventually, the goal of the RBT is to have the replacement behaviors become self-reinforcing for the child, since these behaviors are delivering desired outcomes. When this occurs, the reinforcement system may be faded out and generalization achieved (Maag, 2005).

A couple of studies examining RBT with aggression were identified. Barry and Singer (2001) taught a 10-year-old boy with autism to replace aggressive behavior with social, play, and caregiving skills. The investigators conducted a functional assessment and found that aggression was motivated by access to his younger sibling. These replacement behaviors were taught by using methods such as task analysis, verbal prompting, verbal reinforcement, error correction, and modeling. There was a decrease in aggression toward the younger sibling post intervention. In addition, Kern, Ringdahl, Hilt, and Sterling-Turner (2001) taught three boys who demonstrated aggression how to perform replacement behaviors (requesting attention, break, and tangible items) by self-monitoring. A functional assessment was conducted for both participants and motivating factors for aggression were identified. Replacement behaviors were selected to address these functions, and results found that problem behavior decreased to zero for two participants, and significant decreases were noted for the other participant.

Methodological Limitations

Many studies of social skills interventions indicate little correspondence between the behaviors that have been assessed as deficits and the behaviors being taught in the interventions (Gresham, Cook, & Crews, 2004). For example, Magee Quinn et al. (1999) conducted a meta-analysis and stated that the studies included used "commercially available social skills interventions." These programs teach behaviors that may or may not be assessed as deficits of the participants. Similarly, Gresham et al. (2001a) recommended that interventions target the type of social deficit, skill vs. performance, which the individual child shows, in order to achieve maximum success. Hughes and Sullivan (1988) noted that many studies of social skills interventions do not include a pretreatment level of skill performance before the implementation of interventions. However, one study assessed participants for skill acquisition deficits prior to inclusion in the intervention group (Gresham et al., 2006). This study registered larger effects post-intervention (Gresham et al., 2006) compared to several meta-analyses (Magee Quinn et al., 1999; Mathur, Kavale, Magee Quinn, & Forness, 1998), which only found small-to-moderate effect sizes for social skills interventions.

Another consideration in evaluating studies of social skill training is the reliability and validity of outcome measures that are used. For example, Bulkeley and Cramer (1990) used a social skills questionnaire intended specifically for their study; but no psychometric information was reported. Other studies have also employed methods of measuring social outcomes that have not been psychometrically validated for such purposes. Jamison, Lambert, and McCloud (1986) used voice loudness and Yu, Harris, Solovitz, and Franklin (1986) utilized a subtest from an intelligence test as social outcome measures.

Studies that use direct observations to assess social outcomes also may have questionable reliability and validity (Gresham et al., 2004).

Role-play measures may yield inflated estimates of effectiveness. These types of measures may have questionable validity (Gresham, 1986). Some speculate that role-play assessments assess a participant's knowledge of social skill rather than their behavior in social situations; therefore, a change in behavior may be demonstrated through observation in advance of a change manifested in improved peer or teacher perceptions of the participant. In addition, Gresham (1985) states that outcome measures need to be more socially and clinically valid.

Group assignment to treatment can be based on a child's "unpopularity" which is a more subjective criteria for inclusion. Therefore, it is not clear whether some of the children included in treatment groups actually have deficits regarding target social skills under study. For example, peer nominations are often used to assign children to groups in studies of social skills interventions. These nominations are measures of a child's acceptance or rejection by peers. It is hard to identify specific target social skills that may lead to peer acceptance or rejection. In addition, lack of treatment effects in these studies may be due to the rigidity of peer expectations and stereotypes. For example, any benefits of social skills interventions may not be salient enough to dispel peer attitudes toward rejected children (Bierman, Miller, & Stabb, 1987). Peer and teacher ratings of children's social skills are often utilized as dependent variables in social skills training studies. This method, therefore, relies on the natural occurrence of the behaviors of interest.

Future Directions

Although research on social skills training is plentiful, it is not without flaws. Future research should attempt to address these deficiencies, expand samples used, and investigate individual treatment components. Gresham et al. (2001a) made a number of recommendations regarding how to improve social skills interventions. It was recommended that social skills training be implemented more frequently and intensely than conventional standards. Therefore, future studies should

examine descriptive information concerning the length of the training program and the relationship between length of intervention and treatment effectiveness (Bellini et al., 2007). For example, Gresham et al. (2006) used a 60-hour, 20-week protocol and found larger effects than several meta-analyses (Magee Quinn et al., 1999; Mathur et al., 1998), which included studies with interventions of much shorter duration that noted only small-to-moderate effect sizes. Similarly, McIntosh et al. (1991) noted a relationship between amount of social skills training received and treatment effects.

In a meta-analysis of the effects of social competence training by Beelmann et al. (1994), results showed that these interventions were moderately effective, but long-term effects were weak. Therefore, more longitudinal studies need to be conducted to examine long-term effects and lack thereof. Gresham et al. (2001a) also noted a major weakness of social skills interventions of maintenance and generalization effects. For example, Sawyer et al. (1997) found that children receiving the Rochester program showed some positive effects post-intervention, but results were not maintained at the 1-year follow-up assessment.

Implementation of these programs in more in vivo settings was also recommended by Gresham et al. (2001a). Bellini et al. (2007) conducted a meta-analysis of social skills training in the school setting with children with autism spectrum disorder, which pointed out that maintenance and generalization effects were significantly lower for interventions that were implemented in pullout settings outside the typical classroom. Interventions taking place in the typical classroom not only showed higher generalization across participants, settings, and play stimuli but also higher intervention effects. Therefore, future studies should also be designed to investigate identical training programs in multiple settings to examine which setting shows the highest treatment outcomes. Further recommendations for future studies include designing studies with greater attention to training content, incorporating longer follow-up periods, and investigating the degree to which treatment protocols are actually being correctly implemented (Schneider, 1992).

Many social skills treatment programs are designed for group implementation. According to Magee Quinn et al. (1999), individualized instruction may show better outcomes than group-designed protocols. The fit of the intervention is important, as well as the perceived value of the skills being trained to each student. Schneider and Bryne (1987), however, found that individualized social skills training did not show significantly different effects compared with a nonindividualized intervention.

A meta-analysis by Scruggs and Mastropieri (1998) noted that social skills training showed the lowest treatment effects with preschool groups compared to elementary and secondary students. It has been noted that younger children seem to respond better to monomodal programs compared to multimodal programs (Beelmann et al., 1994). Therefore, researchers may want to investigate this issue further by comparing different interventions with younger populations or testing the effects of modifying current treatment protocols with younger populations.

Since most studies involving social skills interventions include mixed gender samples, it is difficult to draw conclusions about the gender effects of these interventions. There are very few studies of female-only samples. Future studies may include gender- specific issues (Beelmann et al., 1994).

In addition, it may be useful for more studies to utilize attention-placebo control groups. Frequently, social skills training in school settings is done after removing the child/children from their regular school schedule and placing them in small group environments outside of the classroom. The mere act of removing these children from their regular setting may impact how their peers interact with them. In addition, receiving direct positive attention from an adult regularly outside of the classroom setting may also influence that child's social skill set. (Gresham, 1985). Studies with attention-placebo control groups would assist in removing this as a confound.

Because so many of the intervention packages studied utilize several components (modeling, role-playing, problem solving, etc.), it is difficult to identify which components of these treatments are responsible for effects on outcome variables (Gresham, 1985). Therefore, studies which compare the effects of each treatment component would be beneficial in determining which components account for the most behavior change.

Further research should be focused on studying the effects of social skills interventions with samples of children who display challenging behaviors, such as aggression. For example, aggression has been found in the past to be resistant to change (Schneider, 1992). However, special consideration should be taken when designing such studies. Since some children, particularly aggressive children, often associate with peers that share their characteristics (Cairns et al., 1988; Pellegrini, 1998), it may be beneficial to include the peer group as a target for intervention in further research. For example, Vaughn, Lancelotta, and Minnis (1988) conducted a study with a girl with a learning disability. Researchers focused their efforts on assessment, intervention, and outcome evaluation surrounding a significant peer group. Gains in peer status group scores at posttest were significant and were maintained over 12 months which is much longer than other studies have achieved. Focusing on a target peer group promotes entrapment which involves employing communities of reinforcement (McConnell, 1987) in which peers reinforce the participant for performing the target skill. Considering these methods, changes in variables in peer status may be more attainable.

Future studies should also explore the causal relationship between problem behaviors and social skills deficits to determine whether challenging behaviors interfere with the development of social skills or whether children who lack social skills develop challenging behaviors as replacement behaviors. Such an investigation would shed light on what type of treatment approach would be more successful (Matson et al., 2006). Furthermore, studies which incorporated results from a functional assessment of behavior into the design and implementation of social skills training may be beneficial in increasing treatment effects of these interventions with samples of children with challenging behavior.

Conclusion

Research has consistently shown a relationship between social skills deficits and challenging behaviors (Campbell et al., 2006; Matson et al., 2006; 1998). Although, treatment studies have shown short-term effects for social skills interventions (Beelmann et al., 1994), further efforts are needed to modify protocols such as to improve generalization of skills (Gresham et al., 2001a). Further studies need to explore social skills interventions with populations of children with aggressive behavior since some research notes that these samples may be more resistant to change (Schneider, 1992). The role of functional behavior assessment needs to be explored in enhancing the effects of social skills interventions by investigating the function of challenging behaviors and selecting the appropriate replacement behaviors to serve as social skills targets (Maag, 2005).

References

Ager, C., & Cole, C. (1991). A review of cognitive-behavioral interventions for children and adolescents with behavioral disorders. *Behavioral Disorders, 16*, 276–287.

American Psychiatric Association. (2000). *Diagnostic and statistical manual of mental disorders* (4th ed., txt rev.). Washington, DC: Author.

Asarnow, J. R., & Bates, S. (1988). Depression in child psychiatric inpatients: Cognitive and attributional patterns. *Journal of Abnormal Child Psychology, 16*, 601–616.

Baer, R., & Nietzel, M. (1991). Cognitive and behavioral treatment of impulsivity in children: A meta-analytic review of the outcome literature. *Journal of Clinical Child Psychology, 20*, 400–412.

Bannerman, D. J., Sheldon, J. B., Sherman, J. A., & Harchik, A. E. (1990). Balancing the right of habilitation with the right to personal liberties: The rights of people with developmental disabilities to eat too many doughnuts and take a nap. *Journal of Applied Behavior Analysis, 23*, 79–89.

Barkley, R. A., Fischer, M., Smallish, L., & Fletcher, K. (2004). Young adult follow-up of hyperactive children: Antisocial activities and drug use. *Journal of Child Psychology and Psychiatry, 45*, 195–211.

Barry, L. M., & Burlew, S. B. (2004). Using social stories to teach choice and play skills to children with autism. *Focus on Autism and Other Developmental Disabilities, 19*, 45–51.

Barry, L. M., & Singer, G. (2001). A family in crisis: Replacing the aggressive behavior of a child with autism toward an infant sibling. *Journal of Positive Behavior Interventions, 3*, 28–38.

Beelmann, A., Pfingsten, U., & Lösel, F. (1994). Effects of training social competence in children: A meta-analysis of recent evaluation studies. *Journal of Clinical Child Psychology, 23*, 260–271.

Bellini, S. (2003). Social skill deficits and anxiety in high-functioning adolescents with autism spectrum disorder. *Focus on Autism and Other Developmental Disorders, 19*, 78–86.

Bellini, S. (2006). The development of social anxiety in adolescents with autism spectrum disorders. *Focus on Autism and Other Developmental Disorders, 21*, 138–145.

Bellini, S., Peters, J., Benner, L., & Hopf, A. (2007). A meta-analysis of school-based social skills interventions for children with autism spectrum disorders. *Remedial and Special Education, 28*, 153–162.

Berkowitz, L., & Frodi, A. (1977). Stimulus characteristics that can enhance or decrease aggression: Associations with prior positive or negative reinforcements for aggression. *Aggressive Behavior, 3*, 1–15.

Bierman, K., Miller, C., & Stabb, S. (1987). Improving the social behavior and peer acceptance of rejected boys: Effects of social skill training with instructions and prohibitions. *Journal of Consulting and Clinical Psychology, 55*, 194–200.

Bird, F., Dores, P., Moniz, D., & Robinson, J. (1989). Reducing severe aggressive and self-injurious behaviors with functional communication training. *American Journal of Mental Retardation, 4*, 37–48.

Bulkeley, R., & Cramer, D. (1990). Social skills training with young adolescents. *Journal of Youth & Adolescence, 19*, 451–463.

Cairns, R., Cairns, B., Neckerman, H. Gest, S., & Gariépy, J. (1988). Social networks and aggressive behavior: Peer support or peer rejection. *Developmental Psychology, 24*, 815–823.

Campbell, J. (2003) Efficacy of behavioral interventions for reducing problem behaviors in persons with autism: A quantitative synthesis of single subject research. *Research in Developmental Disabilities, 24*, 120–138.

Campbell, S., Spieker, S., Burchinal, M., Poe, M., & The NICHD Early Child Care Research Network. (2006). Trajectories of aggression from toddlerhood to age 9 academic and social functioning through age 12. *Journal of Child Psychology and Psychiatry, 47*, 791–80.

Carr, E. G. (1977). The motivation of self-injurious behavior: A review of some hypotheses. *Psychological Bulletin, 84*, 800–816.

Carr, E. G. (1994). Emerging themes in the functional analysis of problem behavior. *Journal of Applied Behavior Analysis, 27*, 393–399.

Carr, E. G., & Durand, V. M. (1985). Reducing behavior problems through functional communication training. *Journal of Applied Behavior Analysis, 18*, 111–126.

Carr, E. G., Newsome, C. D., & Binkoff, J. A. (1976). Stimulus control of self-destructive behavior in a psychotic child. *Journal of Abnormal Child Psychology, 4*, 139–152.

Casey, S., & Merical, C. (2006). The use of functional communication training without additional treatment procedures in an inclusive school setting. *Behavioral Disorders, 32*, 46–54.

Chang, L. (2003). Variable effects of children's aggression, social withdrawal, and prosocial leadership as functions of teacher beliefs and behaviors. *Child Development, 74*, 535–548.

Chung, H. L., & Steinberg, L. (2006). Relations between neighborhood factors, parenting behaviors, peer deviance, and delinquency among serious juvenile offenders. *Developmental Psychology, 42*, 319–331.

Coie, J., Terry, R., Lenox, K., & Lochman, J. (1995). Childhood peer rejection and aggression as predictors of stable patterns of adolescent disorder. *Development and Psychopathology, 7*, 697–713.

Cone, J. D. (1978). The behavioral assessment grid (BAG): A conceptual framework and taxonomy. *Behavior Therapy, 9*, 882–888.

Dekker, M. C., Koot, H. M., van der Ende, J., & Verhurst, F.C. (2002). Emotional and behavioral problems in children and adolescents with and without intellectual disability. *Journal of Child Psychology and Psychiatry, 43*, 1087–1098.

DeRosier, M. (2004). Building relationships and combating bullying: Effectiveness of a school-based social skills group intervention. *Journal of Clinical Child and Adolescent Psychology, 33*, 196–201.

de Ruiter, K. P., Dekker, M. C., Verhurst, F. C., & Koot, H. M. (2007). Developmental course of psychopathology in youths with and without intellectual disabilities. *Journal of Child Psychology and Psychiatry, 48*, 498–507.

Dodge, K. (1983). Behavioral antecedents of peer social status. *Child Development, 54*, 1386–1399.

Dodge, K. (1985). Attributional bias in aggressive children. In: P. Kendall (Ed.), *Advances in cognitive-behavioral research and therapy* (Vol. 4, pp. 73–110). San Diego, CA: Academic Press.

Douma, J. C., Dekker, M. C., de Ruiter, K., Tick, N., & Koot, H. (2007). Antisocial and delinquent behaviors in youths with mild or borderline disabilities. *American Journal on Mental Retardation, 112*, 207–220.

Duncan, D., Matson, J. L., Bamburg, J. W., Cherry, K. E., & Buckley, T. (1999). The relationship of self-injurious behavior and aggression to social skills in persons with severe and profound learning disability. *Research in Developmental Disabilities, 20*, 441–448.

Durand, V. M., & Crimmins, D. B. (1992). *The motivation assessment scale (MAS) administration guide.* Topeka, KS: Monaco and Associates.

Durlak, J., Fuhrman, T., & Lampman, C. (1991). Effectiveness of cognitive-behavior therapy for maladapting children: A meta-analysis. *Psychological Bulletin, 110*, 204–214.

Dykens, E. M. (2000). Psychopathology in children with intellectual disability. *Journal of Child and Psychiatry, 41*, 407–417.

Dyson, L. (2003). Children with learning disabilities within the family context: a comparison with siblings in global self-concept, academic, self-perceptions, and social competence. *Learning Disabilities Research and Practice, 18*, 1–9.

Emerson, E. (2003). Prevalence of psychiatric disorders in children and adolescents with and without intellectual disability. *Journal of Intellectual Disability Research, 47*, 51–58.

Emerson E., Kiernan, C., Alborz, A., Reeves, D., Mason, H., Swarbrick, R., et al. (2001). The prevalence of challenging behaviors: A total population study. *Research in Developmental Disabilities, 22*, 77–93.

Erdley, C., & Asher, S. (1999). A social goals perspective on children's social competence. *Journal of Emotional and Behavioral Disorders, 7*, 156–167.

Farmer, T., & Hollowell, J. (1994). Social networks in mainstream classrooms: Social affiliations and behavioral characteristics of students with EBD. *Journal of Emotional and Behavioral Disorders, 2*, 143–155.

Frankel, F., & Simmons, J. (1976). Self-Injurious Behavior in Schizophrenic and Retarded Children. *American Journal of Mental Deficiency, 80*, 512–22.

Fussell, J., Macias, M., & Saylor, C. (2005). Social skills and behavior problems in children with disabilities with and without siblings. *Child Psychiatry & Human Development, 36*, 227–241.

Garber, J., Weiss, B., & Shanley, N. (1993). Cognitions, depressive symptoms, and development in adolescents. *Journal of Abnormal Psychology, 102*, 47–57.

Goldstein, A., & Glick, B. (1987). *Aggression replacement training: A comprehensive intervention for aggressive youth.* Champaign, IL: Research Press.

Goldstein, A., Glick, B., Irwin, M., Pask, C., & Rubama, I. (1989). *Reducing delinquency: Intervention in the community.* New York: Pergamon Press.

Gray, C., & Garand, J. (1993). Social stories: Improving responses of students with autism with accurate social information. *Focus on Autistic Behavior, 8*, 1–10.

Gresham, F. M. (1985). Behavior disorder assessment: Conceptual, definitional, and practical considerations. *School Psychology Review, 14*, 495–509.

Gresham, F. (1986). Conceptual issues in the assessment of social competence in children. In P. S. Strain, M. J. Guralnick, & H. M. Walker (Eds.), *Children's social behavior: Development, assessment and modification* (pp. 143–179). Orlando, FL: Academic Press.

Gresham, F. (1997). Social competence and students with behavior disorders: Where we've been, where we are, and where we should go. *Education & Treatment of Children, 20*, 233–249.

Gresham, F., Bao Van, M., & Cook, C. (2006). Social skills training for teaching replacement behaviors: Remediating acquisition deficits in at-risk students. *Behavioral Disorders, 31*, 363–377.

Gresham, F., Cook, C., & Crews, S. (2004). Social skills training for children and youth with emotional and behavioral disorders: Validity considerations and future directions. *Behavioral Disorders, 30*, 32–46.

Gresham, F., & Elliott, S. N. (1990). Social skills as a primary learning disability. *Journal of Learning Disabilities, 22*, 120–124.

Gresham, F. M., & Elliott, S. N. (1991). *Social skills rating system.* Circle Pines, MN: American Guidance Service.

Gresham, F. M., Sugai, G., & Horner, R. H. (2001a). Interpreting outcomes of social skills training for students with high-incidence disabilities. *The Council for Exceptional Children, 67*, 331–344.

Gresham, F. M., Watson, T. S., & Skinner, C. H. (2001b). Functional behavioral assessment: Principles, procedures, and future directions. *School Psychology Review, 2*, 156–172.

Gundersen, K., & Svartdal, F. (2006). Aggression replacement training in Norway: Outcome evaluation of 11 Norwegian student projects. *Scandinavian Journal of Educational Research, 50*, 63–81.

Hannesdottir, D. K., & Ollendick, T. H. (2007). Social cognition and social anxiety among Icelandic schoolchildren. *Child and Family behavior Therapy, 29*, 43–58.

Herzinger, C., & Campbell, J. (2006). Comparing functional assessment methodologies: A quantitative synthesis. *Journal of Autism and Developmental Disorder, 37*, 1430–1445.

Hollinger, J. (1987). Social skills for behaviorally disordered children as preparation for mainstreaming: Theory, practice, and new directions. *Remedial & Special Education*, 8, 17–27.

Horner, R. H. (1980). The effects of an environmental "enrichment" program on the behavior of institutionalized profoundly retarded children. *Journal of Applied Behavior Analysis*, 13, 473–491.

Horner, R. H., & Carr, E. G. (1997). Behavior support for students with severe disabilities: Functional assessment and comprehensive intervention. *Journal of Special Education*, 31, 84–104.

Horner, R., Sprague, J., O'Brien, M., & Heathfield, L. (1990). The role of response efficiency in the reduction of problem behaviors through functional equivalence training: A case study. *Journal of the Association for Personas with SevereHandicaps*, 15, 91–97.

Hughes, J., & Sullivan, K. (1988). Outcome assessment in social skills training with children. *Journal of School Psychology*, 26, 167–183.

Iwata, B. A., Dorsey, M. F., Slifer, K. J. Bauman, K. E., & Richman G. S. (1994). Toward a functional analysis of self-injury. *Journal of Applied Behavior Analysis*, 27, 197–209

Jamison, R., Lambert, E., & McCloud, D. (1986). Social skills training with hospitalized adolescents: An evaluative experiment. *Adolescence*, 21, 55–65.

Kahn, S., Iwata, B., & Lewin, A. (2002). The impact of functional assessment on the treatment of self-injurious behavior. In S. R. Schroeder. M. L. Oster-Granite, & T. Thompson (Eds.), *Self-injurious behavior: Gene-brain-behavior relationships* (pp. 119–131). Washington, DC: American Psychological Association.

Kauffman, J. M. (2004). *Characteristics of emotional and behavioral disorders of children* (8th ed.). Columbus, OH: Merrill-Prentice Hall.

Kazdin, A., Esveldt-Dawson, K., French, N., & Unis, A. (1987). Problem-solving skills training and relationship therapy in the treatment of antisocial child behavior. *Journal of Consulting and Clinical Psychology*, 55, 76–85.

Keltikangas-Järvinen, L. (2001). Aggressive behaviour and social problem-solving strategies: A review of the findings of a seven-year follow-up from childhood to late adolescence. *Criminal Behaviour and Mental Health*, 11, 236–250.

Kern, L., Ringdahl, J., Hilt, A., & Sterling-Turner, H. (2001), Linking self-management procedures to functional analysis results. *Behavioral Disorders*, 26, 214–226.

Kupersmidt, J., Griesler, P., DeRosier, M., Patterson, C., & Davis, P. (1995). Childhood aggression and peer relations in the context of family and neighborhood factors. *Child Development*, 66, 360–375.

Landau, S. L., Milich, R., & Diener, M. B. (1998). Peer relations of children with attention deficit hyperactivity disorder. *Reading and Writing Quarterly*, 14, 83–105.

Lochman, J., Phillips, N., & Barry, T. (2003). Aggressive and nonaggressive boys' physiological and cognitive processes in response to peer provocations. *Journal of Clinical Child and Adolescent Psychology*, 32, 568–576.

Lochman, J., & Wayland, K. (1994). Aggression, social acceptance, and race as predictors of negative adolescent outcomes. *Journal of the American Academy of Child & Adolescent Psychiatry*, 33, 1026–1035.

Maag, J. (2005). Social skills training for youth with emotional and behavioral disorders and learning disabilities: Problems, conclusions, and suggestions. *Exceptionality*, 13, 155–172.

Maag, J., & Kemp, S. (2003). Behavioral intent of power and affiliation: Implications for functional analysis. *Remedial and Special Education*, 24, 57–64.

Maag, J., & Webber, J. (1995). Promoting children's social development in general educational classrooms. *Preventing School Failure*, 39, 13–19.

Mace, F. (1994). The significance and future of functional analysis methodologies. *Journal of Applied Behavior Analysis*, 27, 385–392.

Magee Quinn, M., Kavale, K., Mathur, S., Rutherford, R., & Forness, S. (1999). A meta-analysis of social skill interventions for students with emotional or behavioral disorders. *Journal of Emotional and Behavioral Disorders*, 7, 54–64.

Mansell, J. A., Macdonald, B., & Beadle-Brown, J. (2002). Residential care in the community for adults with intellectual disabilities: Needs, characteristics and services. *Journal of Intellectual Disability Research*, 46, 625–633.

Margalit, M. (1989). Academic competence and social adjustment of boys with learning disabilities and boys with behavior disorders. *Journal of Learning Disabilities*, 22, 41–45.

Mathur, S., Kavale, K., Magee Quinn, M., & Forness, S. (1998). Social skills interventions with students with emotional and behavioral problems: A quantitative synthesis of single-subject research. *Behavioral Disorders*, 23, 193–201.

Matson, J. L. (1995a). *Manual for the Matson Evaluation of Social Skills in Individuals with Severe Retardation (MESSIER)*. Baton Rouge, Louisiana: Scientific Publishers Incorporated.

Matson, J. L. (1995b). *The Diagnostic Assessment for the Severely Handicapped Revised (DASH-II)*. Baton Rouge, LA: Disability Consultants, LLC.

Matson, J. L., Mayville, E. A., & Lott, J. D. (2002). The relationship between behaviour motivation and social functioning in persons with intellectual impairment. *British Journal of Clinical Psychology*, 41, 175–1184.

Matson, J. L., Minshawi, N. F., Gonzales, M. L., & Mayville, S. B. (2006). The relationship of comorbid problem behaviors to social skills in persons with profound mental retardation. *Behavior Modification*, 30, 496–506.

Matson, J. L., Smiroldo, B. B., & Bamburg, J. W. (1998). The relationship of social skills to psychopathology for individuals with severe or profound mental retardation. *Journal of Intellectual and Developmental Disability*, 23, 137–145.

Matson, J. L., & Vollmer, T. (1995). *User's guide Questions About Behavioral Function*. Baton Rouge, LA: Disability Consultants, LLC.

McConnell, S. (1987). Entrapment effects and the generalization and maintenance of social skills training for elementary school students with behavioral disorders. *Behavioral Disorders*, 12, 252–263.

McIntosh, R., Vaughn, S., & Zaragoza, N. (1991). A review of social interventions for students with learning disabilities. *Journal of Learning Disabilities*, 24, 451–458.

Mikami, A. Y., Huang-Pollock, C. L., Pfiffner, L. J., McBurnett, K., & Hangai, D. (2007). Social skills differences among Attention-Deficit/Hyperactivity disorder types in chat room assessment tasks. *Journal of Abnormal Child Psychology, 35*, 509–521.

Miller-Johnson, S., Cole, J., Maumary-Gremaud, A., Lochman, J., & Terry, R. (1999). Relationship between childhood peer rejection and aggression and adolescent delinquency severity and type among African American youth. *Journal of Emotional and Behavioral Disorders, 7*, 137–146.

Myers, S. M., & Plauche-Johnson, C. (2007). Management of children with autism spectrum disorders. *American Academy of Pediatrics, 120*, 11621182.

Neel, R., & Cessna, K. (1993). Behavioral intent: Instructional content of students with behaviour disorders. In K.K. Cessna (Ed.), *Instructionally differentiated programming: A needs-based approach for students with behavior disorders* (pp. 31–39). Denver, Colorado: Department of Education.

Ollendick, T. H., & Schimdt, C. R. (1987). Social learning constructs in the prediction of peer interaction. *Journal of Clinical Child Psychology, 16*, 80–87.

O'Neill, R., Horner, R. H., Albin, R. W., Sprague, J. E., Storey, K., & Newton, J. S. (1999). *Functional assessment and program development for problem behavior: A practical handbook* (2nd ed.). Pacific Grove, CA: Brooks/Cole.

Parkhurst, J. T., & Hopmeyer, A. (1998). Sociometric popularity and peer perceived popularity. Two distinct dimensions of peer status. *Journal of Early Adolescence, 18*, 125–144.

Patterson, G., Reid, J., & Dishion, T. (1992). *Antisocial boys.* Eugene, OR: Castalia.

Pellegrini, A. (1998). Bullies and victims in school: A review and call for research. *Journal of Applied Developmental Psychology, 19*, 165–176.

Puig-Antich, J., Kaufman, J., Ryan, N. D., Williamson, D., Dahl, R. E., Lukens, E., et al. (1993). The psychosocial functioning and family environment of depressed adolescents. *Journal of American Academy of Child and Adolescent Psychiatry, 32*, 244–253.

Reddy, L., & Goldstein, A. (2001). Aggression replacement training: A multimodal intervention for aggressive adolescents. *Residential Treatment for Children & Youth, 18*, 47–62.

Reid, D. H., & Parson, M. B. (1991). Making choice a routine part of mealtimes for persons with profound mental retardation. *Behavioral Residential Treatment, 6*, 249–261.

Reynhout, G., & Carter, M. (2007). Social story efficacy with a child with autism spectrum disorder and moderate intellectual disability. *Focus on Autism and other Developmental Disabilities, 22*, 173–182.

Rincover, A. (1978). Sensory extinction: A procedure for eliminating self-stimulatory behaviour in psychotic children. *Journal of Abnormal Child Psychology, 6*, 299–310.

Rincover, A., & Devany, J. (1982). The application of sensory extinction procedures to self-injury. *Analysis & Intervention in Developmental Disabilities, 2*, 67–81.

Salamivalli, C., Huttunen, A., & Lagerspetz, K. (1997). Peer networks and bullying in schools. *Scandinavian Journal of Psychology, 38*, 305–312.

Sawyer, M., Macmullen, C., Graetz, B., Said, J., Clark, J., & Baghurst, P. (1997). Social skills training for primary school children: A 1-year follow-up study. *Journal of Pediatric Child Health, 33*, 378–383.

Scattone, D., Tingstrom, D., & Wilczynski, S. (2006). Increasing appropriate social interactions of children with autism spectrum disorders using social stories. *Focus on Autism and Other Developmental Disabilities, 21*, 211–222.

Schneider, B. (1992). Didactic methods for enhancing children's peer relations: A quantitative review. *Clinical Psychology Review, 12*, 363–382.

Schneider, B., & Bryne, B.(1987). Individualized social skills training for behavior-disordered children. *Journal of Consulting and Clinical Psychology, 55*, 444–445.

Scruggs, E. T., & Mastropieri, M. A. (1998). The effectiveness of generalization training: A quantitative synthesis of single subject research. In T. E. Scruggs & M. A. Mastropieri (Eds.), *Advances in learning and behavioral disabilities* (Vol. 8, pp. 259–280). Greenwich, CT: JAI Press.

Slaby, R. G., & Guerra, N. G. (1988). Cognitive mediator of aggression in adolescent offenders: 1. Assessment. *Developmental Psychology, 24*, 580–588.

Spence, S. H. (2003). Social skills training with children and young people: Theory, evidence, and practice. *Child and Adolescent Mental Health, 8*, 84–96.

Stone, W. L., & Le Greca, A. M. (1984). Comprehension of nonverbal communication: A reexamination of the social competencies of learning-disabled children. *Journal of Abnormal Child Psychology, 12*, 505–518.

Swaggert, B., & Gagnon, E. (1995). Using social stories to teach social and behavioral skills to children with autism. *Focus on Autistic Behavior, 10*, 1–16.

Synder, J., Horsch, E., & Childs, J. (1997). Peer relationships of young children: Affiliative choices and shaping of aggressive behavior. *Journal of Clinical Child Psychology, 26*, 145–156.

Toro, P. A., Weissberg, R. P., Guare, J., & Liebenstein, N. L. (1990). A comparison of children with and without learning disabilities on behavior, and family background. *Journal of Learning Disabilities, 23*, 115–120.

Vaughn, S., Lancelotta, G., & Minnis, S. (1988). Social strategy training and peer involvement: Increasing peer acceptance of a female, LD student. *Learning Disabilities Focus, 4*, 32–37.

Vaughn, S., Ridley, C., & Bullock, D. (1984). Interpersonal problem-solving skills training with aggressive young children. *Journal of Applied Developmental Psychology, 5*, 213–223.

Vaughn, S., Zaragoza, N, Hogan, A., & Walker, J. (1993). A four-year longitudinal investigation of the social skills and behavior problems of students with learning disabilities. *Journal of Learning Disabilities, 26*, 404–412.

Verduyn, C., Lord, W., & Forrest, G. (1990). Social skills training in schools: An evaluation study. *Journal of Adolescence, 13*, 3–16.

Vickerstaff, S., Heriot, S., Wong, M., Lopes, A., & Dossetor, D. (2007). Intellectual ability, self-perceived social competence, and depressive symptomology in children with high-functioning autism spectrum disorders. *Journal of Autism and Developmental Disorders, 37*, 1647–1164.

Vitaro, F., Brendgen, M., Pagani, L., Tremblay, R., & McDuff, P. (1999). Disruptive behavior, peer association, and conduct disorder: Testing the developmental links through early intervention. *Development and Psychopathology*, *11*, 287–304.

Vollmer, T., & Northup, J. (1996). Some implications of functional analysis for school psychology. *School Psychology Quarterly*, *11*, 76–92.

Wacker, D., Steege, J., Sasso, G., Berg, W., Reimers, T., Cooper, L., et al. (1990). A component analysis of functional communication training across three topographies of severe behavior problems. *Journal of Applied Behavior Analysis*, *23*, 417–423.

Walker, H. M., Block-Pedego, A., Todis, B., & Severson, H. (1991). *School archival records search (SARS): User's guide and technical manual.* Longmont, CO: Sopris West.

Weissberg, R., Cowen, E., Lotyczewski, B., & Gesten, E. (1983). The primary mental health project: Seven consecutive years of program outcome research. *Journal of Consulting and Clinical Psychology*, *51*, 100–107.

Wieseler, N. A, Hanzel, T. A., Chamberlain, T. P., & Thompson, T. (1985). Functional taxonomy of stereotypic and self-injurious behavior. *Mental Retardation*, *23*, 230–234.

Witt, J., Daly, E., & Noelle, G. (2000). *Functional assessments: A step-by-step guide to solving academic and behavior problems.* Longmont, CO: Sopris West.

Yu, P., Harris, G., Solovitz, B., & Franklin, J. (1986). A social problem-solving intervention for children at high risk for later psychopathology. *Journal of Clinical Child Psychology*, *15*, 30–40.

Chapter 7
Social Skills in Autism Spectrum Disorders

Dennis R. Dixon, Jonathan Tarbox, and Adel Najdowski

Autism Spectrum Disorders

Autism was first described by Kanner in 1943 and identified as a disorder characterized by impaired development in language and socialization, as well as the presence of repetitive behaviors and restricted interests. The DSM-IV (APA, 2000) currently classifies Autistic Disorder within the Pervasive Developmental Disorders, which also include Asperger's Disorder, Rett's Disorder, Childhood Disintegrative Disorder, and PDD-Not Otherwise Specified (PDD-NOS). In recent years, researchers have begun to refer to these disorders as autism spectrum disorders (ASD) due to the continuous nature of symptoms with few clear boundaries upon which to differentiate disorders within the spectrum (Matson & Boisjoli, 2007).

While many researchers have attempted to further describe the cluster of symptoms comprising ASDs, these efforts have typically resulted in simply reiterating Kanner's (1943) original description, albeit, with a greater degree of precision. As such, deficits in language, social skills, and repetitive behaviors or restricted interests remain the core deficits upon which ASDs are diagnosed. In this chapter we discuss the assessment and treatment of social skills in children with an ASD.

Assessment of Social Skills in Individuals with Autism Spectrum Disorders

The assessment of social skills in children enjoys a long history of development and attention from researchers and clinicians alike. In a recent review (Matson and Wilkins (2009) identified 48 assessments developed to measure social skills in children. A review of each of these instruments is beyond the scope of this chapter. For an excellent review of the broader topic of assessment of social skills in children, see Boisjoli and Matson (Chapter 4, this volume).

While social skills in typically developing children have garnered much attention, the development of scales specifically for the assessment of social skills in children with an ASD has not received similar attention (Matson & Wilkins, 2007). This is surprising given that deficits in social interactions are one of the core symptoms of ASD. However, it is likely that efforts to develop measures of social skills for this population have focused primarily on developing diagnostic instruments.

A distinction has been made between narrowband and broad-band assessments (Rojahn, Aman, Matson, & Mayville, 2003) wherein broadband assessments are developed to measure a number of areas and typically measure the behavior in more general terms. Diagnostic instruments such as the Autism Diagnostic Interview-Revised (ADI-R; Lord, Rutter, & Le Couteur, 1994) and the Autism Spectrum Disorders – Diagnostic (ASD-D; Matson & González, 2007) would fall into this category. Narrowband assessments on the other hand are those that focus exclusively on one area or a particular

D.R. Dixon (✉)
Manager, Research and Development, Center for Autism and Related Disorders Inc., Tarzana, CA 91356, USA
e-mail: d.dixon@centerforautism.com

J.L. Matson (ed.), *Social Behavior and Skills in Children*, DOI 10.1007/978-1-4419-0234-4_7,
© Springer Science+Business Media, LLC 2009

domain. This distinction may be somewhat arbitrary though as terms like "broad" and "narrow" are relative. For instance, the ADI-R may be considered narrowband when contrasted with the Structured Clinical Interview for DSM Disorders (SCID; First, Gibbon, Spitzer, Williams, & Benjamin, 1997), which is a screening instrument for DSM-IV psychiatric disorders. However, this distinction remains a useful tool for discussing the impact of an assessment's purpose and how it is used.

Diagnostic instruments are developed to focus on symptoms that are indicative of a disorder. An emphasis is made on measuring variables that are relatively stable over time and present in a number of contexts. Further, an emphasis is made on items that differentiate between diagnostic groups. Many items that may offer useful information regarding a child's social skills may be removed if the items do not add to the overall ability of the scale to differentiate among disorders. While information about a child's social skills are lost through this process, this practice is proper given the overall purpose of developing an instrument that diagnoses validly and reliably in the most efficient manner (Matson, Nebel-Schwalm, & Matson, 2007).

In contrast to diagnostic instruments, scales designed primarily for treatment planning or measuring specific domains require a greater emphasis on measuring the domain in depth. These narrowband assessments thus focus on the specific target domain. While diagnostic instruments may be helpful in guiding initial treatment planning, this is not their primary purpose. Assessments for treatment planning need to place a focus on areas of intervention, not symptoms indicative of autism. A recent study by Matson, Dempsey, and LoVullo (2009) is a good example of this, wherein the Matson Evaluation of Social Skills for Individuals with Severe Retardation (MESSIER) was used to evaluate social skill differences among different diagnostic groups. These authors found a number of items that were specific to the ASD groups and offered a much more focused examination of social skills. These observations would not have been possible if a strictly diagnostic instrument had been used.

A third category may also be defined as instruments designed for measuring treatment outcomes. Few instruments have been developed specifically for this purpose. However, the use of the instrument for this purpose should guide the development of both diagnostic and treatment instruments. Scales used for this purpose must yield quantifiable information regarding the target symptoms. Further, the instruments must measure the symptoms in such a manner that researchers can detect treatment changes. Scales with restricted score ranges or simple categorical classifications make this difficult. Overall, the ASD treatment literature has been hindered by a lack of appropriate outcome measures (Matson, 2007).

There are a number of well-developed diagnostic tools for assessing ASD symptoms (Matson et al., 2007). As social skills are one of the primary areas evaluated for a diagnosis, each of these scales is designed to measure this area as a component in their overall assessment process. Due to the significant overlap among diagnostic scales and scales designed to specifically measure social skills, these scales will be discussed together. While each of these scales has received attention regarding their psychometric properties, a focus is made upon those studies that address the measurement of social skills in particular.

Autism Diagnostic Interview-Revised

The ADI-R is a semi-structured interview of caregivers of individuals with autism. Rutter, Le Couteur, and Lord (2003) report that the uses of the ADI-R are to aid in the diagnosis of autism, treatment planning, and differential diagnosis among other developmental disabilities The ADI-R is the second edition of the Autism Diagnostic Interview (Le Couteur et al., 1989). Administration time for the ADI-R is reported to be 1.5–2.5 hours.

The ADI-R provides an algorithm for making a diagnosis of autism. Item domains included in the algorithm that measure social skills include measurements of failure to use direct eye-to-eye gaze, facial expression, body posture, failure to develop peer relationships, lack of social-emotional reciprocity and modulation to context, and seeking to share own enjoyment (Lord et al., 1994). Each of these domains has been shown to have overall interrater reliability agreement above 0.9 (Lord et al., 1994). In addition to these items, the ADI-R also includes nonalgorithm items. These items assess the areas of direct gaze, separation anxiety, social smiling, seeking out others, and greeting others. Each of these items have also been shown to have interrater agreement above 0.89 (Lord et al., 1994). The stability of ADI-R diagnostic scores have been evaluated by a number of researchers (Charman et al., 2005; Cox et al., 1999; Lord et al., 2006; Moore & Goodson, 2003). Each of these studies found scores to be stable over a number of years. However, while these studies report on the stability of the social skills domain, they do so on the group level. Thus the stability of an individual's social skills score is not addressed.

Lord et al. (1994) report on the validity of the social area of the ADI-R in terms of diagnostic differences. However, the data are only relevant in regard to diagnoses made from the algorithm. While this is important for differential diagnosis, it does not address the adequacy of sampling the domain of social skills and the validity of the inferences made regarding a child's social skills. Some evidence of the construct validity of the ADI-R reciprocal social interactions domain has been reported by Mildenberger, Sitter, Noterdaeme, and Amorosa (2001), who contrasted children with autism to children with a receptive language disorder. They found a clear differentiation among groups, with the vast majority of children with receptive language disorder scoring well below the cutoff score.

Autism Diagnostic Observation Schedule – Generic

The Autism Diagnostic Observation Schedule – Generic (ADOS-G; Lord, Rutter, DiLavore, & Risi, 1999) is a semi-structured assessment of ASD symptoms. The assessment uses direct observation and a series of interactions with the individual that are designed to elicit a wide range of social responses that the examiner can use to determine the presence or absence of ASD symptoms. The ADOS-G provides domain scores for social, communication, social communication, and restricted-repetitive behavior.

Lord et al. (2000) report on the reliability and validity of the ADOS-G. Concerning the social and social communication domain scores, they found excellent interrater reliability and acceptable test-retest reliability. As with the ADI-R, validity is reported in terms of diagnostic classification. Lord et al. (2000) found significant differences among diagnostic groups for the social domain and social-communication domain scores. Similar results have been reported for the PL-ADOS (DiLavore, Lord, & Rutter, 1995). Noterdaeme, Sitter, Mildenberger, and Amorosa (2000) contrasted children with autism to children with a receptive language disorder. They found a clear differentiation among groups on the reciprocal social interaction scores, with the vast majority of children with receptive language disorder scoring well below the cutoff score.

Both the ADI-R and ADOS-G have been well developed and thoroughly evaluated regarding reliability and diagnostic accuracy. However, in spite of the substantial research on these scales, little has been done to evaluate the validity of these scales apart from diagnostic accuracy. Considering the widespread use of these scales and their prominence as the "gold standard" for making a diagnosis of autism, further research is warranted on the construct validity regarding the overall measurement of social skills.

Autism Spectrum Disorders – Diagnostic

The ASD-D is the diagnostic component of a larger battery of assessments that include the diagnostic instrument, an assessment for comorbid disorders (ASD-C), and an assessment for problem behaviors (ASD-PB). The ASD-D is a caregiver-completed rating scale that may be administered directly by a trained test user to an informant or it may be given to the parent or caregiver to complete independently (Matson & González, 2007). The ASD-D takes approximately 30–45 minutes to complete. Each of the components of the battery has versions developed specifically for use with children. The ASD-D provides subscale scores for social, communication, and repetitive behaviors/restricted interests domains (Matson, Wilkins, & González, 2007).

A number of studies have been conducted to evaluate the psychometric properties of the ASD-D (Matson, González, & Wilkins, 2009; Matson, González, Wilkins, & Rivet, 2008; Matson, Wilkins,

Boisjoli, & Smith, 2008; Matson et al., 2007; Matson, Boisjoli, González, Smith and Wilkins, 2007). Support for the construct validity of the ASD-D is reported by Matson et al. (2008), who found the ASD-D total score to be significantly correlated with the MESSIER, as well as the socialization domain of the Vineland Adaptive Behavior Scales (VABS). Matson et al. (2007) further report on the reliability of the ASD-D. Overall, kappa values for individual items fell in the acceptable range for both interrater and test-retest reliability. Matson et al. (2008) have similarly evaluated the child version of the ASD-D and found good interrater and test-retest reliability for items included on the social subscale.

Overall, the ASD-D shows good psychometric properties, particularly for a newly developed scale. Not only has the scale been evaluated in terms of differential diagnosis, but also in regard to how well the scale measures the overall construct of social skills in persons with an ASD.

Children's Social Behavior Questionnaire

The Children's Social Behavior Questionnaire (CSBQ; Luteijn, Jackson, Volkmar, & Minderaa, 1998) is a 96-item caregiver-completed questionnaire. The primary purpose of the CSBQ is to describe a broad range of PDD symptoms. Initial development steps are reported by Luteijn et al. (1998), who describe differences among children with PDDNOS and typically developing children. Reliability is discussed only in regard to internal consistency of the item groups, which showed acceptable alpha coefficients (0.73–0.91). The development sample included children 6–12 years of age, but the authors state that the scale is "probably suitable for children up to 18."

A refined version of the CSBQ is described by Luteijn, Luteijn, Jackson, Volkmar, and Minderaa (2000). The previous 135-item version was refined by removing unsatisfactory items resulting in a 96-item version. The refined CSBQ consists of items grouped into five subscales as described by Luteijn et al. (2000). These scales include acting out, social contact problems, social insight problems, anxious/rigid, and stereotypical. Interrater reliability fell in the acceptable range for all scales of

the CSBQ. Test-retest reliability was measured over a period of approximately 4 weeks, calculating intraclass correlation coefficients (ICC). The total score (ICC = 0.9), Acting-Out scale (ICC = 0.85), Social Contact Problems scale(ICC = 0.87), and the Anxious/Rigid scale (ICC = 0.85) were all acceptably high. The Social Insight Problems (ICC = 0.62) and Stereotypical scale (ICC = 0.32) showed less robust test-retest reliability. The validity of the CSBQ was examined by contrasting subscale scores to scores on The Child Behavior Checklist (CBCL; Achenbach, 1991) and the Autism Behavior Checklist (ABC; Krug, Arick, & Almond, 1980). The CSBQ subscales showed a good pattern of correlations with similar subscales on the CBCL and ABC (Luteijn et al., 2000).

The CSBQ has been used to study social problems among children with PDDNOS and ADHD (Luteijn, Serra et al., 2000). In this study, the CSBQ was part of a larger battery of assessments chosen to evaluate differences betweeen these two groups. These authors found the CSBQ to be a useful tool to describe subtle social differences between these groups, particularly in regard to social interactions and communication. The utility of the CSBQ to detect subtle social skills differences between groups with and without autism has further been reported by de Bildt et al. (2005).

Most recently, the CSBQ has undergone additional refinement to reduce the total items to 49 and reexamine the psychometric properties (Hartman, Luteijn, Serra, & Minderaa, 2006). Hartman et al. (2006) present data on a much larger sample of children than previously discussed (N = 3407). Results of a factor analysis showed that the best fit was a 6-factor solution. These 6 factors were titled as follows: 1. behavior/emotion not optimally tuned to the social situation, 2. reduced contact and social interest, 3. orientation problems in time, place, or activity, 4. difficulties in understanding social information, 5. stereotyped behavior, and 6. fear of and resistance to changes. Internal consistency was good for each of these subscales. Likewise, interrater reliability and test-retest reliability were good for all of the new subscales.

These studies, particularly the more recent evaluation by Hartman et al. (2006), show the CSBQ to be emerging as a useful tool with sound psychometric properties. While reliability has been well examined, issues of validity have not been as well discussed. A more direct examination of this scale's construct validity would be beneficial. This scale has undergone a series of revisions, which makes the continuity of its use in research studies somewhat confusing. The 96-item version has been shown to be useful and offers a more thorough evaluation of social skills in ASD than typical measures such as the VABS (de Bildt et al., 2005). While it is likely that this holds true for the 49-item version, this is an empirical question that remains untested.

Matson Evaluation of Social Skills with Youngsters

The Matson Evaluation of Social Skills with Youngsters (MESSY; Matson, Rotatori, & Helsel, 1983) is a 64-item questionnaire designed to assess social behaviors in children. Two factors have been identified, Inappropriate Assertiveness/Impulsiveness and Appropriate Social Skills. Scale scores are norm-referenced and considered "problematic" if they fall below one standard deviation from the mean.

The MESSY has a long history of development and evaluation of its psychometric properties and represents one of the earliest efforts to develop an instrument to measure social skills in children with developmental disabilities. Initial psychometric properties were evaluated by Matson, Macklin, and Helsel (1985) in a sample of children with hearing impairments and intellectual disabilities. Regarding reliability, they found inter-item, split-half, and internal consistency to be high. The usefulness of the MESSY has been demonstrated across a number of areas, including children with hearing impairments (Matson et al., 1985), visual impairments (Matson, Heinze, Helsel, Kapperman, & Rotatori, 1986), psychiatric disorders (Kazdin, Esveldt-Dawson, & Matson, 1983), and intellectual disabilities (Matson et al., 1983).

The MESSY has also received significant attention in regard to translation and establishing local psychometrics and norms outside of the United States (Matson & Wilkins, 2009). The MESSY has been adapted for use in Australia (English; Spence & Liddle, 1990), Belgium (French; Verté, Roeyers, & Buysse, 2003), China (dialect not reported; Chou, 1997), India (Hindi;

Sharma, Sigafoos, & Carroll, 2000), Israel (Hewbrew; Pearlman-Avnion, & Eviator, 2002), Japan (Japanese; Matson & Ollendick, 1988), the Netherlands (Dutch; Meijer, Sinnema, Bijstra, Mellenbergh and Wolters, 2000a, 200b), Spain (Andalusian & Spanish; Landazabal, 2006; Méndez, Hidalgo, & Inglés, 2002; Torres, Cardelle-Elawar, Mena, & Sanchez, 2003), Turkey (Turkish; Bacanli & Erdoğan, 2003), and the United Kingdom (English; Dogra & Parkin, 1997).

While children with autism were included in the general development sample, the MESSY has not been developed specifically to measure social skills within this population but rather within developmental disabilities as a whole. However, Matson, Compton, and Sevin (1991) reported on the use of the MESSY to evaluate social skills and deficits in children with autism or typical development. An item analysis of the MESSY items found that it was useful to identify areas of particular weakness in children with autism, such as rarely smiling at familiar people.

The MESSY has a long history of use and is a well-established measure of social skills in children. The scale has received tremendous attention internationally and is available in numerous languages. Further evaluation of the psychometric properties in children with autism would be beneficial. However, given the good psychometric properties demonstrated across these various studies, it is likely that these properties would also be replicated in larger samples of children with autism.

PDD Behavior Inventory

The PDD Behavior Inventory (PDDBI; Cohen & Sudhalter, 1999) is a parent- or teacher-completed rating scale. According to the authors, the purpose of creating the PDDBI was due to limitations in the existing assessment instruments, most particularly in the area of measuring changes over time (Cohen & Sudhalter, 1999). Further, the PDDBI was developed to measure both adaptive and maladaptive behaviors, not simply focus upon behavior deficits or excesses. As such, the PDDBI is one of the few scales developed to measure treatment effects in children with an ASD

(Cohen, Schmidt-Lackner, Romanczyk, & Sudhalter, 2003). Administration time for the standard form is reported to be 20–30 minutes. Two subscales of the PDDBI address social skills: the Social Pragmatic Problems (SOCPP) and Social Approach Behaviors (SOCAPP).

Cohen and Sudhalter (1999) report on the test-retest reliability of the PDDBI. The SOCPP and SOCAPP subscales showed good stability, with higher coefficients found for the SOCAPP scale over a 12-month period. Similar results were also found for a shorter 2-week interval. Interrater reliability among teachers was low for the SOCPP scale but good for the SOCAPP score, suggesting that the PDDBI is more reliable for measuring the presence of abilities than the presence of problems.

Concerning validity, the PDDBI has been evaluated by Cohen et al. (2003) and Cohen (2003). Cohen et al. (2003) primarily discuss validity in terms of the factor structure of the PDDBI and its subscales. Results of their principal components analyses supported the apriori structure of the SOCPP and SOCAPP subscales. Cohen (2003) discussed the criterion-related validity of the PDDBI. He reported that the PDDBI subscales were significantly correlated with all of the subscales of the VABS but that the social subscales showed the highest correlations with the social subscales of the VABS (Daily Living Skills and Socialization).

The PDDBI has undergone a thorough development as reported in its manual (Cohen & Sudhalter, 1999). As a scale designed specifically to measure treatment outcomes, the PDDBI fills a much-needed role in the ASD treatment literature. Further research is needed though addressing its psychometric properties apart from the original development sample.

The Social Responsiveness Scale

The Social Responsiveness Scale (SRS; Constantino & Gruber, 2005) is a 65-item questionnaire that covers social awareness, social cognition, social communication, social motivation, and autistic mannerisms. Constantino and Gruber (2005) have centered the distinguishing characteristics of ASD on reciprocal social behaviors and posited that reciprocal social behaviors are the *sine qua non* of all autism spectrum conditions. As such, the SRS has been developed primarily as a diagnostic instrument even though it is heavily focused on measuring social behavior. The scale is appropriate for use with children 4–18 years of age and places an emphasis on measuring symptoms across the full spectrum, particularly in the sub threshold for autistic disorder range. Administration time is reported to be 15–20 minutes.

Psychometric evaluation of the SRS has almost exclusively focused on evaluating the measure as a diagnostic scale. Regarding its general psychometric properties, Constantino and Gruber (2005) reported a fairly large development sample ($N = 1636$), which was a combination of five studies conducted throughout North America. The SRS showed good reliability and agreement with other diagnostic scales (ADI-R). The utility of the SRS as a tool for the rapid assessment of ASD symptoms has recently been demonstrated (Constantino et al., 2007). A preschool version of the SRS has also been developed for children 36–48 months of age (Pine, Luby, Abbacchi, & Constantino, 2006).

As noted, there have been few studies conducted that evaluate the use of the SRS for purposes other than diagnosis. Regarding the SRS's ability to measure the construct of social skills, Pine et al. (2006) found the SRS to have good agreement with the VABS adaptive behavior composite score ($r = -0.86$) and the social impairment scores from the ADI-R ($r = 0.63$). Constantino and Gruber (2005) report slightly higher correlation coefficients ($r = 0.74$) between the SRS total score and social impairment scores from the ADI-R.

A number of studies have been conducted in which the SRS was included as a dependent variable (e.g. Constantino & Todd, 2003; 2005; Constantino et al., 2004; 2006). Recently Tse, Strulovitch, Tagalakis, Meng & Fombonne (2007) included the SRS as a dependent variable to measure social skills treatment outcomes. They found significant changes in SRS scores between pretreatment and posttreatment scores. While the scale has been included in many research studies, few have specifically examined the psychometric properties of the scale in regard to measuring social skills. Studies such as that conducted by Tse et al. (2007) do, however, offer indirect support for the construct validity of the scale.

The Social Skills Rating System

The Social Skills Rating System (SSRS; Gresham & Elliott, 1990) is a standardized questionnaire used to evaluate child social behaviors at home and at school. It includes the areas of social skills (cooperation, assertion, responsibility, empathy, self-control), problem behaviors (external, internal, hyperactivity), and academic competence. The SSRS is a norm-referenced instrument designed for use in children and adolescents (3–18 years). The reported administration time is approximately 25 minutes (Gresham & Elliott, 1990). Gresham and Elliott (1984) define social skills as socially acceptable learned behaviors that enable a person to interact effectively with others and to avoid socially unacceptable responses. This definition has guided the construction of the SSRS. Gresham and Elliott (1990) state that the intended uses of the SSRS are for screening, classifying, or making intervention plans.

The manual provides information regarding item development, standardization, and initial examination of the scale's reliability and validity (Gresham & Elliott, 1990). Data presented in the manual show the SSRS to have good internal consistency and good temporal stability. However, interrater reliability was not examined. The authors give the rationale that different reporters will have different perspectives and samples of the child's behavior and as such it should not be expected to have high agreement, hence the reason for a multirater assessment. While this rationale makes sense for contrasts between parent and teacher or teacher and child it fails to address differences among reporters with similar perspectives, such as contrasting two teacher's ratings or ratings among parents. Examining reliability among these reporters is meaningful though and should show some level of consistency. Regarding validity, Gresham and Elliott (1990) report on the content, social, criterion-related, and construct validity. Overall, the data presented support the validity of the SSRS.

As with the MESSY, the SSRS has also received efforts in regards to translation and establishing local psychometrics and norms (Matson & Wilkins, 2009). These countries include Iran (Persian; Shahim, 2001, 2004), the Netherlands (Dutch; Van der Oord et al., 2005), and Puerto Rico (Spanish; Jurado, Cumba-Avilés, Collazo and Matos, 2006).

A longitudinal analysis of the SSRS in 4345 children has recently been reported by Van Horn, Atkins-Burnett, Karlin, Ramey & Snyder (2007). In their study, children were tested from kindergarten through the third grade. Results of this study showed the same general factor structure as described by Gresham and Elliott (1990). However, Van Horn et al. (2007) found that the SSRS appears to not measure the same construct over time. Further, they note that scores are differentially effected by ethnicity, particularly the scores for Hispanic students in their sample.

Two studies were identified that used the SSRS for persons with ASD. Koning and Magill-Evans (2001) used the SSRS to evaluate the social skill differences among boys with Asperger's and matched controls. They found significant differences between the two groups, with the Asperger's group showing particular deficits in the areas of self-control and assertiveness. Macintosh and Dissanayake (2006) used the SSRS to evaluate social skills among children with high-functioning autism, Asperger's disorder, and typical development. They found the HFA and Asperger's groups to be indistinguishable from one another but significantly more impaired than the typical development group.

Since publication, the SSRS has been widely researched and frequently included in research studies. Construct validity has been reported a number of times (Merrell & Popinga, 1994; Stage, Cheney, Walker, & LaRocque, 2002; Stuart, Gresham, & Elliott, 1991). Reliability between teacher and parent ratings have also been evaluated (Fagan, & Fantuzzo, 1999; Manz, Fantuzzo, & McDermott, 1999; Merrell & Popinga, 1994; Powless & Elliott, 1993). The overall conclusion these authors have reached is that the SSRS is a valid measure of social skills but that the context in which it is measured matters significantly and that ratings between parents and teachers will generally not be equivalent.

General Review of Assessments

All of the instruments discussed have been well examined and shown to be reliable instruments. However, not all have been equally examined in regard to assessment of social skills in children with an ASD. A relatively large number of studies have been conducted on the psychometric properties of the SSRS; however these studies have almost exclusively evaluated its use with typically developing children within the school system. The SSRS has been used to examine social skills in children with an ASD, however, reporting on the use of an instrument with a certain population is not the same as evaluating its psychometric properties within that population. Studies that evaluate the reliability and validity of the SSRS specifically for use with children with an ASD are needed. Likewise, the MESSY has received considerable attention for use in children with developmental disabilities. While this is arguably a closer approximation to ASD than typically developing children, further evaluations of the psychometric properties for use with individuals with ASD are warranted.

Diagnostic instruments have the benefit of being developed specifically for use in ASD. As such, these scales have been constructed in such a way as to elicit information concerning the specific social skills and deficits observed in children with an ASD. However, as previously noted, these items have been developed to detect and quantify symptoms warranting a diagnosis. Thus, the vast majority of studies on these scales have evaluated these scales in terms of how well they classify. The adequacy of these scales to measure social skills in general and specifically as they relate to children with an ASD have largely gone unexamined. More attention needs to be given to examining the construct and content validity of these scales as they relate to measuring social skills.

Further, among the diagnostic scales we observed a focus on measuring deficits or peculiarities in social interactions. We would argue that being skilled socially is not simply lacking deficits or problem behavior. An emphasis must be placed upon measuring strengths and abilities as well. Both the MESSY and SSRS provide measurements of social abilities. Thus, test users can identify areas for intervention, as well as identify areas of strength that can be built upon. This is a particular area of strength for these instruments.

Both the SRS and the CSBQ have been developed as diagnostic instruments for ASD symptoms in the PDDNOS range. Further, items on these instruments show a tendency to measure social behavior as a component on almost all of their subscales. As such, the content of these scales include items to measure subtle differences in social skills that children with an ASD exhibit. However, both of these scales lack studies that have specifically examined their validity in regard to measuring social skills. Yet, researchers have used these scales as measures of social skills for their studies. While these measures do show differences in their scores among groups, this cannot be substituted for a demonstration of construct validity. Steps such as expert review of item-content are helpful to guide the development process, but other constructs than social skills may account for a significant portion of item variance. The degree to which social items actually are influenced by other factors though is unknown until examined. Thus, even diagnostic instruments that have been developed with the assumption that the distinguishing feature of autism is social behavior still need to establish that what they measure is actually social skills if inferences about social functioning are to be made from their results.

Overall, researchers have continued to develop and examine the psychometric properties of these scales. This area has received increased attention from researchers, particularly in the past 10 years (Matson & Wilkins, 2009). Scales such as the MESSY and SSRS appear to be well developed to measure this construct, particularly if the intention is to evaluate how well children with ASD compare with typically developing children. The diagnostic scales though offer an assessment of social skills as they are specifically expressed in children with an ASD. There is the possibility though that the diagnostic scales have underrepresented the construct of social skills as a whole. Further exploration of these scales in regards to validity for measuring social skills is needed.

Treatments for Social Skills in Individuals with Autism Spectrum Disorders

Enhancement of social skills in individuals with ASDs is of central concern to treatment of ASDs, given that social deficits are a defining feature of the disorders. Fortunately, a substantial amount of research has been published that has evaluated the efficacy of such efforts. Several thorough reviews of the social skills treatment literature have been published in recent years (Maston, Matson, & Rivet, 2007; McConnell, 2002; Rogers, 2000; Weiss & Harris, 2001; White, Keonig, & Scahill, 2007). Given the substantial size of the empirical literature and the quality of the recently published reviews, it would appear to be both unnecessary, as well as beyond the scope of this chapter, to review every treatment article ever published. Rather, in what follows, we describe major themes in research on social skills interventions for individuals with ASDs and provide a critical analysis of the literature and directions for future research. We also take care to augment the general discussion with highlights from articles published in very recent years.

Social Behaviors Addressed

A wide variety of behaviors or skills which can reasonably be said to fall under the purview of social skills have been addressed in the treatment literature, ranging from very simple behaviors (e.g., greetings) to complex cognitive skills (e.g., perspective-taking). In what follows, we illustrate the wide range of behaviors addressed with examples.

Social Initiations

Social initiations are typically defined as behaviors that are not in response to the social behavior of someone else. These behaviors are often described as "spontaneous" or "unprompted." A variety of studies have demonstrated various behavioral procedures to be effective for increasing social initiations. Examples of social initiations taught in the treatment literature include teaching children with ASDs to say things such as "hi," "look what I'm doing," "look what I have," etc. For example, Taylor, Levin, and Jasper (1999) used video-modeling to teach children with autism to make comments during play (e.g., "This car goes fast!") with siblings. The study demonstrated an increase in appropriate commenting during play, across a variety of play activities. Some studies have focused on teaching children with ASDs to initiate play by requesting others to play, for example, "Let's

play" (Nikopolous & Keenan, 2004). Several studies measure and intervene upon general classes of initiations, rather than discrete topographical definitions. For example, Davis, Brady, Hamilton, and McEvoy (1994) defined social initiations as "any motor or verbal behavior directed to a peer that could occasion a social response" (p. 622).

Responses

A relatively common measure of social behavior in treatment studies is responses to the social initiations of others. The goal in such studies is to increase the extent to which children with autism respond in a social appropriate and successful manner when someone else makes a social initiation to them. For example, Maione and Mirenda (2006) targeted social responses, including language that acknowledged what another said, repeated what another said, agreements with what another said, answering peer questions, comments about ongoing activities, questions about peers' comments, and clarifications of questions asked by peers. L. K. Koegel, Koegel, Hurley & Frea (1992) included the following relatively broad definition of appropriate responses to the verbal initiations of others: "any verbal response or appropriate attempt at a response that was related to the stimulus (question) and occurred within 3 s of the stimulus" (p. 346).

Conversational Behaviour

A significant number of studies have successfully enhanced conversational behavior in children with ASDs. For example, Sarakoff, Taylor, and Poulson (2001) used written scripts to teach children with ASDs to engage one another in conversation about preferred items and objects that were present. The scripts were successfully faded out and large increases in non-scripted conversational statements were observed as well. In another study, video-modeling was used to teach conversational behavior in the form of replying to conversational questions and then asking a question appropriate to the topic (Charlop-Christy, Le, & Freeman, 2000). The targeted conversational behavior improved substantially and generalization was observed across stimuli, people, and settings.

Reciprocal Interactions

Several studies have examined behavioral methods for establishing reciprocal social interactions with children with autism. Reciprocal interactions consist of an initiation on the part of one child and a response on the part of another. For example, McGee, Almeida, Sulzer-Azaroff, & Feldman (1992) used peer-mediated incidental teaching to improve reciprocal interactions between children with autism and their peers. Reciprocal interactions were defined as the occurrence of a child initiation to or from a child with autism or his/her peer, followed by a positive child response from or to the child with autism. That is, the bidirectional interaction between the two children was measured, rather than simply the occurrence of a particular behavior on the part of a particular child.

Sociodramatic Play

Research has been conducted on using behavioral methods for teaching children with autism to engage in sociodramatic play. Sociodramatic play typically consists of two or more children acting out roles together in common themes, such as "cops and robbers," etc. For example, Thorp, Shahmer, and Schreibman (1995) used PRT to teach three boys with autism to engage in sociodramatic play, using child-selected materials and games, and shaping via adult prompting and reinforcement. Goldstein and Cisar (1992) used scripts to teach children with autism to engage in sociodramatic play with typically developing peers. Treatment progressed in a multiple baseline across pet shop, magic shop, and carnival play scenarios. In each scenario, there were three assigned roles. For example, the pet shop scenario included a "salesperson," an "animal caretaker," and a "customer" role. Each role involved 10 behaviors. During teaching, teachers praised correct responding, and praise included expansions and rewordings of behaviors being praised in an attempt to promote variability and generalization. In order to assess whether a generalized ability to play in the

three sociodramatic scenarios was taught, rather than rote memorization of particular behaviors, untrained behaviors which were directly related to the scenario were also measured pretreatment and posttreatment and during tests for generalization to other peers. Results demonstrated robust increases in targeted and untargeted behaviors and substantial generalization across people (children displayed their newly learned play skills with other peers who were not present during training).

Offering Help

In a relatively novel application of behavioral procedures, Harris, Handleman, and Alessandri (1990) taught three adolescent boys with autism to offer assistance to others who were having difficulty with mundane tasks, such as buttoning a button, opening a jar, and putting a key in a lock. The boys were taught to offer help when someone else stated they could not complete a task, and generalization to other people in the training setting was observed.

Perspective-Taking

Much has been made of "theory of mind" in individuals with autism in recent years. Theory of Mind (ToM) refers to one's ability to understand the mental states of others. Such abilities are also sometimes referred to as "social cognition" or "perspective-taking," the term which we will use for the remainder of this chapter. Perspective-taking can be important for social competence because the particular behaviors which are likely to be socially successful often depend on the current mental state of the person with whom one is interacting. For example, the manner in which one might greet a friend who is sad might be quite different from how you might greet the same person when he/she is happy. Similarly, successful conversational behavior likely depends at least partially on detecting what conversational topics are of interest to the person with whom you are interacting (e.g., failing to detect boredom on the part of your conversational partner will likely be detrimental to others' desires to converse with you in the future). In addition, empathy is also likely related to one's perspective-taking ability, in that empathizing with another's mental state presumably depends on one's ability to detect the other's mental state.

Despite the apparent importance of perspective-taking to social skills, few studies have attempted to teach perspective-taking to children with ASDs. In an early attempt to do so, Ozonoff and Miller (1995) taught 5 children with autism and normal intelligence perspective-taking skills and other social skills using a 4.5-long month training program. Results indicated improvements in tasks of perspective-taking but no increases in parent and teacher ratings of social competence. In a series of two studies, Charlop-Christy and colleagues (Charlop-Christy & Daneshvar, 2003; LeBlanc et al., 2003) used a video-modeling procedure to teach children with autism to identify the beliefs and false beliefs of others during the "Sally Anne Task," a common test of perspective-taking. Although these studies demonstrate the potential utility of behavioral procedures for teaching perspective-taking, further research is needed on establishing more comprehensive and nuanced repertoires of perspective-taking, as well as on the effects of doing so on social competence in general.

Intervention Formats

Naturalistic Behavioral Approaches

Naturalistic behavioral teaching formats go by many names, including Pivotal Response Training (PRT), natural language paradigm, incidental teaching, and milieu teaching, just to name a few. While each of these approaches is distinct in some regard from the others, all share some common features: (1) teaching takes place in a less-structured setting, such as during play, (2) learning opportunities are child-initiated, and (3) prompting, reinforcement, and prompt-fading are used. Naturalistic teaching formats can be advantageous for teaching social skills because they involve less structured settings, which are generally the settings in which many social skills should eventually be demonstrated, for example, conversational skills during snack time, sharing skills during free play, turn-taking skills while playing board games, etc. Therefore, naturalistic teaching strategies can be utilized in the environment in which the eventual skill is to be displayed, thereby lessening the disconnect between

the intervention setting and real-life setting. In a recent review, Cowen and Allen (2007) summarized results of studies on using naturalistic behavioral approaches to enhancing social competence and play skills in children with ASDs and conclude that a variety of skills have been enhanced, across clinical and public education settings.

Self-Management

Several studies have demonstrated the successful use of social skills interventions that include self-management components. Self-management procedures, in general, include some or all of the following components: (1) teaching the child awareness of his/her own behavior, (2) recording occurrences of desirable behavior (e.g., initiating, sharing, etc.), (3) tracking progress toward a goal of some kind, (4) reporting to a caregiver, and (5) recruiting or self-administering reinforcement of some kind. For example, Koegel et al. (1992) used a self-management teaching procedure to teach children with autism to increase their responsiveness to others. Four boys were taught to use a wrist tallier to record the occurrence of their own responses to verbal initiations by others. Positive results found in the clinic and generalization were demonstrated across home, community, and school settings. Similarly, Koegel and Frea (1993) used self-management interventions to teach children with autism to monitor and improve their own verbal and nonverbal social behaviors. Shearer, Kohler, Buchan, & McCullough (1996) introduced a self-monitoring procedure for the purpose of helping 5-year-old children with autism to monitor their own activity engagement and social interaction. Finally, Morrison, Kamps, Garcia, and Parker (2001) evaluated a multicomponent intervention, which included a self-monitoring component, for increasing requesting, commenting, and sharing behaviors in the context of game play. Treatment effects were robust, although follow-up data revealed that maintenance was less so.

Social Skills Groups

Social skills groups are a relatively common approach to treatment for individuals with ASDs. Such groups typically have a small number of children on the spectrum and often a small number of typically developing children; they typically meet approximately once per week for approximately an hour. Despite their popularity, there is little sound scientific research demonstrating their effectiveness. White et al. (2007) reviewed published studies on the effects of social skills groups for individuals with ASDs. Of 14 identified studies, only 5 included control groups – one of which was an unpublished dissertation. Of these, only one published study reported significant effects on the social behavior of participants (Yang, Schaller, Huang, Wang, & Tsai, 2003). Interventions in group format have the obvious advantage of having peers present from the outset and of being relatively low cost. However, it is possible that the social deficits of individuals with ASDs are sufficiently severe such that one-to-one intervention may be necessary for some or most individuals, at least at the start of treatment. Further research on individual components of social skills groups, including necessary staffing levels and the utility of combining social skills groups with smaller-format interventions, is needed.

Procedural Components

The vast majority of published research on treatment of social skills in individuals with ASDs has evaluated treatments which are behavioral in orientation. Therefore, it is no surprise that most treatments comprise well-validated behavioral treatment components. For example, most studies involve prompting of some kind, such as vocal, modeling, gestural, etc. (Matson et al., 2007). Many studies also involve the explicit use of contrived positive reinforcement of some kind, typically with the short-term goal of thinning or completely eliminating the reinforcement, while the newly taught behavior continues to occur with little or no adult support.

Scripts

A significant amount of research has evaluated the use of scripts to increase social language with individuals with ASDs. The use of scripts is somewhat controversial outside of the behavioral field, because, the very

nature of successful social interaction is something that is not rote, scripted, or repetitive. The ways in which children play, the comments that are made during play, the topics of conversation, and so on, change from time A to time B, and this natural fluidity and variability is presumably a necessary part of successful social interaction. On this basis then, one might assume that using scripts to teach social interaction might be contraindicated. However, this assumption is better addressed empirically, rather than theoretically, and this assumption has not been borne out by the treatment literature. We will briefly describe examples of social skills interventions which employ scripts below.

Most treatment studies which have employed scripts have done so by providing scripts with appropriate social language written out that the child is then directly prompted to read during appropriate circumstances. The use of prompting and the presence of scripts are then faded out, with the goal of establishing unprompted, spontaneous social language (McClannahan & Krantz, 2005). For example, Goldstein and Cisar (1992) used scripts to teach the language involved in sociodramatic play, in a pet shop, magic shop, and carnival play scenarios, and substantial increases in novel social communication, as well as generalization across peers was observed, as described earlier. Krantz and McClannahan (1998) used scripts to teach three boys with autism to initiate to adults for the adults' attention and found that the behaviors remained high after the scripts were faded. Further, generalization was observed across targets that were not the topic of intervention. Krantz and McClannahan (1993) used a script intervention to increase initiations to peers. Again, initiations remained high after the scripts were faded and the children were noted to combine elements from the scripts in novel ways, thereby demonstrating a generalized effect (i.e., the children were not rotely repeating what was taught). The state of the empirical evidence at the current time suggests that using scripts to teach social skills typically results in generalization to novel, unscripted communication.

Video Modeling

Video modeling is a relatively new procedural component which has been the subject of an increasing number of studies in recent years. Generally, video-modeling proceeds by producing a video that depicts either a peer or an adult engaging in the desired behavior. The participant is then asked to watch the video and often is prompted to talk about the important components of the video as it is playing. The participant is then given the opportunity to rehearse what he/she saw on the video, typically resulting in some kind of positive feedback for appropriate responding. For example, Charlop and Milstein (1989) used video-modeling to teach three boys with high-functioning autism to engage in conversations with adults. The intervention produced increases in appropriate conversational behavior, and the effects were demonstrated to generalize across settings and people and maintenance was observed. In another study, video-modeling was compared to in vivo modeling for teaching a variety of skills, including spontaneous greetings, cooperative play, and conversational behavior (Charlop-Christy et al., 2000). The study found that video-modeling generally led to faster acquisition than in vivo modeling and results generalized. In an attempt to identify the best person to serve as the model in video-modeling, one study compared the use of videos depicting the child, himself/herself, engaging in the desired behavior, versus videos depicting someone else engaging in the behavior (Sherer et al., 2001). The videos were used to teach children with ASDs to answer conversational questions (e.g., "What's your favorite TV show?"). Three of five children readily acquired the skills with both approaches, and the procedures were equally ineffective for two participants, suggesting that the particular person serving as the model in video-modeling may not be critical.

Surreptitious Tactile Prompting

One challenge in prompting social behavior is the fact that it often involves intrusion of an adult into the interaction of a child with his/her peers. One innovative solution to this problem is the use of devices such as hidden vibrating "pager" prompts. Taylor and Levin (1998) used a "Gentle Reminder" pager prompt placed in the pocket of a 9-year-old boy with autism to prompt social initiations in the context of play and cooperative learning contexts.

The device is a vibrating pager that can be set to vibrate at various intervals. The boy was taught to make initiations whenever he felt the device vibrate. Results demonstrated increases in initiations and suggest that the use of a hidden pager prompt can be an effective and unobtrusive procedure for prompting social initiations. A similar procedure was replicated across three additional children with autism, and similar results were found, although fading of the prompt was only successful for one of three children (Shabani et al., 2002). More research on the use of surreptitious vibrating pager prompts is needed, particularly on how to fade their use, but the initial evidence is encouraging.

Social Stories

Social Stories are something akin to fables, in that they are short stories about particular behaviors or practices and the results that they may produce. Social Stories are short in duration (e.g., typically take less than a minute to read) and often include pictures or comic strips depicting the contents of the stories. Individual Social Stories are typically constructed to address particular needs of a given child. For example, a child may have one Social Story that addresses his difficulties with sharing, one that addresses his conversational skills, etc. A clinician typically reads the story with the client and reviews the pictures with him or her on some regular basis (e.g., at the beginning of each day). The primary purpose of Social Stories is reported to be to increase an individual's understanding of a social situation, thereby allowing him/her to behave more effectively (Gray, 2000). Social Stories are a popular treatment approach for addressing the social skills deficits of individuals with ASDs. For example, in a web-based survey of 108 treatments used by parents of children with ASDs, 36% of parents reported that their children were currently being treated with Social Stories, making the approach the 5th most popular of the 108. The popularity of Social Stories is interesting, in that there is very little scientific evidence for their effectiveness. Most studies which have evaluated Social Stories have done so in combination with other procedural components which are already empirically validated. For example, Thiemann and Goldstein (2001) used social stories in combination with verbal and gestural prompting and video-review feedback to improve securing attention, initiating comments, and responding to others' comments in five children with autism. Results were favorable, but it is not possible to determine the contribution, if any, that social stories made to the treatment effect. In a review of research on social stories, Reynhout and Carter (2006) identified 12 published studies which included Social Stories, of which 7 evaluated the use of Social Stories alone. Upon closer examination, the effects demonstrated by these studies are in some cases dubious and in other cases suffer from inadequate experimental designs (Rogers, 2000). For example, Kuoch and Mirenda (2003) used a reversal design to evaluate Social Stories for decreasing challenging behaviors in three boys. The treatment appeared to produce an effect; however, the effect did not deteriorate when Social Stories were discontinued, thereby calling into question the internal validity of the study. A more recent experiment evaluated the effects of parent-mediated social stories in isolation on sportsmanship, maintaining conversation, and social engagement of three boys with Asperger's disorder (Sansosti & Powell-Smith, 2006). Treatment was evaluated in a multiple baseline across the three boys and appeared to have a substantial effect for one boy, a somewhat lesser effect for a second and had no effect for the third.

Despite the currently inconclusive status of social stories research, it stands to reason that enhancing an individual's understanding of the prevailing contingencies in a social situation may indeed help that person adapt to that situation, provided that the contingencies are meaningful to that individual. Therefore, further research into which conditions, if any, provide for effective implementation of Social Stories appears to be warranted.

Locus of Intervention

Several options have been researched regarding the locus of the intervention, that is, who, where, or what is the source of the intervention. There are presumably many options but the most researched

options are peer-mediated, adult-mediated, and ecological manipulations. Each are briefly reviewed below.

Adult-Mediated Interventions

The majority of social skills treatment studies have employed adult-mediated interventions, meaning that one or more adults implement the various components of the intervention (e.g., modeling, prompting, praise, etc.). An obvious advantage of adult-mediated interventions is that adult interventionists can presumably be trained to ensure high degrees of treatment integrity. A clear disadvantage of adult-mediated interventions is that, given that the primary purpose of social skills interventions is to enhance child interactions with peers, these interventions, by definition, provide influence from an outside and unwanted source. Therefore, a critical component of any adult-mediated intervention must be successful fading of adult intervention as quickly as possible, while still retaining treatment effects. That is, although adults may be effective at implementing social skills interventions, the results of these interventions are largely meaningless unless the need for adult presence can be eliminated. It is encouraging to note, however, that technologies of prompt-fading and reinforcement thinning produced by the general applied behavior analytic treatment literature appear to be successfully implemented in the case of social skills training for individuals with ASDs. Few studies report difficulties with fading adult intervention, although it is possible that such studies are never submitted for publication or are rejected when they are submitted.

Peer-mediated interventions. A large number of studies have demonstrated that peer-mediated social skills interventions can be effective with individuals with ASDs. Most peer-mediated intervention approaches explicitly train peers in particular intervention components. Such approaches may involve training peers to prompt and reinforce simple social behaviors (Odom & Strain, 1984). One area of peer-mediated interventions that has been the subject of a significant amount of research is peer-mediated PRT. For example, Pierce and Schreibman (1995) trained peers in a multicomponent PRT intervention approach to increase social behaviors in children with ASDs, using role-playing, modeling, and other components.

The initiations of both children with autism in the study increased significantly, and the results were maintained during follow-up. These results were generally replicated in two subsequent studies by the same research group (Pierce & Schreibman, 1997a, b).

A potential advantage of peer-mediated intervention is that the active variables of the intervention inhere in the social environment with which one wants the client to interact, that is, the client's peers. Therefore, it seems possible that fading intentional treatment out and transferring control of treatment effects to the natural environment might occur more easily, although this is an empirical question to which little or no research has actually been directed. Two potential disadvantages of peer-mediated intervention are that (1) it may be more difficult to train children to implement interventions with a high degree of fidelity and (2) peers' parents may not consent to involving their children in the social skills interventions of other children. More research is needed, then, on the practical factors related to the implementation of peer-mediated interventions in real-life settings.

Ecological Manipulations

Ecological manipulations involve changing features of the larger environment in which social behavior occurs, rather than manipulating antecedent and consequent stimuli which directly affect behavior. Ecological manipulations for increasing social skills in individuals with ASDs have several advantages. They tend to require relatively low effort and low cost, are unobtrusive, and do not necessitate direct intervention by a caregiver during social interactions. Several studies have reported effectiveness. For example, Lord and Magill-Evans (1995) found that mere daily exposure to typical peers produced increases in social engagement, responsiveness, and constructive play for children with autism. However, researchers have not always observed these results. Schleien, Mustonen, and Rynders (1995) found that including children with ASDs in art classes with typically developing peers increased the peers' initiations toward the children with ASDs but did not affect initiations by children with ASDs. In another study on ecological manipulations, DeKlyen and Odom (1989) found that increased structure during social circumstances

produced improved social interactions of children with ASDs. However, these strengths are also the primary limitations, in that ecological variations do not involve direct intervention on social behavior and may therefore be less robust or reliable in their effectiveness. Others (McConnell, 2002) have concluded that ecological manipulations may well produce modest effects but that such manipulations are not likely sufficient to remediate significant social deficits. More research is, therefore, needed on how ecological manipulations can be combined most effectively with other more robust treatment components.

Comparison Studies

Remarkably few studies have been published which directly compare outcomes produced by two or more different social skills treatment approaches. In one exception, Odom et al. (1999) compared 5 conditions: (1) control condition, (2) environmental arrangements, (3) child-specific intervention, (4) peer-mediated intervention, and (5) comprehensive intervention (social skills training and prompts and praise for target children and peers during free play) in 22 classrooms, containing 98 children with disabilities of various varieties, many of whom had ASDs. After 55–60 days, the environmental arrangements, child-specific, and peer-mediated interventions demonstrated positive effects on social interactions. Only the effects of the peer-mediated condition maintained after 1 year. The authors postulated that the comprehensive intervention may not have been implemented with high procedural integrity due to its complex nature. As others (Matson et al., 2007) have noted, there is a clear need for a greater number of studies comparing the many interventions that have proven effective. In addition, and perhaps more importantly, more research is needed to determine how clinicians might identify which procedures are most likely to be effective for which clients.

Intervention for Older Children with ASDs

Research on social skills interventions for individuals with ASDs has included participants of a wide range of ages, but the primary focus has been on preschool and elementary aged children. Accordingly, the majority of treatment research described in this chapter was conducted with children of these ages. However, it is worth noting that treatment research has demonstrated that a variety of behavioral intervention procedures have been shown to be effective in improving a variety of social skills in older children with ASDs. Space does not permit a thorough review of the research, but we will describe a few such studies here. Nikopolous and Keenan (2003) used video-modeling to enhance the social initiations and play behavior of four boys with autism, aged 9–15. Treatment effects were observed to generalize across settings, peers, and toys, and were maintained at 1- and 2-month follow-up periods. Stevenson, Krantz, and McClannahan (2000) used audio-taped scripts to enhance the social interactions of four boys with autism, aged 10–15. Audio-taped scripts were presented to increase the interactions of the boys with adult conversation partners. The scripts were successfully faded, and increases in unscripted interactions were observed, as well as maintenance of treatment gains. In an interesting procedural variation, Jahr, Eldevick, and Eikeseth (2000) enhanced the effectiveness of modeling by requiring participants to actively describe what they observed the model doing before being given the opportunity to imitate it. Boys of various ages, including one 10-year-old and one 12-year-old, were taught to improve turn-taking, initiations, and responding to others' initiations, and treatment effects generalized across play partners, settings, and time.

Generalization

A large number of the treatment studies described in this chapter attempted to assess generalization in at least some way. Further, a large number of the studies that assessed generalization found that it occurred, at least to some degree. As earlier in multiple places above, both stimulus generalization (e.g., exhibiting trained skills in the presence of people or settings not included in initial training) and response generalization (exhibiting new, untrained behaviors as a result of intervention)

have been found. This is encouraging, given that the issue of generalization tends to be under-addressed in applied research (Stokes & Baer, 1977). Nevertheless, relatively little research has addressed generalization across larger repertoires of behavior or the formation of larger, flexible, general classes of social behavior. This issue will be addressed in greater depth shortly.

Maintenance

Relatively few treatment studies have addressed maintenance of skills to any large degree. Many of the studies addressed short-term maintenance, by assessing the presence of treatment effects after a small number of weeks or months following treatment. Failing to address maintenance to an adequate degree is a common shortcoming of treatment research in general (Foxx, 1999), so it is not surprising to find it in the social skills treatment literature. Particularly in the case of adult-mediated interventions, contrived intervention procedures must be eliminated early in the treatment process in order for a meaningful treatment effect to be obtained. Therefore, maintenance in the very short term is a necessary precondition of such interventions to be considered effective at all. Ideally, after new social skills are established and contrived prompts are faded, children with ASDs should come in contact with naturally maintaining contingencies of reinforcement, thereby producing maintenance of the skills taught. Indeed, it might not be unreasonable to posit that if the naturally occurring contingencies do not maintain treatment effects then the skills established by the treatment may have not been appropriate to the child's social context to begin with. In any case, further research is clearly needed on long-term maintenance of the effects of social skills treatments.

Social Validity

The concept of social validity refers to the degree to which the goals, procedures, or effects of an intervention are important to society (Wolf, 1978). This is an inherently subjective construct but is of obvious interest to anyone engaging in applied science or clinical practice. Estimates of social validity in behavioral research typically consist of experimenters asking others for their opinions regarding the importance or acceptability of the goals, procedures, or effects of an intervention. There are many variables which are likely to influence the accuracy of caregiver opinion, and even if caregiver opinion is accurately reported, there is no reason to believe any particular report will be representative of societal viewpoints in general. Despite the inherent shortcomings of such measures, they are the commonly used estimate of the social validity of interventions, and it is generally agreed that they should be solicited as a regular part of treatment research. In their recent review of social skills treatments for individuals with ASDs, Matson et al. (2007) noted that less than 10% of reviewed studies assessed the social validity of their interventions. Furthermore, criticisms of behavioral interventions for ASDs are often based upon the claim that the interventions address behaviors of little or no importance (a claim for which there is also no empirical evidence). Future research on behavioral (and indeed, any) interventions for social skills in individuals with ASDs would, therefore, be greatly enhanced by including measures of social validity. Such measures should include soliciting the opinions of individuals who are least likely to be biased toward the discipline from which the intervention comes (e.g., experts from other disciplines, parents, teachers, etc.).

Directions for Future Research on Treatment of Social Skills

One potential limitation which is common to most psychoeducational treatment research is that it evaluates change across a relatively short period of time. The goal of social skills intervention in ASDs is often broad improvements in the overall social repertoire and overall social lifestyle of the individual being treated. Given how complex the social repertoire of even a young child is, meaningful change inevitably entails far more than an increase or decrease in a small number of specific behaviors. That is, a fully developed social skills repertoire, at virtually any age, is presumably comprised of thousands of behaviors, where

subtle features of the behaviors are virtually always relevant, and the current context is critical to the success or failure of social interaction at any given time. In other words, teaching a child to successfully socialize with his/her peers is an incredibly complex affair, one that, almost by its very nature, cannot be substantially altered in a period of a few weeks or months. This is not to say that intervention studies which focus on changing a small number of behaviors over a short period of time (e.g., teaching a child to say "Let's play" to peers) are irrelevant to the overall job of improving whole repertoires. Indeed, these studies presumably identify procedures which are effective in establishing the building blocks of larger repertoires. However, very little research has evaluated how many such interventions are "put together," to form a comprehensive social skills intervention for an individual, over the course of several months or years. For example, there are many studies which have demonstrated how to teach simple solitary play skills, many other studies which have demonstrated how to teach parallel or cooperative play, many others which have taught sociodramatic play, many others which have taught reciprocal conversational exchanges, but very little research has attempted to establish and track the development of entire social repertoires over time by combining many or all such approaches in a serial or simultaneous manner.

One area of research that has attempted to establish global social repertoires is that of early intensive behavioral intervention (EIBI). EIBI programs are typically initiated as early as possible (e.g., under the age of 5), are conducted at a high degree of intensity (e.g., 25 or more hours per week of one-to-one intervention), and are typically continued for 2–4 years. The purpose of EIBI programs is to address all areas of skill deficits with which a client presents. Because delayed social development is a core feature of ASDs, good-quality EIBI programs have always allocated a significant amount of intervention time to addressing social skills deficits. The format that is commonly employed in EIBI programs is comprehensive, in that it utilizes most of the intervention approaches and components described in this chapter and implements social skills treatment across a large proportion of the client's life and for a long duration of time (e.g., 2 years).

The purpose of outcome studies of EIBI is to evaluate EIBI as a treatment for autism in general, not for social skills in particular. Perhaps for that reason, early outcome studies of EIBI did not include measures of social development (e.g., Lovaas, 1987), and this was a significant limitation. However, more recent studies evaluating the outcomes of EIBI have included measures of socialization and have demonstrated substantial improvements in socialization. Controlled studies have demonstrated increases in standard scores on the socialization subscale of the VABS of 10 points (Sallows & Graupner, 2005), 14 points (Remington et al., 2007), and 15 points (Cohen, Amerine-Dickens, & Smith, 2006). Although this initial evidence is encouraging, more research is needed on the social skills intervention component of EIBI programs, in terms of effectiveness, social validity, and in terms of identifying the most effective combination of procedural components.

Social Skill Versus Social Motivation

A potential area of concern in social skills treatments for individuals with ASDs that has received relatively little discussion in the treatment literature is the distinction between individuals' ability to interact socially versus their desire to do so. For example, on one hand, the quality of an individual's social life may suffer because he does not know how to engage others in lively conversation, despite the fact that he would enjoy doing so if he could. On the other hand, the quality of another individual's social life may also suffer due to a lack of interaction with others, not because he lacks the skills to do so, but rather because he chooses not to. Although this distinction is not often addressed in the behavioral literature, the behavioral perspective lends itself nicely to an interpretation of this distinction. In the first case, the skill of engaging others in conversation may be conceptualized as a behavioral repertoire that has not yet been acquired (and could likely be acquired through one of the many intervention procedures described in this chapter, e.g., prompting, reinforcement, etc.). In the second case, the skill of engaging others in conversation is present in the repertoire of the individual, but the consequences that conversational engagement produces are not positively reinforcing for the person (e.g., attention or approval

from others may not be a source of reinforcement for that individual).

What we often see in the course of clinical practice is that very young children who have no interest at all in playing with others come to actually enjoy doing so, and indeed eagerly seek it out, after a prolonged period of behavioral social skills intervention. As described earlier, most behavioral social skills interventions involve the presentation of positive reinforcement of some kind, immediately following the display of positive social behavior. However this behavior-reinforcer relation does not take place in a vacuum. Each time positive reinforcement is delivered, other social stimuli are present, such as praise, eye contact, physical contact (e.g., high fives, pats on the back), toys, and other play materials. It is possible that the thousands or tens-of-thousands of repeated pairings of positive reinforcers with social stimuli of various sorts result in those stimuli acquiring conditioned reinforcing functions, through the behavioral process of respondent conditioning. Thus, the repeated reinforcement of positive social behaviors may actually have a highly desirable respondent side-effect; turning previously neutral social stimuli into conditioned positive reinforcers. If social stimuli become positive reinforcers, then the child would be more likely to seek them out and to do other things that produce them (e.g., ask other children to play).

Little or no research has directly addressed the outcome of intensive behavioral intervention described above, but it is one that is not uncommon, according to the anecdotal report of many clinicians. The positive results that have been observed in measures of socialization in outcome studies of EIBI lend indirect evidence in support of this possibility. Assuming that improvement in measures of socialization reflect improved social engagement, it would seem at least somewhat unlikely that children would be socially engaged to a significant degree if social interaction were not a source of positive reinforcement. However, this interpretation must be considered purely speculative until further research is available which examines it directly. Future researchers will likely be highly challenged in designing studies that can evaluate this process experimentally. By its very nature, the process is slow (i.e., it may take months or years), and most intervention research is conducted over short periods of time. In addition, single-subject methodology may not be suited to addressing this topic because of the lengthy durations of time required to produce the effect, and because it would presumably be unethical to reverse the effect, once produced. Much additional research is needed to investigate the possibility that behavioral intervention makes children with ASDs actually want to interact socially to a greater degree, and such research will need to be innovative. However, the topic is worthy of investigation, at least partially because it addresses the treatment of social skills at a level which is rarely touched upon – the level of basic behavioral mechanisms.

Conclusion

A large number of studies have evaluated the effectiveness of various approaches to social skills interventions for individuals with ASDs, and this research has been briefly outlined here. The vast majority of intervention studies have been behavioral in conceptual and procedural orientation. Most published studies involve some variation of prompting and reinforcement (Matson et al., 2007). The particular social behaviors addressed range from relatively simple (e.g., social initiations) to relatively complex (e.g., reciprocal interactions), and intervention formats vary, including more and less-structured approaches, and including peer and adult-mediated treatments. A general conclusion that can be gleaned from this body of literature is that behavioral approaches to social skills interventions for individuals with ASDs can be highly effective on a wide variety of social skills and that their effects can be generalized. However, much further research is needed to examine the effects of these interventions on a broader scale, both in terms of the repertoires being developed, across larger swaths of participants' social lives and across larger spans of time.

Another observation is that there has been a general disconnect between the development of assessment methods for measuring social skills in ASD and the use of these scales in treatment studies. The standard practice has been to use these scales to either confirm diagnosis or to describe differences in social skills among various diagnostic groups. However, treatment studies have almost exclusively relied upon operational definitions of specific social skills. One implication is that this may show a general dissatisfaction among applied researchers and treatment providers with the existing scales. Another explanation may be that these studies generally use a single-subject design to teach a few discrete behaviors. In these situations, it is simply more practical to measure changes in the specific target behavior relative to baseline. Further, assessment instruments may simply represent too generalized of a behavior repertoire to be considered useful. Bridging the gap between single-subject design studies that use operationally defined target behaviors and larger group-design studies that use psychometrically reliable and valid instruments is a necessary step in the development of a treatment program (Hayes, Barlow, & Nelson-Gray, 1999). Nonetheless, this step is woefully neglected not simply in the area of social skills but treatments for ASD in general.

Future work must address the divide between assessment methods for measuring social skills in ASD and the use of these scales in treatment studies. Also, as we noted earlier, while treatment studies that refine specific approaches to discrete social behaviors are helpful, at some point this must be broadened to more generalized repertoires of social skills. This has been addressed to some extent in the EIBI literature. Changes in these studies though are typically measured on a broadband level with scales that have not been developed for that purpose. The validity of the inferences made from these scales has generally gone unexamined. Employing more focused assessment tools such as the MESSY and SSRS within studies that target generalized repertoires of social skills in children with ASDs may serve to bridge the divide.

References

Achenbach, T. M. (1991). *Manual for the Child Behavior Checklist/ 4–18 and 1991 profile*. Burlington: University of Vermont Department of Psychiatry.

American Psychiatric Association. (2000). *Diagnostic and statistical manual of mental disorders-fourth edition text revision (DSM-IV-TR)*. Washington, DC: Author.

Bacanli, H., & Erdoğan, F. (2003). Adaptation of the matson evaluation of social skills with youngsters (MESSY) to

Turkish. *Education Sciences: Theory and Practice*, *3*, 368–379.

Charlop, M. H., & Milstein, J. P. (1989). Teaching autistic children conversational speech using video modeling. *Journal of Applied Behavior Analysis*, *22*, 275–285.

Charlop-Christy, M. H., & Daneshvar, S. (2003). Using video modeling to teach perspective taking to children with autism. *Journal of Positive Behavior Interventions*, *5*, 12–21.

Charlop-Christy, M. H., Le, L., & Freeman, K. A. (2000). A comparison of video-modeling with in-vivo modeling for teaching children with autism. *Journal of Autism and Developmental Disorders*, *30*, 537–552.

Charman, T., Taylor, E., Drew, A., Cockerill, H., Brown, J., & Baird, G. (2005). Outcome at 7 years of children diagnosed with autism at age 2: predictive validity of assessments conducted at 2 and 3 years of age and pattern of symptom change over time. *Journal of Child Psychology and Psychiatry*, *46*, 500–513.

Chou, K. (1997). The matson evaluation of social skills with youngsters: Reliability and validity of a Chinese translation. *Personality and Individual Differences*, *22*, 123–125.

Cohen, H., Amerine-Dickens, M., & Smith, T. (2006). Early intensive behavioral treatment: Replication of the UCLA model in a community setting. *Developmental and Behavioral Pediatrics*, *2*, 145–157.

Cohen, I. L. (2003). Criterion-related validity of the PDD behavior inventory. *Journal of Autism and Developmental Disorders*, *33*, 47–53.

Cohen, I. L., Schmidt-Lackner, S., Romanczyk, R., & Sudhalter, V. (2003). The PDD behavior inventory: A rating scale for assessing response to intervention in children with pervasive developmental disorder. *Journal of Autism and Developmental Disorders*, *33*, 31–45.

Cohen, I. L., & Sudhalter, V. (1999). *PDD behavior inventory: Professional manual*. Lutz, FL: Psychological Assessment Resources.

Constantino, J. N., & Gruber, C. P. (2005). *The social responsiveness scale manual*. Los Angeles: Western Psychological Services.

Constantino, J. N., Gruber, C. P., Davis, S., Hayes, S., Passanante, N., & Przybeck, T. (2004). The factor structure of autistic traits. *Journal of Child Psychology and Psychiatry*, *45*, 719–726.

Constantino, J. N., Lajonchere, C., Lutz, M., Gray, T., Abbacchi, A., McKenna, K., et al. (2006). Autistic social impairment in the siblings of children with pervasive developmental disorders. *American Journal of Psychiatry*, *163*, 294–296.

Constantino, J. N., LaVesser, P. D., Zhang, Y., Abbacchi, A. M., Gray, T., & Todd, R. D. (2007). Rapid quantitative assessment of autistic social impairment by classroom teachers. *Journal of the American Academy of Child and Adolescent Psychiatry*, *46*, 1668–1676.

Constantino, J. N., & Todd, R. D. (2003). Autistic traits in the general population: A twin study. *Archives of General Psychiatry*, *60*, 524–530.

Constantino, J. N., & Todd, R. D. (2005). Intergenerational transmission of subthreshold autistic traits in the general population. *Biological Psychiatry*, *57*, 655–660.

Cowen, R. J., & Allen, K. D. (2007). Using naturalistic procedures to enhance learning in individuals with autism: A focus on generalized teaching within the school setting. *Psychology in the Schools*, *44*, 701–715.

Cox, A., Klein, K., Charman, T., Baird, G., Baron-Cohen, S., Swettenham, J. et al. (1999). Autism spectrum disorders at 20 and 42 months of age: Stability of clinical and ADI-R diagnosis. *Journal of Child Psychology and Psychiatry*, *40*, 719–732.

Davis, C. A., Brady, M. P., Hamilton, R., McEvoy, M. A. (1994). Effects of high-probability requests on the social interactions of young children with severe disabilities. *Journal of Applied Behavior Analysis*, *27*, 619–637.

de Bildt, A., Serra, M., Luteijn, E., Kraijer, D., Sytema, S., & Minderaa, R. (2005). Social skills in children with intellectual disabilities with and without autism. *Journal of Intellectual Disability Research*, *49*, 317–328.

DeKlyen, M., & Odom, S. L. (1989). Activity structure and social interactions with peers in developmentally integrated play groups. *Journal of Early Intervention*, *13*, 342–352.

DiLavore, P., Lord, C., & Rutter, M. (1995). Pre-linguistic autism diagnostic observation schedule. *Journal of Autism and Developmental Disorders*, *25*, 355–379.

Dogra, N., & Parkin, A. (1997). Young person's social interaction group. *Clinical Child Psychology and Psychiatry*, *2*, 297–306.

Fagan, J., & Fantuzzo, J. W. (1999). Multirater congruence on the social skills rating system: Mother, father, and teacher assessments of urban head start children's social competencies. *Early Childhood Research Quarterly*, *14*, 229–242.

First, M. B., Gibbon, M., Spitzer R. L., Williams, J. B. W., & Benjamin, L. S.(1997). *Structured clinical interview for DSM-IV Axis II personality disorders (SCID-II)*. Washington, DC: American Psychiatric Press, Inc.

Foxx, R. M. (1999). Long term maintenance of language and social skills. *Behavioral Interventions*, *14*, 135–146.

Goldstein, H., & Cisar, C. L. (1992). Promoting interaction during sociodramatic play: Teaching scripts to typical preschoolers and classmates with disabilities. *Journal of Applied Behavior Analysis*, *25*, 265–280.

Gray, C. (2000). *The new Social Story*[TM] *book. (Illustrated edition)*. Arlington, TX: Future Horizons Inc.

Gresham, F. M., & Elliott, S. N. (1984). Assessment and classification of children's social skills: A review of methods and issues. *School Psychology Review*, *13*, 292–301.

Gresham, F. M., & Elliott, S. N. (1990). *Social skills rating system*. Circle Pines, MN: American Guidance Service.

Harris, S. L., Handleman, J. S., & Alessandri, M. (1990). Teaching youths with autism to offer assistance. *Journal of Applied Behavior Analysis*, *23*, 297–305.

Hartman, C. A., Luteijn, E., Serra, M., & Minderaa, R. (2006). Refinement of the children's social behavior questionnaire (CSBQ): An instrument that describes the diverse problems seen in milder forms of PDD. *Journal of Autism and Developmental Disorders*, *36*, 325–342.

Hayes, S. C., Barlow, D. H., & Nelson-Gray, R. (1999). *The scientist practitioner: Research and accountability in the age of managed care* (2nd Ed.). London: Allyn & Bacon.

Jahr, E., Eldevick, S., & Eikeseth, S. (2000). Teaching children with autism to initiate and sustain cooperative play. *Research in Developmental Disabilities*, *21*, 151–169.

Jurado, M., Cumba-Avilés, E., Collazo, L. C., & Matos, M. (2006). Reliability and validity of a Spanish version of the social skills rating system-teacher form. *Journal of Psychoeducational Assessment, 24*, 195–209.

Kanner, L. (1943). Autistic disturbance of affective contact. *Nervous Child, 2*, 217–250.

Kazdin, A. E., Esveldt-Dawson, K., & Matson, J. L. (1983). The effects on instructional set on social skills performance among psychiatric inpatient children. *Behavior Therapy, 14*, 413–423.

Koegel, R. L., & Frea, W. D. (1993). Treatment of social behavior in autism through the modification of pivotal social skills. *Journal of Applied Behavior Analysis, 26*, 369–377.

Koegel, L. K., Koegel, R. L., Hurley, C., & Frea, W. (1992). Improving social skills and disruptive behavior in children with autism through self-management. *Journal of Applied Behavior Analysis, 25*, 341–353.

Koning, C., & Magill-Evans, J. (2001). Social and language skills in adolescent boys with asperger syndrome. *Autism, 5*, 23–36.

Krantz, P. J., & McClannahan, L. E. (1993). Teaching children with autism to initiate to peers: Effects of a script-fading procedure. *Journal of Applied Behavior Analysis, 26*, 121–132.

Krantz, P. J., & McClannahan L. E. (1998). Social interaction skills for children with autism: A script-fading procedure for beginning readers. *Journal of Applied Behavior Analysis, 31*, 191–202.

Krug, D. A., Arick, J., & Almond, P. (1980). Behavior checklist for identifying severely handicapped individuals with high levels of autistic behavior. *Journal of Child Psychology and Psychiatry, 21*, 221–229.

Kuoch, H., & Mirenda, P. (2003). Social story interventions for young children with autism spectrum disorders. *Focus on Autism and Other Developmental Disabilities, 18*, 219–228.

Landazabal, M. G. (2006). Psychopathological symptoms, social skills and personality traits: A study with adolescents. *The Spanish Journal of Psychology, 9*, 182–192.

LeBlanc, L. A., Coates, A. M., Daneshvar, S., Charlop-Christy, M. H., Morris, C., & Lancaster, B. M. (2003). Using video modeling and reinforcement to teach perspective-taking skills to children with autism. *Journal of Applied Behavior Analysis, 36*, 253–237.

Le Couteur, A., Rutter, M., Lord, C., Rios, P., Robertson, S., Holdgrafer, M. et al. (1989). Autism diagnostic interview: A semistructured interview for parents and caregivers of autistic persons. *Journal of Autism and Developmental Disorders, 19*, 363–387.

Lord, C., & Magill-Evans, J. (1995). Peer interactions of autistic children and adolescents. *Development and Psychopathology, 7*, 611–626.

Lord, C., Risi, S., DiLavore, P. S., Shulman, C., Thurm, A., & Pickles, A. (2006). Autism from 2 to 9 years of age. *Archives of General Psychiatry, 63*, 694–701.

Lord, C., Risi, S., Lambrecht, L., Cook, E. H., Leventhal, B. L., DiLavore, P. C. et al. (2000). The autism diagnostic observation schedule – Generic: A standard measure of social and communication deficits associated with the spectrum of autism. *Journal of Autism and Developmental Disorders, 30*, 205–223.

Lord, C., Rutter, M., DiLavore, P. C., & Risi, S. (1999). *Autism diagnostic observation schedule.* Los Angeles: Western Psychological Services.

Lord, C., Rutter, M., & Le Couteur, A. (1994) Autism diagnostic interview-revised: A revised version of a diagnostic interview for caregivers of individuals with possible pervasive developmental disorders. *Journal of Autism and Developmental Disorders, 24*, 659–686.

Lovaas, I. O. (1987). Behavioral treatment and normal educational and intellectual functioning in young autistic children. *Journal of Consulting and Clinical Psychology, 55*, 3–9.

Luteijn, E. F., Jackson, A. E., Volkmar, F. R., & Minderaa, R. B. (1998). The development of the children's social behavior questionnaire: preliminary data. *Journal of Autism and Developmental Disorders, 28*, 559–565.

Luteijn, E. F., Luteijn, F., Jackson, S., Volkmar, F., & Minderaa, R. (2000). The children's social behavior questionnaire for milder variants of PDD problems: Evaluation of the psychometric characteristics. *Journal of Autism and Developmental Disorders, 30*, 317–330.

Luteijn, E. F., Serra, M., Jackson, S., Steenhuis, M. P., Althaus, M., Volkmar, F. et al. (2000). How unspecified are disorders of children with a pervasive developmental disorder not otherwise specified? A study of social problems in children with PDD-NOS and ADHD. *European Child & Adolescent Psychiatry, 9*, 168–179.

Macintosh, K., & Dissanayake, C. (2006). Social skills and problem behaviours in school aged children with high-functioning autism and asperger's disorder. *Journal of Autism and Developmental Disorders, 36*, 1065–1076.

Maione, L., & Mirenda, P. (2006). Effects of video modeling and video feedback on peer-directed social language skills of a child with autism. *Journal of Positive Behavior Interventions, 8*, 106–118.

Manz, P. H., Fantuzzo, J. W., & McDermott, P. A. (1999). The parent version of the preschool social skills rating scale: An analysis of its use with low-income, ethnic minority children. *The School Psychology Review, 28*, 493–504.

Matson, J. L. (2007). Determining treatment outcome in early intervention programs for autism spectrum disorders: A critical analysis of measurement issues in learning based interventions. *Research in Developmental Disabilities, 28*, 207–218.

Matson, J. L., & Boisjoli, J. A. (2007). Differential diagnosis of PDD-NOS in children. *Research in Autism Spectrum Disorders, 1*, 75–84.

Matson, J., Boisjoli, J., González, M., Smith, K., & Wilkins, J. (2007). Norms and cut off scores for the autism spectrum disorders diagnosis for adults (ASD-DA) with intellectual disability. *Research in Autism Spectrum Disorders, 1*, 330–338.

Matson, J. L., Compton, L. S., & Sevin, J. A. (1991). Comparison and item analysis of the MESSY for autistic and normal children. *Research in Developmental Disabilities, 12*, 361–369.

Matson, J. L., Dempsey, T., & LoVullo, S. V. (2009). Characteristics of social skills for adults with intellectual disability, autism and PDD-NOS. *Research in Autism Spectrum Disorders, 3*, 207–213.

Matson, J. L., & González, M. (2007). *Autism spectrum disorders – child version: Administrator's manual.* Baton Rouge, LA: Disability Consultants.

Matson, J. L., González, M. L., & Wilkins, J. (2009). Validity study of the autism spectrum disorders-diagnostic for children (ASD-DC). *Research in Autism Spectrum Disorders, 3,* 196–206.

Matson, J. L., González, M. L., Wilkins, J., & Rivet, T. T. (2008). Reliability of the autism spectrum disorders-diagnostic for children (ASD-DC). *Research in Autism Spectrum Disorders, 2,* 533–545.

Matson, J. L., & Wilkins, J. (2009). Psychometric testing methods for children's social skills. *Research in Developmental Disabilities, 30,* 249–274.

Matson, J. L., Wilkins, J., Boisjoli, J. A., & Smith, K. R. (2008). The validity of the autism spectrum disorders diagnosis for intellectually disabled adults (ASD-DA). *Research in Developmental Disabilities, 29,* 537–546.

Matson, J. L., Heinze, A., Helsel, W. J., Kapperman, G., & Rotatori, A. F. (1986). Assessing social behaviors in the visually handicapped: The matson evaluation of social skills with youngsters (MESSY). *Journal of Clinical Child Psychology, 15,* 78–87.

Matson, J. L., Macklin, G. F., & Helsel, W. J. (1985). Psychometric properties of the matson evaluation of social skills with youngsters (MESSY) with emotional problems and self concept in deaf children. *Journal of Behavior Therapy and Experimental Psychiatry, 16,* 117–123.

Matson, J., Matson, M., & Rivet, T. (2007). Social-skills treatments for children with autistic spectrum disorders: An overview. *Behavior Modification, 31,* 682–707.

Matson, J. L., Nebel-Schwalm, M. S., & Matson, M. L. (2007). A review of methodological issues in the differential diagnosis of autism spectrum disorders in children. *Research in Autism Spectrum Disorders, 1,* 38–54.

Matson, J. L., & Ollendick, T. H. (1988). *Enhancing children's social skills: Assessment and training (Japanese translation).* Tokyo: UNI Agency Inc.

Matson, J. L., Rotatori, A. F., & Helsel, W. J. (1983). Development of a rating scale to measure social skills in children: The matson evaluation of social skills with youngsters (MESSY). *Behaviour Research and Therapy, 21,* 335–340.

Matson, J. L., & Wilkins, J. (2007). A critical review of assessment targets and methods for social skills excesses and deficits for children with autism spectrum disorders. *Research in Autism Spectrum Disorders, 1,* 28–37.

Matson, J. L., Wilkins, J., & González, M. (2007). Reliability and factor structure of the autism spectrum disorders – Diagnosis scale for intellectually disabled adults (ASD-DA). *Journal of Developmental and Physical Disabilities, 19,* 565–577.

McClannahan, L. E., & Krantz, P. J. (2005). *Teaching conversation to children with autism: Scripts and script fading.* Bethesda, MD: Woodbine House.

McConnell, S. (2002). Interventions to facilitate social interaction for young children with autism: Review of available research and recommendations for educational intervention and future research. *Journal of Autism and Developmental Disorders, 32,* 351–372.

McGee, G., Almeida, C., Sulzer-Azaroff, B., & Feldman, S. (1992). Promoting reciprocal interactions via peer incidental teaching. *Journal of Applied Behavior Analysis, 25,* 117–26.

Meijer, S. A., Sinnema, G., Bijstra, J. O., Mellenbergh, G. J., & Wolters, W. H. G. (2000a). Peer interaction in adolescents with a chronic illness. *Personality and Individual Differences, 29,* 799–813.

Meijer, S. A., Sinnema, G., Bijstra, J. O., Mellenbergh, G. J., & Wolters, W. H. G. (2000b). Social functioning in children with a chronic illness. *The Journal of Child Psychology and Psychiatry and Allied Disciplines, 41,* 309–317.

Méndez, F. X., Hidalgo, M. D., & Inglés, C. J. (2002). The matson evaluation of social skills with youngsters. *European Journal of Psychological Assessment, 18,* 30–32.

Merrell, K. W., & Popinga, M. R. (1994). Parent-teacher concordance and gender differences in behavioral ratings of social skills and social-emotional problems of primary age children with disabilities. *Diagnostique, 19,* 1–14.

Mildenberger, K., Sitter, S., Noterdaeme, M., & Amorosa, H. (2001). The use of the ADI-R as a diagnostic tool in the differential diagnosis of children with infantile autism and children with receptive language disorder. *European Child & Adolescent Psychiatry, 10,* 248–255.

Moore, V., & Goodson, S. (2003). How well does early diagnosis of autism stand the test of time? *Autism, 7,* 47–62.

Morrison, L., Kamps, D., Garcia, J., & Parker, D. (2001). Peer mediation and monitoring strategies to improve initiations and social skills for students with autism. *Journal of Positive Behavior Interventions, 3,* 237–250.

Nikopolous, C. K., & Keenan, M. (2003). Promoting social initiation in children with autism using video modeling. *Behavioral Interventions, 18,* 87–108.

Nikopolous, C. K., & Keenan, M. (2004). Effects of video modeling on social initiations by children with autism. *Journal of Applied Behavior Analysis, 37,* 93–96.

Noterdaeme, M., Sitter, S., Mildenberger, K., & Amorosa, H. (2000). Diagnostic assessment of communicative and interactive behaviours in children with autism and receptive language disorder. *European Child & Adolescent Psychiatry, 9,* 295–300.

Odom, S. L., McConnell, S. R., McEvoy, M. A., Peterson, C., Ostrosky, M., Chandler, L. et al. (1999). Relative effects of interventions supporting the social competence of young children with disabilities. *Topics in Early Childhood Special Education, 19,* 75–91.

Odom, S. L., & Strain, P. S. (1984). Peer mediated approaches to promoting children's social interactions: A review. *American Journal of Orthopsychiatry, 54,* 544–557.

Ozonoff, S., & Miller, J. N. (1995). Teaching theory of mind: A new approach to social skills training for individuals with autism. *Journal of Autism and Developmental Disorders, 25,* 415–433.

Pearlman-Avnion, S., & Eviator, Z. (2002). *Irony understanding preservation in nonverbal learning disabilities.* Haifa, Israel: University of Haifa.

Pierce, K., & Schreibman, L. (1995). Increasing complex social behaviors in children with autism: Effects of peer-implemented pivotal response training. *Journal of Applied Behavior Analysis, 28,* 285–295.

Pierce, K., & Schreibman, L. (1997a). Multiple peer use of pivotal response training social behaviors of classmates with autism: Results from trained and untrained peers. *Journal of Applied Behavior Analysis, 30*, 157–160.

Pierce, K., & Schreibman, L. (1997b). Using peer trainers to promote social behavior in autism: Are they effective at enhancing multiple social modalities? *Focus on Autism and Other Developmental Disabilities, 12*, 207–218.

Pine, E., Luby, J., Abbacchi, A., & Constantino, J. N. (2006). Quantitative assessment of autistic symptomatology in preschoolers. *Autism, 10*, 344–352.

Powless, D. L., & Elliott, S. N. (1993). Assessment of social skills of Native American preschoolers: Teachers' and parents' ratings. *Journal of School Psychology, 31*, 293–307.

Remington, B., Hastings, R. P., Kovshoff, H., Espinosa, F. E., Jahr, E., Brown, T. et al. (2007). Early intensive behavioral intervention: Outcomes for children with autism and their parents after two years. *American Journal on Mental Retardation, 112*, 418–438.

Reynhout, G., & Carter, M. (2006). Social stories for children with disabilities. *Journal of Autism and Developmental Disorders, 30*, 445–469.

Rogers, S. (2000). Interventions that facilitate socialization in children with autism. *Journal of Autism and Developmental Disorders, 30*, 399–409.

Rojahn, J., Aman, M. G., Matson, J. L., & Mayville, E. (2003). The aberrant behavior checklist and the behavior problems inventory: Convergent and divergent validity. *Research in Developmental Disabilities, 24*, 391–404.

Rutter, M., Le Couteur, A., & Lord, C. (2003). *Autism diagnostic interview revised: WPS edition manual.* Los Angeles: Western Psychological Services.

Sallows, G. O., & Graupner, T. D. (2005). Intensive behavioral treatment for children with autism: Four-year outcome and predictors. *American Journal on Mental Retardation, 110*, 417–438.

Sansosti, F. J., & Powell-Smith, K. A. (2006). Using social stories to improve the social behavior of children with asperger syndrome. *Journal of Positive Behavior Interventions, 8*, 43–57.

Sarakoff, R. A., Taylor, B. A., & Poulson, C. L. (2001). Teaching children with autism to engage in conversational exchanges: Script fading with embedded textual stimuli. *Journal of Applied Behavior Analysis, 34*, 81–84.

Schleien, S., J., Mustonen, T., & Rynders, J. E. (1995). Participation of Children with Autism and Nondisabled Peers in a Cooperatively Structured Community Art Program. *Journal of Autism and Developmental Disorders, 25*, 397–413.

Shabani, D. B., Katz, R. C., Wilder, D. A., Beauchamp, K., Taylor, C. R., & Fischer, K. J. (2002). Increasing social initiations in children with autism: Effects of a tactile prompt. *Journal of Applied Behavior Analysis, 35*, 79–83.

Shahim, S. (2001). Reliability of the social skills rating system in a group of Iranian children. *Psychological Reports, 89*, 566–570.

Shahim, S. (2004). Reliability of the social skills rating system for preschool children in Iran. *Psychological Reports, 95*, 1264–1266.

Sharma, S., Sigafoos, J., & Carroll, A. (2000). Social skills assessment of Indian children with visual impairments. *Journal of Visual Impairments and Blindness, 94*, 172–176.

Shearer, D., Kohler, F., Buchan, K., & McCullough, K. (1996). Promoting independent interactions between preschoolers with autism and their nondisabled peers: An analysis of self-monitoring. *Early Education and Development, 7*, 205–220.

Sherer, M., Pierce, K. L., Peredes, S., Kisacky, K. L., Ingersoll, B., & Schreibman, L. (2001). Enhancing conversation skills in children with autism via video technology: Which is better, "Self" or "Other" as model?. *Behavior Modification, 25*, 140–158.

Spence, S. H., & Liddle, B. (1990). Self-report measures of social competence for children: An evaluation of the matson evaluation of social skills for youngsters and the list of social situation problems. *Behavioral Assessment, 12*, 317–336.

Stage, S. A., Cheney, D., Walker, B., & LaRocque, M. (2002). A preliminary discriminant and convergent validity study of the teacher functional behavioral assessment checklist. *School Psychology Review, 31*, 71–93.

Stevenson, C. L., Krantz, P. J., McClannahan, L. E. (2000). Social interaction skills for children with autism: A script-fading procedure for nonreaders. *Behavioral Interventions, 15*, 1–20.

Stokes, T. F., & Baer, D. M. (1977). An implicit technology of generalization. *Journal of Applied Behavior Analysis, 10*, 249–267.

Stuart, D. L., Gresham, F. M., & Elliott, S. N. (1991). Teacher ratings of social skills in popular and rejected males and females. *School Psychology Quarterly, 61*, 16–26.

Taylor, B. A., & Levin, L. (1998). Teaching a student with autism to make verbal initiations: Effects of a tactile prompt. *Journal of Applied Behavior Analysis, 31*, 651–654.

Taylor, B. A., Levin, L., & Jasper, S. (1999). Increasing play-related statements in children with autism toward their siblings: Effects of video modeling. *Journal of Developmental and Physical Disabilities, 11*, 253–264.

Thiemann, K. S., & Goldstein, H. (2001). Social stories, written text cues, and video feedback: Effects on social communication of children with autism. *Journal of Applied Behavior Analysis, 34*, 425–446.

Thorp, D. M., Shahmer, A. C., & Schreibman, L. (1995). Effects on sociodramatic play training on children with autism. *Journal of Autism and Developmental Disorders, 25*, 265–282.

Torres, M. V. T., Cardelle-Elawar, M., Mena, M. J. B., & Sanchez, A. M. M. (2003). Social background, gender and self-reported social competence in 11- and 12-year-old Andalusian children. *Electronic Journal of Research in Educational Psychology, 1*, 37–56.

Tse, J., Strulovitch, J., Tagalakis, V., Meng, L., & Fombonne, E. (2007). Social skills training for adolescents with asperger syndrome and high-functioning autism. *Journal of Autism and Developmental Disorders, 37*, 1960–1968.

Van der Oord, S., Van der Meulen, E. M., Prins, P. J. M., Oosterlaan, J., Buitelaar, J. R., & Emmelkamp, P. M. G. (2005). A psychometric evaluation of the social skills rating system in children and adolescents with attention deficit hyperactivity disorder. *Behaviour Research and Therapy, 43*, 733–746.

Van Horn, M. L., Atkins-Burnett, S., Karlin, E., Ramey, S. L., & Snyder, S. (2007). Parent ratings of children's social skills:

Longitudinal psychometric analyses of the Social Skills Rating System. *School Psychology Quarterly*, *22*, 162–199.

Verté, S., Roeyers, H., & Buysse, A. (2003). Behavioural problems, social competence and self-concept in siblings of children with autism. *Child: Care, Health and Development*, *29*, 193–205.

Weiss, M. J., & Harris, S. L. (2001). Teaching social skills to people with autism. *Behavior Modification*, *25*, 785–802.

White, S., Keonig, K., & Scahill, L. (2007). Social skills development in children with autism spectrum disorders: A review of the intervention research. *Journal of Autism and Developmental Disorders*, *37*, 1858–1868.

Wolf, M. M. (1978). Social validity: The case for subjective measurement or how applied behavior analysis is finding its heart. *Journal of Applied Behavior Analysis*, *11*, 203–214.

Yang, N. K., Schaller, J. L., Huang, T., Wang, M. H., & Tsai, S. (2003). Enhancing appropriate social behaviors for children with autism in general education classrooms: An analysis of six cases. *Education and Training in Developmental Disabilities*, *38*, 405–416.

Chapter 8
Intellectual Disability and Adaptive-Social Skills

Giulio E. Lancioni, Nirbhay N. Singh, Mark F. O'Reilly, and Jeff Sigafoos

Definitions of Intellectual Disability

Definitions of intellectual disability are available from the three most widely recognized classification systems, namely, the ICD 10 (i.e., the 10th edition of *The International Classification of Functioning, Disability and Health [ICF]*; World Health Organization, 2001), the DSM-IV-TR (i.e., the textual revision of the 4th edition of the American Psychiatric Association's *Diagnostic and Statistical Manual of the Mental Disorders*; American Psychiatric Association, 2000), and the AAMR 10 (i.e., the 10th revision of the American Association for Mental Retardation's manual – *Mental Retardation: Definition, Classification and Systems of Support*; Luckasson et al., 2002).

All three systems define intellectual disability on the basis of two main factors: (a) significantly subaverage intellectual functioning generally determined through intelligence tests and (b) concurrent deficits in adaptive behavior functioning, that is, difficulties with the skills required for everyday living (see Carr & O'Reilly, 2007; for a thorough comparison of the three systems). The presence of both these factors should be identified in the developmental period prior to adulthood (i.e., prior to 18 years of age) (Brown, 2007; Brown, Parmenter, & Percy, 2007; Matson, 2007).

Intellectual Functioning

Significantly subaverage intellectual functioning is typically defined as an IQ score that falls two standard deviations or more below the mean on a standardized and individually administered intelligence test (Carr & O'Reilly, 2007; Sigafoos, O'Reilly, & Lancioni, in press). Since most intelligence tests have a mean of 100 and a standard deviation of 15 or 16, the implications of the aforementioned definition is that the cutoff score for intellectual disability is generally considered to be an IQ of 70–75 (MacLean, Miller, & Bartsch, 2001; Matson, 2007). This 5-point range allows for measurement error and acknowledges that the diagnosis of intellectual disability is not exclusively based on IQ scores but also requires the concurrent presence of deficits in adaptive behavior functioning (Carr & O'Reilly, 2007; Tylenda, Beckett, & Barrett, 2007).

Adaptive Behavior Functioning

The second major distinctive element in a diagnosis of intellectual disability is the presence of substantial deficits in adaptive behavior functioning (Carr & O'Reilly, 2007; MacLean et al., 2001; Sigafoos et al., in press). Adaptive behavior functioning is generally defined (see also the DSM-IV-TR) as the extent to which the individual copes with the demands of everyday living. For a diagnosis of intellectual disability to be made, DSM-IV-TR criteria require the presence of deficits in adaptive behavior functioning in at least two of the following skill

G.E. Lancioni (✉)
Department of Psychology, University of Bari, Bari, Italy
e-mail: g.lancioni@psico.uniba.it

J.L. Matson (ed.), *Social Behavior and Skills in Children*, DOI 10.1007/978-1-4419-0234-4_8,
© Springer Science+Business Media, LLC 2009

areas: Communication, self-care, home living, social/interpersonal skills, use of community resources, self-direction, functional academic skills, work, leisure, health, and safety (American Psychiatric Association, 2000). Any assessment of adaptive behavior functioning needs to consider the individual's age and sociocultural background, as well as the environmental context (e.g., home, school, or community) in which the individual is supposed to function (cf. Cory, 2006; Embregts,Dattilo, & Williams, 2002).

Classification of Intellectual Disability

Intellectual disability may be classified in different ways depending upon the purpose of the classification and the context in which this operation is conducted (Carr & O'Reilly, 2007; MacLean et al., 2001; Sigafoos et al., in press). For practical reasons, the three classification criteria taken into consideration here are the etiology (causes) of the disability, the severity of the disability, and the levels of support required by the disability (Carr & O'Reilly, 2007; Luckasson et al., 2002).

Etiology

With respect to the etiology, a basic consideration needs to be made at the outset. Although classification of the causes of intellectual disability can be considered very useful in drawing an overall picture of the developmental/performance characteristics of the individuals and their specific intervention needs, such causes remain not infrequently unknown. At present, an etiology can generally be identified in approximately 75% of cases of moderate-to-profound intellectual disability. Yet, only up to 40% of cases of mild intellectual disability have a known cause (Harris, 2005). These percentages are likely to improve with the expected advances in genetic and biomedical research.

The most recognizable causes usually considered are those linked to genetic syndromes (Carr & O'Reilly, 2007; Udwin & Kuczynski, 2007). Among them, one can find the Cri-du-chat

syndrome, Angelman syndrome, Cornelia de Lange syndrome, Down syndrome, Fragile X syndrome, Lesch-Nyhan syndrome, Prader-Willi syndrome, Williams syndrome, and Rett syndrome. All these syndromes are associated with particular/distinctive physical features and a number of cognitive and behavioral characteristics. Knowledge of these features and characteristics can help educational personnel and parents prepare about the difficulties that are likely to be encountered and the intervention requirements (Udwin & Kuczynski, 2007).

A second set of potential causes include (a) metabolic disorders such as phenylketonuria and congenital hypothyroidism (Carr & O'Reilly, 2007), (b) maternal illness such as hepatitis, rubella, diabetes, cytomegalovirus, and toxoplasmosis or exposure to toxins or radiation (Udwin & Kuczynski, 2007), (c) possible perinatal complications such as hypoxia and brain hemorrhage (Carr & O'Reilly, 2007), and (d) possible postnatal events such as traumatic brain injury (Carr & O'Reilly, 2007; Udwin & Kuczynski, 2007).

Another set of potential causes relate to social and educational factors. Among those factors one could include (a) maternal malnutrition and lack of access to prenatal and perinatal care, (b) combinations and abuses of drugs, smoking, and alcohol during pregnancy, and (c) disturbed interaction between the child and love figures, environmental deprivation, and lack of access to educational opportunities (Carr & O'Reilly, 2007; Udwin & Kuczynski, 2007).

Severity of the Intellectual Disability

Clinical psychologists and educational personnel have found it practically helpful to classify intellectual disability in terms of levels of severity. The levels of severity typically referred to in this context are: Mild, Moderate, Severe, and Profound. This type of classification is used in both the ICD 10 and the DSM-IV-TR but is not explicitly adopted in AAMR 10 (see below). The most immediate implication of this classification is that it provides a reference frame within which each severity level has a corresponding range of educational and leisure/occupational opportunities for the individual involved. Obviously, the educational and leisure/occupational needs of individuals with mild intellectual disability would be very different from the needs of individuals with severe and profound intellectual disability. Even so, it must be emphasized that there is considerable variability in cognitive and adaptive behavior functioning and learning potential among the individuals within each of the four disability levels (Harris, 2005; Matson, 2007; Sigafoos et al., in press).

The mild intellectual disability level is associated with IQ scores ranging from 50–55 to approximately 70. Although mild intellectual disability is occasionally attributed to cultural-familial factors (cf. Carr & O'Reilly, 2007; Tylenda et al., 2007), its etiology may include the full range of known causes (e.g., genetic syndromes, maternal illness, and perinatal complications). Cases of mild intellectual disability may go undetected until the child enters school and begins to fail academically. Such a delay in diagnosis and the negative implications of it in educational and social (familiar) terms would emphasize either a lack of usually prescribed developmental checks or lack of rigor within those checks (see Carr & O'Reilly, 2007).

The moderate intellectual disability level is associated with IQ scores that range from 34–40 to 50–55. Thus an individual with an IQ score of 50 or 55 could be classified as having mild or moderate intellectual disability depending on the extent of his or her adaptive behavior deficits. Generally, cases of moderate intellectual disability are more likely to (a) have a known etiology than is expected for cases with mild intellectual disability (Carr & O'Reilly, 2007; Tylenda et al., 2007), (b) require more carefully designed educational plans, and (c) benefit more extensively from educational programs not relying on conventional school (academic) activities. Given the more complex picture and the usually more obvious developmental delays, moderate intellectual disability is commonly recognized during early childhood.

The severe and profound intellectual disability levels are associated with IQ scores of 20–25 to 35–40 and below 20 or 25, respectively. Virtually all of these individuals are identified in infancy on the basis of known etiology and significant, easily observable developmental delay. Their learning and behavior deficits are usually quite substantial

and the possibility of finding a reliable score on an IQ test is quite difficult. Individuals with severe and profound intellectual disability frequently present with major health-related problems (e.g., epilepsy) as well as sensory and physical impairments, which complicate assessment and educational intervention. Educational programs need to concentrate on issues such as self-help skills, augmentative and alternative communication, and constructive engagement with environmental and social stimuli rather than on school activities.

Levels of Support Required

The American Association on Intellectual and Developmental Disabilities has moved away from a simple and specific classification in terms of severity of intellectual disability based largely on IQ scores. Rather, it has primarily focused on a classification based on the types and amount of support required by the individual (Luckasson et al., 2002). Four levels/categories of support have been identified: Intermittent, Limited, Extensive, and Pervasive. These categories represent a continuum. This ranges from brief periods of targeted intervention at specific times, such as establishing specific self-care skills prior to the transition to a new phase of the educational plan (Intermittent) to more constant, ongoing, and life-sustaining assistance across all areas of functioning (Pervasive) (Carr & O'Reilly, 2007; Green, Sigafoos, O'Reilly, & Arthur-Kelly, 2006; Sigafoos et al., in press; Tylenda et al., 2007). Levels of support do not necessarily or consistently correspond to severity of intellectual disability. Instead, the level of required support would be expected to reflect the perceived range of needs at the time of the assessment, which may change over time (Harris, 2005). For example, a child with mild mental retardation might require extensive support for a short period of time to address emerging problem behaviors (e.g., aggression). After that particular period of time, however, only intermittent supports might be necessary to maintain the behavioral improvements obtained.

Tools for Assessing Adaptive-Social Skills

Adaptive-social skills can be defined as an assortment of behavioral expressions and activities that make an individual fairly satisfactorily adjusted (positively connected) to his or her environment, constructively engaged with objects and people, and easily recognized as acceptable to the social context in which he or she lives (Luiselli, 1998; O'Reilly, Cannella, Sigafoos, & Lancioni, 2006; Saloviita & Pennanen, 2003; Vermeer, Lijnse, & Lindhout, 2004; Wilkins & Matson, 2007). Obviously, the adaptive-social skills can include different ranges of behaviors and activities depending upon the age of the individual and his or her level of intellectual disability, which could also be combined with the presence of other disabilities (e.g., sensory or motor disabilities) (cf. Carr & O'Reilly, 2007). For example, the adaptive-social skills of a 7-year-old child with moderate- to-severe intellectual disability and motor impairment may be reflected by his or her use of assistive technology devices to control environmental stimulation and call for the attention of and contact with a parent or other caregiver (Lancioni et al., 2008a, 2008b). The adaptive-social skills of a 9-year-old child with mild intellectual disabilities may include, among others, conversational aspects that the child displays in connection with peers (with or without disabilities) in different daily contexts, and social problem-solving abilities allowing positive adjustments within interpersonal interactions (i.e., by adopting solutions not previously practiced or not satisfactorily managed) (Brady, 2000; Carter & Maxwell, 1998; Cory et al., 2006; Wilkins & Matson, 2007).

A variety of tools exist for the evaluation (i.e., for drawing a general picture) of an individual's social-adaptive skills. They mainly include sociometric techniques, direct observations, behavioral interviews, and rating scales. Rating scales are very popular approaches and can be administered directly to the individual with intellectual disability who would then be required to provide the responses directly or to people such as teachers and caregivers who are highly familiar with the condition of the individual they are responsible for. A number of the most popular rating scales used in the area are presented below.

Matson Evaluation of Social Skills for Individuals with Severe Retardation (MESSIER)

The MESSIER is a questionnaire containing 85 items designed to measure social strength and weaknesses in individuals with severe and profound intellectual disability from childhood to adulthood (Matson, Wilkins & Matson, 1995; 2007). The items are compiled from the communication and socialization domains of the Vineland Adaptive Behavior Scales (see below), from the Matson Evaluation of Social Skills for Youngsters (see below), and from nomination by experts (Wilkins & Matson, 2007). The scale involves six clinically derived dimensions, namely, positive nonverbal (e.g., discriminates between persons and addresses persons), positive verbal (e.g., thanks others), general positive (e.g., responds properly when meets others), negative nonverbal (e.g., withdraws and isolates self), negative verbal (e.g., makes awkward comments), and general negative (e.g., has difficulties waiting to satisfy own needs). Compared to intelligence tests and some of the other diagnostic tools available, the MESSIER is deemed helpful in underlining individual strengths and weaknesses and thus in providing the basis for developing an intervention plan.

Matson Evaluation of Social Skills for Youngsters (MESSY)

The MESSY is a psychometric alternative to role-play tests, which are generally quite unreliable (Matson, Rotatori, & Helsel, 1983) and covers an age range extending from 7 to 15 years. It involves 64 items that concern positive as well as negative aspects of the individual's behavior, that is, appropriate social skills (e.g., helps a friend who is hurt or walks to people to start a conversation) and inappropriate social behavior (e.g., wants to get even with someone who hurt him/her). The MESSY includes a teacher-report form and a self-report form. Scores on the MESSY were reported to be positively correlated with the results of teachers' ratings, with the children's popularity within the classroom, and with the children's ability to solve social dilemmas. The same scores were reported to be negatively correlated with symptoms of psychopathology such as anxiety and depression.

Vineland Adaptive Behavior Scales (VABS)

The VABS represent a very popular tool for measuring personal and social skills used for everyday living from birth to adulthood (Sparrow, Balla, & Cicchetti, 1984). These scales are suited for evaluating individuals across the spectrum from typical development to different types of disability. The scales are divided into different domains and sub-domains. The four basic domains are: communication, daily living skills, socialization, and motor skills. The sub-domains for communication include receptive, expressive, and written communication forms. The sub-domains for daily living skills cover personal, domestic, and community living skills. The sub-domains for socialization concern interpersonal relationships, play and leisure time, and coping skills. The sub-domains for motor skills concern both fine and gross response abilities.

The second (Vineland II) edition of the scales also includes an optional fifth domain (i.e., maladaptive behavior index) with sub-domains such as "internalizing, externalizing, and other" (Sparrow, Balla, & Cicchetti, 2005). This new edition has four different forms. The first "Survey Interview Form" relies on a survey carried out with a parent or caregiver using a semi-structured interview format. The second "Parent/Caregiver Rating Form" corresponds to the first form in terms of content but depends on a rating-scale format. This format may be seen as (a) an alternative to the first when there is no time for a survey interview and (b) a valuable complement to the first as the rating-scale format could be regularly applied to monitor the individual's progress in relation to a first survey-interview level. The third "Expanded Interview Form" yields a more comprehensive assessment information than the first form and consequently can also be quite helpful in arranging educational intervention programs to improve the situation of the individual evaluated. The fourth "Teacher Rating Form" is an option available for assessing children in school, preschool, or day care centers. Teachers, caregivers, or other educational personnel are asked to complete a questionnaire. The questionnaire covers the same domains as the survey forms (see above) but involves details and information that the special raters may be able to detect within their daily educational contexts.

AAMR Adaptive Behavior Scale-School Second Edition

This tool is applicable for individuals from 3 to 21 years of age (Lambert, Nihira, & Leyland, 1993). Assessment through this tool is expected to (a) determine the strengths and weaknesses of individuals among adaptive domains representing the level of independence and responsibility in daily living, (b) identify individuals who are significantly below their peers in those domains, and (c) document the progress of individuals involved in intervention programs aimed at improving their status within those domains. The first part of the scale focuses on personal independence and is aimed at evaluating coping skills essential to such independence. To this end, nine behavior domains are available: independent functioning, physical development, economic activity, language development, numbers and time, prevocational/vocational activity, self-direction, responsibility, and socialization. The second part of the scale is focused on social maladaptation in general. For the assessment of this social aspect, seven behavior domains are available, that is, social behavior, conformity, trustworthiness, stereotyped behavior, hyperactive behavior, self-abusive behavior, and disturbing interpersonal behavior.

Checklist of Adaptive Living Skills (CALS)

The CALS is a criterion-referenced measure of adaptive living skills with direct implications for development and intervention programming (Bruininks & Moreau, 2004). The CALS may be used for determining the skills that an individual has mastered and needs to acquire for functioning within a certain context. Based on this, it can be adopted as an instrument that helps caregivers (parents and staff personnel) identify instructional needs, formulate individual training objectives, and monitor progress toward those objectives. It is aimed for use with a wide variety of individuals, with and without intellectual disability, from infancy to adulthood. Each behavior in CALS has a corresponding instructional unit (instructional activity) in a parallel intervention curriculum known as the Adaptive Living Skills Curriculum (ALSC) (Bruininks, Moreau, Gilman, & Anderson, 2004). CALS and ALSC consider approximately 800 specific behavioral responses divided into 24 modules and four broad domains. The domains consist of personal living skills, home living skills, community living skills, and employment skills.

Intervention for Promoting Adaptive-Social Skills

Assessment scales and behavioral observation strategies can help provide a clear picture regarding the two broad types of problems that negatively affect individuals with intellectual disability in the context of adaptive-social skills. Those problems have been conceptualized in terms of behavioral deficits and behavioral excesses (Lovaas, 2003). Deficits are generally present in relation to communication, social interaction, daily living, play and leisure, and fine and gross motor skills (cf. Sparrow et al., 2005). Behavioral excesses can be characterized as self-injury, aggression, property destruction, tantrums, hyperactivity, stereotyped movements, and inadequate postures (Braithwaite & Richdale, 2000; Lancioni et al., 2004; Lancioni, O'Reilly et al., 2006; Luiselli, 1998; Saloviita & Pennanen, 2003). It is important to note here that (a) the areas of major concern and the nature and extent of the problems can vary considerably from individual to individual even when the individuals fall within the same level of disability and (b) behavioral deficits and excesses will tend to be more obvious and significant as the severity of intellectual disability increases (Harris, 2005; Schroeder, Tessel, Loupe, & Stodgell, 1997).

Based on the characteristics of the individual and the peculiarity of his or her problems, intervention programs may be quite different in terms of specific objectives targeted and rationale. For example, for a child with apparently severe/profound intellectual disability and minimal engagement with the immediate environment, the objective initially envisaged may consist of increasing his play and leisure skills (see above). The rationale for it may be that play and leisure are essential for development and provide the child a much more adaptive-social look that would contrast with his or her typically passive/withdrawn behavior (Lancioni, Singh et al., 2006; Sigafoos, O'Reilly, & Green, 2007). This new (more positive) look in turn could prompt new caregivers' attention and social engagement (Lancioni et al., 2008a, 2008b; Sigafoos, Arthur-Kelly, & Butterfield, 2006).

For a child with severe intellectual disability and lack of communication means, the objective may be to build basic forms of request for attention or items that could enable the child to be actively engaged with the environment and the persons around him or her. The rationale would be that this objective (which might be pursued through the use of assistive technology) is critical for general development with wide implications in terms of communication, as well as in terms of adaptive-social skills (Sigafoos et al., 2006, 2007; Sparrow et al., 2005). Reaching such an objective would also determine an interactive form of relationship between child and caregiver in substitution of the possibly unidirectional (caregiver-to-child) rapport previously available (Lancioni, O'Reilly et al., 2007; Lancioni et al., 2008a, 2008b).

For a child with mild intellectual disability, an important objective envisaged could be that of learning to ask for desired items and pay independently for them in community settings (O'Reilly et al., 2006). The rationale would be that the possibility of reaching this objective could have important implications in terms of communication, social interaction, and independence and responsibility in daily living. The rest of this section is directed at presenting a number of examples of intervention strategies for promoting adaptive-social skills in children. Those examples (all published studies) illustrate different situations involving different participants, different objectives/rationales, and different strategies. The aim of their presentation is to provide the reader a broad picture of the general issue and its various aspects.

Example 1: A program to promote adaptive (leisure) engagement and improve mood in children with severe/profound intellectual and other disabilities. Lack of constructive engagement with the immediate environment (i.e., lack of play and leisure behavior) and lack of any apparent sign of enjoyment (i.e., a neutral, unengaged look) convey an image of very poor adaptive-social behavior functioning (Favell, Realon, & Sutton, 1996; Green & Reid, 1999a). The image becomes even more serious (more problematic) if signs of unhappiness, such as frowning and crying, appear instead of the aforementioned neutral, unengaged look (Green & Reid, 1999b). The main objective of the intervention program developed for these cases is to establish engagement (e.g., basic object manipulation). To ensure that engagement responses are maintained and possibly strengthened, clearly positive consequences (i.e., preferred stimuli) need to be arranged for them. The availability of these positive consequences and the child's opportunity to control their timing may represent important variables that can improve the child's self-determination, quality of life, and mood (Algozzine, Browder, Karvonen, Test, & Wood, 2001; Tota et al., 2006).

In a study by Lancioni, Singh et al. (2006), two children of 7.3 and 7.5 years of age were provided with different types of balls, which covered a wobble microswitch (i.e., a technical device allowing the child to control environmental events with minimal responses). The manipulation of the ball activated the microswitch and caused the occurrence of brief periods of preferred stimulation. The design used for the children included a simple AB sequence or an ABABAB sequence (Barlow, Nock, & Hersen, 2009). The A represented the baseline condition (i.e., sessions with the availability of the ball and microswitch but no stimuli for the manipulation of the ball) and the B represented the intervention condition (i.e., sessions that also included the stimulation for the manipulation responses). The children's mean frequencies of responses during baseline were 6 and 14. Their mean frequencies during intervention were 15 and 24. The mean frequencies of intervals with indices of happiness (first child) were two and seven across the two conditions, respectively. The mean frequencies of intervals with indices of unhappiness (second child) were six during baseline and one (with a declining trend), during intervention.

Example 2: A program to promote adaptive (leisure) engagement and requests of social attention in children with severe/profound intellectual and other disabilities. Programs with microswitches and positive stimulation contingent on engagement responses can be quite useful in helping individuals with severe/profound intellectual and other disabilities develop leisure activities with important implications from an adaptive-social standpoint (see Example 1). The possibility of using multiple microswitches can lead the individuals to engage in different forms of responses/activities and choose through them among various sets of stimuli (Lancioni et al., 2002). Enriching these activities with the possibility of requesting social attention from (direct contact with) the caregiver can make a significant difference in the individuals' achievement with important implications also for the perception of their adaptive-social skills by the environment at large (Sigafoos et al., 2006).

An intervention program aimed at building activity engagement and requests of social interaction was recently reported with two participants with severe/profound intellectual and other disabilities (Lancioni et al., 2008b). Each of the two participants, who were 10 and 11 years old, was provided with two microswitches and one Vocal Output Communication Aid (VOCA; see Lancioni, O'Reilly et al., 2007). The microswitches allowed them to engage in simple adaptive/leisure activities (e.g., object manipulation) and consequently to access brief periods of preferred stimulation. The VOCA, which could be activated through a simple movement of one hand over the other (covering an optic sensor placed on it), allowed them to call for social attention. That is, it produced the emission of specific verbal requests for attention. Those requests were answered by the caregiver either verbally (i.e., with complimentary/support sentences) or verbally and physically (i.e., talking to and touching/caressing or kissing the participant briefly). The program was successful with both participants. They acquired (a) high levels of responding to each of the two microswitches, (b) increased their overall level of engagement when the two microswitches were simultaneously available, (c) used the VOCA successfully when it was alone and when it was combined with the microswitches, and (d) maintained the use of microswitches and VOCA over time.

Example 3: A program to promote functional communication and reduce problem behaviors in children with moderate or severe intellectual and other disabilities. Absence of formal communication skills and presence of problem behaviors, such as self-injurious behavior or aggression, can be often observed in children with intellectual disabilities. Both these characteristics can make their adaptive-social situation look largely inadequate, create a high level of anxiety within the environment, limit the opportunities of positive social-physical interaction, and prevent successful development (Carter & Maxwell, 1998; Casey & Merical, 2006). A very important line of research has suggested that (a) the problem behavior may be far from accidental and rather serves as a form of communication which produces important environmental effects and (b) building easy (acceptable/alternative) forms of communication to ask for and obtain the same effects may represent a highly desirable intervention strategy (i.e., a strategy that would improve a deficit area such as communication and curb an excess area such as problem behavior) (Lovaas, 2003; Reeve & Carr, 2000; Sparrow et al., 2005).

A compelling example of this approach was reported by Durand (1999). The work was conducted with four children, who were between 3.5 and 11.5 years of age and presented with moderate-to-severe intellectual disability, which could be combined with motor impairment or autism. The children's problem behavior consisted of hand biting and screaming, hand biting and object throwing, physical aggression, and face slapping and hand banging, respectively. Initially, a functional analysis of the problem behavior was carried out to assess possible links between its occurrence and environmental events. Based on this analysis, it was suggested that the problem behavior of the first and the last of the four children was more likely during difficult tasks, which would then be interrupted. The problem behavior of the second child was more likely when followed by tangible consequences, and the problem behavior of the third child was more likely when followed by attention. In the second study, the children were taught to use VOCA devices in their school setting to request access to the variables presumably maintaining their problem behavior (i.e., those identified through the functional analysis). For

example, the teaching range adopted with the last child included among others a meal-preparation task with a very difficult step. In relation to this step, the teacher helped the child to use the VOCA to produce a verbal request for help. Responding to such a request (i.e., helping the child manage the difficult step) was thought to be effective in preventing the occurrence of problem behavior. In the third study, the use of the VOCA devices was extended to community situations. The findings of the second and third studies were largely comparable. All children showed relatively high levels of problem behavior during the baseline phases (i.e., when the VOCA devices were not available). However, the level of such behavior dropped during the intervention period in concomitance with the use of the VOCA device to make functional requests.

Example 4: A program to promote requests of preferred items/activities by children with mild/moderate intellectual disability. Helping nonspeaking children to find ways of requesting preferred items/activities can have critical effects in terms of communication, social interaction, and constructive leisure engagement. Consequently, it can be considered fundamental for building adaptive-social skills in general. One of the procedures to help them in this direction is the use of VOCA (see above). A potentially functional alternative to the VOCA as tool for making requests may be represented by the Pictorial Exchange Communication System (PECS) (Bondy & Frost, 1998, 2001). With this system the participant (communicator) uses pictures to convey request messages.

Bock, Stoner, Beck, Hanley, and Prochnow (2005) compared both these strategies (i.e., PECS and VOCA) to teach six 4-year-old children (boys) to make requests. Although the authors did not provide a specific level of disability for the children, it is likely that they were around the mild or, more probably, the moderate range of intellectual disability. The comparison was carried out according to an alternating treatments design (Barlow et al., 2009). Moreover, parallel intervention phases were devised for the strategies. The three phases adopted for the PECS corresponded to those described by Bondy and Frost (2001). The first phase was aimed at teaching the child to exchange a picture for the preferred item that was in full view but not accessible in any other way than by handing such a picture to the communication partner. The second phase served to enable the child to find a picture from a book before him and to hand it to a communication partner that was not necessarily in the immediate proximity. The third phase was aimed at teaching the child to discriminate between pictures and thus to use (give the communication partner) the correct one, that is, the one corresponding to the preferred item that he intended to request. The first phase devised for the VOCA was to activate the section of the VOCA board containing the picture of the item to be requested. The second phase mirrored that used for the PECS; thus the child was to bring the VOCA with him and use it where the communication partner was. The third phase involved the presence of two pictures on the VOCA board, and the child was to press the one corresponding to the item that he wanted to request. Prior to the start of the intervention, none of the children used either of the systems to make requests. During the 5.5 intervention weeks, all children were able to move to the second phase of the PECS and VOCA programs. Three children required more sessions to complete the first phase of the VOCA as opposed to the first phase of the PECS. Five children completed the second phase of the PECS and moved to the third phase of it. By contrast, only two of them completed the second phase of the VOCA. Two children completed the third phase of the PECS and one completed the third phase of the VOCA.

Example 5: A program to promote adaptive (leisure) engagement and reduce problem (stereotyped) behavior in children with severe/profound intellectual and other disabilities. As mentioned above, the situation of some participants may be characterized by low levels of adaptive-leisure behavior as well as by the presence of problem behavior (e.g., stereotyped behavior such as hand or object mouthing or forms of withdrawal). The latter behavior hinders the social image of the child quite heavily and thus requires attention within any intervention program (Lovaas, 2003; Luiselli, 1998; Saloviita & Pennanen, 2003; Sparrow et al., 2005). An approach to this complex situation has recently been developed that (a) begins with an increase in adaptive-leisure responding through technological assistance and automatic delivery of stimulation on such responding and (b) continues with the delivery of stimulation only for the adaptive-leisure responses that occur free from the problem behavior.

For example, Lancioni, Singh et al. (2007) used this approach with two children of 7.6 and 12.3 years of age who presented with minimal play and leisure behavior and considerable levels of stereotyped behavior (hand or object mouthing). This combination, rooted in a condition of profound intellectual disability and other motor and sensory impairments, made the children's adaptive-social condition look very poor and unattractive for the context and caregivers in general (cf. Lancioni, Singh, O'Reilly, & Oliva, 2003; Luiselli, 1998). The intervention program started with the identification and strengthening of a play (engagement) activity that consisted of manipulating/moving an object connected to a wobble microswitch or knocking objects on the table to activate a vibration microswitch. Strengthening was based on the occurrence of brief periods of preferred stimulation contingent on the play/engagement responses. Once these responses had increased and consolidated, the intervention program was also directed at reducing the stereotyped behavior. Specifically, two procedural variations were introduced. First, the play/engagement responses caused the occurrence of the preferred stimulation only if those responses were performed independent of the stereotyped behavior. Second, the aforementioned stimulation would be interrupted prematurely if the stereotyped behavior appeared during its presentation. The results showed that the first part of the intervention program was effective in increasing by two or three times the baseline levels of play/engagement responses. The second part of the intervention program increased further the frequency of responding and reduced to minimal levels the incidence of the stereotyped behavior during responding, during the stimulation, and during the rest of the session. These positive data were maintained at the post-intervention checks carried out 3 months after the end of the program.

Example 6: A program to reduce sleep problems in children with mild-to-severe intellectual disability. Sleep problems are frequent in children with developmental disabilities and can have serious consequences for the families and the children themselves (Lancioni, O'Reilly, & Basili, 1999). Families have to endure a heavy cost in terms of time commitment, alterations of their habits and rearrangements of their schedules, loss of own sleep, and feelings of social frustration toward their children and of social inadequacy toward their neighbors. Children typically experience high levels of uncertainty and unhappiness that interfere with their quality of life, their development of an acceptable adaptive-social condition, and their quality of interaction with parents (Robinson & Richdale, 2004). Given the range of negative implications, sleep problems are generally targeted for intervention.

A number of intervention procedures have been devised and assessed and the choice of one or the other is based on considerations about the reasons maintaining the problems as well as environmental/practical issues concerning their implementation. If one assumes that the sleep problems are largely due to variables such as unclear bed scheduling, excessively long time planned in bed, and positive attention following the occurrence of the problems, the intervention package may include a clear bedtime routine applied rigorously, reduction in the amount of time planned in bed, and basic extinction procedures (i.e., removal of all positive attention following the behavior problems). Such a package was adopted by Weiskop, Richdale, and Matthews (2005) in a study involving seven children with Fragile X syndrome. The children, whose mean age was about 5 years, presented with mild-to-severe intellectual disability. Initially, parents were exposed to a careful preparation program tackling issues such as (a) the goals of the study, basic principles of learning theory, bedtime routine and reinforcement procedures for compliance, partner support strategies aimed at cementing parenting consistency, and extinction techniques. The study was conducted according to a multiple baseline design across children (Barlow et al., 2009) and included follow-up checks. The study was completed with five of the seven children and abandoned (for family reasons or illness) with the other two. The overall outcome for the first five children was quite positive with drastic reductions in the number of pre-sleep disturbances as well as the number of nights per week in which they slept with parents, and increases in the number of nights they fell asleep alone in their own bed. The effects of the intervention were typically maintained over time.

Example 7: A program to reduce behavior tantrums in children with moderate intellectual disability. Recurrent tantrums may be considered a serious problem that interferes with the development of adaptive-social skills, namely, with constructive play and leisure behavior, positive communication, and positive social/physical interaction (Garland, Augustyn, & Stein, 2007; Wilder, Chen, Atwell, Pritchard, & Weinstein, 2006). Given these harmful consequences, as well as the unpleasant social image connected to tantrums, action is definitely required to confront such a situation. A desirable course of action would involve an assessment of possible links between tantrums and environmental events and intervention programs aimed at reducing the tantrums.

An example of this course of action was reported by O'Reilly, Lacey, and Lancioni (2001) with two children of 3.4 and 5.7 years of age, who had spent long periods of time in Romanian orphanages before being adopted by Irish families. Both children were considered to function in the moderate range of intellectual disability. They engaged in severe tantrums several times a day. Tantrums were similar for the two children and included screaming, hitting persons, throwing items, self-hitting, self-biting, and property destruction. An assessment of the children's tantrums was conducted by exposing the children to four analogue conditions designed for functional analysis of the behavior (cf. Iwata et al., 1994). The four conditions involved attention, demand, noncontingent attention, and free play. Each condition was implemented during 10-min sessions, according to a multielement design (Barlow et al., 2009). The mother served as the therapist and implemented the assessment. Aggression was blocked during the sessions. Based on the results of the assessment, which showed high levels of tantrums during the attention condition, an intervention program was devised that relied on the use of noncontingent attention (i.e., attention provided independent of the tantrums). The program was applied within the children's homes during two 1-hour periods in which they were more likely to display their tantrums. Initially, parents were to provide noncontingent attention every 10 s. Subsequently, noncontingent attention was delivered at intervals of 30 s, and finally, it was shifted to intervals of 60 s. Tantrums decreased dramatically during the intervention and remained low when attention became less frequent. At a 6-month follow-up, parents indicated that tantrums were no longer a concern for them.

Example 8: A program to reduce food refusal in a child with moderate intellectual disability. Food refusal creates concerns about the individual's health and obvious problems with regard to his or her adaptive-social condition. Research literature suggests that food refusal in the absence of organic causes may be primarily maintained by negative reinforcement (i.e., by the opportunity to escape the mealtime situation) for children with intellectual disability (Kuhn, Girolami, & Gulotta, 2007; Luiselli, 2006; Sturmey, Reyer, Mayville, & Matson, 2007). Based on this indication, one of the main intervention strategies has relied on the extinction of the escape response, with the child required to remain at the eating place and continue to be guided by the therapist to accept bites (Luiselli, 2006). This type of intervention is usually carried out by experts within pediatric hospitals.

In an attempt to overcome this situation, O'Reilly and Lancioni (2001) assessed the possibility of having a mother perform as therapist within the home setting. The intervention program was directed at a child of 4.9 years of age who was diagnosed with Williams syndrome and was reported to function in the moderate range of intellectual disability. The program was carried out over the meals with most severe food refusal (i.e., breakfast and lunch). Recording concerned the number of bites the child consumed (i.e., portions of food that the child swallowed without spitting) and the percentage of intervals with aberrant/oppositional behavior (i.e., with behaviors such as throwing the food on the floor, leaving or attempting to leave the table, screaming, and complaining about being sick). The intervention was carried out according to a multiple baseline design across meals. Initially, baseline conditions were implemented in connection with both meals. Then, intervention started in connection with breakfast. During the intervention, the mother prevented the child from leaving the table until a 20-min period had elapsed, ignored aberrant behavior, and presented verbal praise each time the child consumed a bite. When the child's breakfast behavior improved, intervention was extended to lunch as well. The results of the study showed

that the number of bites consumed per session increased from baseline averages of about 1.5 to intervention averages of about 12 and 16 during breakfast and lunch, respectively. The aberrant behaviors decreased very drastically in both meal situations. The aforementioned improvements were maintained during follow-up checks carried out over a period of 3 months.

Example 9: A program to promote self-care skills (hand washing) in children with moderate/severe intellectual disability. Acquiring self-care skills, such as washing and dressing, can be considered highly relevant for the adaptive-social development of all children irrespective of their intellectual condition (Wilkins & Matson, 2007). The ability to become independent in the performance of some of these tasks can provide the child a sense of self-fulfillment with positive implications for his or her general confidence, mood, and interpersonal relation. At the same time, parents and caregivers are also likely to respond positively to any achievements in the area with social approval and other forms of reinforcement favorable for building stronger and more pleasant emotional ties (Lancioni et al., 2008a).

An intervention program to promote hand washing in children with moderate-to-severe intellectual disability was reported by Parrott, Schuster, Collins, and Gassaway (2000). Their study included five children of 6 to 8 years of age. The intervention program was carried out through individual sessions taking place in the restroom near the children's classroom. The task analysis for hand washing had indicated a sequence of 16 steps. During the intervention sessions, a simultaneous prompting procedure was used (Kurt, & Tekin-Iftar, 2008; Morse & Schuster, 2004). Each step instruction was immediately followed by the controlling prompt, that is, a physical prompt ensuring the full and adequate performance of the step. After completion of the step, the therapist delivered descriptive verbal praise and, when fitting, also the instructive feedback about the material used and the performance. Task acquisition was tested during probe sessions in which no instructions and prompts were applied. Once an error or no response occurred, the session was terminated. The program was by and large effective in improving the hand-washing performance of all five children. Three of them reached a 100% level of correct performance and were exposed to maintenance and generalization probes (i.e., across therapists) to which they responded successfully. The other two participants did not manage the 100% level of correct performance and thus did not receive the aforementioned probes.

Example 10: A program to promote appropriate social interaction responding in children with mild intellectual and other disabilities. Promoting appropriate forms of responding toward others during interactive situations, such as meals, educational activities, and recreation, may represent a critical objective in programs for children with mild intellectual disabilities (Hersen & Reitman, 2008; Parmenter, Harman, Yazbeck, & Riches, 2007). In fact, failures within these areas (which become even more likely when the intellectual disability is combined with other developmental/behavioral problems) may severely interfere with the children's possibility of mainstream integration and their social prospect in general (Davies & Witte, 2000).

An elaborate intervention program to promote positive developments in the social interaction behavior of five children was conducted by Embregts (2002). The children were between 10.8 and 12.8 years of age and were reported to be functioning within the mild intellectual disability range and also to have a diagnosis of attention deficits and hyperactivity disorders. The social interaction problems for four of the children consisted of inability to wait for their turns, tendency to interrupt other persons, shouting, hitting, and making provocative gestures or uttering insults and threats. The main problems of the fifth child were his limited initiative toward interaction. Data were collected during lunch, dinner, and tea times, within the group setting that the children shared with others (i.e., a total of 12 children and two direct-care staff members usually frequented that setting). Data collection was carried out by videotaping the aforementioned lunch, dinner and tea events, which had mean durations of 14, 23, and 15 min, respectively. All children received a baseline-intervention sequence according to a multiple baseline design across participants (Barlow et al., 2009). During baseline, no feedback was provided to the children or the staff regarding their social interaction behavior. Intervention included two components: one exclusively directed

to the children and the other to both children and staff. The intervention was carried out with each child individually in a therapy room during school hours. During the initial phase, the therapist prompted the child to generate accurate examples of appropriate and inappropriate social interaction behavior. Then, the child was to rate examples of interaction role-played by the therapist. Eventually, the child was to rate (a) videotaped examples of unknown individuals and (b) videotaped examples of himself while in the group setting. During the next phase, therapist and child sat next to each other and watched videotaped segments of the previous lunch, dinner or tea times. For each segment, the child was to say whether his behavior on the segment was appropriate or inappropriate and was also to record it on a sheet of paper. When the behavior was inappropriate, the child was required to provide an appropriate example. When the behavior was appropriate, the child received one point. At the end of the session, the points were added, and if their number met the preset criterion, the child received a token. The final phase started with staff training and proceeded with staff becoming responsible for carrying out the sessions with the children and providing graphic feedback. Data indicated that the program promoted strong positive changes for three of the children and minor ones for the other two.

Example 11: A program to promote play with typical peers in a child with moderate intellectual disability. Teaching a child to play games with other children is one of the most easily recognizable (and widely agreed) objectives in programs for establishing social skills. Such an objective encompasses constructive engagement, social contact, communication, and ability to follow rules and achieve a common goal (i.e., cooperation). The possibility of achieving such an objective is largely dependent on levels of intellectual disability in the mild to moderate range and on the arrangement of careful intervention conditions.

One study dealing with this objective was reported by Arntzen, Halstadtrø, and Halstadtrø (2003). The study included a 5-year-old boy who was apparently between the moderate and mild levels of intellectual disability. The study took place in the playroom of the integrated school setting the child attended. The sessions involved the presence of four typically functioning peers. Three games usually played by children of this age were selected for assessment and intervention. Within each game, the child was taught both to be the leader and to be a participant. The first game "red light/green light" involved (a) the role of controlling the movement of the peers and ordering them to go back to the wall when they were caught moving and (b) the role of moving away from the wall to return to it if ordered. The second game "Simon says" involved telling the other children to move to him with big or small steps or to follow the same instructions given by another child. The third game "spin the bottle" involved the children sitting in circle and one of them twirling the bottle and giving an instruction to the child who was pointed to by the bottle at the end of its movement. A task analysis was made for each game so a list of steps was identified for measuring performance and arranging the intervention. During the intervention sessions, the typically functioning peers provided positive social consequences to the child when he performed correct responses. At the end of each game, tokens exchangeable for small/preferred items were provided to the child as well as to the peers. The results indicated that the child learned to play all three games as a leader (through an average of about 20 training trials per game) and as a participant (through an average of about 35 training trials per game). The results were maintained during the post-intervention checks carried out over a 3-week period.

Conclusions

In this chapter, we reviewed a series of rating scales used for assessment of adaptive-social skills in children with intellectual disabilities and also presented examples of intervention strategies for promoting adaptive-social skills with these children. The examples (all published studies) served to illustrate different situations involving different participants, different objectives/rationales, and different strategies. The aim was to provide the reader a broad picture of the general issue and its various aspects.

The first consideration one can make in relation to the examples reported is that several of them

could hardly have been identified as illustrative of intervention on social skills ahead of time (i.e., based on the title and general behavioral objectives). Yet, if convincing explanations were provided as to why those examples were considered fitting and relevant, the general view and definition of social skills or adaptive-social behavior may become more flexible. Indeed for a child with minimal engagement with the outside world, the first objective may consist of increasing his adaptive and enjoyable engagement with his immediate environment (i.e., a reasonable equivalent of play and leisure behavior; see above). Play and leisure are essential for development and provide the child a much more adaptive-social look that would contrast with his or her typically passive/withdrawn or unhappy behavior (Di Carlo, Reid, & Stricklin, 2003; Lancioni, Singh, O'Reilly, Oliva, & Basili, 2005; Lancioni, Singh et al., 2006; Sigafoos et al., 2007). This new, positive look in turn could prompt fresh caregivers' attention and social engagement with wide-ranging implications (Crawford & Schuster, 1993; Lancioni et al., 2008a, 2008b; Sigafoos et al., 2006).

Similarly, for children with severe or profound intellectual and other disabilities and minimal opportunities of engagement, communication, and choice, one might seek to develop chances of adaptive-social behavior through the use of augmentative and alternative communication solutions (see Examples 2 and 3). Those solutions in fact would allow the individual to interact with the caregiver on his or her own initiative. The interaction with (attention from) the caregiver may be targeted as a specific objective (see Example 2) or may be a by-product of the mediation role that the caregiver is required to play (see Example 3). In both cases, (a) the child's situation is socially enriched, (b) the interaction is no longer a simple caregiver's initiative, and (c) the overall appearance of the child improves with potentially important implications for an upgraded perception of his or her adaptive-social skills by the context at large (Durand, 1999; Lancioni et al., 2008a, 2008b; Reeve & Carr, 2000; Sigafoos et al., 2006; Wilkins & Matson, 2007).

A second consideration about the examples reported (i.e., particularly those including children with severe or profound intellectual and other disabilities) concerns the fact that assistive technology may be a necessary resource to target developmental goals in general and adaptive-social skills in particular (Henderson, Skelton, & Rosenbaum, 2008; Jans & Scherer, 2006; Lancioni et al., 2008a, 2008b; Tota et al., 2006). It would be difficult to envisage an intervention program to promote constructive/enjoyable engagement (i.e., play and leisure behavior) in children with severe, profound, and multiple disabilities without the help of microswitch-based technology (Lancioni et al., 2002). It would be impossible to enable individuals with intellectual and motor disabilities to make effective communication requests without the availability of VOCA devices. It would be unthinkable to pursue leisure engagement together with (a) requests for social attention or (b) reduction of problem behavior without advanced technological solutions (Lancioni, Singh et al., 2007; Lancioni et al., 2008a, 2008b).

A third consideration is concerned with obvious differences in intervention emphasis among the examples reported. In particular, some of the examples underlined the acquisition of positive behaviors (see Examples 9, 10, and 11) while others specifically emphasized the reduction of problem behaviors (see Examples 6, 7 and 8). Essentially, the two positions are responding to the two types of problems that negatively affect individuals with intellectual disability in the context of adaptive-social skills, that is, the problems of behavioral deficits and the problems of behavioral excesses (Harris, 2005; Lovaas, 2003; Luiselli, 1998, 2006; Sigafoos et al., 2006; Sparrow et al., 2005). Acquiring positive behaviors, such as improved social-interaction responding or advanced play behavior, would counter the problem of adaptive-social deficits and so improve the person's overall status. Limiting (eliminating) aggressive behavior or sleep troubles would alleviate the problem of negative behavioral excesses (see above) and again improve the person's status.

A fourth consideration is concerned with new possible developments regarding intervention technology for improving the adaptive-social skills of individuals with intellectual disabilities. Such developments would most specifically relate to individuals with severe/profound disabilities. These individuals, in fact, more than others depend on the availability of technology to acquire initiative and successful engagement and eventually establish

forms of interaction with the caregiver and overcome problem behaviors. The two forms of technology that might be hypothesized as innovative and useful for these individuals could include (a) VOCA devices that can be activated with minimal motor responses available to most individuals and (b) new microswitch arrangements (i.e., new microswitch clusters; see Lancioni, Singh et al., 2007) to allow the intervention to focus on different combinations of leisure responding and problem behavior.

References

Algozzine, B., Browder, D., Karvonen, M., Test, D. W., & Wood, W. M. (2001). Effects of intervention to promote self-determination for individuals with disabilities. *Review of Educational Research, 71*, 219–277.

American Psychiatric Association (2000). *Diagnostic and statistical manual of mental disorders* (4th ed., text revision). Washington, DC: Author.

Arntzen, E., Halstadtrø, A.-M., & Halstadtrø, M. (2003). Training play behavior in a 5-year-old boy with developmental disabilities. *Journal of Applied Behavior Analysis, 36*, 367–370.

Barlow, D. H., Nock, M., & Hersen, M. (2009). *Single-case experimental designs* (3rd ed.). New York: Allyn & Bacon.

Bock, S. J., Stoner, J. B., Beck, A. R., Hanley, L., & Prochnow, J. (2005). Increasing functional communication in non-speaking preschool children: comparison of PECS and VOCA. *Education and Training in Developmental Disabilities, 40*, 264–278.

Bondy, A., & Frost, L. (1998). The picture exchange communication system. *Seminars in Speech and Language, 19*, 373–389.

Bondy, A., & Frost, L. (2001). The picture exchange communication system. *Behavior Modification, 25*, 725–744.

Brady, N. C. (2000). Improved comprehension of object names following voice output communication aid use: Two case studies. *Augmentative and Alternative Communication, 16*, 197–204.

Braithwaite, K. L., & Richdale, A. L. (2000). Functional communication training to replace challenging behaviors across two behavioral outcomes. *Behavioral Interventions, 15*, 21–26.

Brown, I. (2007). What is meant by intellectual and developmental disabilities. In I. Brown & M. Percy (Eds.), *A comprehensive guide to intellectual and developmental disabilities* (pp. 3–15). Baltimore: Paul H. Brookes Publishing Co.

Brown, I., Parmenter, T. R., & Percy, M. (2007). Trends and issues in intellectual and developmental disabilities. In I. Brown & M. Percy (Eds.), *A comprehensive guide to intellectual and developmental disabilities* (pp. 45–57). Baltimore: Paul H. Brookes Publishing Co.

Bruininks, R. H., & Moreau, L. (2004). *Checklist of adaptive living skills (CALS)*. Chicago: Riverside Publishing Company.

Bruininks, R. H., Moreau, L., Gilman, C. J., & Anderson, J. L. (2004). *Adaptive living skills curriculum (ALSC)*. Chicago: Riverside Publishing Company.

Carr, A., & O'Reilly, G. (2007). Diagnosis, classification and epidemiology. In A. Carr, G. O'Reilly, P. Noonan Walsh, & J. McEvoy (Eds.), *The handbook of intellectual disability and clinical psychology practice* (pp. 3–49). London: Routledge.

Carter, M., & Maxwell, K. (1998). Promoting interaction with children using augmentative communication through a peer-directed intervention. *International Journal of Disability, Development and Education, 45*, 75–96.

Casey, S. D., & Merical, C. L. (2006). The use of functional communication training without additional treatment procedures in an inclusive school setting. *Behavioral Disorders, 32*, 46–54.

Cory, L., Dattilo, J., & Williams, R. (2006). Effects of a leisure education program on social knowledge and skills of youth with cognitive disabilities. *Therapeutic Recreation Journal, 40*, 144–164.

Crawford, M. R., & Schuster, J. W. (1993). Using microswitches to teach toy use. *Journal of Developmental and Physical Disabilities, 5*, 349–368.

Davies, S., & Witte, R. (2000). Self-management and peer-monitoring within a group contingency to decrease uncontrolled verbalizations of children with attention-deficit/hyperactive disorder. *Psychology in the Schools, 37*, 135–147.

Di Carlo, C. F., Reid, D. H., & Stricklin, S. B. (2003). Increasing toy play among toddlers with multiple disabilities in an inclusive classroom: A more-to-less, child-directed intervention continuum. *Research in Developmental Disabilities, 24*, 195–209.

Durand, V. M. (1999). Functional communication training using assistive devices: Recruiting natural communities of reinforcement. *Journal of Applied Behavior Analysis, 32*, 247–267.

Embregts, P. J. C. M. (2002). Effect of resident and direct-care staff training on responding during social interactions. *Research in Developmental Disabilities, 23*, 353–366.

Favell, J. E., Realon, R. E., & Sutton, K. A. (1996). Measuring and increasing the happiness of people with profound mental retardation and physical handicaps. *Behavioral Interventions, 11*, 47–58.

Garland, A., Augustyn, M., & Stein, M. T. (2007). Disruptive and oppositional behavior in an 11-year old boy. *Journal of Developmental and Behavioral Pediatrics, 28*, 406–408.

Green, C. W., & Reid, D. H. (1999a). A behavioral approach to identifying sources of happiness and unhappiness among individuals with profound multiple disabilities. *Behavior Modification, 23*, 280–293.

Green, C. W., & Reid, D. H. (1999b). Reducing indices of unhappiness among individuals with profound multiple disabilities during therapeutic exercise routines. *Journal of Applied Behavior Analysis, 32*, 137–147.

Green, V. A., Sigafoos, J., O'Reilly, M., & Arthur-Kelly, M. (2006). People with extensive to pervasive support needs.

In I. Dempsey & K. Nankervis (Eds.), *Community disability services: An evidence-based approach to practice* (pp. 145–190). Sydney: University of New South Wales Press.

Harris, J. C. (2005). *Intellectual disability: Understanding its development, causes, classification, evaluation and treatment*. New York: Oxford University Press.

Henderson, S., Skelton, H., & Rosenbaum, P. (2008). Assistive devices for children with functional impairments: Impact on child and caregiver function. *Developmental Medicine and Child Neurology, 50*, 89–98.

Hersen, M., & Reitman, D. (Eds.) (2008). *Handbook of clinical psychology, Vol. 2: Children and adolescents*. Hoboken, NJ: John Wiley & Sons.

Iwata, B., Pace, G., Dorsey, M., Zarcone, J., Vollmer, T., Smith, R., et al. (1994). The functions of self-injurious behavior: An experimental-epidemiological analysis. *Journal of Applied Behavior Analysis, 27*, 215–240.

Jans, L. H., & Scherer, M. J. (2006). Assistive technology training: Diverse audiences and multidisciplinary content. *Disability and Rehabilitation: Assistive Technology, 1*, 69–77.

Kuhn, D. E., Girolami, P. A., & Gulotta, C. S. (2007). Feeding disorders. In J. L. Matson (Ed.), *Handbook of assessment in persons with intellectual disability* (pp. 387–414). San Diego: Academic Press.

Kurt, O., & Tekin-Iftar, E. (2008). A comparison of constant time delay and simultaneous prompting within embedded instructions on teaching leisure skills to children with autism. *Topics in Early Childhood Special Education, 28*, 53–64.

Lambert, N., Nihira, K., & Leyland, H. (1993). *Adaptive behavior scale-school version* (2nd ed.). Washington DC: American Association on Mental Retardation.

Lancioni, G. E., O'Reilly, M. F., & Basili, G. (1999). Review of strategies for treating sleep problems in persons with severe or profound mental retardation or multiple handicaps. *American Journal on Mental Retardation, 104*, 170–186.

Lancioni, G. E., O'Reilly, M. F., Singh, N. N., Oliva, D., Piazzolla, G., Pirani, P., et al. (2002). Evaluating the use of multiple microswitches and responses for children with multiple disabilities. *Journal of Intellectual Disability Research, 46*, 346–351.

Lancioni, G. E., O'Reilly, M. F., Cuvo, A. J., Singh, N. N., Sigafoos, J., & Didden, R. (2007). PECS and VOCA to enable students with developmental disabilities to make requests: An overview of the literature. *Research in Developmental Disabilities, 28*, 468–488.

Lancioni, G. E., O'Reilly, M. F., Singh, N. N., Sigafoos, J., Oliva, D., Baccani, S., et al. (2006). Microswitch clusters promote adaptive responses and reduce finger mouthing in a boy with multiple disabilities. *Behavior Modification, 30*, 892–900.

Lancioni, G. E., O'Reilly, M. F., Singh, N. N., Sigafoos, J., Oliva, D., & Severini, L. (2008a). Enabling two persons with multiple disabilities to access environmental stimuli and ask for social contact through microswitches and a VOCA. *Research in Developmental Disabilities, 29*, 21–28.

Lancioni, G. E., O'Reilly, M. F., Singh, N. N., Sigafoos, J., Oliva, D., & Severini, L. (2008b). Three persons with multiple disabilities accessing environmental stimuli and asking for social contact through microswitch and VOCA technology. *Journal of Intellectual Disability Research, 52,* 327–336.

Lancioni, G. E., Singh, N. N., O'Reilly, M. F., La Martire, M. L., Stasolla, F., Smaldone, A., et al. (2006). Microswitch-based programs as therapeutic recreation interventions for students with profound multiple disabilities. *American Journal of Recreation Therapy, 5,* 15–20.

Lancioni, G. E., Singh, N. N., O'Reilly, M. F., & Oliva, D. (2003). Some recent research efforts on microswitches for persons with multiple disabilities. *Journal of Child and Family Studies, 12,* 251–256.

Lancioni, G. E., Singh, N. N., O'Reilly, M. F., Oliva, D., & Basili, G. (2005). An overview of research on increasing indices of happiness of people with severe/profound intellectual and multiple disabilities. *Disability and Rehabilitation, 27,* 83–93.

Lancioni, G. E., Singh, N. N., O'Reilly, M. F., Oliva, D., Scalini, L., Vigo, C. M., et al. (2004). Microswitch clusters to support responding and appropriate posture of students with multiple disabilities: Three case evaluations. *Disability and Rehabilitation, 26,* 501–505.

Lancioni, G. E., Singh, N. N., O'Reilly, M. F., Sigafoos, J., Oliva, D., Severini, L., et al. (2007). Microswitch technology to promote adaptive responses and reduce mouthing in two children with multiple disabilities. *Journal of Visual Impairment and Blindness, 101,* 628–636.

Lovaas, O. I. (2003). *Teaching individuals with developmental delays: Basic intervention techniques.* Austin, TX: Pro-Ed.

Luckasson, R. A., Schalock, R. L., Spitalnik, D. M., Spreat, S., Tasse, M., Snell, M. E., et al. (2002). *Mental retardation: Definition, classification, and systems of support.* Washington, DC: American Association on Mental Retardation.

Luiselli, J. K. (1998). Treatment of self-injurious hand-mouthing in a child with multiple disabilities. *Journal of Developmental and Physical Disabilities, 10,* 167–174.

Luiselli, J. K. (2006). Pediatric feeding disorders. In J. K. Luiselli (Ed.), *Antecedent assessment and intervention* (pp. 165–185). Baltimore: Paul H. Brookes Publishing Co.

MacLean Jr., W. E., Miller, M. L., & Bartsch, K. (2001). Mental retardation. In C. E. Walker & M. C. Roberts (Eds.), *Handbook of clinical child psychology* (3rd ed., pp. 542–560). New York: John Wiley & Sons.

Matson, J. L. (1995). *The Matson evaluation of social skills for individuals with severe retardation.* Baton Rouge, LA: Scientific Publishers, Inc.

Matson, J. L. (Ed.) (2007). *Handbook of assessment in persons with intellectual disability.* San Diego: Academic Press.

Matson, J. L., Rotatori, A., & Helsel, W. J. (1983). Development of a rating scale to measure social skills in children: The Matson evaluation of social skills with youngsters (MESSY). *Behaviour Research and Therapy, 21,* 335–340.

Morse, T., & Schuster, J. W. (2004). Simultaneous prompting: A review of the literature. *Education and Training in Developmental Disabilities, 39,* 153–168.

O'Reilly, M., Lacey, C., & Lancioni, G. E. (2001). A preliminary investigation of the assessment and treatment of tantrums with two post-institutionalized Romanian adoptees. *Scandinavian Journal of Behaviour Therapy, 30,* 179–187.

O'Reilly, M. F., Cannella, H. I., Sigafoos, J., & Lancioni, G. (2006). Communication and social skills intervention. In J. K. Luiselli (Ed.), *Antecedent assessment and intervention* (pp. 187–206). Baltimore: Paul H. Brookes Publishing Co.

O'Reilly, M. F., & Lancioni, G. E. (2001). Treating food refusal in a child with Williams syndrome using the parent as therapist in the home setting. *Journal of Intellectual Disability Research, 45,* 41–46.

Parmenter, T. R., Harman, A. D., Yazbeck, M., & Riches, V. C. (2007). Life skills training for adolescents with intellectual disabilities. In A. Carr, G. O'Reilly, P. Noonan Walsh, & J. McEvoy (Eds.), *The handbook of intellectual disability and clinical psychology practice* (pp. 687–728). London: Routledge.

Parrott, K. A., Schuster, J. W., Collins, B. C., & Gassaway, L. J. (2000). Simultaneous prompting and instructive feedback when teaching chained tasks. *Journal of Behavioral Education, 10,* 3–19.

Reeve, C. E., & Carr, E. G. (2000). Prevention of severe behavior problems in children with developmental disorders. *Journal of Positive Behavior Interventions, 2,* 144–160.

Robinson, A. M., & Richdale, A. L. (2004). Sleep problems in children with an intellectual disability: Parental perceptions of sleep problems, and views of treatment effectiveness. *Child: Care, Health and Development, 30,* 139–150.

Saloviita, T., & Pennanen, M. (2003). Behavioural treatment of thumb sucking of a boy with fragile X syndrome in the classroom. *Developmental Disabilities Bulletin, 31,* 1–10.

Schroeder, S. R., Tessel, R. E., Loupe, P. S., & Stodgell, C. J. (1997). Severe behavior problems among people with developmental disabilities. In W. E. MacLean, Jr. (Ed.), *Ellis' handbook of mental deficiency, psychological theory and research* (3rd ed., pp. 439–464). Mahwah, NJ: Lawrence Erlbaum.

Sigafoos, J., Arthur-Kelly, M., & Butterfield, N. (2006). *Enhancing everyday communication for children with disabilities.* Baltimore: Paul H. Brookes Publishing Co.

Sigafoos, J., O'Reilly, M. F., & Green, V. A. (2007). Communication difficulties and the promotion of communication skills. In A. Carr, G. O'Reilly, P. Noonan Walsh, & J. McEvoy (Eds.), *The handbook of intellectual disability and clinical psychology practice* (pp. 606–642). London: Routledge.

Sigafoos, J., O'Reilly, M. F., & Lancioni, G. E. (in press). Mental retardation. In J. Thomas & M. Hersen (Eds.), *Handbook of clinical psychology competencies (HCPC): Volume III: Intervention and treatment for children and adolescents.* New York: Springer.

Sparrow, S. S., Balla, D. A., & Cicchetti, D. V. (1984). *Vineland adaptive behavior scales: Interview edition survey form.* Circle Pines, MN: American Guidance Service.

Sparrow, S. S., Balla, D. A., & Cicchetti, D. V. (2005). *Vineland-II adaptive behavior scales* (2nd ed.). Minneapolis: Pearson.

Sturmey, P., Reyer, H., Mayville, S. B., & Matson, J. L. (2007). Feeding difficulties and eating disorders. In A. Carr, G. O'Reilly, P. Noonan Walsh, & J. McEvoy (Eds.), *The handbook of intellectual disability and clinical psychology practice* (pp. 488–528). London: Routledge.

Tota, A., Lancioni, G. E., Singh, N. N., O'Reilly, M. F., Sigafoos, J., & Oliva, D. (2006). Evaluating the applicability of optic microswitches for eyelid responses in students with profound multiple disabilities. *Disability and Rehabilitation: Assistive Technology, 1*, 217–223.

Tylenda, B., Beckett, J., & Barrett, R. P. (2007). Assessing mental retardation using standardized intelligence tests. In J. L. Matson (Ed.), *Handbook of assessment in persons with intellectual disability* (pp. 27–97). San Diego: Academic Press.

Udwin, O., & Kuczynski, A. (2007). Behavioural phenotypes in genetic syndromes associated with intellectual disability. In A. Carr, G. O'Reilly, P. Noonan Walsh, & J. McEvoy (Eds.), *The handbook of intellectual disability and clinical psychology practice* (pp. 447–487). London: Routledge.

Vermeer, A., Lijnse, M., & Lindhout, M. (2004). Measuring perceived competence and social acceptance in indivi-duals with intellectual disabilities. *European Journal of Special Needs Education, 19*, 283–300.

Weiskop, S., Richdale, A., & Matthews, J. (2005). Behavioural treatment to reduce sleep problems in children with autism or fragile X syndrome. *Developmental Medicine and Child Neurology, 47*, 94–104.

Wilder, D. A., Chen, L., Atwell, J., Pritchard, J., & Weinstein, P. (2006). Brief functional analysis and treatment of tantrums associated with transitions in preschool children. *Journal of Applied Behavior Analysis, 39*, 103–107.

Wilkins, J., & Matson, J. L. (2007). Social skills. In J. L. Matson (Ed.), *Handbook of assessment in persons with intellectual disability* (pp. 321–363). San Diego: Academic Press.

World Health Organization (2001). *The international classification of functioning, disability and health (ICF).* Geneva: Author.

Chapter 9
Attention-Deficit/Hyperactivity Disorder

Amori Yee Mikami, Allison Jack, and Matthew D. Lerner

Attention-Deficit/Hyperactivity Disorder (ADHD) is one of the most prevalent disorders of childhood, characterized by a persistent, impairing pattern of inattention and/or hyperactivity/impulsivity. Youth with ADHD are known to be at high risk for adjustment problems, including academic underachievement and school failure, disruptive and oppositional behaviors, substance abuse problems, internalizing behaviors, and poor social relationships with adults and with peers (Barkley, 2002; Hinshaw, Owens, Sami, & Fargeon, 2006; Mannuzza & Klein, 2000). Each domain of impairment merits attention, but for the purposes of this chapter we primarily focus on the difficulties in peer relationships faced by youth with ADHD. The magnitude of the problems is so profound that, although peer relationship difficulties are not currently part of the diagnostic criteria for ADHD, some scholars have argued that they should be included (Whalen & Henker, 1985; Wheeler & Carlson, 1994). Because peer rejection is known to increase the risk for future maladjustment in this population, the public health significance of interventions for social competence is high.

In this chapter, we first provide a brief background on the diagnostic criteria, prevalence, and etiology of ADHD. We then summarize the current state of knowledge about assessment of social skills, peer relationship problems, and existing social competence interventions for youth with ADHD. We conclude with some theoretical implications and directions for future research and practice.

Definition of the Population

The key symptoms of ADHD fall along two dimensions: (a) inattention and (b) hyperactivity/impulsivity. Children must display six of nine possible symptoms of inattention and/or six of nine possible symptoms of hyperactivity/impulsivity to meet DSM-IV-TR criteria for the disorder (American Psychiatric Association, 2000). In addition, symptoms must appear early in development (before age seven), be persistent (official criterion is over six months), and impair functioning in more than one setting (for instance, both home and school). Note that these criteria have varied somewhat in previous editions of the DSM. In neither the DSM-III nor the DSM-III-R, for example, was symptom expression across settings a requirement for diagnosis, and differences in the required number of symptoms existed (American Psychiatric Association, 1980, 1987). For further details beyond the cursory review herein, please see Barkley (1998).

DSM-IV-TR further categorizes three subtypes of ADHD, based on the predominant pattern of symptoms. Children with ADHD-Combined Type (ADHD-C) surpass clinical thresholds for both inattention and hyperactivity/impulsivity. Those with ADHD-Inattentive Type (ADHD-I) present with inattention but do not display clinically significant hyperactivity/impulsivity. Those with ADHD-Hyperactive Impulsive Type (ADHD-HI) present

A.Y. Mikami (✉)
Department of Psychology, University of Virginia, Charlottesville, VA 29904-4400, USA
e-mail: mikami@virginia.edu

J.L. Matson (ed.), *Social Behavior and Skills in Children*, DOI 10.1007/978-1-4419-0234-4_9,
© Springer Science+Business Media, LLC 2009

with hyperactivity/impulsivity but do not cross thresholds for inattention. It has been argued that ADHD-I may represent a qualitatively distinct disorder from ADHD-C/HI, because some of these youth display a drowsy, hypoactive behavioral style referred to as sluggish cognitive tempo, which markedly differs from youth with the other subtypes of ADHD (McBurnett, Pfiffner, & Frick, 2001; Milich, Balentine, & Lynam, 2001).

Clinically, the impairing inattentive symptoms of elementary school-age children with ADHD often present as a difficulty completing their morning routine without repeated prompts from parents, beyond what would be typical for a child their age. Parents report that these children cannot remember a sequence of events such as "get dressed, brush your teeth, and get your backpack" independently. In school, children are likely to daydream during instruction or be distracted by almost any noise in the classroom and have a harder time, relative to their peers, re-centering their attention to the task at hand. They forget homework assignments, lose important materials, and keep a messy and disorganized backpack. With peers, inattention may lead children to miss important social cues and game rules and to have difficulty breaking into conversations at the appropriate time.

The impairing hyperactive/impulsive symptoms of children this age often present as difficulty sitting still in the classroom during seatwork or at home at the dinner table. Children will run or climb on things at the store when it is inappropriate to do so and when other youth their age would not. These children will blurt out answers before people can finish asking the question, sometimes answering incorrectly because they did not wait to hear the full instruction. Commonly, they also interrupt or intrude into ongoing conversations, which can disrupt peer relationships. More details about the peer relationships of youth with ADHD are discussed later in this chapter.

A key reason for the controversy surrounding the disorder is that ADHD is a categorical diagnosis applied to symptoms presenting on a continuum among all youth. The core ADHD behaviors are ubiquitous among toddlers, with a societal expectation that the majority of youth will grow out of these behaviors progressively as they age. Thus, for diagnosis, a clinical judgment must be made about whether the ADHD symptoms are extreme and impairing relative to what would be expected given the child's age and situation. The cutoff score for diagnosable ADHD is, as in the case of many other disorders, somewhat arbitrary.

The recommended diagnostic procedure involves soliciting both parent and teacher ratings of the DSM-IV-TR ADHD symptoms on a normed scale, supplemented by clinician's observation and assessment of other medical and psychological conditions that mimic ADHD (see Hinshaw, March, et al., 1997). Children are thought to be poor informants of their own ADHD symptoms (Loeber, Green, Lahey, & Stouthamer-Loeber, 1991). As is the case with all rating scales, the biases, perceptions, and expectations among adult informants may influence their ratings of the child's behavior (Mikami, Chi, & Hinshaw, 2004). Behaviors may also fluctuate day to day and depending on the setting, meaning that there is no uniform, definitive test that can assess whether or not a child has ADHD.

Prevalence

Prevalence rates for ADHD vary dramatically depending on whether community or clinical samples are considered. In community samples, epidemiological studies suggest that about 3–7% of elementary school-age children in the United States meet diagnostic criteria for ADHD (American Psychiatric Association, 2000; Jensen et al., 1995). The most common subtype is ADHD-I, followed by ADHD-C (Wolraich, Hannah, Pinnock, Baumgaertel, & Brown, 1996). ADHD-HI is largely salient for preschoolers, the majority of whom become ADHD-C when they reach school-age and the demands for sustained attending increase (Lahey et al., 1994, 1998). Boys are estimated to outnumber girls 3:1 among school-age children (Lahey, Miller, Gordon, & Riley, 1999), although sex ratios vary by ADHD subtype; the lowest male to female ratio, 2:1, exists among children with the Inattentive subtype of ADHD (Carlson & Mann, 2000). In clinical samples, by contrast, ADHD is the most common reason for referral of school-age children (Steele & Roberts, 2005). The most prevalent subtype in clinical samples is ADHD-C, most likely because of the higher rates of aggressive behaviors among children with ADHD-C relative to ADHD-I (Milich et al., 2001). Sex ratios in clinical samples are commonly 9:1 male to female (Lahey et al., 1999), again presumably because youth with comorbid aggression—more common in males—have a greater likelihood of being referred to treatment (Mikami & Hinshaw, 2008).

The high male predominance in ADHD raises the question of whether sex-specific diagnostic criteria should be applied. Current DSM-IV-TR criteria are sex neutral, leading to more males than females surpassing diagnostic criteria for ADHD. Consequently there is lessened awareness that ADHD exists in girls (Quinn, 2005), which may explain why a smaller proportion of girls who do meet criteria for ADHD have been formally diagnosed and treated relative to boys who meet criteria for ADHD (Barbaresi et al., 2006; Quinn, 2005; Robison, Sclar, Skaer, & Galin, 2004). In addition, the comorbidity, impairment, and longitudinal adjustment of girls with ADHD may also be poorer than that of their male counterparts (Dalsgaard, Mortensen, Frydenberg, & Thomsen, 2002; Mikami, Hinshaw, Patterson, & Lee, 2008), perhaps because to receive a diagnosis of ADHD, a girl must behave far more atypically relative to her peers (Eme, 1992).

Although there has been debate about whether ADHD is a Western cultural construct (Bird, 2002; Timimi & Taylor, 2004), a recent meta-analysis of 102 international studies found few statistically significant differences between overall prevalence rates in the West and elsewhere in the world (Polanczyk, de Lima, Horta, Biederman, & Rohde, 2007). Any variability in reported prevalence rates appeared to be driven by differences in investigators' methodology, particularly with regard to the diagnostic criteria employed. Overall, the worldwide pooled prevalence estimate derived from this study was a little over 5%, a number similar to the estimated North American prevalence rate. Such findings suggest that ADHD is a cross-culturally valid diagnostic construct.

The vast majority of research on ADHD has focused on school-age, preadolescent children; however, 50–80% of youth diagnosed with ADHD in childhood continue to display impairing

symptoms in adolescence and adul-thood (Barkley, Fischer, Smallish, & Fletcher, 2002; Hinshaw et al., 2006; Mannuzza & Klein, 2000). Commonly, hyperactive and impulsive symptoms attenuate with age, but inattention remains (Hart et al., 1995), such that many youth previously diagnosed with ADHD-C in preadolescence instead meet criteria for ADHD-I in adolescence or adulthood (Hinshaw et al., 2006). The male to female ratio in community samples (although not clinical samples) may also become more equal in adolescence and approach 1:1 in adulthood (DuPaul et al., 2001). Despite findings that fewer adolescents and adults meet criteria for ADHD relative to school-age children, it has been argued that the symptoms are not disappearing but rather that the DSM-IV-TR criteria for ADHD are not sensitive to symptom manifestations among adults (Wolraich et al., 2005). For example, hyperactivity expressed as running about or climbing on things is rare among adults but may instead be more commonly expressed in fast, reckless driving (Barkley et al., 2002; Cox et al., 2006). Girls with ADHD-C in childhood appear at risk for impulsive disorders such as bulimia nervosa in adolescence, even when they no longer meet criteria for an ADHD diagnosis (Mikami et al., 2008).

Comorbidity among youth with ADHD is more the rule than the exception (Barkley, 2003). About half of school-age youth with ADHD display comorbid externalizing problems, most commonly Oppositional Defiant Disorder or Conduct Disorder (Jensen, Martin, & Cantwell, 1997). Comorbid internalizing problems, such as depression or anxiety, are present in about a quarter to a third of youth with ADHD (Jensen et al., 1997). These high rates of comorbidity present challenges for assessment, prognosis, and treatment. It is important to determine whether ADHD symptoms of distraction and restlessness, for example, are not better explained by a comorbid condition. In addition, although it is clear that children with ADHD are at elevated risk for a wide range of adjustment problems in adolescence/adulthood, it is important to distinguish between the contribution ADHD makes to these future difficulties relative to that of the other conditions comorbid with ADHD.

Etiology

The etiology of ADHD, like that of most psychiatric disorders, is best understood from an interactive and transactional perspective (Hinshaw, 2002b) that considers multiple levels of influence—from genes and prenatal conditions to school and family environment—as well as the ways in which these levels reciprocally interact. A distinct genetic liability lies at the heart of this disorder, but different environmental factors may influence its expression. Twin, family, and adoption studies provide evidence that both individual classes of symptoms, such as hyperactivity (Goodman & Stevenson, 1989; Price, 2001) and inattention (Alberts-Corush, Firestone, & Goodman, 1986; Goodman & Stevenson, 1989), and the disorder as a whole (Sherman, McGue, & Iacono, 1997; Sprich, Biederman, Crawford, Mundy, & Faraone, 2000) have a significant genetic component. A recent meta-analysis pooling the results of 20 twin studies places the heritability of ADHD at approximately 75% (Faraone et al., 2005), a number that makes ADHD "among the most heritable of psychiatric disorders" (p. 1313).

The high heritability estimates for this disorder have made identifying genes associated with ADHD a research priority. Observing that effective stimulant medication treatments for ADHD act to increase the amount of available extracellular dopamine (Madras, Miller, & Fischman, 2005), researchers have focused on investigating genes that regulate the dopaminergic system, with notable success (Brookes et al., 2006; Faraone, Doyle, Mick, & Biederman, 2001). The dopamine D4 receptor gene (DRD4) has been associated with novelty-seeking behavior (Benjamin et al., 1996; Ebstein et al., 1996); specifically, the 7-repeat allele of this gene is found more often in individuals with ADHD than in controls (LaHoste et al., 1996), and is associated with a more persistent form of the disorder (El-Faddagh, Laucht, Maras, Vöhringer, & Schmidt, 2004; Langley et al., 2008), though one less prone to cognitive symptoms (Swanson et al., 2000). Hinshaw (2002b) has suggested that while behavioral symptoms of ADHD may have a significant genetic component, cognitive features often associated with ADHD (i.e., sluggish cognitive tempo, impaired executive functions) may be more influenced by environmental risk factors, particularly those that impinge upon prenatal development. Considerable work remains to understand exactly how allelic variations of this gene and others confer risk, and, as Hinshaw (2002b) astutely observes, exploration of the wider context in which the individual lives will aid in this investigation.

Low birth weight (Hultman et al., 2007; Mick, Biederman, Prince, Fischer, & Faraone, 2002; Nigg & Breslau, 2007) and maternal smoking during pregnancy (Milberger, Biederman, Faraone, & Jones, 1998; Thapar et al., 2003) are factors in the prenatal environment that may be associated with the disorder. It is important to note that the majority of children with ADHD never encounter these risk factors; however, children who do experience these stressors are more likely to develop ADHD (Barkley, 2003). These early-life events may confer risk selectively depending on the setting in which a child is raised. Breslau and Chilcoat (2000) reported that low birth weight is significantly associated with ADHD in urban but not suburban settings. Similarly, Laucht et al. (2007) found that children experiencing multiple psychosocial risks (e.g., living in overcrowded conditions, born as the result of an unwanted pregnancy, cared for by a parent with a psychiatric disorder, etc.) were more likely to develop ADHD, but only if they were also genetically predisposed to the condition.

As these findings demonstrate, the etiology of ADHD cannot be understood without considering the interaction and transaction of multiple levels of influence on the individual. Although ADHD is often targeted by critics in the popular media who argue that its origins are cultural, it is inappropriate to construe ADHD as a manufactured diagnosis of convenience. ADHD has been conceived of as the result of overindulgent or otherwise "inadequate" parenting (Bailly, 2005), ingestion of sugar and artificial additives (Bateman et al., 2004; Feingold, 1975), and overexposure to television (Christakis, Zimmerman, DiGiuseppe, & McCarty, 2004); yet empirical evidence suggests that the influence of such factors on ADHD has been largely overblown (for more detailed critiques, see Coghill, 2005; Eigenmann & Haenggeli, 2004; Mehmet-Radji, 2004). Most critically, although parents' behaviors can influence the social competence of their children with ADHD (as we discuss in the treatment section below), poor parenting does not cause this disorder.

Assessment of Social Skills

Social competence is defined as the ability to respond adaptively and skillfully to various interpersonal demands in peer interactions (Bierman & Welsh, 2000). Children high in social competence are presumed to (a) possess a strong repertoire of socially skilled behaviors and (b) have their competence reflected in acceptance and friendships within their peer group. Because youth with ADHD are at high risk for difficulties in their peer relationships, it is important to consider the different aspects of social competence and dysfunction in this population, and accordingly, how each facet is assessed. Below we review the assessment methods for social competence most widely used for ADHD populations. We note that the majority of these methods—including their pros and cons—are parallel to those used to assess social competence in typically developing youth (see Bierman & Welsh, 2000), but we raise some issues that may uniquely pertain to an ADHD population.

Adult Informants

The most common method for assessing social competence involves soliciting ratings of the child's skilled behavior from adult informants, typically teachers or parents. Many standardized and well-normed questionnaires exist for this purpose; some of the most common used in the ADHD literature are the Social Skills Rating System (Gresham & Elliott, 1990) and the social problems subscale from the Child Behavior Checklist (Achenbach, 1991a, 1991b). Questionnaires often have broadband scores corresponding to an overall level of social skills (converted to a percentile ranking relative to the population), and narrow-band subscales corresponding to specific types of social skills (e.g., cooperation, assertion) that can help identify the child's pattern of interpersonal strengths and weaknesses. Indeed, in some cases it has been theorized that one particular type of social skill will be most impaired for ADHD youth or most responsive to intervention (see, for example, Antshel & Remer, 2003).

There is some question about whether teachers or parents present the most accurate information about a child's social competence. It is generally thought that teachers are better informants than parents because teachers have more opportunities to view the child interacting with his or her peers (see, for example, Dishion, 1990). However, parents may also bring unique knowledge about children's social skills with siblings (Mikami & Pfiffner, 2007) or with close friends in dyadic playdates that occur at home (Frankel & Myatt, 2003). Best practice in research and clinical work typically involves soliciting both parents and teachers as informants, because their correspondence when rating the same child's behavior is low (Achenbach, McConaughy, & Howell, 1987). Once youth reach adolescence, though, more peer interactions take place outside of the classroom and home, decreasing the usefulness of both teachers and parents as informants.

Self-Report Strategies

An alternative strategy is to have youth self-report on their social competence. Self-report versions of the Social Skills Rating System and the Child Behavior Checklist have been normed in typically developing populations for adolescents, who are thought to have more self-awareness than children and for whom adult report is thought to be less valid. For some aspects of peer relationships such as receipt of bullying, self-report has commonly been used because of the theory that adolescents are the best aware of covert victimization experiences (Olweus, 1992)—but note that the heavy reliance on self-report measures in the bullying literature has also been criticized (Cornell, Sheras, & Cole, 2006).

Although self-report of social competence has sometimes been used for typically developing youth, characteristics unique to youth with ADHD likely make this assessment strategy less viable. Elementary school-age children with ADHD are known to overestimate their social competence with peers (Hoza et al., 2004; Hoza, Waschbusch, Pelham, Molina, & Milich, 2000), a phenomenon termed "positive illusory bias"; by contrast, typically developing youth appear to be accurate in their self-assessment. Longitudinal evidence suggests that youth with ADHD maintain their over-inflated estimates of their social skills as they reach adolescence, such that the gap in accuracy between youth with ADHD versus typically developing youth persists (Hoza, Murray-Close, Arnold, Hinshaw, & MTA Cooperative Group, 2008)

Peers as Informants

Peers can also be informants about a child's social competence. In the sociometric procedure (Coie, Dodge, & Coppotelli, 1982), peers nominate children in their peer group who fit particular behavioral descriptions. Sociometric procedures have typically been used with classroom peers of children in elementary school but can be successfully modified for adolescents whose peer interactions take place outside of a single classroom (see, for example, Allen, Porter, McFarland, Marsh, & McElhaney, 2005).

The most common use of the sociometric nomination procedure is to assess peer rejection, which is an indication of how disliked a child is in his or her peer group. For this purpose, peers nominate the children whom they most and least like. Each child then has a "social preference score" that is derived by taking the proportion of "most liked" nominations he received from peers, minus the proportion of "least liked" nominations received, controlling for the number of peers who made nominations. Children who are peer-rejected, typically comprising about 15% of a peer group, receive many negative nominations and few positive nominations. By contrast, popular children have many positive and few negative nominations, controversial children have a high frequency of both positive and negative nominations, and neglected children have few nominations of either the positive or negative type.

Other aspects of social competence can also be assessed using sociometric nomination procedures. Friendship, for instance, involves a reciprocal relationship between two children. Children can have a close friend without being well-liked overall in their peer group and vice versa, although the constructs are correlated (Parker & Asher, 1993). In order to assess friendship, peers nominate children whom they consider to be friends, noted to be distinct from children whom they like. A friendship is considered to exist only if both children nominate each other as friends. Finally, sociometric nomination procedures can assess children's social behaviors by having peers nominate those children who "say nice things to other kids," "help other children out," "are shy and are alone a lot," or other descriptors of specific social skills, as opposed to or in addition to nominations of whom they like and dislike (Coie et al., 1982).

Sociometrically assessed peer rejection has been found to be moderately, but not strongly, correlated with parent and teacher ratings of children's social skills in an ADHD sample (Milich & Landau, 1982). Some of the inconsistency between methods may occur because the behaviors that adults find skillful may not matter to children for determining whom they like and dislike. For example, a common item on social skills questionnaires is "offers to help out around the house without being asked," a skill that may be appreciated by parents but is unlikely to affect the appraisal of peers. Furthermore, adults commonly rate whether or not a child compliments others as an indication of social competence, but evidence suggests that peer-rejected children with ADHD may not actually be impaired in compliment-giving (Mikami, Huang-Pollock, Pfiffner, McBurnett, & Hangai, 2007). Ultimately, it is notable that peer-assessed rejection better predicts future adjustment than do adult-rated social skills (Landau & Moore, 1991), suggesting that whether or not children are liked by their peers, regardless of what social skills adults think they possess, is perhaps the most sensitive indicator of their social competence.

Observational Assessment Techniques

A strength of informant report measures is that they assess the child's behavior in naturalistic social settings. A weakness of these measures, however, is that they all rely on the informant's impressions of the child's global behavior (Chi & Hinshaw, 2002; Mikami et al., 2004). In addition, ratings of children's social skills are not suited to capturing the child's micro-behaviors in peer interactions.

Observational assessment of children's social skills can address some of these limitations. In a typical observational procedure, children are placed with unfamiliar peers in a social interaction. The rationale for peers not knowing each other is so that children's behaviors will not be influenced by previous interactions or reputations. Observers, typically not privy to background information about the children, are trained to code children's molecular social behaviors. A great deal of training for observers is required, and a proportion of interactions are double coded by observers to yield calculations of inter-rater reliability.

Observational procedures vary in degree of structure. In some cases, children are left to engage in whatever interaction they choose with their peers (see Erhardt & Hinshaw, 1994; Hodgens, Cole, & Boldizar, 2000; Mikami & Hinshaw, 2003). In other cases, children are given a structured task to do with their peers, such as to verbally communicate instructions about how to land a lunar cruiser in a simulation (Whalen, Henker, Collins, McAuliffe, & Vaux, 1979). Peer rejection from sociometric nominations in these procedures has been found to correlate 0.50–0.74 with sociometric status at school (Bierman & Welsh, 2000), which supports the validity of observational assessment techniques. Observational procedures have been used successfully with children who have ADHD, and social skills differences between ADHD and comparison children have reliably emerged within the first few hours of interaction (Erhardt & Hinshaw, 1994; Hodgens et al., 2000). Similar procedures have also been successfully modified for use with adolescents (Allen, Porter, & McFarland, 2006; Dishion, McCord, & Poulin, 1999).

One important downside of observing interactions with peers is that this methodology cannot account for the extent to which a child's behavior is influenced by other peers in the group (see Kraemer & Jacklin, 1979 for discussion). For instance, a child's social skills may appear better in a group of peers who are similar to that child in behavior, personality, or ethnicity (Chang, 2004; Kao & Joyner, 2004; Stormshak et al., 1999) or are simply more disposed to be friendly to that child. Thus, the uncontrolled factor of other peers' behaviors in the group introduces variance in a child's display of social competence.

Novel directions that may address some of the concerns about the existing measures involve standardizing observations so that children are provided the same stimulus from a peer but are free to respond to it in their own way (Bierman & Welsh, 2000). One method is to train a peer confederate to interact with the child in a prescribed manner and then observe and code the child's responses (see Hoza et al., 2000; Sandstrom, Cillessen, & Eisenhower, 2003). Another method is to place children in a "chat room" with a standardized computer program simulating confederate peers; the child's responses to the computer can then be recorded and coded (Mikami et al., 2007; Ohan & Johnston, 2007). As increasing numbers of children are interacting with their peers online, this procedure is an ecologically valid means of assessing social behaviors.

Summary

The gold standard for assessing social competence relies on multiple measures from multiple informants. A battery of parent and teacher ratings of social skills, peer sociometric nominations, and observational procedures is considered ideal to reduce problems associated with shared method variance. Realistically, however, clinicians who want to assess the social skills of their client with ADHD will be hard pressed to incorporate all these measures. It is understandably more feasible for clinicians to rely solely on parent and teacher report for this purpose. However, if clinicians can make observations of the child's behavior with peers or if assessment techniques such as the chat room computer program can be provided for clinicians to install on their office computer, these tools may assist clinicians in gaining a broader picture of the child's social functioning not available from adult informant report alone.

Social Skills Problems Unique to ADHD

A robust and consistent finding is that youth with ADHD, on average, struggle profoundly in their social relationships relative to comparison youth.

Although in this chapter we primarily focus on the difficulties youth with ADHD have with their peers, we note that this population additionally has trouble in social relationships with their parents (Johnston & Mash, 2001; Peris & Hinshaw, 2003) and siblings (Mikami & Pfiffner, 2007) as well as with non-related adults such as teachers (Rucklidge & Tannock, 2001; Stormont, 2001) and camp counselors (Mikami & Hinshaw, 2003). In fact, the presence of youth with ADHD may also generate discord in the marital relationships of their parents (Wymbs, Pelham, Molina, & Gnagy, 2008). For these reasons, youth with ADHD have been called "negative social catalysts" for their frequent role in disruptive social relationships (Whalen & Henker, 1992).

In the sections below, we first review the findings about social dysfunction in ADHD, with particular attention to the different assessment methodologies used and the domain of functioning captured by each method. We then review what is known about ways in which sex, ADHD subtype, and comorbidity influence the social profiles of this population. Finally, we review empirical literature suggesting reasons why youth with ADHD struggle so much socially.

Magnitude of Social Impairment

Deficits in social functioning have been consistently found using a wide variety of measurement techniques from diverse informants: parent and teacher ratings (Landau, Milich, & Diener, 1998; Landau & Moore, 1991), sociometric nominations from peers (Hoza, Mrug, et al., 2005), behavioral observation in playgroups with peers (Hodgens et al., 2000; Hubbard & Newcomb, 1991), and observation in controlled confederate paradigms (Mikami et al., 2007; Ohan & Johnston, 2007). Only ADHD youth themselves may not self-report poorer social functioning, or, if they do report poorer functioning, it is not to the extent suggested by the other adult-informant, peer-informant, and observational assessment measures; this positive illusory bias has been suggested to be a defense mechanism against the reality of their impairment (Hoza et al., 2004).

The magnitude of the difference in social competence between ADHD and comparison youth appears to be about one standard deviation on adult informant rating scales of social skills, such that the average comparison youth is rated to have better social skills than 84% of youth with ADHD (Bagwell, Molina, Pelham, & Hoza, 2001; Greene et al., 2001; Hinshaw et al., 2006). This finding is consistent across both parent and teacher ratings. This is considered a large effect size (Cohen, 1988), with the magnitude being about equivalent to the mean differences in cognitive skill and academic achievement found between ADHD and comparison youth (Hinshaw, 1992, 2002a). Parent and teacher reports have largely assessed the child's demonstration of skillful behaviors but, notably, parent and teacher ratings of the child's peer rejection also suggest youth with ADHD are impaired relative to comparison youth (Bagwell et al., 2001; Mikami & Hinshaw, 2003).

Studies using sociometric nominations from peers have been equally consistent in their findings that children with ADHD are highly rejected by their peers. Children with ADHD receive more negative nominations and fewer positive nominations from peers than do comparison children—differences similarly about one standard deviation in magnitude—although the impairment of children with ADHD may be more pronounced for negative nominations than positive nominations (Hinshaw, 2002a). In one study, 82% of a sample of 49 children with ADHD received negative nominations one standard deviation above the class mean of negative nominations, and 60% of the children with ADHD scored two standard deviations above the class mean (e.g., in the top 2.5% of their class) (Pelham & Bender, 1982). Other research suggests that more than half of children with ADHD are peer-rejected, relative to under 15% of children without ADHD (Hoza, Mrug, et al., 2005; Stormont, 2001). Furthermore, children with ADHD show impairment in friendship in addition to popularity (Blachman & Hinshaw, 2002; Hoza, Mrug, et al., 2005). They have fewer dyadic friendships, and those friendships they do have are likely to be of lower quality.

Evidence suggests that children with ADHD may be more rejected by peers than are youth with any other disorder (Asarnow, 1988); peers are often more tolerant of youth with mental retardation, learning disorders, aggression, or depression alone, when not comorbid with ADHD. In addition, peer rejection happens quickly, within the first few hours of meeting unfamiliar peers (Erhardt & Hinshaw, 1994; Hodgens et al., 2000). Once rejection occurs, it is relatively stable for this population (Hinshaw & Melnick, 1995), in particular for negative peer nominations relative to positive nominations (Blachman & Hinshaw, 2002).

Interestingly, children with ADHD do not, in general, appreciably differ from children without ADHD in the choices of whom they like and do not like. In fact, in sociometric nomination procedures both children with ADHD and typically developing children tend to pick peers without ADHD as those they like most and peers with ADHD as those they like least (Blachman & Hinshaw, 2002; Hoza, Mrug, et al., 2005). Thus, if children with ADHD are more likely to socialize with other children with ADHD, it may be that their shared low social status in the peer group leaves few others as potential friends.

Behavioral observation paradigms in both free play and controlled settings have commonly documented more aggressive and hostile behaviors among children with ADHD relative to comparison children, again with effect sizes of about one standard deviation of difference (Hinshaw, 2002a; Hinshaw, Zupan, Simmel, Nigg, & Melnick, 1997; Ohan & Johnston, 2007). More social withdrawal has sometimes been found for children with ADHD relative to comparison children, but the effect is not as robust as that for aggression, and social withdrawal may also vary depending on ADHD subtype as discussed in more detail in the section below (Hodgens et al., 2000; Mikami et al., 2007). In two studies using controlled settings that allowed examination on specific conversational skills, one with a naïve peer and one with a confederate, youth with ADHD displayed elevated rates of irrelevant conversation and lower sensitivity to the peer's needs (Mikami et al., 2007; Whalen et al., 1979).

Social Impairment in Adolescence

The majority of research on ADHD, including research on social impairment in this population, has been conducted with school-age children.

However, prospective longitudinal work consistently demonstrates that youth with ADHD in childhood continue to display impairment as adolescents on parent and teacher ratings of social skills and friendship (Bagwell et al., 2001; Greene, Biederman, Faraone, Sienna, & Garcia-Jetton, 1997; Hinshaw et al., 2006; Mannuzza & Klein, 2000). In addition, provocative work finds that college students with ADHD may have more difficulty in romantic relationships than do comparison students (Canu & Carlson, 2003). Although more research needs to be conducted using developmentally sensitive measures of social competence for individuals in adolescence and adulthood, the sum of the evidence to date is that social problems do not go away for this population as they age.

Interestingly, findings of social impairment often hold among adolescents who had ADHD in childhood but no longer meet diagnostic criteria for ADHD (see, for example, Hinshaw et al., 2006). It is unclear whether this is because youth who are peer-rejected in childhood lose opportunities for social interaction and thus fail to learn social skills in formative years (Ladd & Mize, 1982), leading to the persistence of social problems independent from ADHD symptoms. An alternative explanation is that DSM-IV criteria for ADHD are not sensitive to the manifestation of ADHD symptoms past puberty, meaning that many individuals who meet criteria for ADHD in childhood but not adolescence may not in fact be experiencing diminution of symptoms (Barkley, 2002). Finally, it may be that maladaptive cognitive or emotional processing biases or comorbidities associated with ADHD remain even when symptoms of ADHD become subclinical.

ADHD Subtype, Comorbidity, and Sex Considerations

Certain populations remain understudied in the ADHD literature: youth with ADHD-I relative to those with ADHD-C, ADHD youth with comorbid internalizing problems relative to those with comorbid oppositional and conduct problems, and girls relative to boys. The relationship between these understudied populations is not accidental. Boys with ADHD-C and comorbid oppositional and conduct disorders are the most common referrals to clinics (and thus the easiest population to recruit for research studies). By contrast, girls are relatively better represented in the ADHD-I subtype than in the ADHD-C subtype (Carlson & Mann, 2000; Lahey et al., 1994; Milich et al., 2001). In addition, youth with ADHD-I are relatively less likely to have comorbid oppositional and conduct problems and relatively more likely to have comorbid internalizing problems than are youth with ADHD-C (Carlson & Mann, 2000; Milich et al., 2001; but for an exception, see Power, Costigan, Eiraldi, & Leff, 2004). Similarly, some evidence suggests that girls with ADHD are both less likely to have comorbid conduct problems and more likely to have internalizing problems than are boys with ADHD (Gershon, 2002).

Evidence from several studies suggests that parents and teachers rate children with ADHD-I as less aggressive and disruptive, but more passive and withdrawn, than children with ADHD-C (Barkley, DuPaul, & McMurray, 1990; Edelbrock, Costello, & Kessler, 1984; Maedgen & Carlson, 2000), although in other samples adults have rated children with ADHD-C and ADHD-I as equally impaired in social behaviors relative to comparison children (Gadow et al., 2004; Hinshaw et al., 2006). In three observational studies of peer interactions, two where children interacted freely with previously unfamiliar peers (Hinshaw, 2002a; Hodgens et al., 2000) and one where children interacted with a computer program simulating peers (Mikami et al., 2007), children with ADHD-I were found to be more shy, withdrawn, and reserved relative to children with ADHD-C and comparison children, who did not differ from one another. Children with ADHD-C, however, were found to be more aggressive, to start more fights, and to make many more off-topic statements, relative to children with ADHD-I and comparison children. These differences in behavioral style may explain why children with ADHD-I may be less rejected by their peers than children with ADHD-C and may be more likely to instead be neglected by their peers (Carlson & Mann, 2000; Hinshaw, 2002a). Sluggish cognitive tempo—a syndrome of low alertness and slow processing thought to characterize up to 30% of children with ADHD-I but not youth with ADHD-C—may also account for ADHD subtype differences in social impairment

(Hartman, Willcutt, Rhee, & Pennington, 2004; McBurnett et al., 2001). One study using an all-ADHD-I sample found that sluggish cognitive tempo predicted higher levels of teacher-reported withdrawn behavior and lower levels of aggressive behavior (Carlson & Mann, 2002). In an observational study, sluggish cognitive tempo was also found to predict poor memory for the peer's conversation and lower hostility, above and beyond the effect of ADHD subtype (Mikami et al., 2007).

Regarding comorbidity, it is important to separate the core symptoms of ADHD from the oppositional and conduct problems that are often associated with ADHD but not required for the disorder (Hinshaw, 1987). Crucially, the higher likelihood for comorbid aggression does not completely explain the peer relationship problems of children with ADHD: Children with ADHD and no comorbid conduct problems remain more peer-rejected than either conduct-disordered children without ADHD (Asarnow, 1988) or typically developing children (Landau & Moore, 1991). That said, children with ADHD and comorbid oppositional and conduct disorders do have poorer social functioning than children with ADHD alone (Mikami & Pfiffner, 2007; Pfiffner, Calzada, & McBurnett, 2000). In one study, aggressive behavior displayed by ADHD boys explained 46% of the variance in peer acceptance (Erhardt & Hinshaw, 1994), and peers commonly attribute their dislike of youth with ADHD to the aggression of these youth (Hinshaw, Zupan, et al., 1997). There is some indication that aggression in children with ADHD and comorbid conduct disorders may be qualitatively different from aggression in children with oppositional defiant disorder or conduct disorder alone, without ADHD. While both ADHD and non-ADHD children may use instrumental, proactive aggression, children with ADHD may be more likely to also use hostile, reactive aggression (Atkins & Stoff, 1993), a type of aggression that more strongly predicts peer rejection (Dodge & Coie, 1987; Kempes, Matthys, de Vries, & van Engeland, 2005).

It remains largely unknown how the social profile of children with ADHD and internalizing comorbidities might differ from that of children with ADHD and oppositional or conduct problems, or children with ADHD and no comorbidities (Pfiffner et al., 2000). Although it is theorized that internalizing comorbidities may lead to social impairment based on research about social withdrawal and its association with peer rejection (Hymel, Bowker, & Woody, 1993), aggression may also more clearly predict poor social functioning than does withdrawal (Boivin, Hymel, & Burkowski, 1995; although see Chang, 2003).

Girls with ADHD are clearly known to be socially impaired relative to comparison girls, based on parent and teacher ratings of social skills, peer sociometrically assessed rejection and friendship, and observations of social behaviors (Biederman et al., 1999; Blachman & Hinshaw, 2002; Hinshaw, 2002a; Hinshaw et al., 2006; Mikami & Hinshaw, 2003; Zalecki & Hinshaw, 2004). However, evidence has been mixed regarding how the social dysfunction among girls with ADHD compares to that among boys with ADHD. Some studies have found girls with ADHD to be less socially impaired relative to their male ADHD counterparts (Johnston, Pelham, & Murphy, 1985), whereas others suggest girls with ADHD may in fact be more peer-rejected than boys with ADHD (Carlson, Tamm, & Gaub, 1997). Still, the most comprehensive study comparing peer relationships of both sexes to date, involving children with ADHD-C from the Multimodal Treatment Study of ADHD (MTA), found no sex differences in the high level of rejection associated with ADHD (Hoza, Mrug, et al., 2005).

The contradictory findings about how the social competence of girls with ADHD compares to that of boys with ADHD may partly result from a failure to account for differing rates of ADHD subtypes and comorbidities between the sexes. To the extent that girls with ADHD may be more likely to have ADHD-I and lack externalizing comorbidities, relative to their male counterparts, the absence of hyperactivity/impulsivity and disruptive, aggressive behaviors may lead to relatively better peer relationships. Thus, differences in social competence may not be attributable to sex so much as to the particular pattern of symptomotology more common among girls. This may partly explain why, in the MTA sample of youth, all of whom had ADHD-C, there were no sex differences in social dysfunction. Yet the core symptoms of ADHD are more unusual in a sex-normative sense when displayed by girls, and likely more disruptive within female peer groups, given the strong focus on verbal give-and-take for females (Maccoby, 1998). It may be that girls with ADHD who have matched levels of hyperactive-impulsive symptoms and aggressive behaviors as boys will appear more socially impaired than boys in the peer domain.

ADHD Symptomotology

Now that we have established the magnitude of the social problems faced by youth with ADHD, in the next sections we review empirical evidence for reasons that may explain why this population struggles socially. First and foremost, the core symptoms of inattention, hyperactivity, and impulsivity characteristic of ADHD probably impede social relationships. Inattention can contribute to children with ADHD having trouble following conversations, picking up on subtle social cues, or engaging and withdrawing from peer groups at the correct time (Landau et al., 1998; Nixon, 2001; Whalen & Henker, 1992). A social problem probably unique to the ADHD-I subtype and related to the sluggish cognitive tempo symptoms associated with ADHD-I is that some children appear apathetic during games or peer interactions, not excited to play, and content to daydream off to the side by themselves (Pfiffner, 2003), behaviors which interfere with the formation of deep social relationships.

Hyperactive and impulsive behaviors further disrupt peer relationships. Such behaviors contribute to difficulties waiting in line or waiting one's turn in a game. Impulsivity also results in children with ADHD interrupting and intruding into ongoing conversations (Whalen & Henker, 1992). When playing games, it is common for these children to change the rules to ensure that they win, to tell peers how they should act or where they should move their game pieces, and to argue and react angrily when they lose; these behaviors are likely related to impulsivity as these children have difficulty inhibiting their immediate reactions and controlling impatience (Barkley, 1997, 2003).

Other Cognitive and Emotional Biases

In addition to the core symptoms of ADHD, other maladaptive cognitive and emotional biases characteristic of children with ADHD may also impede their peer relationships. It is possible that such cognitive and emotional patterns remain even when ADHD symptoms become subclinical, and this explains the persistence of social problems among youth who had ADHD in childhood but no longer meet criteria for the disorder in adolescence.

Examples of cognitive biases involve errors in social information processing and goal-setting. Youth with social information processing biases attribute hostile intentions to the ambiguous behaviors of peers and generate ineffective solutions to social problems (Crick & Dodge, 1994; Dodge, 1980). Such biases have been most commonly studied among highly aggressive youth and have been found to be predicted by early experiences of peer rejection, as well as to predict future social dysfunction (Dodge et al., 2003; Lansford et al., 2006). Work in ADHD samples has found that boys with ADHD and comorbid conduct problems may display more social information processing biases than boys with ADHD only (Matthys, Cuperus, & van England, 1999; Murphy, Pelham, & Lang, 1992), who, in turn, display more biases than comparison boys. In addition, adolescent girls with ADHD may have more social information processing biases than comparison girls (Mikami, Lee, Hinshaw, & Mullin, 2008). In this study, comorbid conduct problems did not explain the prevalence of social information processing problems in the ADHD group. However peer rejection was associated with social information processing problems for comparison girls only and not girls with ADHD (Mikami et al., 2008).

Further evidence exists that boys with ADHD may choose maladaptive goals (e.g., more "trouble-seeking," less focus on fairness) in their peer interactions relative to comparison boys (Hinshaw & Melnick, 1995; Melnick & Hinshaw, 1996). This may particularly occur among highly aggressive boys with ADHD, and Melnick and Hinshaw (1996) suggest that maladaptive goal selection may be more related to comorbid oppositional and conduct disorders than to ADHD per se. Holding positive social goals (or at least *appearing* to hold

these goals according to adult observers) such as wanting to be liked or to exhibit good sportsmanship was positively correlated with social acceptance among comparison boys but appeared uncorrelated with acceptance for boys with ADHD (Melnick & Hinshaw, 1996). Other research with girls, however, suggests that girls with ADHD, regardless of whether or not they have comorbid conduct problems, may choose the same goals as do comparison girls, but offer ineffective strategies to meet these goals (e.g., more aggression, less negotiation) (Thurber, Heller, & Hinshaw, 2002).

Other biases common in ADHD relate to difficulties with accurately perceiving, mirroring, and regulating emotional states. In multiple experimental paradigms, youth with ADHD have demonstrated impairment relative to comparison youth in interpreting facial affect (Boakes, Chapman, Houghton, & West, 2008; Singh et al., 1998), as well as speech intonation (Corbett & Glidden, 2000), although for an exception see Guyer et al. (2007). Errors among youth with ADHD have sometimes appeared independent from the contribution of comorbid conduct problems (Cadesky, Mota, & Schachar, 2000). Crucially, youth with ADHD appear to demonstrate a selective impairment in recognizing emotional facial expressions; their difficulties in this domain do not generalize to the recognition of non-emotional information (Yuill & Lyon, 2007). Further, impairment in emotion recognition has been found to be correlated with peer relationship problems only among youth at risk for ADHD and not related to peer relationships among comparison youth (Kats-Gold, Besser, & Priel, 2007). Perhaps stemming from their difficulties in recognizing emotions, youth with ADHD also appear less likely than comparison youth to mirror the existing emotion of a character in a story, which has been suggested to reflect poor empathy (Braaten & Rosen, 2000).

An inability to regulate one's own emotions has been well established to predict peer rejection in typically developing samples (Cooper, Shaver, & Collins, 1998; Southam-Gerow & Kendall, 2002). The research that does exist in ADHD samples suggests that impairment in emotion regulation is salient for youth with ADHD and may contribute to their peer relationship problems. In two different studies using tasks designed to elicit frustration, boys with ADHD demonstrated more difficulty regulating their emotions than did comparison boys (Melnick & Hinshaw, 2000; Walcott & Landau, 2004). It was further found that emotion regulation problems were correlated with responses on a well-established measure of impulsivity, the stop signal reaction time task (Walcott & Landau, 2004). Consistent with the hypothesis that emotion regulation problems are an extension of impulsivity, difficulties with emotion regulation have been found to be more salient for youth with ADHD-C, relative to youth with ADHD-I (Maedgen & Carlson, 2000). Emotion regulation problems in the laboratory task were also subsequently found to predict noncompliance and (marginally) predict peer rejection in a naturalistic summer camp setting (Melnick & Hinshaw, 2000).

The problems youth with ADHD have in accurately interpreting both the behaviors and emotional states of peers may be attributable to an overarching difficulty with organizing and encoding information. In experimental tasks, children with ADHD from preschool to early adolescence have repeatedly been found to fail to conceptually link facts presented in fiction stories so as to be able to make accurate causal inferences and interpretations (Flory et al., 2006; Lorch, Milich, Astrin, & Berthiaume, 2006). These organizing and encoding deficits have been hypothesized to explain the difficulties in peer relationships among children with ADHD (Milch-Reich, Campbell, Pelham, Connelly, & Geva, 1999), although the direct link has yet to be empirically tested.

Stigma and Reputational Bias

Although social skills deficits in children with ADHD no doubt contribute to the social impairment of this population, accepted peers may also influence the predominant rejection of youth with ADHD. Development of positive peer relationships requires complex, reciprocal interactions that do not occur in a vacuum where only the behavior of the child with ADHD child's behavior is important (McElwain & Volling, 2002). Attitudes, behaviors,

and prejudices of accepted peers have been understudied in a research literature that predominantly focuses on skills deficits within disliked children to explain their reject-ion (Bierman, 2004).

The stigma associated with ADHD can impede accepted peers' willingness to befriend children with this disorder. In experimental paradigms, merely labeling a target child as "ADHD" (even if the target does not in fact have ADHD) has been shown to elicit negative judgments among unfamiliar peers about the target that extend far beyond the specific behavioral information provided (Whalen, Henker, Dotemoto, & Hinshaw, 1983). Further, naïve peers report greater unwillingness to be friends with the target (Canu, Newman, Morrow, & Pope, 2008; Martin, Pescosolido, Olafsdottir, & McLeod, 2007). In a study by Harris, Milich, and McAninch (1998), the label of ADHD evoked a negative self-fulfilling prophecy. When peers were told that a target had ADHD, even though this information was false and the target was not aware of what the peer had been told, peers behaved poorly toward that target, who then responded with negative, socially unskilled behavior that confirmed the peers' expectations.

Finally, it is important to note that the widespread findings of parents and teachers rating children with ADHD as more socially deficient than comparison children may at least be partly explained by the tendency for adults to be biased in their ratings against youth with ADHD. Because ratings from adult informants require a social judgment, they are susceptible to interpretive biases on the part of the informant (Hart & Lahey, 1999). For instance, adults must determine whether a child is aggressively abusing a peer or just standing up for himself. Research in an ADHD sample has found that adults tend to like comparison youth better than children with ADHD, and adult informants in turn overestimated the problem behavior of children who were disliked by adults, relative to more objective findings from a molecular behavioral observation system (Mikami et al., 2004). Similarly, mothers who were depressed—also more common among youth with ADHD—were found to overestimate the problem behavior of their children with ADHD (Chi & Hinshaw, 2002).

Summary

As a group, children with ADHD have profound difficulties in peer relationships as assessed via multiple measures and informants. Evidence suggests that these social difficulties persist from childhood through adolescence and young adulthood, across sexes, and across ADHD subtypes. However, youth with ADHD-I may be less aggressive and more withdrawn than are youth with ADHD-C, leading to them more often being neglected, as opposed to rejected, by peers. Youth with ADHD and comorbid conduct problems have poorer social functioning than do youth with ADHD and no disruptive comorbidities, although importantly, conduct problems alone do not fully account for the social dysfunction common to ADHD. More research, however, is needed to examine the impact of comorbid internalizing conditions on peer relationships. Research about the peer relationships of girls with ADHD compared to that of boys with ADHD has yielded mixed findings about which sex is more impaired. However, it is important to separate the impact of sex from ADHD subtype and comorbidity patterns more commonly found among boys than girls with ADHD. Finally, the factors of core ADHD symptomotology and cognitive and emotional biases (both among youth with ADHD and among their peers) may be potential explanations for the social struggles of youth with ADHD.

Treatment for Social Dysfunction

The high frequency of social dysfunction in ADHD populations is of concern, because evidence suggests that peer rejection and ADHD each independently predict problems later in life: depression and suicide, drug abuse, school dropout and academic failure, juvenile delinquency, adult criminality, and lower job attainment (Mannuzza & Klein, 2000; Parker, Rubin, Price, & DeRosier, 1995). Thus, children with ADHD are already at high risk for poor adjustment, and some evidence suggests that the risk increases if they are additionally rejected by their peers (Greene et al., 1997; Mikami & Hinshaw, 2006). In fact, peer rejection may be a major mediator of the relationship between ADHD and

negative long-term outcomes (Marshal, Molina, & Pelham, 2003). Collectively, these findings demonstrate the urgency of developing interventions to encourage social competence among children with ADHD. In this section, we open by reviewing the first-line treatments for ADHD symptoms—stimulant medication and behavioral therapy—and findings about their impact on social dysfunction. We then discuss social skills training and other novel interventions that directly target social problems, with consideration of particular adaptations relevant for ADHD youth.

First-Line Treatments for ADHD

Stimulant medication and behavioral contingency management techniques, both independently and in combination, are demonstrated to be effective for reducing the core symptoms of ADHD; their usefulness for increasing children's social competence is considerably less conclusive, however. Data pooled from multiple studies suggest that around 60–80% of children with ADHD show a beneficial response to stimulant medication as demonstrated by reduced inattentive, hyperactive, and impulsive behaviors (Barbaresi et al., 2006; Barkley, 1989; Swanson, McBurnett, Christian, & Wigal, 1995). In the classroom, children given stimulant preparations produce more on-task behavior, compliance, and completion of work relative to children taking placebo. Stimulant medication is the most common treatment for ADHD, and prescription rates have been increasing (Robison et al., 2004; Robison, Skaer, Sclar, & Galin, 2002).

Behavioral contingency management approaches are also demonstrated effective for reducing ADHD symptoms (Pelham, Wheeler, & Chronis, 1998). They are typically recommended to supplement stimulant medication treatments. However, some children do not respond to stimulant medication, experience intolerable side effects from the medication, or have families who are opposed to pharmacological treatment, making exclusive treatment with behavioral techniques the most viable option. In behavioral contingency management approaches, the child's expected behaviors are made explicit, and a highly structured system of reinforcements and punishments are instituted to shape appropriate conduct (Pelham & Hoza, 1996). It is typically recommended that parents and teachers collaborate together to institute a consistent behavior plan reinforcing the same expectations, so as to maximize effectiveness.

The MTA Study, a multi-site trial funded by the National Institute of Mental Health, is the most comprehensive study of treatment effectiveness in ADHD to date. The trial enrolled 579 children aged 7.0–9.9, all of whom had ADHD-C (no other subtypes). Children were randomly assigned to one of four treatment conditions: multi-component behavior therapy, medication management (almost exclusively with stimulant medications), the combination of behavior therapy and medication management, or referral to self-selected usual community care. Treatments for the first three conditions were administered by study personnel for 14 months, after which families proceeded to naturalistic follow-up (for further details, see Greenhill et al., 1996; Wells et al., 2000). At the conclusion of the 14-month active treatment period, medication management and combined medication management plus behavioral therapy were the most effective in reducing the core ADHD symptoms by parent, teacher, and observer ratings (M.T.A. Cooperative Group, 1999a).

Further analyses in the MTA sample suggested that children with ADHD and comorbid oppositional defiant and conduct disorders responded equally well to medication management alone and combined treatment, but children with ADHD and comorbid anxiety had the best response when provided combined treatment relative to the other three conditions (Jensen et al., 2001; M.T.A. Cooperative Group, 1999b). In addition, on average, children receiving combined treatment were stabilized on lower doses of stimulants than were children on medication management alone, while still achieving the same overall therapeutic effect (M.T.A. Cooperative Group, 1999a).

Unfortunately, little evidence exists overall for maintenance of gains after either treatment is stopped. Children typically return to their former level of ADHD symptoms when their medication wears off, as well as if the structured contingency management plans are removed (Barkley, 1989; Mrug, Hoza, & Gerdes, 2001). In the MTA study,

once the provision of treatment by study personnel concluded after the 14-month active period (although families were allowed to continue the same medication dose and behavioral plans in community care), the effect for the superiority of the medication and combined treatment groups reduced in size by 10 months post-treatment (M.T.A. Cooperative Group, 2004) and completely dissipated by 22 months after treatment ended (Jensen et al., 2007).

Although stimulant medication preparations and behavioral contingency management techniques are optimally effective in reducing the core symptoms of ADHD, their usefulness for improving these children's peer relationships is considerably more circumscribed. At the conclusion of the 14-month active MTA treatment period—when treatment group effects were strongest for ADHD symptoms—children in the medication, behavioral therapy, and combined treatment groups did not differ significantly from one another in their parent- and teacher-rated social skills, and only combined treatment appeared to be better than community care (M.T.A. Cooperative Group, 1999a). Even so, this improvement in social skills ratings had a much smaller effect size than the demonstrated improvements in ADHD symptom reduction. In other research, stimulant medication as well as the combination of medication and behavioral contingency management has been shown to reduce displayed aggressive and disruptive behaviors, noted by observers, in peer social interactions (Hinshaw, Henker, Whalen, Erhardt, & Dunnington, 1989; Hinshaw et al., 2000; Klein & Abikoff, 1997; Murphy et al., 1992). However, medication may not increase prosocial behaviors or reduce social withdrawal, which are other behaviors that may also be important for positive peer relationships (Hinshaw et al., 1989).

Despite some evidence that these first-line treatments for ADHD may improve adaptive social behaviors with peers (at least, as rated by adult informants and in observation), these treatments probably do not affect peer ratings of the child's competence as assessed by sociometric nominations. In the MTA study at the end of the 14-month treatment period, despite suggestions that children receiving combined treatment had higher parent- and teacher-rated social skills, there were no effects for any treatment modality on peer sociometrically assessed rejection and friendship (Hoza, Gerdes, et al., 2005). Relative to a matched sample of comparison children, the children with ADHD remained profoundly impaired on every sociometric measure, no matter which of the four treatment conditions they had just completed. As discussed by the authors, it is notable that the state-of-the-art, first-line treatments for ADHD, delivered in ideal conditions, could not reduce the severe rejection faced by this population (Hoza, Gerdes, et al., 2005). In other research, even children who have improved in fewer negative nominations from peers after receiving intensive behavioral contingency management nonetheless continue to be rejected by their classmates, just less so (Pelham & Bender, 1982).

It is intriguing that, even though medication and behavioral treatments may reduce the core symptoms of ADHD and the aggressive and noncompliant behavior common in this population, associated gains in peer acceptance do not follow. This finding supports the notion that other factors must contribute to the peer rejection of youth with ADHD beyond their symptoms alone. Because sociometrically assessed peer rejection is superior to other measures of social competence in predicting future adjustment difficulties (Landau & Moore, 1991; Parker & Asher, 1987), the importance of change on this construct cannot be underestimated.

Social Skills Training

One obvious limitation to medication and behavior therapy is that they in no way specifically target social behaviors with peers. Social skills training interventions, by contrast, operate on the assumption that peer-rejected children lack the skills needed for making interpersonal connections and that didactic instruction in such skills will result in improved social competence. Such social skills training approaches attempt to remediate these skill deficits by teaching children a particular social behavior, giving repeated opportunities to practice that behavior, and then providing feedback on their performance (Beelman, Pfingsten, & Losel, 1994; Ladd, 1985). Common skills taught to youth with ADHD

are starting conversations, listening to peers, giving compliments, and good sportsmanship.

Evidence for the effectiveness of social skills training in ADHD populations has not been strong. Notably, in general, social skills training programs have shown mixed effectiveness for improving the popularity of rejected children who may not have ADHD. Research pooling findings from multiple studies suggest that fewer than half of programs produce any gains in children's social competence (Beelman et al., 1994; Moote, Smith, & Wodarski, 1999). In addition, most social skills training programs have not used peer sociometric measures of rejection to assess effects and have instead relied on parent and teacher ratings of social skills. As established above, achieving change on sociometric measures is likely more difficult, but also more valuable.

There is some suggestion, however, that the efficacy of social skills training approaches may be even weaker for the population of peer-rejected youth with ADHD than for the general population of peer-rejected youth (Landau et al., 1998; Mikami & Pfiffner, 2006; Mrug et al., 2001). There are several theories regarding why this might occur. First, peer-rejected children can be conceptualized as having deficits either in social knowledge or in performance. For instance, is it that children do not know the correct behavior for a specific social situation, or is it that they know what they should do but are unable to control competing unskilled behaviors, particularly in the heat of the moment? Social skills training programs rely on the assumption that knowledge deficits are a significant part of the problem. However, although knowledge deficits may interfere with peer relationships to a greater extent for peer-rejected children without ADHD, it is thought that the primary barrier for children with ADHD-C is performance deficits (Barkley, 1997; Pfiffner et al., 2000). Note that this may be less true for youth with ADHD-I who might specifically need instruction on active participation, engagement, and assertion (Antshel & Remer, 2003; Pfiffner et al., 2000). A second potential reason is that children with ADHD may be more likely to have cognitive and emotion regulation biases, as discussed in the section on social skills problems above, that are not well addressed in existing didactic social skills training paradigms and thus remain to impede peer relationships.

Related to the issue of performance deficits, another common problem is children's difficulty in generalizing the skills they have learned to situations either outside of the treatment context or once treatment has concluded. Clinically, children with ADHD have been observed to walk out of a social skills training session for which the topic was "negotiation during conflicts" and then fight with one another about seating arrangements while boarding the bus for the ride back home. It is as if these children do not recognize that the current interpersonal situation is the same as the one they have just been discussing in group. Overall, there is remarkably little evidence for generalization of social skills training among ADHD samples, particularly in follow-up once the treatment ends (Chronis, Jones, & Raggi, 2006; Mrug et al., 2001). Important exceptions may occur when parents and teachers also receive concurrent instruction with the children's social skills groups. In such cases, adult informants report that treated children display short-term generalization of social skills, perhaps because adult training allows parents and teachers to help reinforce the skills taught (Frankel, Myatt, Cantwell, & Feinberg, 1997; Pfiffner & McBurnett, 1997; Pfiffner et al., 2007). However, none of these studies has incorporated peer sociometric nominations as an index of change.

Novel Directions for Treatment

Given the limitations of the existing interventions to reduce peer rejection, researchers are considering novel ways to improve the social competence of youth with ADHD. Several investigators have issued calls for friendship interventions, the idea being that if changing popularity is too difficult or impractical, developing friendships may be a good alternative (Asher, Parker, & Walker, 1996; Mrug et al., 2001). Crucially, research suggests that having a friend reduces a child's relative risk for negative outcomes in adolescence, even if the child remains unpopular in the larger peer group (Bagwell, Newcomb, & Bukowski, 1998). Hoza, Mrug, and Pelham (2003) conducted a pilot intervention that paired children with ADHD together as "buddies," noting that the children involved appeared to develop friendships; however, the intervention's effectiveness was not evaluated relative to a control group. Frankel et al. (1997) reported that children both with and without ADHD benefited equally from a friendship intervention. However, results were assessed using parent and teacher ratings, not peer sociometrics or observational measures. In sum, interventions focused on building friendships appear promising for ADHD populations; yet further study is needed.

A second avenue involves interventions for peer rejection that change the attitudes or behaviors of accepted peers in the dominant peer group, in addition to or instead of changing the rejected child's behaviors. The prevailing conceptualization of peer rejection as resulting from social skills deficits inside the rejected child ignores the importance of social context in encouraging the display of skillful behavior (Mikami, Boucher, & Humphreys, 2005; Mikami & Pfiffner, 2006). Children with ADHD may appear more socially skilled, for example, with friendly peers or in peer group contexts that are highly structured, which could explain the low cross-situational correspondence on child behavior ratings across settings (Achenbach et al., 1987). As discussed above in the section about social dysfunction, accepted peers have been demonstrated to hold prejudices against youth with ADHD, and these biases impede social relationships. A useful intervention might encourage classroom peers to be more tolerant of children with ADHD, which is an understudied technique (Bierman, 1989, 2004).

A promising strategy involves using cooperative learning instructional strategies in the classroom, such that children must work together to achieve common goals (Bierman & Furman, 1984; Cohen & Lotan, 1995; Mikami et al., 2005). This process is parallel to that documented in social psychology literature in which cooperative learning, but not contact alone, fosters positive interpersonal relationships between the dominant majority group and ethnic minority individuals (Aronson & Patnoe, 1997). A recent meta-analysis corroborated this effect, demonstrating that cooperative goal structures were associated with positive social relationships among group members (Roseth, Johnson, & Johnson, 2008). Social competence classroom curricula that provide instruction to all peers uniformly about the importance of cooperation and respect also carry promise for changing accepted peers' biases against children with ADHD (e.g., Conduct Problems Prevention Research Group, 1999; Greenberg & Kusche, 2006).

Summary

Peer relationship problems appear to be the most treatment-resistant domain of impairment in ADHD. Existing medication and behavioral treatments that reduce ADHD symptoms have overall shown disappointing results at normalizing peer status, particularly when assessed by sociometric nomination measures. Social skills training approaches have been limited in reducing peer rejection among children with ADHD with regard to generalization outside of the treatment setting and after completion of treatment. In the next and final section, we further speculate about why intervening in social problems may be so difficult with this population and how the effectiveness of interventions might be increased.

Current Status and Future Directions

It has been well established that youth with ADHD, as a group, have considerable peer relationship problems as assessed via a wide variety of measures. Yet as a field we need to progress further to understand, on a molecular and sequential level, what exactly are the behaviors performed by children with ADHD that are so off-putting to peers. We need to consider the affect associated with these social behaviors, their timing, and the way they unfold in order. Indeed, what is considered a socially skilled behavior depends on a large number of contextual subtleties unique to that specific situation. For instance, in order to competently make eye contact and introduce oneself (a skill commonly taught in social skills training), the actual behaviors and affect vary significantly depending on how formal the context is, what has just occurred in the setting, and what the individual's status is in the particular group. To find the appropriate time to make the introduction, to

assess the verbal and nonverbal behaviors of the group that indicate responsiveness, and to correctly modulate one's own behaviors and emotions in the interaction all require multiple levels of consideration and decision-making. Research that breaks down these complex levels in social interactions will help investigators better understand the nature of the social dysfunction in ADHD, as it is clear that core ADHD symptoms alone do not fully account for the problems faced by this population.

Relatedly, a promising future direction involves examining the social context in which peer rejection occurs, and how accepted peers' behaviors may influence the development of social dysfunction in ADHD. Given the stigma associated with an ADHD diagnosis, and evidence that the social ostracism experienced by this population is furthered by the negative expectations accepted peers develop about children with ADHD, it is critical to determine the role that peers play, relative to the role that the child's behaviors play, in the child's rejection. A vicious cycle likely occurs for many youth in which the child's negative behaviors evoke peer dislike, which in turn further encourages an increase in the rejected child's dysfunctional behavior. Future research can better determine the respective influences of social context versus the child's behaviors by using a methodology of repeatedly placing the same child in different peer groups to investigate the cross-situational correspondence of sociometric status.

The findings yielded by these research advances may prove useful in furthering the treatment of social problems in this population. A better and more nuanced understanding of the sequence of behaviors required for social competence, as well as knowledge about where children with ADHD falter, may provide better direction for social skills training interventions. It may be that the skills being taught in social skills training are not actually the ones that most matter to peers in determining who they like and dislike. Alternatively, it may be that the skills taught are important but are only a subset of the true skills required for social acceptance. For instance, perhaps there are emotional and nonverbal components that go along with the skills that rejected youth with ADHD are failing to master. Directly incorporating these components into instruction and behavioral practice may improve treatment effectiveness. It is also becoming increasingly apparent that investigating the ways in which socially competent (or incompetent) molecular behaviors vary by sex, ADHD subtype, and comorbidity will be key to designing more individualized and effective social skills treatments.

In addition, a comprehensive model including the contribution of social context to rejection generates more options for interventions targeting accepted peers. For instance, helping accepted peers to be more tolerant of children who are behaviorally deviant and to break down negative stereotypes associated with the label of ADHD are essentially untapped targets for intervention in the current literature. Such approaches also have more potential to produce generalization of treatment effects, because they change the group environment in which the child regularly spends time. This type of contextual model further suggests that whereas some children may have social skills deficits in need of remediation, others may simply be in a poor social context; still other children may have both problems. Distinguishing between these populations may allow for treatments to be tailored more carefully towards individuals.

Considerable evidence suggests that increasing social competence leads to better future adjustment among youth with ADHD, making peer relationship dysfunction a problem with high public health significance. Overall, we hope we have clarified the nature of the social difficulties faced by many youth with ADHD, outlined some of the strategies currently in use for remediation of these difficulties, and provided some direction for the next generation of studies designed to improve treatment effectiveness. Although there is certainly a long way to go, the advances in this topic will be exciting to behold, with far-reaching implications for conceptual models and treatment of peer rejection in psychopathology beyond ADHD.

References

Achenbach, T. M. (1991a). *Manual for child behavior checklist and revised child behavior profile*. Burlington, VT: University Associates in Psychiatry.

Achenbach, T. M. (1991b). *Manual for teacher's report form and 1991 profile*. Burlington, VT: University Associates in Psychiatry.

Achenbach, T. M., McConaughy, S. H., & Howell, C. T. (1987). Child/adolescent behavioral and emotional problems: Implications of cross-informant correlations for situational specificity. *Psychological Bulletin, 101,* 213–232.

Alberts-Corush, J., Firestone, P., & Goodman, J. T. (1986). Attention and impulsivity characteristics of the biological and adoptive parents of hyperactive and normal control children. *American Journal of Orthopsychiatry, 56,* 413–423.

Allen, J. P., Porter, M. R., & McFarland, F. C. (2006). Leaders and followers in adolescent close friendships: Susceptibility to peer influence as a predictor of risky behavior, friendship instability, and depression. *Development and Psychopathology, 18,* 155–172.

Allen, J. P., Porter, M. R., McFarland, F. C., Marsh, P., & McElhaney, K. B. (2005). The two faces of adolescents' success with peers: Adolescent popularity, social adaptation, and deviant behavior. *Child Development, 76,* 747–760.

American Psychiatric Association. (1980). *Diagnostic and statistical manual of mental disorders* (3rd ed.). Washington, DC: American Psychiatric Association.

American Psychiatric Association. (1987). *Diagnostic and statistical manual of mental disorders* (3rd rev. ed.). Washington, DC: American Psychiatric Association.

American Psychiatric Association. (2000). *Diagnostic and statistical manual of mental disorders* (4th ed. text rev.). Washington, DC: Author.

Antshel, K. M., & Remer, R. (2003). Social skills training in children with Attention Deficit Hyperactivity Disorder: A randomized-controlled clinical trial. *Journal of Clinical Child and Adolescent Psychology, 32,* 153–165.

Aronson, E., & Patnoe, S. (1997). *The Jigsaw classroom* (2nd ed.). New York: Longman.

Asarnow, J. R. (1988). Peer status and social competence in child psychiatric inpatients: A comparison of children with depressive, externalizing, and concurrent depressive and externalizing disorders. *Journal of Abnormal Child Psychology, 16,* 151–162.

Asher, S. R., Parker, J. G., & Walker, D. L. (1996). Distinguishing friendship from acceptance: Implications for intervention and assessment. In W. M. Bukowski & A. F. Newcomb (Eds.), *The company they keep: Friendship in childhood and adolescence* (pp. 366–405). New York: Cambridge University Press.

Atkins, M. S., & Stoff, D. M. (1993). Instrumental and hostile aggression in childhood disruptive behavior disorders. *Journal of Abnormal Child Psychology, 21,* 165–178.

Bagwell, C., Molina, B. S. G., Pelham, W. E., & Hoza, B. (2001). Attention-deficit hyperactivity disorder and problems in peer relations: Predictions from childhood to adolescence. *Journal of the American Academy of Child and Adolescent Psychiatry, 40,* 1285–1292.

Bagwell, C., Newcomb, A. F., & Bukowski, W. M. (1998). Preadolescent friendship and peer rejection as predictors of adult adjustment. *Child Development, 69,* 140–153.

Bailly, L. (2005). Stimulant medication for the treatment of attention-deficit hyperactivity disorder: Evidence-b(i)ased practice? *Psychiatric Bulletin, 29,* 284–287.

Barbaresi, W. J., Katusic, S. K., Colligan, R. C., Weaver, A. L., Leibson, C. L., & Jacobsen, S. J. (2006). Long-term stimulant medication treatment of attention-deficit/ hyperactivity disorder: Results from a population-based study. *Journal of Developmental and Behavioral Pediatrics, 27,* 1–10.

Barkley, R. A. (1989). Attention deficit-hyperactivity disorder. In E. J. Mash & R. A. Barkley (Eds.), *Treatment of childhood disorders* (pp. 39–72). New York: Plenum Press.

Barkley, R. A. (1997). *ADHD and the nature of self-control.* New York: Guilford.

Barkley, R. A. (1998). *Attention deficit hyperactivity disorder: A handbook for diagnosis and treatment* (2nd ed.). New York: Guilford Press.

Barkley, R. A. (2002). ADHD: Long-term course, adult outcome, and comorbid disorders. In P. S. Jensen & J. R. Cooper (Eds.), *Attention-deficit/hyperactivity disorder: State of the science and best practices* (pp. 4–1–4–12). Kingston, NJ: Civic Research Institute.

Barkley, R. A. (2003). Attention-deficit/hyperactivity disorder. In E. J. Mash & R. A. Barkley (Eds.), *Child psychopathology* (2nd ed., pp. 75–143). New York: Guilford Press.

Barkley, R. A., DuPaul, G. J., & McMurray, M. B. (1990). Comprehensive evaluation of attention deficit disorder with and without hyperactivity as defined by research criteria. *Journal of Consulting & Clinical Psychology, 58,* 775–789.

Barkley, R. A., Fischer, M., Smallish, L., & Fletcher, K. (2002). The persistence of attention-deficit/hyperactivity disorder into young adulthood as a function of reporting source and definition of disorder. *Journal of Abnormal Psychology, 111,* 279–289.

Bateman, B., Warner, J. O., Hutchinson, E., Dean, T., Rowlandson, P., Gant, C., et al. (2004). The effects of a double blind, placebo controlled, artificial food colourings and benzoate preservative challenge on hyperactivity in a general population sample of preschool children. *Archives of Disease in Childhood, 89,* 506–511.

Beelman, A., Pfingsten, U., & Losel, F. (1994). Effects of training social competence in children: A meta-analysis of recent evaluation studies. *Journal of Clinical Child Psychology, 23,* 260–271.

Benjamin, J., Li, L., Patterson, C., Greenberg, B. D., Murphy, D. L., & Hamer, D. H. (1996). Population and familial association between the D4 dopamine receptor gene and measures of Novelty Seeking. *Nature Genetics, 12,* 81–84.

Biederman, J., Faraone, S. V., Mick, E., Williamson, S., Wilens, T. E., Spencer, T. J., et al. (1999). Clinical correlates of ADHD in females: Findings from a large group of girls ascertained from pediatric and psychiatric referral sources. *Journal of the American Academy of Child and Adolescent Psychiatry, 38,* 966–975.

Bierman, K. L. (1989). Improving the peer relationships of rejected children. In B. B. Lahey & A. E. Kadzin (Eds.), *Advances in Clinical Child Psychology* (pp. 53–84). New York: Plenum Press.

Bierman, K. L. (2004). *Peer rejection: Developmental processes and intervention strategies.* New York: Guilford Press.

Bierman, K. L., & Furman, W. (1984). The effects of social skills training and peer involvement on the social adjustment of preadolescents. *Child Development, 55,* 151–162.

Bierman, K. L., & Welsh, J. A. (2000). Assessing social dysfunction: The contributions of laboratory and performance-based measures. *Journal of Clinical Child Psychology, 29,* 526–539.

Bird, H. R. (2002). The diagnostic classification, epidemiology and cross-cultural validity of ADHD. In P. S. Jensen & J. Cooper (Eds.), *Attention deficit hyperactivity disorder: State of the science: Best practices* (pp. 2-1–2-16). Kingston, NJ: Civic Research Institute.

Blachman, D. R., & Hinshaw, S. P. (2002). Patterns of friendship among girls with and without attention-deficit/ hyperactivity disorder. *Journal of Abnormal Child Psychology, 30,* 625–640.

Boakes, J., Chapman, E., Houghton, S., & West, J. (2008). Facial affect interpretation in boys with attention deficit/ hyperactivity disorder. *Child Neuropsychology, 14*(1), 82–96.

Boivin, M., Hymel, S., & Burkowski, W. M. (1995). The roles of social withdrawal, peer rejection, and victimization by peers in predicting loneliness and depressed mood in childhood. *Development & Psychopathology, 7,* 765–785.

Braaten, E. B., & Rosen, L. A. (2000). Self-regulation of affect in attention deficit-hyperactivity disorder (ADHD) and non-ADHD boys: Differences in empathic responding. *Journal of Consulting and Clinical Psychology, 68,* 313–321.

Breslau, N., & Chilcoat, H. D. (2000). Psychiatric sequelae of low birth weight at 11 years of age. *Biological Psychiatry, 47,* 1005–1011.

Brookes, K., Xu, X., Chen, W., Zhou, K., Neale, B., Lowe, N., et al. (2006). The analysis of 51 genes in DSM-IV combined type attention deficit hyperactivity disorder: Association signals in DRD4, DAT1 and 16 other genes. *Molecular Psychiatry, 11,* 934–953.

Cadesky, E. B., Mota, V. L., & Schachar, R. J. (2000). Beyond words: How do problem children with ADHD and/or conduct problems process nonverbal information about affect? *Journal of the American Academy of Child & Adolescent Psychiatry, 39*(9), 1160–1167.

Canu, W. H., & Carlson, C. L. (2003). Differences in heterosocial behavior and outcomes of ADHD-symptomatic subtypes in a college sample. *Journal of Attention Disorders, 6,* 123–133.

Canu, W. H., Newman, M. L., Morrow, T. L., & Pope, D. L. W. (2008). Social appraisal of adult ADHD: Stigma and influences of the beholder's Big Five personality traits *Journal of Attention Disorders, 11,* 700–710.

Carlson, C. L., & Mann, M. (2000). Attention-deficit/hyperactivity disorder, predominantly inattentive subtype. *Child and Adolescent Psychiatric Clinics of North America, 9,* 499–510.

Carlson, C. L., & Mann, M. (2002). Sluggish cognitive tempo predicts a different pattern of impairment in the attention deficit hyperactivity disorder, predominantly inattentive type. *Journal of Clinical Child and Adolescent Psychology, 31,* 123–129.

Carlson, C. L., Tamm, L., & Gaub, M. (1997). Gender differences in children with ADHD, ODD,and co-occurring ADHD/ODD identified in a school population. *Journal of the American Academy of Child and Adolescent Psychiatry, 36*, 1706–1714.

Chang, L. (2003). Variable effects of children's aggression, social withdrawal, and prosocial leadership as functions of teacher beliefs and behaviors. *Child Development, 74*, 535–548.

Chang, L. (2004). The role of classroom norms in contextualizing the relations of children's social behaviors to peer acceptance. *Developmental Psychology, 40*, 691–702.

Chi, T. C., & Hinshaw, S. P. (2002). Mother-child relationships of children with ADHD: The role of maternal depressive symptoms and depression-related distortions. *Journal of Abnormal Child Psychology, 30*, 387–400.

Christakis, D. A., Zimmerman, F. J., DiGiuseppe, D. L., & McCarty, C. A. (2004). Early television exposure and subsequent attentional problems in children. *Pediatrics, 113*, 708–713.

Chronis, A. M., Jones, H. A., & Raggi, V. L. (2006). Evidence-based psychosocial treatments for children and adolescents with attention-deficit/hyperactivity disorder. *Clinical Psychology Review, 26*, 486–502.

Coghill, D. (2005). Attention-deficit hyperactivity disorder: Should we believe the mass media or peer-reviewed literature? *Psychiatric Bulletin, 29*, 288–291.

Cohen, E. G., & Lotan, R. A. (1995). Producing equal-status interaction in the heterogeneous classroom. *American Education Research Journal, 32*, 99–120.

Cohen, J. (1988). *Statistical power analysis for the behavioral sciences* (2nd ed.). Hillsdale, NJ: Lawrence Earlbaum Associates.

Coie, J. D., Dodge, K. A., & Coppotelli, H. (1982). Dimensions and types of social status: A cross-age perspective. *Developmental Psychology, 18*, 557–570.

Conduct Problems Prevention Research Group. (1999). Initial Impact of the Fast Track Prevention Trial for Conduct Problems II: Classroom Effects. *Journal of Consulting and Clinical Psychology, 67*, 648–657.

Cooper, M. L., Shaver, P. R., & Collins, N. L. (1998). Attachment styles, emotion regulation, and adjustment in adolescence. *Journal of Personality and Social Psychology, 74*, 1380–1397.

Corbett, B., & Glidden, H. (2000). Processing affective stimuli in children with attention-deficit hyperactivity disorder. *Child Neuropsychology, 6*(2), 144–155.

Cornell, D. G., Sheras, P. L., & Cole, J. C. M. (2006). Assessment of bullying. In S. R. Jimerson & M. J. Furlong (Eds.), *The handbook of school violence and school safety* (pp. 191–209). Mahwah, NJ: Lawrence Erlbaum Associates.

Cox, D. J., Merkel, R. L., Moore, M., Thorndike, F., Muller, C., & Kovatchev, B. (2006). Relative benefits of stimulant therapy with OROS methylphenidate versus mixed amphetamine salts extended-release in improving the driving performance of adolescent drivers with ADHD. *Pediatrics, 118*, 704–710.

Crick, N. R., & Dodge, K. A. (1994). A review and reformulation of social information-processing mechanisms in children's social adjustment. *Psychological Bulletin, 115*, 74–101.

Dalsgaard, S., Mortensen, P. B., Frydenberg, M., & Thomsen, P. H. (2002). Conduct problems, gender and adult psychiatric outcome of children with attention-deficit hyperactivity disorder. *British Journal of Psychiatry, 181*, 416–421.

Dishion, T. J. (1990). The peer context of troublesome child and adolescent behavior. In P. E. Leone (Ed.), *Understanding troubled and troubling youth: Multiple perspectives.* Thousand Oaks, CA: Sage.

Dishion, T. J., McCord, J., & Poulin, F. (1999). When interventions harm: Peer groups and problem behavior. *American Psychologist, 54*, 755–764.

Dodge, K. A. (1980). Social cognition and children's aggressive behavior. *Child Development, 51*, 162–170.

Dodge, K. A., & Coie, J. D. (1987). Social-information processing factors in reactive and proactive aggression in children's peer groups. *Journal of Personality & Social Psychology, 53*, 1146–1158.

Dodge, K. A., Lansford, J. E., Burks, V. S., Bates, J. E., Pettit, G. S., Fontaine, R., et al. (2003). Peer rejection and social information-processing factors in the development of aggressive behavior problems in children. *Child Development, 74*, 374–393.

DuPaul, G. J., Schaughency, E. A., Weyandt, L. J., Tripp, G., Kiesner, J., Ota, K., et al. (2001). Self-report of ADHD symptoms in university students: Cross-gender and cross-national prevalence. *Journal of Learning Disabilities, 34*, 370–379.

Ebstein, R. P., Novick, O., Umansky, R., Priel, B., Osher, Y., Blaine, D., et al. (1996). Dopamine D4 receptor (DRD4) exon III polymorphism associated with the human personality trait of Novelty Seeking. *Nature Genetics, 12*, 78–80.

Edelbrock, C. S., Costello, A. J., & Kessler, M. D. (1984). Empirical correlation of the attention deficit disorders. *Journal of the American Academy of Child Psychiatry, 23*, 285–290.

Eigenmann, P. A., & Haenggeli, C. A. (2004). Food colourings and preservatives – allergy and hyperactivity. *The Lancet, 364*, 823–824.

El-Faddagh, M., Laucht, M., Maras, A., Vöhringer, L., & Schmidt, M. H. (2004). Association of dopamine D4 receptor (DRD4) gene with attention-deficit/hyperactivity disorder (ADHD) in a high-risk community sample: A longitudinal study from birth to 11 years of age. *Journal of Neural Transmission, 111*, 883–889.

Eme, R. F. (1992). Selective female affliction in the developmental disorders of childhood: A review. *Journal of Child Clinical Psychology, 21*, 354–364.

Erhardt, D., & Hinshaw, S. P. (1994). Initial sociometric impressions of hyperactive and comparison boys: Predictions from social behaviors and from nonverbal variables. *Journal of Consulting and Clinical Psychology, 62*, 833–842.

Faraone, S. V., Doyle, A. E., Mick, E., & Biederman, J. (2001). Meta-analysis of the association between the 7-repeat allele of the dopamine D4 receptor gene and attention deficit hyperactivity disorder. *American Journal of Psychiatry, 158*, 1052–1057.

Faraone, S. V., Perlis, R. H., Doyle, A. E., Smoller, J. W., Goralnick, J. J., Holmgren, M. A., et al. (2005).

Molecular genetics of attention-deficit/hyperactivity disorder. *Biological Psychiatry, 57*, 1313–1323.

Feingold, B. F. (1975). Hyperkinesis and learning disabilities linked to artificial food flavors and colors. *The American Journal of Nursing, 75*, 797–803.

Flory, K., Milich, R., Lorch, E. P., Hayden, A. N., Strange, C., & Welsh, R. (2006). Online story comprehension among children with ADHD: Which core deficits are involved. *Journal of Abnormal Child Psychology, 34*, 853–864.

Frankel, F., & Myatt, R. (2003). *Children's friendship training*. New York: Brunner-Routledge.

Frankel, F., Myatt, R., Cantwell, D. P., & Feinberg, D. (1997). Parent-assisted transfer of children's social skills training: Effects on children with and without attention-deficit hyperactivity disorder. *Journal of the American Academy of Child and Adolescent Psychiatry, 36*, 1056–1064.

Gadow, K. D., Drabick, D. A. G., Loney, J., Sprafkin, J., Salisbury, H., Azizian, A., et al. (2004). Comparison of ADHD symptom subtypes as source-specific syndromes. *Journal of Child Psychology & Psychiatry, 45*, 1135–1149.

Gershon, J. (2002). A meta-analytic review of gender differences in ADHD. *Journal of Attention Disorders, 5*, 143–154.

Goodman, R., & Stevenson, J. (1989). A twin study of hyperactivity – II. The aetiological role of genes, family relationships and perinatal adversity. *Journal of Child Psychology and Psychiatry, 30*, 691–709.

Greenberg, M. T., & Kusche, C. (2006). Building social and emotional competence: The PATHS curriculum. In S. R. Jimerson & M. J. Furlong (Eds.), *Handbook of school violence and school safety* (pp. 395–412). Mahwah, NJ: Lawrence Erlbaum Associates.

Greene, R. W., Biederman, J., Faraone, S. V., Monuteaux, M., Mick, E., DuPre, E. P., et al. (2001). Social impairment in girls with ADHD: Patterns, gender comparisons, and correlates. *Journal of the American Academy of Child and Adolescent Psychiatry, 40*, 704–710.

Greene, R. W., Biederman, J., Faraone, S. V., Sienna, M., & Garcia-Jetton, J. (1997). Adolescent outcome of boys with Attention Deficit Hyperactivity Disorder and social disability: Results from a 4-year longitudinal follow-up study. *Journal of Consulting and Clinical Psychology, 65*, 758–767.

Greenhill, L. L., Abikoff, H. B., Arnold, L. E., Cantwell, D. P., Conners, C. K., Elliott, G., et al. (1996). Medication treatment strategies in the MTA: Relevance to clinicians and researchers. *Journal of the American Academy of Child and Adolescent Psychiatry, 35*, 1304–1313.

Gresham, F. M., & Elliott, S. N. (1990). *Social skills rating system*. Circle Pines, MN: Assistance Service.

Guyer, A. E., McClure, E. B., Adler, A. D., Brotman, M. A., Rich, B. A., Kimes, A. S., et al. (2007). Specificity of facial expression labeling deficits in childhood psychopathology. *Journal of Child Psychology and Psychiatry, 48*(9), 863–871.

Harris, M. J., Milich, R., & McAninch, C. B. (1998). When stigma becomes self-fulfilling prophecy: Expectancy effects and the causes, consequences, and treatment of peer rejection. In J. Brophy (Ed.), *Advances in research on teaching* (pp. 243–272). Greenwich, CT: JAI Press.

Hart, E. L., & Lahey, B. B. (1999). General child behavior ratings. In D. Shaffer, C. P. Lucas, & J. E. Richters (Eds.), *Diagnostic assessment in child and adolescent psychopathology* (pp. 65–90). New York: Guilford Press.

Hart, E. L., Lahey, B. B., Loeber, R., Applegate, B., Green, S. M., & Frick, P. J. (1995). Developmental change in attention-deficit hyperactivity disorder in boys: A four-year longitudinal study. *Journal of Abnormal Child Psychology, 23*, 729–749.

Hartman, C. A., Willcutt, E. G., Rhee, S. H., & Pennington, B. F. (2004). The relation between Sluggish Cognitive Tempo and DSM-IV ADHD. *Journal of Abnormal Child Psychology, 32*, 491–503.

Hinshaw, S. P. (1987). On the distinction between attentional deficits/hyperactivity and conduct problems/aggression in child psychopathology. *Psychological Bulletin, 101*, 443–463.

Hinshaw, S. P. (1992). Academic underachievment, attention deficits, and aggression: Comorbidity and implications for intervention. *Journal of Consulting & Clinical Psychology, 60*, 893–903.

Hinshaw, S. P. (2002a). Preadolescent girls with attention-deficit/hyperactivity disorder: I. Background characteristics, comorbidity, cognitive and social functioning, and parenting practices. *Journal of Consulting and Clinical Psychology, 70*, 1086–1098.

Hinshaw, S. P. (2002b). Process, mechanism, and explanation related to externalizing behavior in developmental psychopathology. *Journal of Abnormal Child Psychology, 30*, 431–446.

Hinshaw, S. P., Henker, B., Whalen, C. K., Erhardt, D., & Dunnington, R. E. (1989). Aggressive, prosocial, and nonsocial behavior in hyperactive boys: Dose effects of methylphenidate in naturalistic settings. *Journal of Consulting and Clinical Psychology, 57*, 636–643.

Hinshaw, S. P., March, J. S., Abikoff, H., Arnold, L. E., Cantwell, D. P., Conners, C. K., et al. (1997). Comprehensive assessment of childhood attention-deficit hyperactivity disorder in the context of a multisite, multimodal clinical trial. *Journal of Attention Disorders, 1*, 217–234.

Hinshaw, S. P., & Melnick, S. M. (1995). Peer relationships in children with attention-deficit hyperactivity disorder with and without comorbid aggression. *Development and Psychopathology, 7*, 627–647.

Hinshaw, S. P., Owens, E. B., Sami, N., & Fargeon, S. (2006). Prospective follow-up of girls with attention-deficit/hyperactivity disorder into adolescence: Evidence for continuing cross-domain impairment. *Journal of Consulting & Clinical Psychology, 74*, 489–499.

Hinshaw, S. P., Owens, E. B., Wells, K. C., Kraemer, H. C., Abikoff, H. B., Arnold, L. E., et al. (2000). Family processes and treatment outcomes in the MTA: Negative/ineffective parenting practices in relation to multimodal treatment. *Journal of Abnormal Child Psychology, 28*, 555–568.

Hinshaw, S. P., Zupan, B. A., Simmel, C., Nigg, J. T., & Melnick, S. (1997). Peer status in boys with and without attention-deficit hyperactivity disorder: Predictions from overt and covert antisocial behavior, social isolation, and authoritative parenting beliefs. *Child Development, 68*, 880–896.

Hodgens, J. B., Cole, J., & Boldizar, J. (2000). Peer-based differences among boys with ADHD. *Journal of Child Clinical Psychology*, *29*, 443–452.

Hoza, B., Gerdes, A. C., Hinshaw, S. P., Arnold, L. E., Pelham, W. E., Molina, B. S. G., et al. (2004). Self-perceptions of competence in children with ADHD and comparison children. *Journal of Consulting & Clinical Psychology*, *72*, 382–391.

Hoza, B., Gerdes, A. C., Mrug, S., Hinshaw, S. P., Bukowski, W. M., Gold, J. A., et al. (2005). Peer-assessed outcomes in the Multimodal Treatment Study of children with Attention Deficit Hyperactivity Disorder. *Journal of Clinical Child and Adolescent Psychology*, *34*, 74–86.

Hoza, B., Mrug, S., Gerdes, A. C., Bukowski, W. M., Kraemer, H. C., Wigal, T., et al. (2005). What aspects of peer relationships are impaired in children with attention-deficit/hyperactivity disorder? *Journal of Consulting & Clinical Psychology*, *73*, 411–423.

Hoza, B., Mrug, S., & Pelham, W. E. (2003). A friendship intervention for children with attention-deficit/hyperactivity disorder: Preliminary findings. *Journal of Attention Disorders*, *6*, 87–98.

Hoza, B., Murray-Close, D., Arnold, L. E., Hinshaw, S. P., & MTA Cooperative Group. (2008). *Time-dependent changes in positive illusory self-perceptions of children with ADHD: A developmental psychopathology perspective*. Unpublished manuscript.

Hoza, B., Waschbusch, D. A., Pelham, W. E., Molina, B. S. G., & Milich, R. (2000). Attention-deficit/hyperactivity disordered and control boys' responses to social success and failure. *Child Development*, *71*, 432–446.

Hubbard, J. A., & Newcomb, A. F. (1991). Initial dyadic peer interaction of attention deficit-hyperactivity disorder and normal boys. *Journal of Abnormal Child Psychology*, *19*, 179–195.

Hultman, C. M., Torrång, A., Tuvblad, C., Cnattingius, S., Larsson, J. O., & Lichtenstein, P. (2007). Birth weight and attention-deficit/hyperactivity symptoms in childhood and early adolescence: A prospective Swedish twin study. *Journal of the American Academy of Child and Adolescent Psychiatry*, *46*, 370–377.

Hymel, S., Bowker, A., & Woody, E. (1993). Aggressive versus withdrawn unpopular children: Variations in peer and self-perceptions in multiple domains. *Child Development*, *64*, 879–896.

Jensen, P. S., Arnold, L. E., Swanson, J. M., Vitiello, B., Abikoff, H. B., Greenhill, L. L., et al. (2007). 3-year follow-up of the NIMH MTA study. *Journal of the American Academy of Child and Adolescent Psychiatry*, *46*, 989–1002.

Jensen, P. S., Hinshaw, S. P., Kraemer, H. C., Lenora, N., Newcorn, J. H., Abikoff, H. B., et al. (2001). ADHD comorbidity findings from the MTA study: Comparing comorbid subgroups. *Journal of the American Academy of Child and Adolescent Psychiatry*, *20*, 147–158.

Jensen, P. S., Martin, D., & Cantwell, D. P. (1997). Comorbidity in ADHD: Implications for research, practice, and DSM-V. *Journal of the American Academy of Child and Adolescent Psychiatry*, *36*, 1065–1079.

Jensen, P. S., Watanabe, H. K., Richters, J. E., Cortes, R., Roper, M., & Liu, S. (1995). Prevalence of mental disorder in military children and adolescents: A two-stage community survey. *Journal of the American Academy of Child and Adolescent Psychiatry*, *34*, 1514–1524.

Johnston, C., & Mash, E. J. (2001). Families of children with attention-deficit/hyperactivity disorder: Review and recommendations for future research. *Clinical Child and Family Psychology Review*, *4*, 183–207.

Johnston, C., Pelham, W. E., & Murphy, H. A. (1985). Peer relationships in ADDH and normal children: A developmental analysis of peer and teacher ratings. *Journal of Abnormal Child Psychology*, *13*, 89–100.

Kao, G., & Joyner, K. (2004). Do race and ethnicity matter among friends? Activities among interracial, interethnic, and intraethnic adolescent friends. *Sociological Quarterly*, *45*, 557–573.

Kats-Gold, I., Besser, A., & Priel, B. (2007). The role of simple emotion recognition skills among school aged boys at risk of ADHD. *Journal of Abnormal Child Psychology*, *35*(3), 363–378.

Kempes, M., Matthys, W., de Vries, H., & van Engeland, H. (2005). Reactive and proactive aggression in children: A review of theory, findings and the relevance for child and adolescent psychiatry. *European Journal of Child and Adolescent Psychiatry*, *14*, 11–19.

Klein, R. G., & Abikoff, H. (1997). Behavior therapy and methylphenidate in the treatment of children with ADHD. *Journal of Attention Disorders*, *2*, 89–114.

Kraemer, H. C., & Jacklin, C. N. (1979). Statistical analysis of dyadic social behavior. *Psychological Bulletin*, *82*, 217–224.

Ladd, G. W. (1985). Documenting the effects of social skills training with children. In B. H. Schneider, K. H. Rubin, & J. E. Ledingham (Eds.), *Children's peer relations: Issues in assessment and intervention* (pp. 243–269). New York: Springer-Verlag.

Ladd, G. W., & Mize, J. (1982). Social skills training and assessment with children: A cognitive-social learning approach. *Child and Youth Services*, *5*, 61–74.

Lahey, B. B., Applegate, B., McBurnett, K., Biederman, J., Greenhill, L. L., Hynd, G. W., et al. (1994). DSM-IV field trials for attention deficit/hyperactivity disorder in children and adolescents. *American Journal of Psychiatry*, *151*, 1673–1685.

Lahey, B. B., Miller, T. L., Gordon, R. A., & Riley, A. W. (1999). Developmental epidimiology of the disruptive behavior disorders. In H. C. Quay & A. E. Hogan (Eds.), *Handbook of disruptive behavior disorders* (pp. 23–48). New York: Kluwer Academic/Plenum.

Lahey, B. B., Pelham, W. E., Stein, M. A., Loney, J., Trapani, C., Nugent, K., et al. (1998). Validity of DSM-IV attention-deficit/hyperactivity disorder for younger children. *Journal of the American Academy of Child and Adolescent Psychiatry*, *37*, 695–702.

LaHoste, G. J., Swanson, J. M., Wigal, S. B., Glabe, C., Wigal, T., King, N., et al. (1996). Dopamine D4 receptor gene polymorphism is associated with attention deficit hyperactivity disorder. *Molecular Psychiatry*, *1*, 121–124.

Landau, S. L., Milich, R., & Diener, M. B. (1998). Peer relations of children with attention-deficit hyperactivity disorder. *Reading and Writing Quarterly*, *14*, 83–105.

Landau, S. L., & Moore, L. A. (1991). Social skills deficits in children with attention-deficit hyperactivity disorder. *School Psychology Review, 20*, 235–251.

Langley, K., Fowler, T., Grady, D. L., Moyzis, R. K., Holmans, P. A., van den Bree, M. B. B., et al. (2008). Molecular genetic contribution to the developmental course of attention-deficit hyperactivity disorder. *European Child and Adolescent Psychiatry*.

Lansford, J. E., Malone, P., Dodge, K. A., Crozier, J. C., Pettit, G. S., & Bates, J. E. (2006). A 12-year prospective study of patterns of social information processing problems and externalizing behaviors. *Journal of Abnormal Child Psychology, 34*, 709–718.

Laucht, M., Skowronek, M. H., Becker, K., Schmidt, M. H., Esser, G., Schulze, T. G., et al. (2007). Interacting effects of the dopamine transporter gene and psychosocial adversity on attention-deficit/hyperactivity disorder symptoms among 15-year-olds from a high-risk community sample. *Archives of General Psychiatry, 64*, 585–590.

Loeber, R., Green, S. M., Lahey, B. B., & Stouthamer-Loeber, M. (1991). Difference and similarities between children, mothers, and teachers as informants on disruptive child behavior. *Journal of Abnormal Child Psychology, 19*, 75–95.

Lorch, E. P., Milich, R., Astrin, C. C., & Berthiaume, K. S. (2006). Cognitive engagement and story comprehension in typically developing children and children with ADHD from preschool to elementary school. *Developmental Psychology, 42*, 1206–1219.

M.T.A. Cooperative Group. (1999a). A 14-month randomized clinical trial of treatment strategies for attention-deficit/hyperactivity disorder. *Archives of General Psychiatry, 56*, 1073–1086.

M.T.A. Cooperative Group. (1999b). Moderators and mediators of treatment response for children with attention-deficit/hyperactivity disorder, *Archives of General Psychiatry, 56*, 1088–1096.

M.T.A. Cooperative Group. (2004). The NIMH MTA follow-up: 24-month outcomes of treatment strategies for attention-deficit/hyperactivity disorder (ADHD). *Pediatrics, 113*, 754–761.

Maccoby, E. E. (1998). *The two sexes: Growing up apart, coming together*. Cambridge, MA: Harvard University Press.

Madras, B. K., Miller, G. M., & Fischman, A. J. (2005). The dopamine transporter and attention-deficit/hyperactivity disorder. *Biological Psychiatry, 57*, 1397–1409.

Maedgen, J. W., & Carlson, C. L. (2000). Social functioning and emotional regulation in the attention deficit hyperactivity disorder subtypes. *Journal of Clinical Child Psychology, 29*, 30–42.

Mannuzza, S., & Klein, R. G. (2000). Long term prognosis in attention-deficit/hyperactivity disorder. *Child and Adolescent Psychiatric Clinics of North America, 9*, 711–726.

Marshal, M. P., Molina, B. S. G., & Pelham, W. E. (2003). Childhood ADHD and adolescent substance use: An examination of deviant peer group affiliation as a risk factor. *Psychology of Addictive Behaviors, 17*, 293–302.

Martin, J. K., Pescosolido, B. A., Olafsdottir, S., & McLeod, J. D. (2007). The construction of fear: Americans' preferences for social distance from children and adolescents with mental health problems. *Journal of Health and Social Behavior, 48*, 50–67.

Matthys, W., Cuperus, J. M., & van England, H. (1999). Deficient social problem-solving in boys with ODD/CD, with ADHD, and with both disorders. *Journal of the American Academy of Child and Adolescent Psychiatry, 38*, 311–321.

McBurnett, K., Pfiffner, L. J., & Frick, P. J. (2001). Symptom properties as a function of ADHD type: An argument for continued study of sluggish cognitive tempo. *Journal of Abnormal Child Psychology, 29*, 207–213.

McElwain, N. L., & Volling, B. L. (2002). Relating individual control, social understanding, and gender to child-friend interaction: A relationships perspective. *Social Development, 11*, 362–385.

Mehmet-Radji, O. (2004). Review of "Early television exposure and subsequent attentional problems in children". *Child: Care, Health and Development, 30*, 559–560.

Melnick, S. M., & Hinshaw, S. P. (1996). What they want and what they get: The social goals of boys with ADHD and comparison boys. *Journal of Abnormal Child Psychology, 24*, 169–185.

Melnick, S. M., & Hinshaw, S. P. (2000). Emotion regulation and parenting in AD/HD and comparison boys: Linkages with social behaviors and peer preference. *Journal of Abnormal Child Psychology, 28*, 73–86.

Mick, E., Biederman, J., Prince, J., Fischer, M. J., & Faraone, S. V. (2002). Impact of low birth weight on attention-deficit hyperactivity disorder. *Journal of Developmental and Behavioral Pediatrics, 23*, 16–22.

Mikami, A. Y., Boucher, M. A., & Humphreys, K. (2005). Prevention of peer rejection through a classroom-level intervention in middle school. *Journal of Primary Prevention, 26*, 5–23.

Mikami, A. Y., Chi, T. C., & Hinshaw, S. P. (2004). Behavior ratings and observations of externalizing symptoms in girls: The role of child popularity with adults. *Journal of Psychopathology and Behavioral Assessment, 26*, 151–164.

Mikami, A. Y., & Hinshaw, S. P. (2003). Buffers of peer rejection among girls with and without ADHD: The role of popularity with adults and goal-directed solitary play. *Journal of Abnormal Child Psychology, 31*, 381–397.

Mikami, A. Y., & Hinshaw, S. P. (2006). Resilient adolescent adjustment among girls: Buffers of childhood peer rejection and attention-deficit/hyperactivity disorder. *Journal of Abnormal Child Psychology, 26*, 823–837.

Mikami, A. Y., & Hinshaw, S. P. (2008). Attention-deficit/hyperactivity disorder in girls. In K. McBurnett & L. J. Pfiffner (Eds.), *Attention deficit/hyperactivity disorder: Concepts, controversies, new directions* (pp. 259–272). New York: Informa Healthcare.

Mikami, A. Y., Hinshaw, S. P., Patterson, K. A., & Lee, J. C. (2008). Eating pathology among adolescent girls with Attention-deficit/hyperactivity disorder. *Journal of Abnormal Psychology, 117*, 225–235.

Mikami, A. Y., Huang-Pollock, C. L., Pfiffner, L. J., McBurnett, K., & Hangai, D. (2007). Social skills differences among Attention-deficit/hyperactivity disorder subtypes in a chat room assessment task. *Journal of Abnormal Child Psychology, 35*, 509–521.

Mikami, A. Y., Lee, S. S., Hinshaw, S. P., & Mullin, B. C. (2008). Relationships between social information processing and aggression among adolescent girls with and without ADHD. *Journal of Youth and Adolescence, 37*, 761–771.

Mikami, A. Y., & Pfiffner, L. J. (2006). Social skills training for youth with disruptive behavior disorders: A review of best practices. *Emotional and Behavioral Disorders in Youth, 6*, 3–23.

Mikami, A. Y., & Pfiffner, L. J. (2007). Sibling relationships among children with Attention-deficit/hyperactivity disorder. *Journal of Attention Disorders, 11*, 1–11.

Milberger, S., Biederman, J., Faraone, S. V., & Jones, J. (1998). Further evidence of an association between maternal smoking during pregnancy and attention deficit hyperactivity disorder: Findings from a high-risk sample of siblings. *Journal of Clinical Child Psychology, 27*, 352–358.

Milch-Reich, S., Campbell, S. B., Pelham, W. E., Connelly, L. M., & Geva, D. (1999). Developmental and individual differences in children's on-line representations of dynamic social events. *Child Development, 70*, 413–431.

Milich, R., Balentine, A., & Lynam, D. (2001). ADHD combined type and ADHD predominantly inattentive type are distinct and unrelated disorders. *Clinical Psychology: Science and Practice, 8*, 463–488.

Milich, R., & Landau, S. L. (1982). Socialization and peer relations in hyperactive children. In K. D. Gadow & I. Bialer (Eds.), *Advances in learning and behavioral disabilities* (Vol. 1, pp. 283–339). Greenwich, CT: JAI.

Moote, G. T., Smith, N. J., & Wodarski, J. S. (1999). Social skills training with youth in school settings: A review. *Research on Social Work Practice, 9*, 427–465.

Mrug, S., Hoza, B., & Gerdes, A. C. (2001). Children with attention-deficit/hyperactivity disorder: Peer relationships and peer-oriented interventions. In D. W. Nangle & C. A. Erdley (Eds.), *The role of friendship in psychological adjustment. New directions for child and adolescent development.* San Francisco: Jossey-Bass/Pfeiffer.

Murphy, D. A., Pelham, W. E., & Lang, A. R. (1992). Aggression in boys with attention-deficit/hyperactivity disorder: Methylphenidate effects on naturalistically observed aggression, provocation, and social information processing. *Journal of Abnormal Child Psychology, 20*, 451–466.

Nigg, J. T., & Breslau, N. (2007). Prenatal smoking exposure, low birth weight, and disruptive behavior disorders. *Journal of the American Academy of Child and Adolescent Psychiatry, 46*, 362–369.

Nixon, E. (2001). The social competence of children with Attention Deficit Hyperactivity Disorder: A review of the literature. *Child Psychology and Psychiatry Review, 6*, 172–180.

Ohan, J. L., & Johnston, C. (2007). What is the social impact of ADHD in girls? A multi-method assessment. *Journal of Abnormal Child Psychology, 35*, 239–250.

Olweus, D. (1992). Bullying among schoolchildren: Intervention and prevention. In R. D. Peters, R. J. McMahon, & V. L. Quinsey (Eds.), *Aggression and violence throughout the life span* (pp. 100–125). Thousand Oaks: Sage Publications.

Parker, J. G., & Asher, S. R. (1987). Peer relations and later personal adjustment: Are low-accepted children at risk? *Psychological Bulletin, 102*, 357–389.

Parker, J. G., & Asher, S. R. (1993). Friendship and friendship quality in middle childhood: Links with peer group acceptance and feelings of loneliness and social dissatisfaction. *Developmental Psychology, 29*, 611–621.

Parker, J. G., Rubin, K. H., Price, J. M., & DeRosier, M. E. (1995). Peer relationships, child development, and adjustment: A developmental psychopathology perspective. In D. Cicchetti & D. J. Cohen (Eds.), *Developmental psychopathology, Vol. 2: Risk, disorder, and adaptation* (pp. 96–161). New York: John Wiley & Sons.

Pelham, W. E., & Bender, M. E. (1982). Peer relationships in hyperactive children: Description and treatment. In K. D. Gadow & I. Bailer (Eds.), *Advances in learning and behavioral disabilities* (Vol. 1, pp. 365–436). Greenwich, CT: JAI Press.

Pelham, W. E., & Hoza, B. (1996). Intensive treatment: A summer treatment program for children with ADHD. In E. Hibbs & P. S. Jensen (Eds.), *Psychosocial treatments for child and adolescent disorders: Empirically based strategies for clinical practice* (pp. 311–340). New York: APA Press.

Pelham, W. E., Wheeler, T., & Chronis, A. M. (1998). Empirically supported psychosocial treatments for attention deficit hyperactivity disorder. *Journal of Child Clinical Psychology, 27*, 190–205.

Peris, T. S., & Hinshaw, S. P. (2003). Family dynamics and preadolescent girls with ADHD: The relationship between expressed emotion, ADHD symptomatology, and comorbid disruptive behavior. *Journal of Child Psychology & Psychiatry, 44*, 1177–1190.

Pfiffner, L. J. (2003). Psychosocial treatment for ADHD-Inattentive Type. *The ADHD Report, 11*, 1–8.

Pfiffner, L. J., Calzada, E., & McBurnett, K. (2000). Interventions to enhance social competence. *Child and Adolescent Psychiatric Clinics of North America, 9*, 689–709.

Pfiffner, L. J., & McBurnett, K. (1997). Social skills training with parent generalization: Treatment effects for children with attention deficit disorder. *Journal of Consulting & Clinical Psychology, 65*, 749–757.

Pfiffner, L. J., Mikami, A. Y., Huang-Pollock, C. L., Easterlin, B., Zalecki, C. A., & McBurnett, K. (2007). A randomized controlled trial of integrated home-school behavioral treatment for ADHD, Predominantly Inattentive Type. *Journal of the American Academy of Child and Adolescent Psychiatry, 46*, 1041–1050.

Polanczyk, G., de Lima, M. S., Horta, B. L., Biederman, J., & Rohde, L. A. (2007). The worldwide prevalence of ADHD: A systematic review and metaregression analysis. *American Journal of Psychiatry, 164*, 942–948.

Power, T. J., Costigan, T. E., Eiraldi, R. B., & Leff, S. S. (2004). Variations in anxiety and depression as a function of ADHD subtypes defined by DSM-IV: Do subtype differences exist or not? *Journal of Abnormal Child Psychology, 32*, 27–37.

Price, T. S. (2001). Hyperactivity in preschool children is highly heritable. *Journal of the American Academy of Child and Adolescent Psychiatry, 40*, 1362–1364.

Quinn, P. Q. (2005). Treating adolescent girls and women with ADHD: Gender-specific issues. *Journal of Clinical Psychology*, *61*, 579–587.

Robison, L. M., Sclar, D. A., Skaer, T. L., & Galin, R. S. (2004). Treatment modalities among U.S. children diagnosed with attention-deficit hyperactivity disorder: 1995–1999. *International Clinical Psychopharmacology*, *19*, 17–22.

Robison, L. M., Skaer, T. L., Sclar, D. A., & Galin, R. S. (2002). Is attention deficit hyperactivity disorder increasing among girls in the US? Trends in diagnosis and the prescribing of stimulants. *CNS Drugs*, *16*, 129–137.

Roseth, C. J., Johnson, D. W., & Johnson, R. T. (2008). Promoting early adolescents' achievement and peer relationships: The effects of cooperative, competitive, and individualistic goal structures. *Psychological Bulletin*, *134*, 223–246.

Rucklidge, J. J., & Tannock, R. (2001). Psychiatric, psychosocial, and cognitive functioning of female adolescents with ADHD. *Journal of the American Academy of Child and Adolescent Psychiatry*, *40*, 530–540.

Sandstrom, M. J., Cillessen, A. H. N., & Eisenhower, A. (2003). Children's appraisal of peer rejection experiences: Impact on social and emotional adjustment. *Social Development*, *12*, 530–550.

Sherman, D. K., McGue, M. K., & Iacono, W. G. (1997). Twin concordance for attention deficit hyperactivity disorder: A comparison of teachers' and mothers' reports. *American Journal of Psychiatry*, *154*, 532–535.

Singh, S. D., Ellis, C. R., Winton, A. S. W., Singh, N. N., Leung, J. P., & Oswald, D. P. (1998). Recognition of facial expressions of emotion by children with attention-deficit hyperactivity disorder. *Behavior Modification*, *22*, 128–142.

Southam-Gerow, M. A., & Kendall, P. C. (2002). Emotion regulation and understanding: Implications for child psychopathology and therapy. *Clinical Psychology Review*, *22*, 189–222.

Sprich, S., Biederman, J., Crawford, M. H., Mundy, E., & Faraone, S. V. (2000). Adoptive and biological families of children and adolescents with ADHD. *Journal of the American Academy of Child and Adolescent Psychiatry*, *39*, 1432–1437.

Steele, R. G., & Roberts, M. C. (Eds.). (2005). *Handbook of mental health services for children, adolescents, and families*. New York: Kluwer.

Stormont, M. (2001). Social outcomes of children with AD/HD: Contributing factors and implications for practice. *Psychology in the Schools*, *38*, 521–531.

Stormshak, E. A., Bierman, K. L., Bruschi, C., Dodge, K. A., Coie, J. D., & Conduct Problems Prevention Research Group. (1999). The relation between behavior problems and peer preference in different classroom contexts. *Child Development*, *70*, 169–182.

Swanson, J. M., McBurnett, K., Christian, D. L., & Wigal, T. (1995). Stimulant medication and treatment of children with ADHD. In T. H. Ollendick & R. J. Prinz (Eds.), *Advances in clinical child psychology* (Vol. 17, pp. 265–322). New York: Plenum.

Swanson, J. M., Oosterlaan, J., Murias, M., Schuck, S., Flodman, P., Spence, M. A., et al. (2000). Attention deficit/hyperactivity disorder children with a 7-repeat allele of the dopamine receptor D4 gene have extreme behavior but normal performance on critical neuropsychological tests of attention. *Proceedings of the National Academy of Sciences*, *97*, 4754–4759.

Thapar, A., Fowler, T., Rice, F., Scourfield, J., van den Bree, M., Thomas, H., et al. (2003). Maternal smoking during pregnancy and attention deficit hyperactivity disorder symptoms in offspring. *American Journal of Psychiatry*, *160*, 1985–1989.

Thurber, J. R., Heller, T. L., & Hinshaw, S. P. (2002). The social behaviors and peer expectation of girls with attention deficit hyperactivity disorder and comparison girls. *Journal of Clinical Child and Adolescent Psychology*, *31*, 443–452.

Timimi, S., & Taylor, E. (2004). ADHD is best understood as a cultural construct. *British Journal of Psychiatry*, *184*, 8–9.

Walcott, C. M., & Landau, S. L. (2004). The relation between disinhibition and emotion regulation in boys with Attention Deficit Hyperactivity Disorder. *Journal of Clinical Child and Adolescent Psychology*, *33*, 772–782.

Wells, K. C., Pelham, W. E., Kotkin, R. A., Hoza, B., Abikoff, H. B., Abramowitz, A., et al. (2000). Psychosocial treatment strategies in the MTA study: Rationale, methods, and critical issues in design and implementation. *Journal of Abnormal Child Psychology*, *28*, 483–505.

Whalen, C. K., & Henker, B. (1985). The social worlds of hyperactive (ADDH) children. *Clinical Psychology Review*, *5*, 447–478.

Whalen, C. K., & Henker, B. (1992). The social profile of attention-deficit hyperactivity disorder: Five fundamental facets. *Child and Adolescent Psychiatric Clinics of North America*, *1*, 395–410.

Whalen, C. K., Henker, B., Collins, B. E., McAuliffe, S., & Vaux, A. (1979). Peer interaction in a structured communication task: Comparisons of normal and hyperactive boys and of methylphenidate (Ritalin) and placebo effects. *Child Development*, *50*, 388–401.

Whalen, C. K., Henker, B., Dotemoto, S., & Hinshaw, S. P. (1983). Child and adolescent perceptions of normal and atypical peers. *Child Development*, *54*, 1588–1598.

Wheeler, J., & Carlson, C. L. (1994). The social functioning of children with ADD with hyperactivity and ADD without hyperactivity: A comparison of peer relations and social deficits. *Journal of Emotional and Behavioral Disorders*, *2*, 2–12.

Wolraich, M. L., Hannah, J. N., Pinnock, T. Y., Baumgaertel, A., & Brown, J. (1996). Comparison of diagnostic criteria for attention-deficit/hyperactivity disorder in a county-wide sample. *Journal of the American Academy of Child and Adolescent Psychiatry*, *35*, 319–324.

Wolraich, M. L., Wibbelsman, C. J., Brown, T. E., Evans, S. W., Gotlieb, E. M., Knight, J. R., et al. (2005). Attention-deficit/hyperactivity disorder among adolescents: A review of the diagnosis, treatment, and clinical implications. *Pediatrics*, *115*, 1734–1746.

Wymbs, B. T., Pelham, W. E., Molina, B. S. G., & Gnagy, E. M. (2008). Mother and adolescent reports of interparental discord among parents of adolescents with and without attention-deficit/hyperactivity disorder. *Journal of Emotional and Behavioral Disorders, 16,* 29–41.

Yuill, N., & Lyon, J. (2007). Selective difficulty in recognising facial expressions of emotion in boys with ADHD: General performance impairments or specific problems in social cognition? *European Child & Adolescent Psychiatry, 16*(6), 398–404.

Zalecki, C. A., & Hinshaw, S. P. (2004). Overt and relational aggression in girls with Attention Deficit Hyperactivity Disorder. *Journal of Clinical Child and Adolescent Psychology, 33,* 125–137.

Chapter 10
Evidence-Based Methods of Dealing with Social Deficits in Conduct Disorder

Kimberly Renk, Rachel Wolfe White, Samantha Scott, and Melissa Middleton

Conduct Disorder affects a significant number of children, resulting in serious ramifications for the social relationships as well as the emotional and behavioral functioning of these children. In particular, the incidence of Conduct Disorder in young children may be as high as 35% (Webster-Stratton & Hammond, 1998). A significant percentage of older children and adolescents also are affected (2–3%, Maughan, Rowe, Messer, Goodman, & Meltzer, 2004; 1–10%, APA, 2000), with males showing higher rates of diagnosis than females (6–16% of boys versus 2–9% of girls; APA, 2000). Given the social, emotional, and behavioral difficulties that accompany a diagnosis of Conduct Disorder, it is often cited as the most common reason for referrals for mental health services (e.g., preschoolers, Luby & Morgan, 1997; school-age children, Foster, Kelsch, Kamradt, Sosna, & Yang, 2001). Of most concern, the behaviors associated with Conduct Disorder (e.g., aggression) show significant stability over time (Keenan, Shaw, Delliquadri, Giovannelli, & Walsh, 1998).

Given the prevalence of Conduct Disorder as well as the anticipated long-term trajectory of its related problematic behaviors, understanding this disorder, identifying the most useful means of identifying this disorder, and implementing the treatments with the strongest evidence base are critically important for mental health professionals who work with families who have children with conduct problems. As a result, this chapter will examine the criteria used to diagnose Conduct Disorder from the *Diagnostic and Statistical Manual of Mental Disorders-Fourth Edition-Text Revision* (APA, 2000), briefly survey etiological factors that are linked to conduct problems, highlight relevant assessment instruments for making a diagnosis of Conduct Disorder, and identify treatments that are used to promote the best psychosocial and behavioral outcomes for children who are diagnosed with Conduct Disorder.

Conduct Disorder Criteria

The most recent version of *the Diagnostic and Statistical Manual of Mental Disorders, the Fourth Edition-Text Revision (DSM-IV-TR;* APA, 2000) refers to Conduct Disorder as a repetitive or persistent pattern of behavior in which the basic rights of others or major age-appropriate societal norms or rules are violated. Thus, difficulties in social relationships as well as in emotional and behavioral functioning are inherent in this disorder. In particular, to make a diagnosis of Conduct Disorder, the *DSM-IV-TR* requires that children exhibit at least 3 of 15 criteria that fall into four categories. These categories include aggressive behavior that threatens or causes physical harm to other individuals or animals (e.g., bullying other individuals, initiating physical fights, using weapons, being physically cruel to animals, being physically cruel to other individuals, engaging in confrontational stealing,

K. Renk (✉)
Department of Psychology, University of Central Florida,
Orlando, FL 32816, USA
e-mail: krenk@ucf.edu

forcing another individual into sexual activity), destruction of property (e.g., deliberately setting fires, deliberately destroying others' property), deceitfulness or theft (e.g., breaking into another individual's home, lying to obtain goods or avoid obligations, stealing items without confrontation), and serious violations of rules (e.g., staying out at night despite parental prohibitions, running away from home, being truant from school; APA, 2000). Given these criteria, social difficulties are inherent to this disorder.

In addition to exhibiting these criteria, children must show a persistent course of conduct problems. In particular, to make a diagnosis of Conduct Disorder, each criterion must have occurred in the past 12 months, with at least one criterion occurring in the past 6 months. The *DSM-IV-TR* also states that these problematic behaviors must cause clinically significant problems in social, academic, or occupational functioning for a diagnosis to be made (APA, 2000). Thus, changes in functioning, particularly in the domains of social relationships and academic functioning, from that exhibited by typically developing children will be noteworthy.

In addition to the specific criteria noted above, children's ages should be considered carefully with a diagnosis of Conduct Disorder. First, as part of the diagnostic criteria, the *DSM-IV-TR* states that if the individual is 18 years of age or older the individual being diagnosed with Conduct Disorder must not meet criteria for Antisocial Personality Disorder (i.e., a personality disorder diagnosed in individuals who are 18 years of age and older when behaviors demonstrating a persistent disregard for and violation of the rights of others are present; APA, 2000). Second, children's ages are important when diagnosing particular types of Conduct Disorder. In particular, there are three subtypes of Conduct Disorder. The Childhood-Onset Type is diagnosed when children display at least one criterion prior to the age of 10. In contrast, the Adolescent-Onset Type is diagnosed when children do not exhibit any of the criteria prior to the age of 10. Further, the Unspecified Onset Type is diagnosed when the age of onset for the diagnostic criteria is unknown (APA, 2000). Generally, research suggests that those diagnosed with the Childhood-Onset Type exhibit a more problematic course of symptoms and a poorer outcome over time relative to those

diagnosed with the Adolescent-Onset Type (Frick & Loney, 1999; Moffitt, 1993; Moffitt & Caspi, 2001).

Finally, when diagnosing Conduct Disorder, the severity of the disorder is specified. The disorder is considered to be "mild" if few conduct problems are exhibited in excess of those required to make the diagnosis and if these problems cause only minor harm to other individuals. In contrast, the disorder is considered to be "moderate" if the number of conduct problems and their effect on other individuals are between mild and severe. Finally, the disorder is considered to be "severe" if many conduct problems are exhibited in excess of those required to make the diagnosis or if these problems cause considerable harm to other individuals (APA, 2000). Thus, children's impact on other individuals is critical in determining the degree of severity noted with Conduct Disorder.

The Etiology of Conduct Disorder

Rather than simply diagnosing Conduct Disorder, mental health professionals should seek to uncover the potential causative factors that may be promoting children's conduct problems. Further, given the ramifications of Conduct Disorder symptoms for children's social relationships as well as their emotional and behavioral functioning, researchers are seeking to identify factors that may cause these symptoms. As part of this research endeavor, several biological, individual, and psychosocial risk factors associated with the etiology of Conduct Disorder have been identified (e.g., see Frick, 2004, for a review). It is important to note that the etiology of Conduct Disorder usually involves several interacting factors (Frick & Ellis, 1999), rather than one simple underlying mechanism. The most common etiological factors associated with Conduct Disorder are discussed here.

As part of this discussion, however, it is important to note that etiological factors may interact differentially with children's age at the time of symptom onset and with their gender (Silverthorn & Frick, 1999). In particular, children's biological makeup and individual characteristics (e.g., temperament) as well as psychosocial factors (e.g., familial dysfunction, poverty) are associated with the development of the Childhood-Onset Type of Conduct Disorder (Moffitt & Caspi, 2001). As a result, the behaviors associated with the Childhood-Onset Type of Conduct Disorder are more likely to increase during the adolescent years and to persist into adulthood (Moffitt, 1993; Moffitt & Caspi, 2001). In contrast, the Adolescent-Onset Type of Conduct Disorder is associated with increased socialization with deviant peers and the need to gain autonomy (Frick, 2004; Moffitt, 1993; Moffitt & Caspi, 2001). As a result, children with the Adolescent-Onset Type may particularly benefit from treatment interventions that work to improve their social skills. Further, research suggests that Conduct Disorder is diagnosed rarely in girls during childhood (Silverthorn & Frick, 1999). Although girls may not display behavior that is consistent with Conduct Disorder until adolescence, their risk factors are similar to those of the Childhood-Onset Type (Moffitt & Caspi, 2001). Thus, children's age and gender may hold important information for identifying potentially causative mechanisms, identifying helpful assessment instruments, and selecting the most effective treatments.

Biological Factors

Genetics

Genetic factors are a key component in understanding the etiology of Conduct Disorder. Although it is difficult to separate genetic contributions from psychosocial risk factors, research suggests that genetic factors account for a considerable amount of variance in the development of Conduct Disorder (Arseneault et al., 2003; Holmes, Slaughter, & Kashani, 2001). For example, research examining the Conduct Disorder symptoms of twins indicates that monozygotic twins display more similarities in the level of their conduct problems and antisocial behavior relative to dizygotic twins (Reid, Dorr, Walker, & Bonner, 1986; Rhee & Waldman, 2002). Further, Arseneault and colleagues (2003) report that there is a stronger genetic contribution for the severe, pervasive conduct problems of 5-year old children relative to those of children with an older age of onset. Thus, genetics may make a significant

contribution to the development of early-onset conduct problems.

Neurophysiological Factors

The contribution of neurophysiological factors to the development of conduct problems is also the focus of much research (e.g., Kim-Cohen et al., 2006; Manuck et al., 1999). In particular, the relationship between the neurotransmitter serotonin and varying levels of aggression is of interest. For example, Kruesi and colleagues (1990) report that children who exhibit conduct problems and physical aggression have low levels of 5-hydroxyindoleacetic acid (5-HIAA; a metabolite of 5-HT) in their cerebrospinal fluid (CSF). Further, CSF 5-HIAA levels predict the severity of these children's physically aggressive behavior 2 years later (Kruesi et al., 1992). There are also conflicting results related to CSF 5-HIAA, however, suggesting that serotonin's role in the development of conduct problems may depend on other child-specific factors.

In addition to the findings regarding serotonin, other neurotransmitters may be important in predicting conduct problems as well. For example, low monoamine oxidase A (MAO-A) appears to act as a biological risk factor for the development of conduct problems (e.g., Caspi et al., 2002; Kim-Cohen et al., 2003). MAO-A only is implicated as a risk factor when combined with psychosocial factors such as child abuse or neglect, however (Caspi et al., 2002). Further, research suggests that adrenal androgen functioning may be higher in children who exhibit oppositional behaviors (Van Goozen et al., 2000) that may be related to conduct problems. Thus, the neurophysiological factors that contribute to the etiology of Conduct Disorder likely present a complex picture.

Prenatal Predispositions

Exposure to certain substances in the prenatal environment also is linked to the development of Conduct Disorder (Dodge & Pettit, 2003). For example, research suggests that fetal exposure to opiates or methadone in utero may lead to conduct problems 10 to 13 years later (de Cubas & Field,

1993). Further, exposure to alcohol, marijuana, and/or tobacco during the prenatal period places a fetus at a considerably higher risk for developing Conduct Disorder in the future (relative to those who are not exposed to these substances in the prenatal environment; Day, Richardson, Goldschmidt, & Cornelius, 2000). The effects of such prenatal factors must be considered in relationship to the development of cognitive deficits associated with each substance, however (Dodge & Pettit, 2003). Thus, prenatal factors also present a complex picture for the etiology of Conduct Disorder.

Children's Individual Characteristics

Temperament

Temperamental characteristics, or biologically based behavioral approaches and emotional dispositions that appear early in life (Bates, 2001; Calkins, Hungerford, & Dedmond, 2004), may also be important in relation to Conduct Disorder. For example, research suggests that temperamentally difficult children are at greater risk for developing conduct problems and aggression in the future (see Frick & Morris, 2004, for a review; Shaw, Owens, Giovannelli, & Winslow, 2001). In particular, temperamentally difficult children are characterized as irritable, highly active, rigid, unaffectionate, and aversive (Shaw et al., 2001). Further, the characteristics that are associated with temperamentally difficult children at the ages of 3 and 5 predict adolescent behaviors that are consistent with Conduct Disorder in a 12-year longitudinal study (Caspi, Henry, McGee, Moffitt, & Silva, 1995). Thus, although the link between difficult temperament and later conduct problems may be indirect (i.e., dependent on psychosocial factors, such as parenting practices), these characteristics are continually noted as risk factors for later conduct problems (see Frick & Morris, 2004, for a review).

Callous-Unemotional Traits

Research also suggests that children who exhibit callous-unemotional traits (e.g., a lack of empathy and guilt) are more likely to develop severe conduct problems in childhood. These problems may persist into adolescence and even adulthood (Frick, Cornell, Barry, Bodin, & Dane, 2003). For example, Frick and colleagues (2003) indicate that children who exhibit both conduct problems and callous-unemotional traits show greater levels of conduct problems, aggression, and delinquent acts 1 year later relative to children who exhibit conduct problems alone. Moreover, research examining children as young as 4 years of age indicates that callous-unemotional traits are associated with conduct problems 1 year later (Dadds, Fraser, Frost, & Hawes, 2005). Accordingly, callous-unemotional traits may be a critical factor in the development, severity, and persistence of behaviors accompanying a diagnosis of Conduct Disorder.

Low Verbal Intelligence

Research further indicates that children who are diagnosed with Conduct Disorder exhibit poor performance on standardized tests of verbal ability as well as poor verbal scores on intelligence tests (Moffitt & Lynam, 1994). These performance difficulties extend to more generalized measures as well, with children who have conduct problems exhibiting higher rates of deficits in their general verbal skills (Lynan & Henry, 2001) and pragmatic use of language (Gilmour, Hill, Place, & Skuse, 2004). Research also demonstrates that, when compared to boys without severe conduct problems, boys with conduct problems have the greatest deficits in both verbal skills and verbal memory and are more likely to perform poorly on tests of verbal intelligence beginning at the age of 5 (Moffitt, 1990, 1993). Relative to children who do not exhibit conduct problems, the verbal intelligence scores of children who are diagnosed with Conduct Disorder are notably lower, even when variables such as socioeconomic status, academic achievement, and motivation are controlled (Lynam, Moffitt, & Stouthamer-Loeber, 1993). Thus, although verbal deficits may result from the conduct problems that children exhibit, it may also be the case that such verbal deficits contribute to the development of children's conduct problems.

Comorbid Psychological Factors

Research also suggests that the presence of inattention, impulsivity, and hyperactivity are prominent factors in the development of conduct problems (see Holmes et al., 2001, for a review). Moreover, when compared to children who exhibit conduct problems alone, children who exhibit comorbid conduct problems and ADHD symptoms are at a greater risk for developing more severe and persistent conduct problems (Lynam, 1998). In addition, children who exhibit conduct problems display symptoms commonly associated with anxiety and depressive disorders (Miller-Johnson, Lochman, Coie, Terry, & Hyman, 1998). Thus, identifying and treating comorbid symptomatology in children may be beneficial to the treatment of Conduct Disorder.

Psychosocial Factors

Family

In general, the relationship that children have with their parents is related critically to children's behavior (Patterson, 1982). Such a relationship is also important in the development of Conduct Disorder. For example, positive and proactive parenting (e.g., parents and children spending time playing together) may diminish children's risk of developing conduct problems over time (Gardner, Ward, Burton, & Wilson, 2003). Research also suggests that parenting behaviors including harsh discipline, inconsistency, low warmth, and minimal involvement contribute greatly to the development of Conduct Disorder in children (e.g., Patterson, 1982; Stormshak, Bierman, McMahon, Lengua, & the Conduct Problems Prevention Research Group, 2000). Further, Patterson (1982) indicates that, relative to parents of control children, parents of children with Conduct Disorder are more inconsistent, use more harsh commands, and are less involved in their parenting practices. Patterson (1982) also notes that parents of children with Conduct Disorder are more likely to engage in coercive processes when interacting with their children. In particular, these parents negatively reinforce their children's

conduct problems, thereby maintaining and often exacerbating these problems. Given these findings, it may be that children who have conduct problems may begin experiencing difficulties in their social relationships very early, as their interactions with their parents are often problematic.

In addition, child abuse and neglect contribute to the development of Conduct Disorder. For example, Johnson and colleagues (2002) demonstrate that, at an early age, children who experience child abuse display heightened levels of conduct problems and aggression. Further, research indicates that children who experience abuse or neglect have a 50% increased probability of engaging in future criminal behavior (Widom, 1989, 1997). Other forms of familial discord [e.g., inconsistent parental figures (Ackermann, Brown, D'Eramo, & Izard, 2002), marital conflict (Rutter, Giller, & Hagell, 1998), familial stress (Campbell, Pierce, Moore, Marakowitz, & Newby, 1996)] also place children at a heightened risk for the development of Conduct Disorder.

Further, parents' psychological health is an area of concern when examining the development of Conduct Disorder in children. For example, having a parent who exhibits antisocial behavior greatly increases the likelihood that children will develop Conduct Disorder (Tiet et al., 2001). Research also suggests that parental substance abuse (Loeber, Green, Keenan, & Lahey, 1995) and parental depression (Campbell, 1990) are each associated with conduct problems in children. Thus, familial factors, in addition to children's individual characteristics, should be considered when identifying potential treatments for Conduct Disorder.

Peers

In addition to family characteristics, social relationships with peers are an important factor to consider in the development of Conduct Disorder. In particular, research indicates that the development of conduct problems is associated with early peer rejection and increased socialization with peers who have conduct problems or antisocial behavior (Poulin & Boivin, 2000; Vitaro, Brendgen, & Tremblay, 2000). Consistently, children who are aggressive are more likely to be rejected by their peers and to display increasing conduct problems over time (Vitaro et al., 2000). Further, following rejection from their non-deviant peers, children who are aggressive are more likely to associate with peers who also are aggressive (Poulin & Boivin, 2000). Attention from such peers often acts as a reinforcer for conduct problems (Kiesner, Dishion, & Poulin, 2001). Thus, associations with these peers serve to maintain and exacerbate children's conduct problems (Vitaro et al., 2000). Overall, these problems occur partly because of the rejection that children experience from their non-deviant peers (Vitaro et al., 2000) and partly because of increased socialization with peers who are aggressive. In fact, associations with peers such as those described here are related most closely to the Adolescent-Onset Type of Conduct Disorder (Moffitt, 2003). It is also noteworthy that children who are aggressive tend to interpret ambiguous situations in hostile ways, suggesting that they maintain a hostile attribution bias. Unfortunately, this bias may exacerbate children's aggressive behaviors and negative feelings, resulting in further peer rejection (MacBrayer, Milich, & Hundley, 2003).

Neighborhood

Although peers contribute to the etiology of Conduct Disorder, the neighborhoods in which children reside may make a contribution as well. For example, research suggests that children who live in impoverished neighborhoods with a lower socioeconomic status (SES) are at a heightened risk for developing conduct problems (Leventhal & Brooks-Gun, 2000). In particular, research indicates that these children are more likely to be exposed to neighborhood acts of violence, which are predictors of Conduct Disorder in adolescents (McCabe, Lucchini, Hough, Yeh, & Hazen, 2005). For example, Gorman-Smith and Tolan (1998) examine boys from a low SES neighborhood and report that 65% of these boys report exposure to severe violence during the previous year. These boys also experience a significant increase in their level of aggression (Gorman-Smith & Tolan, 1998). It is important to note that, although poverty is associated with conduct problems in children, it also is associated with familial conflict and parenting

problems (e.g., Pinderhughes et al., 2001). Thus, although neighborhood interventions may be one focus of treatment, interventions targeting the family may be more beneficial.

Etiology Summary

Taken together, there are various etiological factors that may promote the development of Conduct Disorder in children. In fact, many researchers combine these factors into multifactorial models that describe the etiology of conduct problems, as it is unlikely that any single risk factor is a necessary or sufficient cause (Rockhill, Collett, McClellan, & Speltz, 2006). For example, Liaw and Brooks-Gunn (1994) examine 13 risk factors in conjunction with children's behavior problems. The findings of this study suggest that the incidence of behavior problems increases as the number of risk factors increases. Further, Greenberg, Speltz, DeKlyen, and Jones (2001) use many different factors (i.e., child characteristics, parenting practices, parent-child attachment, and family ecology variables) to differentiate families seeking services for boys who meet criteria for Oppositional Defiant Disorder, a diagnosis that is related to Conduct Disorder (Borduin, Henggeler, & Manley, 1995), from those with matched comparison boys with 81% sensitivity and 85% specificity. A dramatic increase in clinic status occurred when three or more risk factors were present. Thus, it appears that an increased number of risk factors is related closely to an increased risk of conduct problems.

Rather than examining only the number of risk factors that children experience, other models are beginning to examine the implications of interactions among etiological factors. For example, McKinney and Renk (2007) propose the Interactional-Developmental-Etiological Approach to understanding the etiology of Disruptive Behavior Disorders. This approach considers a variety of pathways to conduct problems, including genetic factors, dispositional factors, and environmental factors, each of which may interact to promote the occurrence of conduct problems at different stages of development. Given the implications of such a model, it may be more important for future research to examine the manner in which etiological factors interact to promote the development of Conduct Disorder. Further, each of these etiological factors has important implications for the implementation of successful interventions for children who are diagnosed with Conduct Disorder. The following sections will review useful tools for the assessment of Conduct Disorder and interventions that have been designed for children who have been diagnosed with Conduct Disorder.

Rationale for the Assessment and Treatment of Conduct Disorder

Although it is important for mental health professionals to understand the diagnostic criteria and etiological factors related to Conduct Disorder, the practicalities of working with children who are diagnosed with Conduct Disorder will require that mental health professionals have a good understanding of the assessment measures needed to identify the symptoms of Conduct Disorder as well as the means to implement evidence-based treatment interventions. For mental health professionals who work with children, it is likely that they will encounter children who can be diagnosed with Conduct Disorder. As mentioned previously, externalizing behavior problems, such as those involving conduct problems (e.g., defiance, anger, noncompliance), are primary reasons for children to be referred for mental health services (e.g., preschool age: Gadow, Sprafkin, & Nolan, 2001; Renk, 2005). Further, children who have conduct problems are likely to show persistent problems over time. For example, in one study, 73% of boys, compared to 48% of girls, assessed at 4 years of age continued to have persistent and severe symptoms at follow-up at 8 years of age (Christophersen & Mortweet, 2002). Thus, these characteristics of Conduct Disorder suggest the importance of identifying and treating the symptoms of this disorder.

The assessment and effective treatment of Conduct Disorder becomes even more important when the costs to society resulting from this disorder are considered. These costs can be considered in terms of psychosocial and financial expenditures. With regard to psychosocial costs, Conduct Disorder is related to criminal activities, use and abuse of illegal substances (Brook, Whiteman, Finch, & Cohen, 1996), and difficulties related to early sexual activity (e.g., unwanted pregnancy; Capaldi, Crosby, & Stoolmiller, 1996). Certainly, such costs have implications for the social relationships of children with Conduct Disorder as well as their emotional and behavioral functioning. In addition to these psychosocial costs, the financial expenditures of the services provided to children who have conduct problems and who are diagnosed with Conduct Disorder also can be great. In fact, some estimates suggest a cost of $130,000 or more per child over the course of a 6-month period (Foster et al., 2001). Other researchers (e.g., Cohen, 1998) estimate that children who follow a path consistent with the Childhood-Onset Type of Conduct Disorder and who persist in their criminal behavior may cost society at least $1.3 million per child. Thus, the costs of Conduct Disorder to the children who receive the diagnosis and to society in general are quite great.

Another important rationale for improving mental health professionals' knowledge of the effective assessment and treatment of Conduct Disorder is the usual rate of service usage by children who have conduct problems and who are diagnosed with Conduct Disorder. In a study examining the public expenditures of Conduct Disorder, findings suggest that children who are diagnosed with Conduct Disorder have a high rate of service usage (i.e., 5% receive inpatient services, 15% receive outpatient services, 18% receive special education, and 21% have contact with the police; Foster, Jones, & the Conduct Problems Prevention Research Group, 2005). In addition, children who are diagnosed with Conduct Disorder incur a significantly higher average total cost for services by the time they graduate from high school (i.e., exceeding $140,000 for the average child who is diagnosed with Conduct Disorder or a cost that is over six times greater than that for the average child who does not have Conduct Disorder). In particular, inpatient and outpatient mental health costs account for approximately 70% of the difference in costs for those who are diagnosed with Conduct Disorder versus those who are not (Foster et al., 2005). Studies such as those noted here suggest that it is imperative that Conduct Disorder be identified accurately with the assessment instruments that we have available, treated effectively with evidence-based interventions, and prevented when possible.

The Assessment of Conduct Disorder

An evidence-based comprehensive assessment is a crucial first step in diagnosing and effectively treating Conduct Disorder (McMahon & Frick, 2005). In general, evaluations of children who exhibit oppositionality and conduct problems should assess the topography of these children's behavior (Rockhill et al., 2006). The following section aims to describe the overarching goals for the assessment of Conduct Disorder as well as the multiple methods that have utility in the diagnosis of Conduct Disorder. In addition, several diagnostic considerations will be reviewed, including comorbidity, age considerations, gender considerations, risk factors associated with Conduct Disorder, and the effects of the Conduct Disorder label.

Goals of Assessment in the Context of Treatment

Clinical assessment is a tool used for obtaining a clear picture of clients' emotional and behavioral functioning in the context of the complex system in which they live. In general, and as applied to the assessment of Conduct Disorder, the purposes of clinical assessments are to describe clients' current functioning, inform treatment, and confirm clients' diagnoses (Meyer et al., 2001). Further, a comprehensive assessment can provide predictive information regarding prognosis and the likelihood of treatment success (Meyer et al., 2001). As Conduct Disorder develops through several different pathways and manifests in many forms, conceptualization of this disorder is difficult but vital to treatment planning (McMahon & Frick, 2005). When assessing children for Conduct Disorder, the examiner must ask several questions: (1) How many symptoms is the child exhibiting? (2) What types of problematic behaviors is the child exhibiting? (3) To what degree is this child's functioning being

impaired? and (4) How appropriate is this referral (McMahon & Frick, 2005)? Keeping these purposes in mind will help mental health professionals to select appropriate assessment instruments, to include important considerations in their thinking about the assessment of Conduct Disorder, and to plan effectively for future treatment interventions.

Methods of Assessment

Several methods exist for the assessment of conduct problems. These methods include clinical interviews, behavioral rating scales, and behavioral observations, among other methods. It is important to note that, although each method is described here as an independent and distinct tool, the utilization of multiple methods of assessment is the norm in the assessment of Conduct Disorder. Further, the use of multiple methods is particularly important given the complexity of the symptoms described throughout this chapter (McMahon & Frick, 2005).

Clinical Interviews

Clinical interviews provide an important avenue through which mental health professionals can gain a large amount of information regarding children referred for conduct problems. In particular, clinical interviews provide an opportunity to gain important information regarding the types of behaviors that children are manifesting, the severity of these behaviors, the level of impairment in functioning that children are experiencing, and the nature of typical parent–child interactions (McMahon & Frick, 2005). Further, clinical interviews may allow mental health professionals to gain information about children's medical, academic, and social history and facilitate the use of clinical expertise and judgment about the level of children's impairment (Hartung, McCarthy, Milich, & Martin, 2005). In addition, such interviews are useful in obtaining a precise picture of children's clinical diagnosis, its severity, and a description of the clinical course of children's symptoms (Rockhill et al., 2006). It also is noteworthy that interviews can be used for assessing children's social skills (Merrell, 2001). In an effort to collect this information, clinical interviews can be administered to parents, children, and, in some cases, teachers.

Clinical interviews may vary in the level of flexibility allocated for pursuing the information noted above. They can be unstructured, semi-structured, or structured. With regard to structured interviews, they are often helpful because they provide an organized method by which information can be obtained (McMahon & Frick, 2005). Further, structured interviews are designed typically to collect information in such a way that diagnoses consistent with the diagnostic criteria set forth by the *DSM-IV-TR* (APA, 2000) can be made, and they are often comprehensive enough to allow for the assessment of comorbid disorders. Given these characteristics, structured clinical interviews are considered to be the premiere method of assessment for Conduct Disorder because these interviews have adequate convergent validity across informants (e.g., youth and parents) and are considered to have superior reliability and validity when compared to rating scales (Hartung et al., 2005). The *Diagnostic Interview for Children* (Shaffer, Fisher, Lucas, Dulcan, & Schwab-Stone, 2000) and the *Diagnostic Interview for Children and Adolescents* (Reich, 2000) are two widely used structured clinical interviews that prove helpful in the diagnosis of Conduct Disorder. In addition, the *Kiddie Schedule of Affective Disorders and Schizophrenia* (Kaufman, Birmaher, Brent, & Rao, 1997) is a semi-structured interview (i.e., an interview that has more flexibility but one that still thoroughly assesses diagnostic criteria) that is helpful for differential diagnosis. This particular interview can be administered to both children and their parents.

Interviews also may be helpful for assessing the social relationships and social skills of children with Conduct Disorder. In particular, it may be helpful to interview these children about their responses to hypothetical social situations (Renshaw & Asher, 1983). Such an interview would assess children's goals and social strategies for approaching these situations, with the assumption that social objectives and problem-solving techniques would differ for children who are popular versus those who are not (Landau & Milich, 1990). Consistently, children who are more popular tend to have spontaneous social strategies that are more friendly, positive, and outgoing relative to children who hold a lower status among their peers (Landau & Milich, 1990). Interviews regarding social skills can also be useful in collecting information about the environment in which children's behavior problems occur, providing a more direct linkage to intervention (Merrell, 2001).

Although structured clinical interviews are considered a vital part of an assessment for Conduct Disorder, they are not without limitations. Aside from being time-consuming to administer, structured clinical interviews typically do not include normative data. Further, as the interview proceeds, informants tend to report fewer and fewer symptoms (Jensen, Watanabe, & Richters, 1999). In other words, informants tend to report more symptoms earlier in the interview and then decrease in the number of symptoms that are reported later in the interview. This response pattern tends to occur regardless of the order in which symptoms are assessed. It is also important to note that children under the age of 9 are not considered reliable informants when clinical interviews are administered (Loney & Frick, 2003).

Rating Scales

A second method of assessment for Conduct Disorder is the use of behavioral rating scales. McMahon and Frick (2005) identify a number of ways in which behavioral rating scales can be useful in the assessment process. In particular, behavioral rating scales cover an extensive range of conduct problems, including the dimensions described previously. Further, because rating scales tend to be brief, they are helpful as screening devices. They also can assist in the assessment of other adjustment problems and are often accompanied by normative data, allowing for the comparison of children to peers of the same age. In addition, behavioral rating scales generally allow for the inclusion of multiple informants, with parents, children, and teachers being able to complete such scales. For example, the *Child Behavior Checklist, Youth Self-Report,* and *Teacher Report Form* are three premiere broad-based behavioral rating scales that can be administered to parents, children, and teachers, respectively. In addition to measuring broad-based domains of internalizing, externalizing, and total behavior problems, these scales include narrow-band scales and DSM-oriented scales that assess more specific behavior domains relevant to conduct problems as well as scales addressing children's competence (Achenbach & Rescorla, 2001).

In addition to measuring difficulties in emotional and behavioral functioning, rating scales can be used to assess children's social relationships and social skills. In fact, Merrell (2001) suggests that rating scales should be considered a first-line choice for social skills assessment. Although there is less research on the utility of self-reports for social skills assessment (relative to that for self-reports of emotional and behavioral functioning; Merrell, 2001; Renk & Phares, 2004), Gresham and Elliott's (1990) *Social Skills Rating System* is a well-researched measure of children's social skills and includes measures that can be completed by teachers, parents, and children themselves. Certainly, there are a variety of measures that can be used generally to assess children's social skills and competence, such as sociometric measures (Hymel, 1983) and the *Self-Perception Profile for Children* (Harter, 1985). Other measures of children's social skills are designed specifically for assessing performance in school settings. For example, teachers can complete many measures, including the *Social Competence Scale* (Kohn & Rosman, 1972), the *Social Behavior Assessment-Revised* (Byrne & Schneider, 1985), the *Social Competence and Behavior Evaluation Scale* (LaFreniere, Dumas, Capuano, & Dubeau, 1992), the *School Social Behavior Scales* (Merrell, 1993), and the *Walker-McConnell Scales of Social Competence and School Adjustment* (Walker & McConnell, 1995). Given that there is only small-to-moderate agreement across informants in their ratings of children's social skills and competence (Renk & Phares, 2004), there may be occasions when it would be helpful to collect information about children's social skills from multiple informants. In these cases, measures specific to particular informants could be used, such as the *Teacher Rating of Social Skills-Children* (i.e., a measure completed by teachers regarding children's social skills; Clark, Gresham, & Elliott, 1985) or Harter's (1985) *Rating Scale of Actual Behavior* (a measure that can be completed by teachers and/or parents and linked to the *Self-Perception Profile for Children*).

Observations

Finally, behavioral observations allow mental health professionals to observe behavior in a natural or immediate environment (McMahon & Frick, 2005). Such observations may be particularly important for examining social skills, especially when children can be observed in settings where they interact with peers (e.g., school; Merrell, 2001). Thus, observations are beneficial in that mental health professionals are able to draw valuable conclusions about children separately from the reports of other informants (e.g., parents and teachers; McMahon & Frick, 2005). When conducting behavioral observations, it is helpful to use the same observer across multiple observations and to minimize conspicuous recording equipment (Aspland & Gardner, 2003). The *Dyadic Parent-Child Coding System II* (Robinson & Eyberg, 1981) is an example of a structured coding system for behavioral observations in which children and their parents are observed engaging in a series of structured play tasks. For classroom observations, Achenbach and Rescorla (2001) have developed the *Direct Observation Form* to assist in coding teacher–child interactions as well as the amount of time that a student engages in academic activity and on-task versus off-task behaviors.

With regard to observing children's social skills, the *Peer Social Behavior Code* (part of the *Systematic Screening for Behavior Disorders*; Walker & Severson, 1992) can be used to categorize children's social behaviors (e.g., social engagement, parallel play) during free play situations. Further, some may use observations of role-play situations to assess children's social skills. In such situations, children are presented with a standard set of situations that involve social interactions and asked to respond to a provided prompt as if the situations were real. One such role-play situation is the *Role-Play Test* (Hughes et al., 1989).

A possible limitation of behavioral observation is the reactivity (i.e., changes in behaviors resulting from the state of being observed) that children (or parents) may experience during an observation session. As long as the children (or parents) are given ample time to become accustomed to the observational procedure, however, reactivity is typically not a problem (McMahon & Frick, 2005). It also may be difficult or unrealistic for mental health professionals to conduct extensive behavioral observations of the children (or parents) being assessed. To address this particular limitation, adults who have regular conduct with the children being assessed (e.g., parents or teachers) can be trained to make observations of the children. Observing covert behaviors also may be a challenge (McMahon & Frick, 2005) unless special procedures are used. For example, temptation-provocation tasks can be used to measure covert behaviors (Hinshaw, Zupan, Simmel, Nigg, & Melnick, 1997). Otherwise, mental health professionals will have to use alternative assessment methods to gain information regarding covert behaviors.

Important Considerations in the Assessment of Conduct Disorder

Dimensions of Conduct Disorder

There are many important things to consider when assessing children for Conduct Disorder. In order to make a valid diagnosis of Conduct Disorder and in order to most effectively inform treatment, an understanding of the dimensions of Conduct Disorder is helpful (McMahon & Frick, 2005). First, conduct problems manifest themselves in either an overt or covert fashion (or both). Overt behaviors are confrontational in nature and include bullying, arguing with adults, and being aggressive toward other individuals and/or animals, amongst other things. In contrast, covert behaviors are considered non-confrontational (e.g., stealing, truancy). Second, behaviors can be divided into those that are destructive and those that are not destructive. This dimension can be combined with the overt-covert dimension to form four categories: overt-destructive (e.g., physical aggression), overt-nondestructive (e.g., oppositional behaviors), covert-destructive (e.g., destruction of property), and covert-nondestructive (e.g., substance use). See McMahon and Frick (2005) for a comprehensive review of research in this area. Further, Knock, Kazdin, Hiripi, and Kessler (2006) provide an alternative, yet similar, conceptualization that may prove helpful in developing treatment plans. This conceptualization includes five subtypes of Conduct Disorder, three of which are specialized (i.e., rule violations, deceit/theft, and aggression) and two more general but severe subtypes (i.e., severe covert and pervasive).

McMahon and Frick (2005) point out that considering conduct problems along the aforementioned dimensions during assessment is important for several reasons. First, conduct problems are associated strongly with delinquency and the criminal justice system (Moffitt, 1993). These same divisions or dimensions are used in legal systems. Therefore, the congruence between the psychological and criminal justice schools of thought can be helpful in allowing communication to occur across professionals in the mental health and criminal justice fields. Second, it is helpful to note whether children are exhibiting behaviors consistent with only one conduct dimension or are more variable in their pattern of conduct problems. In particular, children who exhibit a more heterogeneous pattern of conduct problems tend to experience worse outcomes than those who only exhibit one dimension of conduct problems (Frick & Loney, 1999; Loeber et al., 1993). Finally, noting these dimensions during assessment can provide important clues regarding the role of genetics in the development of children's difficulties. In particular, research shows that destructive behaviors are likely inherited traits, whereas nondestructive behaviors are not (Simonoff, Pickles, Meyer, Silberg, & Maes, 1998). This distinction may be important as more stable or inherited traits, relative to those that are learned, will likely require different types of treatment.

An equally important dimension to examine when assessing children with conduct problems is whether or not they possess callous-unemotional traits (e.g., lacking empathy or guilt). Such traits are associated with increasingly severe conduct problems and aggression (Frick et al., 2003). Children who exhibit conduct problems and possess callous-unemotional characteristics also tend to experience more life stressors (e.g., peer rejection, family dysfunction, harsh and inconsistent discipline) and a more stable, severe pattern of conduct problems (Frick & Dantagnan, 2005). Interestingly, children with callous-unemotional characteristics tend to associate less with deviant peer groups. This finding may indicate that these children experience a greater level of social rejection than those in other groups (Frick & Dantagnan, 2005). Further, longitudinal research finds that antisocial traits and detachment are moderately stable over time and may be predictive of a more severe life-course persistent pattern of antisocial behavior (Loney, Taylor, Butler, & Iacono, 2007). Thus, it is recommended that callous-unemotional traits be examined early in assessments of Conduct Disorder so that the remainder of the assessment can be structured accordingly (McMahon & Frick, 2005).

Gaining information about these characteristics will allow for the prediction and isolation of later social difficulties and problems in emotional and behavioral functioning. This information also will be important for confirming a diagnosis of Conduct Disorder as well as for planning for treatment interventions (Loney et al., 2007; McMahon & Frick, 2005).

Comorbidity

In addition to assessing the different dimension of Conduct Disorder, it is important to note comorbidity (i.e., the co-occurrence of other disorders along with Conduct Disorder) in the context of assessment. In particular, treatment implications may differ depending on the diagnoses that are comorbid with Conduct Disorder (McMahon & Frick, 2005). Specifically, it is important to assess for Attention Deficit/Hyperactivity Disorder, Anxiety Disorders, and Mood Disorders (i.e., disorders that most commonly co-occur with Conduct Disorder; Waschbusch, 2002). Substance use is also associated highly with Conduct Disorder (Hawkins, Catalano, & Miller, 1992) and should be assessed during the assessment process. Most structured clinical interviews and many behavioral ratings scales (as described previously) can facilitate the assessment of these comorbid disorders in children who present with conduct problems.

Age Considerations

It is also important to note children's age at the onset of the conduct problems that they are exhibiting, as this information can be helpful in the development of assessment guidelines and in designing a treatment plan suitable for their individual needs (McMahon & Frick, 2005). As noted previously, children who begin exhibiting conduct problems before the age of 10 tend to have more severe conduct problems in adolescence and are more likely to continue to display such characteristics into adulthood (Frick & Loney, 1999; Moffitt & Caspi, 2001). These characteristics tend to be associated with children's stable temperament and often lead to criminal behavior and involvement with the criminal justice system. Further, the development of such characteristics before the age of 10 (i.e., the Childhood-Onset Type of Conduct Disorder) is correlated with other stable risk factors as well (e.g., lower intellectual functioning, family dysfunction; McMahon & Frick, 2005). In contrast, children who begin showing such behaviors after the age of 10 (i.e., the Adolescent-Onset Type of Conduct Disorder) are more likely to develop conduct problems as a result of their affiliation with deviant peers and are more likely to be described as conflicting with authority or as being "rebellious" (Moffit & Caspi, 2001; Moffitt, Caspi, Dickinson, Silva, & Stanton, 1996). Given this information, children's age at the onset of their conduct problems can provide helpful information about the measures that should be included in the assessment process, probable components of effective treatment interventions, and a likely prognosis.

Gender Considerations

In addition to children's age at the onset of their conduct problems, it is important to note that boys and girls who are diagnosed ultimately with Conduct Disorder may manifest different types of conduct problems. First, girls are more likely to engage in relational forms of aggression (e.g., gossip, slander) as opposed to overt aggression (e.g., fighting, cruelty; Frick, O'Brien, Wootton, & McBurnett, 1994; Xie, Cairns, & Cairns, 2005). As a result, McMahon and Frick (2005) suggest that a measure of relational aggression should be administered during the assessment process, so as to not "miss" girls who meet the diagnostic criteria for Conduct Disorder. Second, girls with conduct problems are at higher risk for the comorbid disorders of Depression and Anxiety (Fergusson, Horwood, & Ridder, 2005). Therefore, it is important for mental health professionals to closely screen for such disorders so that the most effective and comprehensive treatment intervention can be implemented (McMahon & Frick, 2005). Overall, the gender of the client being assessed for Conduct Disorder should inform the assessment measures that are included.

Risk Factors

The assessment of risk factors is also important for informing future treatment interventions. For example, as discussed previously, language impairments and lower intellectual functioning are two variables related to Conduct Disorder (Lynam & Henry, 2001; Lynam et al., 1993). Given this relationship, it is helpful to administer tests of intellectual functioning (e.g., using the *Wechsler Intelligence Scale for Children-Fourth Edition*; Wechsler, 2003) and academic achievement (e.g., using the *Woodcock Johnson Tests of Academic Achievement-Third Edition*; Woodcock, McGrew, & Mather, 2001) when assessing children for Conduct Disorder. Collecting information regarding children's intellectual and academic functioning may prove useful in predicting a prognosis for children's conduct problems, as lower intellectual functioning is associated with the persistence of conduct problems and is predictive of adolescent delinquency (Frick & Loney, 1999). Further, the presence or absence of callous-unemotional traits may be particularly informative for the type of treatment intervention that is pursued (McKinney & Renk, 2006). Coercive parent–child relationships (Patterson, Reid, & Dishion, 1992), family factors (e.g., marital and financial stress; McMahon & Estes, 1997), and peer relationships (e.g., association with deviant peers; Fergusson, Swain-Campbell, & Horwood, 2002) are several additional factors associated with the development of Conduct Disorder that should be assessed. In particular, observation of the parent–child relationship is vital, as understanding this relationship can help determine whether the focus of treatment interventions should be on children's personal characteristics, the interactions occurring between children and parents, and/or parenting practices (McMahon & Frick, 2005).

The Effects of Labeling

As with any mental health label, the diagnosis of Conduct Disorder may come with a price. Unfortunately, labeling children with antisocial characteristics may lead to unnecessary stigmatization and to adults making punitive decisions regarding these children (e.g., the type of treatment intervention that may be required, the types of punishment that may be warranted in response to conduct problems; Rockett, Murrie, & Boccaccini, 2007). Therefore, Conduct Disorder-related terminology should be used cautiously and conservatively when describing children and should always be presented in the context of children's developmental, social, familial, and academic experiences.

Assessment Summary

Although assessment and treatment are two distinct processes, the assessment process is an essential, therapeutic part of the intervention process (Meyer et al., 2001). For the families of children who present with conduct problems, assessment can be a time when all family members are allowed to provide input. In some situations, the assessment process is the first time when all family members are able to talk about or process their experiences and difficulties in a safe, validating environment. It is also a time when family members can work together with the mental health professional in a collaborative effort to ameliorate the negative effects that their children's conduct problems can have on the children themselves, their family members, and other individuals in the community (McMahon & Frick, 2005). Further, receiving assessment-based feedback often is relieving and therapeutic for these children and their family members, especially if their initial attempts to decrease children's conduct problems have failed (Meyer et al., 2001).

In general, when conducting an assessment with children who are exhibiting conduct problems, the assessment process should be flexible, should use multiple methods of assessment, should use information collected from multiple informants, and should examine the children's conduct problems, comorbid conditions, risk factors, and other characteristics. By conducting assessments in this fashion, treatment interventions can be selected carefully and informatively so that the best possible outcomes can occur for these children and their families.

Treatment of Conduct Disorder

As children who have conduct problems are a challenge for parents, teachers, and mental health professionals as a result of their usual behaviors (e.g., disruptive behavior, noncompliance, defiance, aggression, oppositionality, social deficits), identifying effective treatment interventions for these children is difficult. Further, a lack of replicable findings and generalized treatment effects (Eyberg, Nelson, & Boggs, 2008), as well as a myriad of confounding factors (e.g., comorbid disorders and symptoms, individual differences in presenting symptoms, parental psychopathology, poor parenting practices), interfere with the ability to place one specific treatment modality ahead of the rest (Frick, 2001). Further, some treatment interventions are effective in some studies but not in others, with some resulting in iatrogenic effects (Dishion, McCord, & Poulin, 1999). Thus, even after carefully considering the diagnostic criteria for Conduct Disorder, considering the etiological factors that may be present, and conducting a careful assessment of children who have conduct problems, it may still be difficult for mental health professionals to identify the most beneficial treatment intervention for children who are diagnosed with Conduct Disorder. As a result, this section will review those treatment interventions that have empirical support and provide information about treatment interventions that may prove problematic for children who have conduct problems.

Treatments That Have Empirical Support

To better understand the wide range of possible treatment interventions, a few in-depth studies are noted in the research literature. These studies identify a number of evidence-based psychosocial treatments (EBTs) that address the impairments in social relationships and emotional and behavioral functioning experienced by children who are diagnosed with Conduct Disorder (Brestan & Eyberg, 1998; Eyberg et al., 2008; Frick, 2001). Further review of such studies indicates that identified EBTs are effective for specific age groups and vary based on the method of delivery (i.e., individual versus group treatment and the degree to which the treatment is child-focused versus parent-focused). Although it is clear that more research is needed to better delineate the effectiveness of differing treatment interventions for children who are diagnosed with Conduct Disorder, information that can be useful to mental health professionals in selecting treatment interventions is currently available. Effective interventions may be individualized and applied in different settings.

The most recent review of EBTs for children who have disruptive behavior (Eyberg et al., 2008) identifies 16 EBTs (15 *probably efficacious* and one *well-established)* and nine *possibly efficacious* treatments. This review by Eyberg and colleagues (2008) examines the literature from 1996 to 2007, including a few earlier treatments that were identified previously as efficacious. The EBTs identified in this review are categorized using established criteria for identifying well-established and probably efficacious treatments (for a complete review of the criteria used to identify well-established and probably efficacious treatments, see Chambless & Hollon, 1998, or Chambless & Ollendick, 2001). Further, reviews of the literature identify many moderators that may prove beneficial for mental health professionals when choosing the most appropriate treatment intervention.

In particular, Frick (2001) suggests that the developmental trajectory of conduct problems differs as a function of children's age at the time of their symptom onset. Conduct problems consistent with the Childhood-Onset Type of Conduct Disorder may reflect a more severe and pervasive disturbance, whereas symptoms developing in adolescence (i.e., those consistent with the Adolescent-Onset Type of Conduct Disorder) may reflect a negative exaggeration of typical adolescent behaviors or situational factors (Frick, 2001). Differences in children's ages at the time of their symptom onset may be one reason that parent-focused interventions, or child-focused treatments with accompanying parent components, are effective with younger children (Eyberg et al., 2008; Kazdin & Weisz, 2003). In fact, Eyberg and colleagues (2008) suggest that parent-focused components of treatment be used first with younger children and that more direct cognitive-behavioral approaches be used with adolescents. As children often do not receive immediate services for conduct problems, children's ages when they begin a treatment intervention also should be considered. Various treatment interventions are effective, but their effectiveness is often specific to the ages of the children being treated and to the formats of the treatments that are used (Eyberg et al., 2008). Thus, children's ages will be used to categorize the treatment interventions discussed here.

Treatments for Young Children

When treating young children who have conduct problems, the inclusion of parents in the treatment intervention is vital. One treatment program that has empirical support is *Parent–Child Interaction Therapy* (PCIT; Hembree-Kigin & McNeil, 1995). PCIT is a *probably efficacious* treatment for young children (i.e., children who are 2–7 years old; Eyberg et al., 2008) with a focus on parenting skills and parent–child interactions. Specifically, this program has a basis in both attachment theory (Herschell, Calzada, Eyberg, & McNeil, 2002) and operant conditioning (Shillingsburg, 2005). As a result, this program allows parents the opportunity to incorporate skills of responsive parenting to meet the needs of their young children and to learn to positively attend to positive behaviors and to actively ignore negative behaviors, respectively. Parents and their young children attend sessions together, providing an in-vivo training component. Given this format, parents practice child behavior management skills with their young children while being provided feedback from a mental health professional (Brinkmeyer & Eyberg, 2003; Kazdin, 2005). Parents also are expected to continue practicing these skills at home, allowing for the generalization and mastery of these skills in the home setting (Capage, Foote, McNeil, & Eyberg, 1998).

With PCIT, parents and their young children participate in two sequential treatment modules. First, parents and their young children participate in a Child-Directed module (CDI). As part of this module, parents are coached on how to interact attentively with their young children. This module is similar to play therapy (Eyberg, 2003), in that parents are asked to engage in special playtime with their young children. During this playtime, parents describe, imitate, and praise their young children's appropriate behavior while they reflect appropriate speech, ignore inappropriate behavior, and avoid criticism, commands, and questions (Greco, Sorrell, & McNeil, 2001). Overall, the purpose of this module is to improve interactions between parents and their young children. Second, parents and their young children participate in a Parent-Directed module (PDI). As part of this module, parents are coached in effective contingency management skills that can be used to manage child noncompliance (Hembree-Kigin & McNeil, 1995). In particular, the purpose of this module is to help parents decrease their young children's problematic behavior and increase their young children's prosocial behaviors (Eisenstadt, Eyberg, McNeil, Newcomb, & Funderburk, 1993). Generally, PCIT is designed to improve young children's social relationships (particularly, the parent–young child relationship), improve the parenting skills of mothers and fathers, and improve young children's emotional and behavioral functioning.

Overall, research suggests that PCIT meets these goals. In particular, research shows that PCIT is effective in improving interactions between parents and their young children and in decreasing young children's behavior problems (Eyberg et al., 2001; Eyberg & Robinson, 1982; Herschell et al., 2002). Further, PCIT is effective in decreasing children's conduct problems in a variety of settings (e.g., school; Eyberg, Boggs, & Algina, 1995; McNeil, Eyberg, Eisenstadt, Newcomb, & Funderburk, 1991) and decreasing the likelihood that children will meet criteria for their initially diagnosed disorders upon completing treatment (Boggs et al., 2005). PCIT also results in a reduction in conduct problems over time (i.e., 3–6 years; Hood & Eyberg, 2003). Given this support for PCIT's effectiveness, this treatment intervention would be a beneficial choice for families with young children who have conduct problems.

Another useful treatment intervention is the *Helping the Noncompliant Child* (*HNC*; Forehand & McMahon, 1981) program. Similar to PCIT, HNC is also a *probably efficacious* treatment for addressing the conduct problems of young children between the ages of 3 and 8 years (Eyberg et al., 2008). In addition, HNC focuses on similar parenting behaviors as PCIT (e.g., attending to positive behaviors, ignoring negative behaviors, employing effective discipline strategies). Further, HNC utilizes in vivo treatment strategies, where parents and young children are seen together in the clinic or at home (McMahon & Forehand, 2003). There are two phases included in this program as well. During the first phase, Differential Attention, parents learn to increase the frequency and range of the social attention that they provide to their children, to decrease the frequency of their competing verbal behaviors, and to ignore minor inappropriate behaviors. With these goals, parents are assisted in creating positive and mutually reinforcing relationships with their young children by practicing these skills in session and at home during 10- to 15-min sessions with their young children (i.e., Child's Game; McMahon & Forehand, 2003). During the second phase, Compliance Training, parents are coached in the use of appropriate commands so that the compliance of their young children can be increased (i.e., using the Parent's Game). They are also coached in the use of standing rules as a supplement to clear instructions and in the use of these skills outside of the home (McMahon & Forehand, 2003).

Similar to PCIT, HNC also is designed to improve young children's social relationships (particularly, the parent–young child relationship), improve the parenting skills of mothers and fathers, and improve young children's emotional and behavioral functioning. In support of this treatment intervention, McMahon and Forehand (2003) summarize many of the outcome studies that examine the HNC program. In general, these studies provide support for the HNC program (e.g., Forehand & King, 1974, 1977). For example, previous controlled studies find that HNC is effective in increasing the compliance of young children in response to parental demands and in improving secondary conduct problems (e.g., aggression, tantrums; Wells,

Forehand, & Griest, 1980). Given these findings, the HNC program would also be a beneficial treatment intervention for young children who have conduct problems and their families.

A third treatment intervention, the *Incredible Years* (*IY-CT*; Webster-Stratton & Reid, 2003) program, is also *probably efficacious* for parents and their young children (Eyberg et al., 2008). The Incredible Years program includes several components. Similar to the first two treatment programs described in this section, this program includes a treatment component for parents. In addition, other components can be included for young children (i.e., social skills training) as well as for teachers (Reid & Webster-Stratton, 2001; Webster-Stratton, 2001). The Incredible Years Parent Training (IY-PT) component utilizes videotaped vignettes designed to teach and spur discussion about positive parent–child interactions, effective discipline techniques, and how to foster appropriate problem-solving skills. A supplemental component of IY-PT (ADVANCE) is often offered at the completion of the BASIC parent program. With the ADVANCE component of IY-PT, parents are taught more effective communication, self-control, and problem-solving skills for use in their marital relationship and are encouraged to strengthen their social support network (Webster-Stratton & Reid, 2003). As part of IY-PT, parents view videotaped parent models who engage in appropriate parenting behaviors and then participate in parent discussion groups and complete homework assignments to practice the skills that they see demonstrated by the videotaped models (Webster-Stratton, 1981b). Thus, IY-PT focuses specifically on the parenting behaviors of mothers and fathers.

Although typically administered in conjunction with IY-PT, the *Incredible Years Child Training* (IY-CT; Webster-Stratton & Reid, 2003) component is *probably efficacious* as an individual treatment (as is IY-PT; Eyberg et al., 2008). Similar to IY-PT, IY-CT employs the use of videotaped vignettes; however, with IY-CT, the videotaped vignettes depict social situations that young children are likely to encounter at home and at school. In small groups (i.e., 6–7 children), young children who are between the ages of 3 and 8 years discuss how they would feel during the videotaped situations and provide suggestions of appropriate responses. Modeling and feedback are utilized through a variety of games, activities, and role-playing, with the goal of teaching young children the basic skills of empathy, communication, friendship, anger control, and problem solving (Webster-Stratton & Reid, 2003). Thus, IY-CT focuses specifically on the social deficits that young children who have conduct problems exhibit. When compared to young children participating in other programs (e.g., the *Problem-Solving Curriculum*) and to those serving as wait list controls, young children who participate in IY-CT demonstrate significant improvements in aggressive and noncompliant behavior (Webster-Stratton, Reid, & Hammond, 2001). Further, when used in conjunction with the *Incredible Years Teacher Training* program, young children exhibit more social competence and emotional self-regulation as well as decreased levels of conduct problems (Webster-Strat ton, Reid, & Stoolmiller, 2008).

Further, the combination of IY-PT and IY-CT results in improvements in young children's social competence (Brotman et al., 2005; Drugli, Larsson, & Clifford, 2007) and in reductions in young children's conduct problems over time (i.e., at 1-year follow-up; Webster-Stratton & Hammond, 1997). In particular, results regarding the BASIC IY-PT program indicate that mothers decrease their directive behaviors (Webster-Stratton, 1981b, 1982), demonstrate increased confidence (Webster-Stratton, 1981a), and show more positive and significantly less negative interactions with their young children (Webster-Stratton, 1981b, 1982). With regard to the ADVANCE IY-PT program, significant reductions in the behavior problems of young children and improvements in the prosocial behaviors of young children are related to improvements in parental communication, collaboration, and problem-solving skills. Results further suggest that improvements in parents' marital relationship, as a result of better communication and support skills, is related to improvements in young children's conduct problems (Webster-Stratton & Reid, 2003). In particular, young children whose parents participate in this program exhibit decreases in negative affect and submissive behavior and increases in positive affect (Webster-Stratton, 1981b, 1982). These findings suggest that the Incredible Years

program would provide benefits to young children and their families.

Treatments for Children

Similar to the treatment interventions described previously for young children, treatment interventions for school-age children also include treatments intended to address the parenting strategies used by mothers and fathers. For example, the *Positive Parenting Program* (*Triple P*; Sanders, 1999) offers two parent-focused treatment approaches that are considered to be *probably efficacious* EBTs (Eyberg et al., 2008). In particular, Triple P offers five levels of preventive treatment for children who are 12 years of age and younger. These levels increase in intensity, ranging from the dissemination of basic information on parenting strategies to individual and group training sessions for parents of children who have severe behavior problems. With the availability of these different levels of treatment intervention, mental health professionals could individualize the treatment intervention provided to different families with children who have conduct problems.

For example, the *Triple P Standard Individualized Treatment* (i.e., level 4) is a 10-session program that utilizes modeling, rehearsal, and feedback to teach parents core parenting skills (e.g., managing misbehavior, preventing problematic behavior, teaching and encouraging new and appropriate behaviors, improving the parent–child relationship). This treatment program can also be offered in a group format (*Group Triple P*; Sanders, 1999). In the group format, which is also a *possibly efficacious* treatment intervention (Eyberg et al., 2008), parents practice newly acquired parenting skills in small groups. Further, the *Triple P Enhanced Treatment* is the most intensive level of treatment (i.e., level 5) and incorporates home visits where therapists attempt to improve characteristics of the home environment (e.g., parenting stress, communication, coping, mood management, partner support) as well as increase effective parenting skills (Sanders, 1999). These different levels of Triple P result in fewer child disruptive behaviors, greater parental competence, and less dysfunctional parenting over time (e.g., at 1 year post-treatment, Sanders, Markie-Dadds, Tully, & Bor, 2000; at 3 years post-treatment, Sanders, Bor, & Morawska, 2007). Other studies suggest that Triple P is beneficial in reducing children's problematic behaviors, even when confounding factors (e.g., maternal psychopathology, marital discord) are present (Sanders, 1999). Although the focus of this treatment intervention is on improving the parenting behaviors of mothers and fathers, it is likely that the improvements in children's conduct problems that also result will promote improvements in the social relationships of these children.

Another *well-established* parent-focused treatment intervention (Eyberg et al., 2008) for parents of children who are 12 years of age and younger is the *Parent Management Training Oregon Model* (*PMTO*; Patterson, Reid, Jones, & Conger, 1975). PMTO appears to be a variant of a previously well-established treatment called *Living with Children* (Patterson & Gullion, 1968); this treatment intervention employs behavior modification techniques that are based on operant theoretical principles (Brestan & Eyberg, 1998). PMTO, like other parent training programs, teaches parents basic behavior modification principles. In particular, parents learn how to better monitor their children's behaviors and to implement effective discipline strategies. Based on a long history of research regarding Conduct Disorder and antisocial behavior, PMTO accounts for individualized differences in children's symptoms, children's developmental trajectory, and basic principles of positive and negative reinforcement (Patterson, Reid, & Eddy, 2002). Previous controlled studies indicate that PMTO is effective in reducing deviant behaviors in children who are younger than 12 years of age (Patterson, Chamberlain, & Reid, 1982). Given these findings, PMTO also may have secondary benefits for children's social relationships.

For school-age children, individual and group therapy programs also become an option. For example, *Problem Solving Skills Training* (*PSST*; Kazdin, 2003) is labeled as a *probably efficacious* treatment intervention (Eyberg et al., 2008). PSST is a cognitive approach that targets deficits in accurately perceiving situations. Children who have conduct problems are taught problem-solving skills meant to foster their development of accurate

appraisals of social situations. Treatment strategies include having mental health professionals model appropriate behaviors, games, activities, role-playing, and the use of a token economy reward system (Kazdin, 1996, 2003). The original PSST may also be complemented with an in-vivo component (PSST + Practice); this combination is also labeled as being *probably efficacious* (Eyberg et al., 2008). As part of this combined program (which is also called *Supersolvers*), parents, who learn the problem-solving steps taught to their children, help their children apply these skills in everyday situations (Kazdin, 1996, 2003).

A third variation of PSST includes *Parent Management Training* (PMT; Kazdin, 2003, 2005). PMT uses operant conditioning principles to change children's adaptive functioning, parents' behavior, and parent–child interactions. In particular, parents learn to better identify problem behaviors and implement effective reinforcement and punishment methods of discipline. Randomized control trials of this program suggest that treatment leads to statistically significant changes (Kazdin, 2005), with approximately 79% of clinically referred children and adolescents who complete treatment making changes that parents label as being important (Kazdin & Wassell, 1998). These changes also seem to be maintained for 1–2 years following treatment (Kazdin, 2005). Based on the findings of several controlled studies, PMT is effective (Kazdin, 1996) and is listed as a *probably efficacious* treatment when combined with PSST (i.e., PSST + PMT; Eyberg et al., 2008). In particular, research suggests that the use of PSST and PMT decreases children's antisocial behavior and increases their prosocial behavior. Further, the simultaneous combination of PSST and PMT is superior to either treatment alone (Kazdin, 2003; Kazdin, Siegel, & Bass, 1992). Given these results, PSST would be a beneficial treatment intervention for families with school-age children who have conduct problems.

A number of group treatment interventions also are described as EBTs for the reduction of conduct problems in school-age children. These group treatment interventions vary in the amount of involvement expected from children and their parents. For example, *Anger Control Training* (Lochman, Barry, & Pardini, 2003) is a child-focused group treatment intervention that is labeled as being *probably effica-cious* (Eyberg et al., 2008). Anger Control Training for children in elementary school is a school-based program in which children discuss social situations, identify the potential social cues and motives of the individuals in each situation, and practice appropriate problem-solving strategies. Through discussion, role playing, and the videotaping of practice inter-actions, children learn to identify how they feel in social situations and how to better control their feelings while being provided feedback by a mental health professional (Lochman, 1992; Lochman et al., 2003). In general, anger coping programs decrease future substance use as well as improve self-esteem and problem-solving skills with long-term benefits (i.e., 3 years follow-up; Lochman, 1992). Thus, such treatment interventions directly address the social deficits of children who have conduct problems.

Treatments for Adolescents

Currently, there are no individualized treatment interventions for adolescents who have conduct problems and related social deficits that are estab-lished as EBTs. Some group treatment interventions are labeled as being *probably efficacious* EBTs, how-ever. One group treatment intervention, *Group Assertiveness Training* (Huey & Rank, 1984), is labeled as being *probably efficacious* for African-American adolescents in the Eighth and Ninth Grades (Eyberg et al., 2008). Group Assertiveness Training is a highly structured, short (i.e., eight 1-hour sessions provided over the course of a 4-week period) school-based program. As part of this pro-gram, trained counselors or peers lead reflective group discussions on a variety of topics (e.g., anger, aggression, rules) for adolescents who have conduct problems. These discussions maintain a strong emphasis on emotional awareness and feel-ings (Huey & Rank, 1984). Research suggests that Group Assertiveness Training is more effective than group discussion in reducing classroom aggression (Huey & Rank, 1984).

A second school-based EBT that is labeled as *probably efficacious* for older adolescents (i.e.,

Hispanic and African-American adolescents in the 11th and 12th grades; Eyberg et al., 2008) is the *Rational-Emotive Mental Health Program* (REHM; Block, 1978). REHM is a highly struc-tured and directive cognitive-behavioral group treatment program that is based on the rational-emotive therapy model. In this program, students are taught to be introspective and self-aware as they practice the rational appraisal of social situations. To achieve this goal, REHM utilizes specific cogni-tive-behavioral techniques (e.g., in vivo activities, group discussion, homework assignments). Relative to Group Assertiveness Training, REHM is a longer, more intensive program, with adolescents meeting 5 days per week for 12 weeks (Block, 1978). Research suggests that REHM promotes improvements in adolescents' grade point averages and decreases adolescents' truancy and disruptive behavior over time (i.e., at 4 months follow-up; Block, 1978). Thus, these programs also directly address the social deficits exhibited by adolescents who have conduct problems.

Multisystemic Therapy (*MST*; Henggeler & Lee, 2003) is a third EBT that is used with adolescents who exhibit severe antisocial and delinquent beha-vior and that has been labeled as *probably effica-cious* (Eyberg et al., 2008). MST is a very intensive but flexible treatment program that utilizes a variety of established treatment interventions (e.g., cogni-tive-behavioral therapies, parent training, pharma-cological interventions). MST is based on ecological and family systems theories, supporting the idea that treatment should incorporate and generalize to the myriad of interconnected systems in the envir-onments of children and adolescents (e.g., families, peers, neighborhoods, schools, larger community contexts). Thus, services are often provided in mul-tiple settings (e.g., at home, in the school setting).

The core principles of MST involve tailoring treatment interventions to meet the needs of the children and adolescents being treated based on their presenting symptoms, focusing on positive aspects of family involvement, evaluating treatment gains continually and making modifications as they are needed, and generalizing the positive effects of the treatment interventions that are being used across various settings (Eyberg et al., 2008; Heng-geler & Lee, 2003). Thus, the treatment interven-tions that are used with children and adolescents are selected based on the individualized needs of these children and adolescents and their families. Controlled studies report that MST is more effective than individual therapy in reducing behavior problems, increasing family relationships, and preventing criminal behavior 4 years following treatment (Borduin, Mann, & Cone, 1995). Given the comprehensive nature of MST, it would be a beneficial treatment intervention for children and adolescents who have significant conduct problems.

Other Treatments (Not Based on Age)

A final EBT identified by Eyberg and colleagues (2008) is *Multidimensional Treatment Foster Care* (*MTFC*; Chamberlain & Smith, 2003). MTFC is a community-based program for children of all ages who have disruptive and antisocial behavior problems. This very intensive program includes placing children in foster care for 6–9 months. As part of this program, foster parents are provided training in the use of positive reinforcement, discipline practices, positive feedback for appropriate behavior, and daily behavior management capitalizing on a token economy procedure. These foster parents provide children with a stable environment that models and encourages appropriate behavior. During the foster placement, children in MTFC attend individual therapy sessions designed to improve their anger management, problem solving, and social skills (Chamberlain & Smith, 2003). These children also are given in vivo training in the community, so that they can practice their prosocial behaviors while being provided with direct reinforcement and feedback from a mental health professional. Finally, during foster care placement, biological parents are provided intensive parent management training, in which they learn and practice effective communication, parenting, and disciplining skills (Chamberlain & Smith, 2003). Thus, MTFC is a very intensive program.

Research suggests that several core components of MTFC account for the effectiveness of this treatment intervention. These components include the children being closely supervised by and having a close relationship with an adult, foster parents setting clear limits for the children who are being fostered, and foster parents preventing children's interactions with deviant peers (Chamberlain, Leve, & DeGarmo, 2007). In addition, biological parents are provided with intensive intervention while trained foster parents care for their children. Controlled studies of MTFC indicate that this treatment intervention is more effective than group care for adolescent boys (Chamberlain & Reid, 1998) and girls (Chamberlain et al., 2007), resulting in fewer criminal and delinquent acts in 1 and 2 year follow-ups, respectively. Given these findings, positive outcomes are promoted by providing intensive training to biological parents and addressing the behavioral and social deficits of the children who have conduct problems.

Although many consider *psychotropic medications* to be an effective treatment intervention of children who have conduct problems, less research on the use of these medications for the treatment of Conduct Disorder is available relative to that for the psychosocial treatment interventions described previously (Farmer, Compton, Burns, & Robertson, 2005). Although no psychotropic medications are approved for conduct problems and aggression at this time (Rockhill et al., 2006), psychostimulants are used regularly and are effective in reducing the symptoms of Attention-Deficit/Hyperactivity Disorder (ADHD; Farmer et al., 2005; Pelham, 1993). As there is overlap in the symptoms exhibited by children who are diagnosed with ADHD and those who are diagnosed with Conduct Disorder (e.g., impulsivity, noncompliance, verbal and physical aggression), psychostimulants also may be beneficial in treating these problem behaviors in children who have Conduct Disorder (Frick, 2001). Further, a reduction in such conduct problems may improve other behaviors that are associated tangentially with Conduct Disorder (e.g., poor peer interactions, problem-solving skills; Frick, 2001).

Although psychostimulants may aid in the reduction of some conduct problems, other medications such as alpha-2 adrenoreceptor agonists, mood stabilizers, and antipsychotic medications are sometimes used to treat aggression in children (Steiner, Saxena, & Chang, 2003). For example, Olfson, Blanco, Liu, Moreno, and Laje (2006) examine trends in the usage of antipsychotic medications as part of outpatient visits for children in the United States. This study documents an increase in the use of antipsychotic medications from 1993 to 2003, particularly in visits for males and with regard to Disruptive Behavior Disorders. As these medications are indicated for the treatment of adults only, any use of these medications in children would be considered off label, with limited research noting their utility (Findling, 2003). As some suggest that the more severe symptoms of children who are diagnosed with Conduct Disorder require more intensive psychosocial interventions (Eyberg et al., 2008), psychotropic medications may be beneficial as a supplement to psychosocial interventions for some children or when psychosocial interventions are unsuccessful (Eyberg et al., 2008; Frick, 2001; Pelham, 1993). Given these suggestions, the use of psychotropic medications for the treatment of Conduct Disorder should be examined further.

Finally, there are other treatment interventions that show promise but that require more research regarding their effectiveness for the treatment of Conduct Disorder. For example, other parent training programs are available but do not have as extensive a research basis for their effectiveness. In particular, Barkley (1997; Barkley, Edwards, & Robin, 1999) developed two parent training programs. The *Defiant Children* program (Barkley, 1997) is developed for parents of children up to the age of 12 years and is designed to improve parents' management skills in dealing with their children's behavior problems, improve their knowledge of the potential causes for their children's behavior problems, improve their children's compliance with their commands and rules, and increase family harmony. A second but related program, the *Defiant Teen* program (Barkley et al., 1999), adapts the *Defiant Children* program for use with adolescents and includes problem-solving and communication training. Although these programs do not have extensive outcome research, the skills taught to parents as part of these programs have received an extensive amount of research support (McMahon & Forehand, 2003).

In addition, comprehensive classroom-based interventions may hold promise for the reduction of conduct problems and the improvement of social deficits in children and adolescents over the long term. Most notably, comprehensive preschool programs (e.g., Head Start) are related to decreases in behavior problems and juvenile delinquency (Yoshikawa, 1994). Other research supports classroom-based interventions that include behavioral training and consultation for teachers as well as implementation of token-

ecomony systems and response-cost interventions (Filcheck, McNeil, Greco, & Bernard, 2004). Given these preliminary findings, further research should examine the utility of these school-based treatment interventions for decreasing the conduct problems and improving the social deficits of children and adolescents who have conduct problems.

Prevention

Prevention programs, particularly if they are initiated early enough and are designed to address multiple causes, may also prove useful in the treatment of children who have conduct problems (Bernat, August, Hektner, & Bloomquist, 2007; Slough, McMahon, & the Conduct Problems Prevention Research Group, 2008). The *Fast Track Project*, a multisite, collaborative research project examining a comprehensive, multicomponent intervention for preventing serious conduct problems, is one such prevention program (Slough et al., 2008). Fast Track includes many different components depending on the age and needs of the children, including the provision of a curriculum that promotes social and emotional competence, positive family–school relationships, and effective communication and discipline skills. Thus far, studies indicate that Fast Track promotes positive outcomes for children (e.g., improvements in child behavior, social skills, emotion recognition, social problem solving, and language skills) and for parents (e.g., less use of physical punishment, improvements in parenting behaviors and satisfaction; Slough et al., 2008). Further, Fast Track appears to be cost-effective in terms of reducing the diagnosis of Conduct Disorder in children who are at the highest risk (Foster, Jones, & the Conduct Problems Prevention Research Group, 2006).

A second prevention program that has promising results thus far is *the Early Risers Preventive Intervention* program (Bernat et al., 2007). As part of this program, Kindergartners in 23 elementary schools were screened for aggressive behavior and then were assigned randomly to either the Early Risers program or a control condition. Those who were assigned to the program were provided an intensive intervention in their Kindergarten year through the summer after their Third Grade year and then partici- pated in a booster phase in the Fourth and Fifth Grades. The preventive intervention consists of five components, including a 6-day summer wilderness program emphasizing community building and peer support activities, a "Circle of Friends" group in which children met independently in six monthly groups per year, a Family Skills parent group in which expert speakers presented topics and tips to parents, as well as a Monitoring and Mentoring School Support and Family Support programs (Bernat et al., 2007). Chil- dren who participate experience significant increases in their academic achievement as well as in their cog- nitive competence and concentration (as rated by tea- chers) following the first 2 years of treatment and into the third program year (August, Realmuto, Hektner, & Bloomquist, 2001). At follow-up at the end of the Sixth Grade year, children who participate in the inter- vention show lower rates of conduct problems (Bernat et al., 2007). In particular, participation in this pro- gram appears to decrease nondeviant peer relations and improve social skills. These improvements then are related to decreases in children's symptoms (Ber- nat et al., 2007). Thus, preventive interventions may have benefits for children's social relationships as well as their emotional and behavioral functioning.

Commonalities Among EBTs: Why Are They Effective?

The EBTs described previously for children who have conduct problems may differ in format but overlap greatly in terms of the skills being taught and the behaviors being addressed. For children who have conduct problems, it appears that parents need to take an active role in the treatment inter- ventions provided to their children (Eyberg et al., 2008; Kazdin & Weisz, 2003). Children who have conduct problems may present additional chal- lenges to their mothers and fathers, resulting in poor relationships with their parents. Further, par- ents who have poor parenting skills may have an additional risk of negative interactions with their children (Frick, 1998). Accordingly, all the effective parent-focused treatment interventions described previously teach effective parenting skills while encouraging positive parent–child interactions,

consistency, and structure. They also encourage or implement modeling and active practicing of newly learned behaviors, further creating opportunities for positive parent–child interactions.

Although there are some promising child- focused treatment interventions, the most effective treatment interventions at this time are those that provide parent-focused treatment components and/ or that encourage parent involvement. Further, the child-focused approaches that teach problem sol- ving, anger management, and social skills seem to be enhanced when parents are taught how to foster these skills in their children at home, making them generalizable across settings. Thus, a second com- monality among the EBTs described previously is that they target the identified deficits often found in children who have conduct problems. For example, children who have conduct problems often have difficulty in social situations and with handling con- flict because they lack the cognitive ability to appro- priately appraise these situation and to identify how they, and those with whom they are interacting, are feeling (Kazdin, 2003, 2005). As a result, these chil- dren often are impulsive and unable to predict the consequences of their actions. They subsequently respond with negative problem solving skills (Kaz- din, 2005). Thus, all the child-focused treatment interventions described previously address pro- blem-solving skills. In particular, the important component related to effectiveness may be the inclu- sion of emotional awareness and increasing accu- rate perceptions of social situations.

Potentially Problematic Treatments

As described previously, EBTs for adolescents often utilize a group format and are employed in school settings. These group interventions that incorporate social skills training are considered an effective means of treating adolescents who are diagnosed with Conduct Disorder (Eyberg et al., 2008). There- fore, it would make sense that the most economical and convenient way to conduct treatment interven- tions for adolescents would be to use a group for- mat. The research literature on group treatment interventions provides mixed results, however. Although a meta-analysis by Weiss and colleagues

(2005) suggests that there is little evidence to indicate that group treatments are iatrogenic or that deviancy training underlies iatrogenic effects, other studies suggest that such group treatment interventions may actually cause more harm than benefit to adolescents.

A number of theories explain why many group treatment interventions, especially with older children and adolescents, may have iatrogenic effects. For example, De-Haan and MacDermid (1999) posit that the general stigma of being in treatment and its resulting influence on adolescents' self-concepts may be related to an increase in conduct problems. Iatrogenic effects also may be amplified by "deviancy training," or the reinforcement of deviant behavior by other group members (Dishion et al., 1999). In particular, social skills interventions with high-risk youth may increase the amount of contact that individuals have with other deviant peers, further contributing to their maladjustment (Dishion & Andrews, 1995).

Given the cost-effectiveness and convenience of group treatment interventions, along with the mixed findings regarding their effectiveness and/or potential harm to children who have conduct problems, certain points should be noted when considering group treatment interventions. First, deviancy training is likely to be of utmost concern for adolescents (Dishion et al., 1999), as adolescents are progressing from primarily identifying with their family members to seeking an identity through their relationships with their peers. Second, iatrogenic effects are likely to occur when group treatment interventions are lacking structure (Dodge, 1999). Third, low risk children or children who do not have a history of antisocial behavior are considered the most vulnerable to deviancy training influences (Dishion et al., 1999). These children may have experienced overall rejection by peers but have not associated with deviant peers until participating in such group treatment interventions (Weiss et al., 2005). Further, Mager, Milich, Harris, and Howard (2005) indicate that group treatments that include both high and low risk children may have greater iatrogenic effects and poorer outcomes than group treatment interventions that include only adolescents who are at high risk. It may be that group leaders unknowingly provide a greater amount of preferential treatment and positive reinforcement to those adolescents who are at low risk. This differential treatment may lead adolescents who are at high risk to mentally or emotionally withdraw from the group process and form a minority outgroup in which reinforcement is sought out from other deviant peers (Mager et al., 2005).

In contrast, the treatment interventions described previously are effective with very small groups (i.e., 6–8 adolescents) and with specific targeted populations (e.g., Assertiveness Training for adolescents who are in the Eighth and Ninth Grades; REMH for adolescents in the Eleventh and Twelfth Grades). Further, adolescents may benefit from more direct interventions as opposed to parent training programs (Eyberg et al., 2008). Thus, with these group treatment interventions, it appears that highly structured, very small groups are most effective. It is important, however, to consider children's age at the onset of their symptoms. For those children whose problematic behaviors do not emerge until adolescence, less intense, group treatment interventions may be enough to produce changes in behavior (Eyberg et al., 2008). For adolescents who have a long history of conduct problems, however, early problematic behaviors have the chance to worsen over time, likely resulting in poor parent–child relationships. As a result, incorporating parents into treatment interventions may be necessary to counteract this history of conduct problems, as evidenced by more intensive programs such as MST and MTFC (Eyberg et al., 2008).

Beyond the controversy regarding group treatment interventions, other treatment interventions also have problematic results, such as Scared Straight programs, drug abuse resistance education, and boot camp programs (see Lilienfeld, 2007). Scared Straight programs expose children who are at high risk for conduct problems to prison conditions in the hope that such an experience would be upsetting enough to deter them from committing acts of delinquency and crime in the future. Results indicate that children who take part in this type of program experience a significantly higher likelihood of offending and a significant increase in arrests, however (Lilienfeld, 2007; Petrosino, Turpin-Petrosino, & Buehler, 2003). Similarly, drug abuse resistance education, such as that included in the DARE program, is counterproductive. For example, Werch and Owen (2002) indicate that such programs are ineffective in teaching the necessary social skills to resist peer pressure to use drugs and are related to increased substance intake. Finally, boot camp interventions have mixed results regarding their effectiveness. This particular social skills program emphasizes discipline and obedience. It is associated, however, with a number of deaths and other related problems (e.g., dehydration; Lilienfeld, 2007). Thus, these treatment interventions are not recommended.

Considerations for Successful Intervention

Although effective EBTs are described for children who have conduct problems, many of these treatment interventions are only efficacious with specific age groups and in specific treatment formats. Further, these treatment interventions may decrease, but not always eliminate, conduct problems. Therefore, other confounding factors must be considered when choosing the most appropriate treatment interventions for children who have conduct problems. Age is an important confounding factor to consider. In particular, the developmental trajectories for those who are diagnosed with the Childhood-Onset Type versus those who are diagnosed with the Adolescent-Onset Type of Conduct Disorder vary greatly, resulting in tremendous individual differences in presenting symptoms (Frick, 2001). As noted previously, the Childhood-Onset Type of Conduct Disorder tends to be more chronic in nature and is linked to more severe, disruptive, and antisocial behaviors. Further, early conduct problems, when untreated, are often met with coercive, ineffective parenting strategies, leading to a deterioration of the parent–child relationship and a worsening of children's behavior. Over time, this coercive cycle may be an impetus for more severe antisocial and delinquent behaviors (Reid & Patterson, 1989). Although the Adolescent-Onset Type of Conduct Disorder may be situational or more normative in nature (Frick, 2001), presenting conduct problems still are of concern. Further, adolescence is a period marked by a striving for autonomy as well as a need to belong (Vander Zanden, Crandell, & Crandell, 2006). As such, deviant adolescent peer groups may lead to a worsening of symptoms, including engaging in dangerous, illegal activity with grave repercussions.

Therefore, although the Childhood-Onset Type and the Adolescent-Onset Type of Conduct Disorder may differ in presentation, they both require early, structured intervention to prevent degradation of children's behavior, degradation of the relationships between children and their parents, and the formation of deviant peer networks. As such, the most effective interventions for children who have long histories of conduct problems appear to be those that include a parent-focused component to treatment (Eyberg et al., 2008; Kazdin & Weisz, 2003). In these cases, individualized treatment interventions may be a beneficial supplement to many parent-focused interventions. Finally, when utilized, group treatment interventions should be small, highly structured, and prevent the formation of deviant peer networks and peer reinforcement for negative behavior (Dodge, 1999).

Second, children who have conduct problems vary greatly in their presenting symptoms, with a large number of children experiencing other comorbid disorders (e.g., ADHD, ODD; Kazdin, 1996). As a result, these children often have a myriad of co-occurring symptoms and other behavior problems (e.g., impulsivity, inattention, oppositionality, poor peer relationships) that complicate treatment. By treating only the symptoms of Conduct Disorder and not children's individualized presentation, mental health professionals may fail to treat problematic behaviors and/or may choose an ineffective treatment intervention. As the EBTs described previously are noted to decrease specific conduct problems that are characteristic of Conduct Disorder (e.g., noncompliance, disruptive behavior, aggression, oppositionality, delinquency) rather than addressing multiple diagnoses, these treatment interventions may not always be the most beneficial treatments for children who have comorbid conditions. In contrast, Kazdin and Whitley (2006) examine the effectiveness of PMT, PSST, or both (both categorized as *probably efficacious* treatments by Eyberg et al., 2008) in children who have comorbid conditions. The results of this study indicate that children who are diagnosed with Conduct Disorder or Oppositional Defiant Disorder (ODD) and have up to four additional diagnoses (i.e., are considered to have comorbid conditions) actually have greater behavioral changes relative to children with Conduct Disorder or ODD and no additional diagnoses. Thus, it seems that comorbid conditions may complicate treatment but that positive treatment effects are still possible when an appropriate treatment intervention is used.

Finally, confounding variables related to children's environments may interfere with treatment gains. For example, a number of confounding variables moderate or mediate the effects of psychosocial treatments (e.g., parental psychopathology and substance abuse, parents' marital adjustment, harsh and ineffective parenting practices; Beauchaine, Webster-Stratton, & Reid, 2005). Stressors in the home environment (e.g., low SES, poor educational opportunities, living in high-risk neighborhoods) are also likely related to the effectiveness of various treatments and the generalization of treatment gains across settings (Frick, 1998, 2001). Negative parental attitudes toward treatment also decrease the effectiveness of treatment interventions (Kazdin & Whitley, 2006). Thus, these factors are important to consider, especially with families who exhibit many of these characteristics and who have lost hope that their children's conduct problems will improve.

Conclusions

Based on the various characteristics of children who have conduct problems, the assessment options that are available, and the evidence-based treatment interventions that are beneficial for children who have conduct problems, it appears that no one approach will be best for all families who seek mental health services for their children who have conduct problems. It is clear, however, that children receiving services for conduct problems will benefit from early intervention that is tailored individually to their specific needs and those of their families. As a result, it behooves the field to move in the direction of matching the characteristics of families who present for services in response to their children's conduct problems to the treatments that they are to receive. Research should examine these issues carefully so as to maximize the effectiveness of the treatments that are used. As the research literature continues to develop this area of interest, special considerations should be given to children's age at the onset of their conduct problems, children's age

when their families seek treatment, the presence of comorbid disorders, and other potential barriers to treatment (e.g., parental psychopathology, ineffective parenting, high degree of daily stressors, parental attitude toward treatment) as assessment protocols and subsequent treatment interventions are selected.

Once the most appropriate treatment intervention is identified and implemented, treatment gains should be monitored continually so that mental health professionals can remain flexible and open to alternative and/or supplemental methods of treatment. As part of this endeavor, future research should examine the differential effectiveness of the many components included in the treatment interventions described above as well as the utility of using different intensities of treatment interventions (e.g., intervention length, inclusion of one versus many system levels). Finally, research should continue to develop and examine evidence-based prevention programs so that families and the communities in which they live can foster environments that enrich the experiences of their children. In this way, children who are at risk for or already have conduct problems can show the greatest improvements in their social relationships and their emotional and behavioral functioning with the most suitable but efficient treatment intervention.

References

Achenbach, T. M., & Rescorla, L. A. (2001). *Manual for the ASEBA school-age forms and profiles.* Burlington: University of Vermont, Research Center for Children, Youth, and Families.

Ackerman, B. P., Brown, E. D., D'Eramo, K. S., & Izard, C. E. (2002). Maternal relationship instability and the school behavior of children from disadvantaged families. *Developmental Psychology, 38,* 694–704.

American Psychiatric Association (APA). (2000). *Diagnostic and statistical manual of mental disorders* (4th ed., text rev.). Washington, DC: American Psychiatric Association.

Arseneault, L., Moffitt, T. E., Caspi, A., Taylor, A., Rijsdijk, F. V., Jaffee, S. R., et al. (2003). Strong genetic effects on cross-situational antisocial behavior among 5-year-old children according to mothers, teachers, examiner-observers, and twins' self-reports. *Journal of Child Psychology and Psychiatry, 44,* 832–848.

Aspland, H., & Gardner, F. (2003). Observational measures of parent–child interaction: An introductory review. *Child and Adolescent Mental Health, 8*, 136–143.

August, G. J., Realmuto, G. M., Hektner, J. M., & Bloomquist, M. L. (2001). An integrated components preventive intervention for aggressive elementary school children: The Early Risers program. *Journal of Consulting and Clinical Psychology, 69*, 614–626.

Barkley, R. A. (1997). *Defiant children: A clinician's manual for assessment and parent training* (2nd ed.). New York: The Guilford Press.

Barkley, R. A., Edwards, G. H., & Robin, A. L. (1999). *Defiant teens: A clinician's manual for assessment and family intervention.* New York: The Guilford Press.

Bates, J. E. (2001). Adjustment style in childhood as a product of parenting and temperament. In T. D. Wach & G. A. Kohnstamm (Eds.), *Temperament in context* (pp. 173–200). Mahwah, NJ: Lawrence Erlbaum.

Beauchaine, T. P., Webster-Stratton, C., & Reid, M. J. (2005). Mediators, moderators, and predictors of 1-year outcomes among children treated for early-onset conduct problems: A latent growth curve analysis. *Journal of Consulting and Clinical Psychology, 73*, 371–388.

Bernat, D. H., August, G. J., Hektner, J. M., & Bloomquist, M. L. (2007). The Early Risers Preventive Intervention: Testing for six-year outcomes and mediational processes. *Journal of Abnormal Child Psychology, 35*, 605–617.

Block, J. (1978). Effects of a rational-emotive mental health program on poorly achieving, disruptive high school students. *Journal of Counseling Psychology, 25*, 61–65.

Boggs, S. R., Eyberg, S. M., Edwards, D. L., Rayfield, A., Jacobs, J., Bagner, D., et al. (2005). Outcomes of parent–child interaction therapy: A comparison of treatment completers and study dropouts one to three years later. *Child and Family Behavior Therapy, 26*, 1–22.

Borduin, C. M., Henggeler, S. W., & Manley, C. M. (1995). Conduct and oppositional disorders. In V. B. Van Hasselt & M. Hersen (Eds.), *Handbook of adolescent psychopathology* (pp. 349–383). New York: Lexington Books.

Borduin, C. M., Mann, B. J., & Cone, L. T. (1995). Multisystemic treatment of serious juvenile offenders: Long-term prevention of criminality and violence. *Journal of Consulting and Clinical Psychology, 63*, 569–578.

Brestan, E. V., & Eyberg, S. M. (1998). Effective psychosocial treatments of conduct-disordered children and adolescents: 29 years, 82 studies, and 5,272 kids. *Journal of Clinical Child Psychology, 27*, 180–189.

Brinkmeyer, M. Y., & Eyberg, S. M. (2003). Parent–child interaction therapy for oppositional children. In A. E. Kazdin & J. R. Weisz (Eds.), *Evidence-based psychotherapies for children and adolescents* (pp. 204–223). New York: Guilford.

Brook, J. S., Whiteman, M., Finch, S. J., & Cohen, P. (1996). Young adult drug use and delinquency: Childhood antecedents and adolescent mediators. *Journal of the American Academy of Child and Adolescent Psychiatry, 35*, 1584–1592.

Brotman, L. M., Gouley, K. K., Chesir-Teran, D., Dennis, T., Klein, R. G., & Shrout, P. (2005). Prevention for preschoolers at high risk for conduct problems: Immediate outcomes on parenting practices and child social competence.

Journal of Clinical Child and Adolescent Psychology, 34, 724–734.

Byrne, B. M., & Schneider, B. H. (1985). Factorial validity of Stephens' Social Behavior Assessment. *Journal of Consulting and Clinical Psychology, 53*, 259–260.

Calkins, S. D., Hungerford, A., & Dedmon, S. E. (2004). Mothers' interactions with temperamentally frustrated infants. *Infant Mental Health Journal, 25*, 219–239.

Campbell, S. B. (1990). *Behavior problems in preschool children: Clinical and developmental issues.* New York: Guilford Press.

Campbell, S. B., Pierce, E. W., Moore, G., Marakovitz, S., & Newby, K. (1996). Boys' externalizing problems at elementary school age: Pathways from early behavior problems maternal control, and family stress. *Development and Psychopathology, 8*, 701–719.

Capage, L. C., Foote, R., McNeil, C. B., & Eyberg, S. M. (1998). Parent–child interaction therapy: An effective treatment for young children with conduct problems. *The Behavior Therapist, 21*, 137–138.

Capaldi, D. M., Crosby, L., & Stoolmiller, M. (1996). Predicting the timing of first sexual intercourse for at-risk adolescent males. *Child Development, 67*, 344–359.

Caspi, A., Henry, B., Mcgee, R. O., Moffitt, T. E., & Silva, P. A. (1995). Temperamental origins of child and adolescent behavior problems: From age three to age fifteen. *Child Development, 66*, 55–68.

Caspi, A., Mcclay, J., Moffitt, T., Mill, J., Martin, J., & Craig, I. W. (2002). Role of genotype in the cycle of violence in maltreated children. *Science, 297*, 851–854.

Chamberlain, P., Leve, L. D., & DeGarmo, D. S. (2007). Multidimensional treatment foster care for girls in the juvenile justice system: 2-year follow-up of a randomized clinical trial. *Journal of Consulting and Clinical Psychology, 75*, 187–193.

Chamberlain, P., & Reid, J. B. (1998). Comparison of two community alternatives to incarceration for chronic juvenile offenders. *Journal of Consulting and Clinical Psychology, 66*, 624–633.

Chamberlain, P., & Smith, D. K. (2003). Antisocial behavior in children and adolescents: The Oregon Multidimensional Treatment Foster Care Model. In A. E. Kazdin & J. R. Weisz (Eds.), *Evidence-based psychotherapies for children and adolescents* (pp. 282–300). New York: Guilford.

Chambless, D. L., & Hollon, S. D. (1998). Defining empirically supported therapies. *Journal of Consulting and Clinical Psychology, 66*, 7–18.

Chambless, D. L., & Ollendick, T. H. (2001). Empirically supported psychological interventions: Controversies and evidence. *Annual Review in Psychology, 52*, 685–716.

Christophersen, E. R., & Mortweet, S. L. (2002). *Treatments that work with children: Empirically supported strategies for managing childhood problems.* Washington, DC: American Psychological Association.

Clark, L., Gresham, F. M., & Elliott, S. N. (1985). Development and validation of a social skills assessment measure: The TROSS-C. *Journal of Psychoeducational Assessment, 4*, 347–356.

Cohen, M. A. (1998). The monetary value of saving a high-risk youth. *Journal of Quantitative Criminology, 14*, 5–33.

Dadds, M. R., Fraser, J., Frost, A., & Hawes, D. J. (2005). Disentangling the underlying dimensions of psychopathy and conduct problems in childhood: A community study. *Journal of Consulting and Clinical Psychology, 73,* 400–410.

Day, N. L., Richardson, G. A., Goldschmidt, L., & Cornelius, M. D. (2000). Effects of prenatal tobacco exposure on preschoolers' behavior. *Journal of Developmental and Behavioral Pediatrics, 21,* 180–188.

de Cubas, M. M., & Field, T. (1993). Children of methadone-dependent women: Developmental outcomes. *American Journal of Orthopsychiatry, 63,* 266–276.

De-Haan, L. G., & MacDermid, S. M. (1999). Identity development as a mediating factor between urban poverty and behavioral outcomes for junior high school students. *Journal of Family and Economic Issues, 20,* 123–148.

Dishion, T. J., & Andrews, D. W. (1995). Preventing escalation in problem behaviors with high-risk young adolescents: Immediate and 1-year outcomes. *Journal of Consulting and Clinical Psychology, 63,* 538–548.

Dishion, T. J., McCord, J., & Poulin, F. (1999). When interventions harm: Peer groups and problem behavior. *American Psychologist, 54,* 755–764.

Dodge, K. A. (1999). Cost effectiveness of psychotherapy for child aggression. First, is there cost effectiveness? *Group Dynamics: Theory, Research, and Practice, 3,* 275–278.

Dodge, K. A., & Pettit, G. S. (2003). A biophysiological model of the development of chronic conduct problems in adolescence. *Developmental Psychology, 39,* 349–371.

Drugli, M. B., Larsson, B., & Clifford, G. (2007). Changes in social competence in young children treatment because of conduct problems as viewed by multiple informants. *European Child and Adolescent Psychiatry, 16,* 370–378.

Eisenstadt, T. H., Eyberg, S., McNeil, C. B., Newcomb, K., & Funderburk, B. (1993). Parent–child interaction therapy with behavior problem children: Relative effectiveness of two stages and overall treatment outcome. *Journal of Clinical Child Psychology, 22,* 42–51.

Eyberg, S. M. (2003). Parent–child interaction therapy. In T. H. Ollendick & C. S. Schroeder (Eds.), *Encyclopedia of clinical child and pediatric psychology.* New York: Plenum.

Eyberg, S. M., Boggs, S. R., & Algina, J. (1995). New developments in psychosocial, pharmacological, and combined treatments of conduct disorders in aggressive children. *Psychopharmacology Bulletin, 31,* 83–91.

Eyberg, S. M., Funderburk, B. W., Hembree-Kigin, T. L., Mcneil, C. B., Querido, J. G., & Hood, K. K. (2001). Parent–child interaction therapy with behavior problem children: One and two year maintenance of treatment effects in the family. *Child and Family Behavior Therapy, 23,* 1–20.

Eyberg, S. M., Nelson, M. M., & Boggs, S. R. (2008). Evidence-based psychosocial treatments for children and adolescents with disruptive behavior. *Journal of Child and Adolescent Psychology, 37,* 215–237.

Eyberg, S. M., & Robinson, E. A. (1982). Parent–child interaction training: Effects on family functioning. *Journal of Clinical Child Psychology, 11,* 130–137.

Farmer, E. M. Z., Compton, S. N., Burns, B. J., & Robertson, E. (2005). Review of the evidence base for treatment of childhood psychopathology: Externalizing disorders. *Journal of Consulting and Clinical Psychology, 70,* 1267–1302.

Fergusson, D.M., Horwood, L.J., & Ridder, E.M. (2005). Show me the child at seven: The consequence of conduct problems in childhood for psychological functioning in adulthood. *Journal of Child Physchology and Psychiatry, 46,* 837–849.

Fergusson, D. M., Swain-Campbell, N. R., & Horwood, L. J. (2002). Deviant peer affiliations, crime and substance use: A fixed effects regression analysis. *Journal of Abnormal Child Psychology, 30,* 419–430.

Filcheck, H. A., McNeil, C. B., Greco, L. A., & Bernard, R. S. (2004). Using a whole-class token economy and coaching of teacher skills in a preschool classroom to manage disruptive behavior. *Psychology in the Schools, 41,* 351–361.

Findling, R. (2003). Dosing of atypical antipsychotics in children and adolescents. *Primary Care Companion Journal of Clinical Psychiatry, 5,* 10–13.

Forehand, R., & King, H. E. (1974). Pre-school children's non-compliance: Effects of short-term behavior therapy. *Journal of Community Psychology, 2,* 42–44.

Forehand, R., & King, H. E. (1977). Noncompliant children: Effects of parent training on behavior and attitude change. *Behavior Modification, 1,* 93–108.

Forehand, R., & McMahon, R. J. (1981). *Helping the non-compliant child: A clinician's guide to parent training.* New York: Guilford.

Foster, E. M., Jones, D. E., & the Conduct Problems Prevention Research Group. (2005). The high costs of aggression: Public expenditures resulting from conduct disorder. *American Journal of Public Health, 95,* 1767–1772.

Foster, E. M., Jones, D. E., & the Conduct Problems Prevention Research Group. (2006). Can a costly intervention be cost-effective? An analysis of violence prevention. *Archives of General Psychiatry, 63,* 1284–1291.

Foster, E. M., Kelsch, C. C., Kamradt, B., Sosna, T., & Yang, Z. (2001). Expenditures and sustainability in systems of care. *Journal of Emotional and Behavioral Disorders, 9,* 53–62.

Frick, P. J. (1998). *Conduct disorders and severe antisocial behavior.* New York: Plenum Press.

Frick, P. J. (2001). Effective interventions for children and adolescents with conduct disorder. *Canadian Journal of Psychiatry, 46,* 597–608.

Frick, P. J. (2004). Developmental pathways to conduct disorder: Implications for serving youth who show severe aggressive and antisocial behavior. *Psychology in the Schools, 41,* 823–834.

Frick, P. J., Cornell, A. H., Barry, C. T., Bodin, S. D., & Dane, H. A. (2003). Callous-unemotional traits and conduct problems in the prediction of conduct problem severity, aggression, and self-report of delinquency. *Journal of Abnormal Child Psychology, 31,* 457–470.

Frick, P. J., & Dantagnan, A. L. (2005). Predicting the stability of conduct problems in children with and without callous-unemotional traits. *Journal of Child and Family Studies, 14,* 469–485.

Frick, P. J., & Ellis, M. L. (1999). Callous-unemotional traits and subtypes of conduct disorder. *Clinical Child and Family Psychology Review, 2,* 149–168.

Frick, P. J., & Loney, B. R. (1999). Outcomes of children and adolescents with conduct disorder and oppositional defiant disorder. In H. C. Quay & A. Hogan (Eds.), *Handbook of disruptive behavior disorders* (pp. 507–524). New York: Plenum.

Frick, P. J., & Morris, A. S. (2004). Temperament and developmental pathways to conduct problems. *Journal of Clinical Child and Adolescent Psychology, 33,* 54–68.

Frick, P. J., O'Brien, B. S., Wootton, J. M., & Mcburnett, K. (1994). Psychopathy and conduct problems in children. *Journal of Abnormal Child Psychology, 103,* 700–707.

Gadow, K. D., Sprafkin, J., & Nolan, E. E. (2001). DSM-IV symptoms in community and clinic preschool children. *Journal of the American Academy of Child and Adolescent Psychiatry, 40,* 1383–1392.

Gardner, F., Ward, S., Burton, J., & Wilson, C. (2003). The role of mother-child joint play in the early development of children's conduct problems: A longitudinal observational study. *Social Development, 12,* 361–378.

Gilmour, J., Hill, B., Place, M., & Skuse, D. H. (2004). Social communication deficits in conduct disorder: A clinical and community survey. *Journal of Child Psychology and Psychiatry, 45,* 967–978.

Gorman-Smith, D., & Tolan, P. (1998). The role of exposure to community violence and developmental problems among inner-city youth. *Development and Psychopathology, 10,* 101–116.

Greco, L. A., Sorrell, J. T., & McNeil, C. B. (2001). Understanding manual-based behavior therapy: Some theoretical foundations of parent–child interaction therapy. *Child and Family Behavior Therapy, 23,* 21–36.

Greenberg, M. T., Speltz, M. L., Deklyen, M., & Jones, K. (2001). Correlates of clinic referral for early conduct problems: Variable- and person-oriented approaches. *Development and Psychopathology, 13,* 255–276.

Gresham, F. M., & Elliott, S. N. (1990). *Social skills rating system.* Circle Pines, Minnesota: American Guidance Service.

Harter, S. (1985). *Manual fort he self-perception profile for children.* Denver, CO: University of Denver.

Hartung, C. M., McCarthy, D. M., Milich, R., & Martin, C. A. (2005). Parent-adolescent agreement on disruptive behavior symptoms: A multitrait-multimethod model. *Journal of Psychopathology and Behavioral Assessment, 27,* 159–168.

Hawkins, J. D., Catalono, R. F., & Miller, J. Y. (1992). Risk and protective factors for alcohol and other drug problems in adolescence and early adulthood: Implications for substance abuse prevention. *Psychological Bulletin, 112,* 64–105.

Hembree-Kigin, T. L., & McNeil, C. B. (1995). *Parent–child interaction therapy.* New York: Plenum Press.

Henggeler, S. W., & Lee, T. (2003). Multisystemic treatment of serious clinical problems. In A. E. Kazdin & J. R. Weisz (Eds.), *Evidence-based psychotherapies for children and adolescents* (pp. 301–322). New York: Guilford.

Herschell, A. D., Calzada, E. J., Eyberg, S. M., & McNeil, C. B. (2002). Parent–child interaction therapy: New directions in research. *Cognitive and Behavioral Practice, 9,* 9–16.

Hinshaw, S. P., Zupan, B. A., Simmel, C., Nigg, J. T., & Melnick, S. (1997). Peer status in boys with and without attention-deficit hyperactivity disorder: Predictions from overt and covert antisocial behavior, social isolation, and authoritative parenting beliefs. *Child Development, 68,* 880–896.

Holmes, S. E., Slaughter, J. R., & Kashani, J. (2001). Risk factors in childhood that lead to the development of conduct disorder and antisocial personality disorder. *Child Psychiatry and Human Development, 31,* 183–193.

Hood, K. K., & Eyberg, S. M. (2003). Outcomes of parent–child interaction therapy: Mothers' reports of maintenance three to six years after treatment. *Journal of Clinical Child and Adolescent Psychology, 32,* 419–429.

Huey, W. C., & Rank, R. C. (1984). Effects of counselor and peer-led group assertive training on black adolescent aggression. *Journal of Counseling Psychology, 31,* 95–98.

Hughes, J. N., Boodoo, G., Alcala, J., Maggio, M., Moore, L., & Villapando, R. (1989). Validation of a role-play measure of children's social skills. *Journal of Abnormal Child Psychology, 17,* 633–646.

Hymel, S. (1983). Preschool children's peer relations: Issues in sociometric assessment. *Merrill-Palmer Quarterly, 29,* 237–260.

Jensen, P. S., Watanabe, H. K., & Richters, J. E. (1999). Who's up first? Testing for order effects in structured interviews using a counterbalanced experimental design. *Journal of Abnormal Child Psychology, 27,* 439–445.

Johnson, R. M., Kotch, J. B., Catellier, D. J., Dufort, V., Hunter, W., & Amaya-Jackson, L. (2002). Adverse behavioral and emotional outcomes from child abuse and witnessed violence. *Child Maltreatment, 7,* 179–186.

Kaufman, J., Birmaher, B., Brent, D., & Rao, U. (1997). Schedule for affective disorders and schizophrenia for school-age children-present and lifetime version (K-SADS-PL): Initial reliability and validity data. *Journal of the American Academy of Child and Adolescent Psychiatry, 36,* 980–988.

Kazdin, A. E. (1996). Problem solving and parent management in treating aggressive and antisocial behavior. In E. D. Hibbs & P. S. Jensen (Eds.), *Psychosocial treatments for child and adolescent disorders: Empirically based strategies for clinical practice* (pp. 377–408). Washington, DC: American Psychological Association.

Kazdin, A. E. (2003). Problem-solving skills training and parent management training for conduct disorder. In A. E. Kazdin & J. R. Weisz (Eds.), *Evidence-based psychotherapies for children and adolescents* (pp. 241–262). New York: Guilford.

Kazdin, A. E. (2005). *Parent management training: Treatment for oppositional, aggressive and antisocial behavior in children and adolescents.* New York, NY: Oxford University Press.

Kazdin, A. E., Siegel, T. C., & Bass, D. (1992). Cognitive problem-solving skills training and parent management training in the treatment of antisocial behavior in children. *Journal of Consulting and Clinical Psychology, 60,* 733–747.

Kazdin, A. E., & Wassell, G. (1998). Treatment completion and therapeutic change among children referred for outpatient therapy. *Professional Psychology: Research and Practice, 29,* 332–340.

Kazdin, A. E., & Weisz, J. R. (2003). Introduction: Context and background of evidence-based psychotherapies for children and adolescents. In A. E. Kazdin & J. R. Weisz (Eds.), *Evidence-based psychotherapies for children and adolescents* (pp. 3–20). New York: Guilford.

Kazdin, A. E., & Whitley, M. K. (2006). Comorbidity, case complexity, and effects of evidence-based treatment for children referred for disruptive behavior. *Journal of Consulting and Clinical Psychology, 74*, 455–467.

Keenan, K., Shaw, D., Delliquadri, E., Giovannelli, J., & Walsh, B. (1998). Evidence for the continuity of early problem behaviors: Application of a developmental model. *Journal of Abnormal Child Psychology, 26*, 441–454.

Kiesner, J., Dishion, T. J., & Poulin, F. (2001). A reinforcement model for conduct problems in children and adolescence: Advance in theory and intervention. In J. Hill & B. Maughan (Eds.), *Conduct disorders in childhood and adolescence* (pp. 264–291). Cambridge: Cambridge University Press.

Kim-Cohen, J., Caspi, A., Moffitt, T. E., Harrington, H., Milne, B. J., & Poulton, R. (2003). Prior juvenile diagnoses in adults with mental disorders: Developmental follow-back of a prospective-longitudinal cohort. *Archives of General Psychiatry, 60*, 709–717.

Kim-Cohen, J., Caspi, A., Taylor, A., Williams, B., Newcombe, R., & Craig, I. W. (2006). MAOA, maltreatment, and gene-environment interactions predicting children's mental health: New evidence and a meta-analysis. *Molecular Psychiatry, 11*, 903–913.

Knock, M. K., Kazdin, A. E., Hiripi, E., & Kessler, R. C. (2006). Prevalence, subtypes, and correlates of DSM-IV conduct disorder in the National Comorbidity Survey replication. *Psychological Medicine, 36*, 699–710.

Kohn, M., & Rosman, B. L. (1972). A social competence sale and symptom checklist for the preschool child: Factor dimensions, their cross-instrument generality, and longitudinal persistence. *Developmental Psychology, 6*, 430–444.

Kruesi, M. J. P., Hibbs, E. D., Zahn, T. P., Keysor, T. S., Hamburger, S. D., Bartko, J. J., et al. (1992). A 2-year prospective follow-up study of children and adolescents with disruptive behavior disorders: Prediction by cerebrospinal fluid 5-hydroxyindoleacetic acid, homovanallic acid, and autonomic measures? *Archives of General Psychiatry, 49*, 429–435.

Kruesi, M. J., Rapoport, J. L., Hamburger, S., Hibbs, E., Potter, W. Z., & Lenane, M. (1990). Cerebrospinal fluid monoamine metabolites, aggression, and impulsivity in disruptive behavior disorders of children and adolescents. *Archives of General Psychiatry, 47*, 419–426.

Lafreniere, P. J., Dumas, J., Capuano, F., & Dubeau, D. (1992). The development and validation of the preschool socio-affective profile. *Psychological Assessment: Journal of Consulting and Clinical Psychology, 4*, 442–450.

Landau, S., & Milich, R. (1990). Assessment of children's social status and peer relations. In A. M. LaGreca (Ed.), *Through the eyes of the child: Obtaining self-reports from children and adolescents*. Boston: Allyn and Bacon.

Leventhal, T., & Brooks-Gunn, J. (2000). The neighborhoods they live in: The effects of neighborhood and residence on child and adolescent outcomes. *Psychological Bulletin, 126*, 309–337.

Liaw, F., & Brooks-Gunn, J. (1994). Cumulative familial risks and low birth weight children's cognitive and behavioral development. *Journal of Clinical Child Psychology, 23*, 360–372.

Lilienfeld, S. O. (2007). Psychological treatments that cause harm. *Perspectives on Psychological Science, 2*, 53–70.

Lochman, J. E. (1992). Cognitive-behavioral intervention with aggressive boys: Three-year follow-up and preventive effects. *Journal of Consulting and Clinical Psychology, 60*, 426–432.

Lochman, J. E., Barry, T. D., & Pardini, D. (2003). Anger control training for aggressive youth. In A. E. Kazdin & J. R. Weisz (Eds.), *Evidence-based psychotherapies for children and adolescents* (pp. 263–281). New York: Guilford.

Loeber, R., Green, S. M., Keenan, K., & Lahey, B. B. (1995). Which boys will fare worse? Early predictors of conduct disorder in a six-year longitudinal study. *Journal of the American Academy of Child and Adolescent Psychiatry, 34*, 499–509.

Loeber, R., Wung, P., Keenan, K., Giroux, B., Stouthamer-Loeber, M., Van Kammen, W. B., et al. (1993). Developmental pathways in child disruptive behavior. *Development and Psychopathology, 5*, 101–131.

Loney, B. R., & Frick, P. J. (2003). Structured diagnostic interviewing. In C. R. Reynolds & R. W. Kamphaus (Eds.), *Handbook of educational assessment of children* (2nd ed., pp. 235–247). New York: Guilford.

Loney, B. R., Taylor, J., Butler, M. A., & Iacono, W. G. (2007). Adolescent psychopathy features: 6-year temporal stability and the prediction of externalizing symptoms during the transition to adulthood. *Aggressive Behavior, 33*, 242–252.

Luby, J., & Morgan, K. (1997). Characteristics of an infant/preschool psychiatric clinic sample: Implications for clinical assessment and nosology. *Infant Mental Health Journal, 18*, 209–220.

Lynam, D. R. (1998). Early identification of the fledgling psychopath: Locating the psychopathic child in the current nomenclature. *Journal of Abnormal Psychology, 107*, 566–575.

Lynam, D. R., & Henry, V. (2001). The role of neuropsychological deficits in conduct disorders. In J. Hill & B. Maughan (Eds.), *Conduct disorders in childhood and adolescence*. Cambridge: Cambridge University Press.

Lynam, D. R., Moffitt, T. E., & Stouthamer-Loeber, M. (1993). Expanding the relationship between IQ and delinquency: Class, race, test motivation, school failure, or self-control? *Journal of Abnormal Psychology, 102*, 187–196.

Macbrayer, E. K., Milich, R., & Hundley, M. (2003). Attributional biases in aggressive children and their mothers. *Journal of Abnormal Psychology, 112*, 698–708.

Mager, W., Millich, R., Harris, M. J., & Howard, A. (2005). Intervention groups for adolescents with conduct problems: Is aggregation harmful or helpful? *Journal of Abnormal Child Psychology, 33*, 349–362.

Manuck, S. B., Flory, J. D., Ferrell, R. E., Dent, K. M., Mann, J. J., & Muldoon, M. F. (1999). Aggression and anger-related traits associated with a polymorphism of the tryptophan hydroxylase gene. *Biological Psychiatry*, *45*, 603–614.

Maughan, B., Rowe, R., Messer, J., Goodman, R., & Meltzer, H. (2004). Conduct disorder and oppositional defiant disorder in a national sample: Developmental epidemiology. *Journal of Child Psychology and Psychiatry*, *45*, 609–621.

Mccabe, K. M., Lucchini, S. E., Hough, R. L., Yeh, M., & Hazen, A. (2005). The relation between violence exposure and conduct problems among adolescents: A prospective study. *American Journal of Orthopsychiatry*, *75*, 575–584.

McKinney, C., & Renk, K. (2006). Similar presentations of disparate etiologies: A new perspective on oppositional defiant disorder. *Child and Family Behavior Therapy*, *28*, 37–48.

McKinney, C., & Renk, K. (2007). Emerging research and theory in the etiology of oppositional defiant disorder: Current concerns and future directions. *International Journal of Behavior Consultation and Therapy*, *3*, 349–371.

McMahon, R. J., & Estes, A. M. (1997). Conduct problems. In E. J. Mash & L. G. Terdal (Eds.), *Assessment of childhood disorders* (3rd ed., pp. 130–193). New York: Guilford.

McMahon, R. J., & Forehand, R. L. (2003). *Helping the noncompliant child: Family-based treatment for oppositional behavior* (2nd ed.). New York: Guilford.

McMahon, R. J., & Frick, P. J. (2005). Evidence-based assessment of conduct problems in children and adolescents. *Journal of Clinical Child and Adolescent Psychology*, *34*, 477–505.

McNeil, C. B., Eyberg, S., Eisenstadt, T. H., Newcomb, K., & Funderburk, B. (1991). Parent-child interaction therapy with behavior problem children: Generalization of treatment effects to the school setting. *Journal of Clinical Child Psychology*, *20*, 140–151.

Merrell, K. W. (1993). *School social behavior scales*. Iowa City: Assessment Intervention Resources.

Merrell, K. W. (2001). Assessment of children's social skills: Recent developments, best practices, and new directions. *Exceptionality*, *9*, 3–18.

Meyer, G. J., Finn, S. E., Eyde, L. D., Kay, G. G., Moreland, K. L., Dies, R. R., et al. (2001). Psychological testing and psychological assessment: A review of evidence and issues. *American Psychologist*, *56*, 128–165.

Miller-Johnson, S., Lochman, J. E., Coie, J. D., Terry, R., & Hyman, C. (1998). Comorbidity of conduct and depressive problems at sixth grade: Substance use outcomes across adolescence. *Journal of Abnormal Child Psychology*, *26*, 221–232.

Moffitt, T. E. (1990). The neuropsychology of delinquency: A critical review of theory and research. In M. Morris & M. Tonry (Eds.), *Crime and justice: An annual review of research* (Vol. 12, pp. 99–169). Chicago: University of Chicago Press.

Moffitt, T. E. (1993). Adolescence-limited and life-course persistent antisocial behavior: A developmental taxonomy. *Psychological Review*, *100*, 674–701.

Moffitt, T. E. (2003). Life-course persistent and adolescent-limited antisocial behavior: A 10-year research review and research agenda. In B. B. Lahey, T. E. Moffitt, & A. Caspi (Eds.), *Causes of conduct disorder and juvenile delinquency* (pp. 49–75). New York: Guilford.

Moffitt, T. E., & Caspi, A. (2001). Childhood predictors differentiate life-course persistent and adolescent-limited antisocial pathways in males and females. *Development and Psychopathology*, *8*, 399–424.

Moffitt, T. E., Caspi, A., Dickinson, N., Silva, P., & Stanton, W. (1996). Childhood-onset versus adolescent-onset antisocial conduct problems in males: Natural history from ages 3 to 18 years. *Development and Psychopathology*, *8*, 399–342.

Moffitt, T. E., & Lynam, D. R. (1994). The neuropsychology of conduct disorder and delinquency: Implications for understanding antisocial behavior. In D. Fowles, P. Sutker, & S. Goodman (Eds.), *Psychopathy and antisocial personality: A developmental perspective* (Vol. 18, pp. 233–262). New York: Springer.

Olfson, M., Blanco, C., Liu, L., Moreno, C., & Laje, G. (2006). National trends in the outpatient treatment of children and adolescents with antipsychotic drugs. *Archives of General Psychiatry*, *63*, 679–685.

Patterson, G. R. (1982). *Coercive family process*. Eugene, OR: Castalia.

Patterson, G. R., Chamberlain, P., & Reid, J. B. (1982). A comparative evaluation of a parent-training program. *Behavior Therapy*, *13*, 638–650.

Patterson, G. R., & Gullion, M. E. (1968). *Living with children: New methods for parents and teachers*, Champaign, IL: Research Press.

Patterson, G. R., Reid, J. B., & Dishion, T. J. (1992). Antisocial boys. Eugene, OR: Castalia.

Patterson, G. R., Reid, J. B., & Eddy, J. M. (2002). A brief history of the Oregon model. In J. B. Reid, G. R. Patterson, & J. Snyder (Eds.), *Antisocial behavior in children and adolescents: A developmental analysis and model for intervention* (pp. 3–21). Washington, DC: American Psychological Association.

Patterson, G. R., Reid, J. B., Jones, R. R., & Conger, R. E. (1975). *A social learning approach to family intervention: Families with aggressive children (Vol. 1)*. Eugene, OR: Castalia.

Pelham, W. E. (1993). Pharmocotherapy for children with attention-deficit hyperactivity disorder. *School Psychology Review*, *22*, 199–227.

Petrosino, A., Turpin-Petrosino, C., & Buehler, J. (2003). Scared Straight and other juvenile awareness programs for preventing juvenile delinquency: A systematic review of the randomized experimental evidence. *Annals of the American Academy of Political and Social Science*, *589*, 41–62.

Pinderhughes, E. E., Nix, R., Foster, E. M., Dones, D., Bierman, K. L., Coie, J. D., et al. (2001). Parenting in context: Impact of neighborhood poverty, residential stability, public services, social networks, and danger on parental behaviors. *Journal of Marriage and Family*, *63*, 941–953.

Poulin, F., & Boivin, M. (2000). The role of proactive and reactive aggression in the formation and development of boys' friendships. *Developmental Psychology*, *36*, 233–240.

Reich, W. (2000). Diagnostic interview for children and adolescents (DICA). *Journal of the American Academy of Child and Adolescent Psychiatry*, *39*, 59–66.

Reid, W. H., Dorr, D., Walker, J. I., & Bonner, J. W. (1986). *Unmasking the psychopath: Antisocial personality and related syndromes.* New York: Norton.

Reid, J. B., & Patterson, G. R. (1989). The development of antisocial behavior patterns in childhood and adolescence. *European Journal of Personality, 3,* 107–119.

Reid, M. J., & Webster-Stratton, C. (2001). The Incredible Years parent, teacher, and child intervention: Targeting multiple areas of risk for a young child with pervasive conduct problems using a flexible, manualized treatment program. *Cognitive and Behavioral Practice, 8,* 377–386.

Renk, K. (2005). Reasons young children are referred for psychological services. *Child and Family Behavior Therapy, 27,* 61–71.

Renk, K., & Phares, V. (2004). Cross-informant ratings of social competence in children and adolescents. *Clinical Psychology Review, 24,* 239–254.

Renshaw, P. D., & Asher, S. R. (1983). Children's goals and strategies for social interaction. *Merrill-Palmer Quarterly, 29,* 353–375.

Rhee, S. H., & Waldman, I. D. (2002). Genetic and environmental influences on antisocial behavior: A meta-analysis of twin and adoption studies. *Psychological Bulletin, 128,* 490–529.

Robinson, E. A., & Eyberg, S. M. (1981). The dyadic parent-child interaction coding system: Standardization and validation. *Journal of Consulting and Clinical Psychology, 49,* 245–250.

Rockett, J. L., Murie, D. C., & Boccaccini, M. T. (2007). Diagnostic labeling in juvenile justice settings: Do psychopathy and conduct disorder findings influence clinicians? *Psychological Services, 4,* 107–122.

Rockhill, C. M., Collett, B. R., Mcclellan, J. M., & Speltz, M. L. (2006). Oppositional defiant disorder. In J. L. Luby (Ed.), *Handbook of preschool mental health: Development, disorders, and treatment* (pp. 80–114). New York: The Guilford Press.

Rutter, M., Giller, H., & Hagell, A. (1998). *Antisocial behavior by young people.* New York: Cambridge University Press.

Sanders, M. R. (1999). Triple P-positive parenting program: Towards an empirically validated multilevel parenting and family support strategy for the prevention of behavior and emotional problems in children. *Clinical Child and Family Psychological Review, 2,* 71–90.

Sanders, M. R., Bor, W., & Morawska, A. (2007). Maintenance of treatment gains: A comparison of enhanced, standard, and self-directed Triple P-positive parenting program. *Journal of Abnormal Child Psychology, 35,* 983–998.

Sanders, M. R., Markie-Dadds, C., Tully, L. A., & Bor, W. (2000). The Triple P-parenting program: A comparison of enhanced, standard, and self-directed behavioral family intervention for parents of children with early onset conduct problems. *Journal of Consulting and Clinical Psychology, 68,* 624–640.

Shaffer, D., Fisher, P., Lucas, C. P., Dulcan, M. K., & Schwab-Stone, M. E. (2000). NIMH diagnostic interview schedule for children version IV (NIMH DISC-IV): Description, differences from previous versions, and reliability of some common diagnoses. *Journal*

of the American Academy of Child and Adolescent Psychiatry, 40, 1228–1231.

Shaw, D. S., Owens, E. B., Giovannelli, J., & Winslow, E. B. (2001). Infant and toddler pathways leading to early externalizing disorders. *Journal of the American Academy of Child and Adolescent Psychiatry, 40,* 36–43.

Shillingsburg, M. A. (2005). The use of the establishing operation in parent-child interaction therapies. *Child and Family Behavior Therapy, 26,* 43–58.

Silverthorn, P., & Frick, P. J. (1999). Developmental pathways to antisocial behavior: The delayed-onset pathway in girls. *Development and Psychopathology, 27,* 383–392.

Simonoff, E., Pickles, A., Meyer, J., Silberg, J., & Maes, H. (1998). Genetic and environmental influences on subtypes of conduct disorder behavior in boys. *Journal of Abnormal Child Psychology, 26,* 495–510.

Slough, N. M., Mcmahon, R. J., & the Conduct Problems Prevention Research Group. (2008). Preventing serious conduct problems in school-age youth: The Fast Track Program. *Cognitive and Behavioral Practice, 15,* 3–17.

Steiner, H., Saxena, K., & Chang, K. (2003). Psychopharmacologic strategies for the treatment of aggression in juveniles. *CNS Spectrum, 8,* 298–308.

Stormshak, E. A., Bierman, K. L., McMahon, R. J., Lengua, L. J., & the Conduct Problems Prevention Research Group (2000). Parenting practices and child disruptive behavior problems in early elementary school. *Journal of Clinical Child Psychology, 29,* 17–29.

Tiet, Q. Q., Bird, H. R., Hoven, C. W., Moore, R., Wu, P., & Wicks, J. (2001). Relationship between specific adverse life events and psychiatric disorders. *Journal of Abnormal Child Psychology, 29,* 153–164.

Van Goozen, S. H., Van Den Ban, E., Matthys, W., Chen-Kettenis, P. T., Thijsse, J. H., & Van Engeland, H. (2000). Increased adrenal androgen functioning in children with oppositional defiant disorder: A comparison with psychiatric and normal controls. *Journal of the American Academy of Child and Adolescent Psychiatry, 39,* 1446–1451.

Vander Zanden, J. W., Crandell, T. L., & Crandell, C. H. (2006). *Human development* (8th ed.). New York: McGraw-Hill.

Vitaro, F., Brendgen, M., & Tremblay, R. E. (2000). Influence of deviant friends on delinquency: Searching for moderator variables. *Journal of Abnormal Child Psychology, 28,* 313–326.

Walker, H. M., & Mcconnell, S. (1995). *Walker-McConnell scale of social competence and school adjustment, Elementary version.* San Diego, CA: Singular.

Walker, H. M., & Severson, H. (1992). *Systematic screening for behavior disorders.* Longmont, CO: Sopris West.

Waschbusch, D. A. (2002). A meta-analytic examination of comorbid hyperactive-impulsive-attention problems and conduct problems. *Psychological Bulletin, 128,* 118–150.

Webster-Stratton, C. (1981a). Modification of mothers' behaviors and attitudes through a videotape modeling group discussion program. *Behavior Therapy, 12,* 634–642.

Webster-Stratton, C. (1981b). Videotape modeling: A method of parent education. *Journal of Clinical Child Psychology, 10,* 93–98.

Webster-Stratton, C. (1982). Teaching mothers through videotape modeling to change their children's behavior. *Journal of Pediatric Psychology, 7*, 279–294.

Webster-Stratton, C. (2001). The Incredible Years: Parents, teachers, and children training series. *Residential Treatment for Children and Youth, 18*, 31–45.

Webster-Stratton, C., & Hammond, M. (1997). Treating children with early-onset conduct problems: A comparison of child and parent training interventions. *Journal of Consulting and Clinical Psychology, 65*, 93–109.

Webster-Stratton, C., & Hammond, M. (1998). Conduct problems and level of social competence in Head Start children: Prevalence, pervasiveness, and associated risk factors. *Clinical Child and Family Psychology Review, 1*, 101–124.

Webster-Stratton, C., & Reid, M. (2003). The incredible years parents, teachers, and children training series: A multifaceted treatment approach for young children with conduct problems. In A. E. Kazdin & J. R. Weisz (Eds.), *Evidence-based psychotherapies for children and adolescents* (pp. 224–240). New York: Guilford.

Webster-Stratton, C., Reid, J., & Hammond, M. (2001). Social skills and problem-solving training for children with early-onset conduct problems: Who benefits? *Journal of Child Psychology and Psychiatry, 42*, 943–952.

Webster-Stratton, C., Reid, M. J., & Stoolmiller, M. (2008). Preventing conduct problems and improving school readiness: Evaluation of the Incredible Years Teacher and Child Training Programs in high-risk schools. *Journal of Child Psychology and Psychiatry, 49*, 471–488.

Wechsler, D. (2003). WISC-IV: Wechsler Intelligence Scale for Children-Fourth Edition. San Antonio, Texas: The Psychological Corporation.

Weiss, B., Caron, A., Ball, S., Tapp, J., Johnson, M., & Weisz, J. R. (2005). Iatrogenic effects of group treatment for antisocial youth. *Journal of Consulting and Clinical Psychology, 73*, 1036–1044.

Wells, K. C., Forehand, R. L., & Griest, D. L. (1980). Generality of treatment effects from treated to untreated behaviors resulting from a parent training program, *Journal of Clinical Child Psychology, 9*, 217–219.

Werch, C. E., & Owen, D. M. (2002). Iatrogenic effects of alcohol and drug prevention programs. *Journal of Studies on Alcohol, 63*, 581–590.

Widom, C. S. (1989). Child abuse, neglect, and adult behavior: Research design and findings on criminality, violence, and child abuse. *American Journal of Orthopsychiatry, 59*, 355–367.

Widom, C. S. (1997). Child abuse, neglect, and witnessing violence.In D. Stoff, J. Breiling, & J. D. Maser (Eds.), *Handbook of antisocial behavior* (pp. 159–170). New York: John Wiley & Sons.

Woodcock, R. W., McGrew, K. S., & Mather, N. (2001). Woodcock-Johnson-III. Itasca, IL: Riverside Publishing.

Xie, H., Cairns, B. D., & Cairns, R. B. (2005). The development of aggressive behaviors among girls: Measurement issues, social functions, and differential trajectories. In D. J. Pepler, K. C. Madsen, C. Webster, & K. S. Levene (Eds.), *The development and treatment of girlhood aggression* (pp. 105–136). Mahwah, NJ: Lawrence Erlbaum Associates Publishers.

Yoshikawa, H. (1994). Prevention as cumulative protection: Effects of early family support and education on chronic delinquency and its risks. *Psychological Bulletin, 115*, 28–54.

Chapter 11
Anxiety Disorders and Phobias

Thompson E. Davis III, Melissa S. Munson, and Erin V. Tarcza

Introduction

According to the *Diagnostic and Statistical Manual of Mental Disorders-4th edition* (*DSM-IV-TR*, American Psychiatric Association, 2000) there are more than a dozen anxiety disorders and phobias which can be diagnosed in children. Most of these disorders include a criterion requiring interference in social and academic situations or, as is the case in agoraphobia, interference from embarrassment or the need of a companion (cf. *DSM-IV-TR*). As a diagnostic group, as well, these disorders are associated with a variety of social difficulties including social withdrawal, shyness, problematic peer relations, parent–child interaction difficulties, skills deficits, and cognitive distortions (Elizabeth et al., 2006; Ollendick & Hirshfeld-Becker, 2002; Rapee & Spence, 2004; Spence, Donovan, & Brechman-Toussaint, 1999). Anxiety disorders also cast a negative stigma upon children with these disorders (Jorm & Wright, 2008). Moreover, children with anxiety disorders also suffer from discrimination and victimization (e.g., Storch et al., 2006). As a result, it is surprising that the assessment and treatment of difficulties in social skills and social behavior in anxiety-disordered children have received relatively little attention outside of social phobia. For example, a recent review of evidence-based treatments for child anxiety indicated that social skills training was included in less than 10% of treatment protocols—the least included component of the 18 treatment strategies selected for review (Chorpita & Southam-Gerow, 2006). Thus, this chapter will examine the interplay of anxiety disorders and social skills difficulties with particular focus on social phobia, given its relevance to the theme of this volume and the pertinent research that has occurred in that area. Topics to be reviewed include the unique impact of social skills problems on those with anxiety disorders, as well as the assessment and treatment of social skills deficits in anxiety-disordered children.

Definition of the Population

Describing children with social difficulties and anxiety disorders is best done through a brief discussion of emotion and emotional responding to better appreciate the interplay of anxiety and social behavior. Anxiety is an emotion composed of several theoretical types of information which are tied to one's memory. In essence, when vast associative networks of information contained in long-term memory are stimulated, they cue an "action disposition" or emotion (Lang, Cuthbert, & Bradley, 1998, p. 656). These networks are subdivided into associations between stimulus, response, and meaning units of information (Drobes & Lang, 1995; Foa & Kozak, 1998; Lang et al., 1998). Essentially, emotion is a

T.E. Davis III (✉)
Department of Psychology, Louisiana State University,
Baton Rouge, LA 70803, USA
e-mail: ted@lsu.edu

In J. Matson (Ed.), *Practitioner's guide to social behavior and skills in children*

J.L. Matson (ed.), *Social Behavior and Skills in Children*, DOI 10.1007/978-1-4419-0234-4_11,
© Springer Science+Business Media, LLC 2009

conglomeration of properties which are based on sensations associated with the stimulus, our potential responses, and the meaning attributed to the stimulus or situation which serves to further connect the stimulus and response units. Overall, these associative networks broadly guide our approach or avoidance of stimuli and situations based on the information activated.

Given this, anxiety and fear can be conceived of as a neural program that facilitates emotional responding or changes in physiology, behavior, and cognition (Foa & Kozak, 1986; Lang, 1979). As a result, psychopathology differs from the typical and more normative experience of fear or worry by cueing a pathological network that incorporates exaggerated emotional responses—catastrophic cognitions and inaccurate views of the world, behavioral avoidance, and physiologic discomfort that is problematic and resistant to change (Foa & Kozak, 1986, 1998). Conceived of in this way, children having problems with social difficulties have a pathological response which may incorporate catastrophic thoughts about or interpretations of social situations, avoidance of social situations or people, and panic-like physiological symptoms to social stimuli. These responses, and the prognosis for therapeutic benefit, likely depend upon the child's unique presentation and the potentiation of the associative network (see sections below on etiology and developmental psychopathology). A child with anxiety and social difficulties, then, is a child with emotional difficulties rooted in myriad developmental, biological, environmental, and experiential factors. Further, this process is dynamic and reciprocal (Davis, in press). For example, a socially anxious child may display pathologized responses when entering a new play group (e.g., thinking "other children won't like me," being behaviorally avoidant by hovering awkwardly outside of the group, and experiencing an elevated heart rate). These emotional responses are then observed by the children and often elicit neutral, negative, or even punitive responses from them. The peer group's responses are then taken in by the child and further influence pathologized emotional responding while potentially confirming distorted thinking and expectations about social situations, and so on reciprocally. In addition, the child may be negatively reinforced for future avoidance as social withdrawal

and shyness may allow the child to avoid or reduce aversive physiology and cognition, and the entire experience may be associated with a sense of helplessness and uncontrollability (Mineka & Zinbarg, 2006).

Diagnostically, children with anxiety and fear are likely to experience social difficulties and peer rejection with many of the potential *DSM-IV-TR* anxiety disorder presentations (see Social Skills Problems Unique to the Population below). Most relevant and widely studied, however, is the diagnosis of social phobia (also called social anxiety disorder). In children, social phobia is characterized by a marked and persistent fear of social performance or evaluation when being observed by children and adults alike (i.e., not just fear with authority figures or adults; *DSM-IV-TR*). Exposure typically provokes a pathological emotional response similar to that described above. A physiological response, possibly even a panic attack, may be present; behaviorally, the child may withdraw, cry, throw a tantrum, or avoid social situations or when avoidance is not possible endure exposure with significant discomfort (*DSM-IV-TR*). Cognitively, anxious apprehension or distress must interfere with the child's functioning and social relationships, and the child may believe the fearful response is warranted (i.e., no recognition that the emotional response is severe, excessive, or unreasonable; *DSM-IV-TR*). For a child the fear must endure and be present for at least 6 months to hopefully avoid any transient, developmentally appropriate social fears from being diagnosed. In addition, children presenting with broader social-evaluative anxiety and interference across a number of social situations may be further specified as having the "generalized" type as opposed to more specific and circumscribed social fears (e.g., public speaking; *DSM-IV-TR*).

While social phobia may seem to be the most pertinent diagnostic consideration, social concerns related to other anxiety disorders should be examined as well. With separation anxiety disorder, a child is overly concerned about separation from a parent, a guardian, or the home and may experience social disruption from embarrassment at leaving friends houses or needing close proximity to caregivers; such a child not only suffers from the symptoms of the disorder, but also is denied positive socialization experiences (*DSM-IV-TR*). In cases of generalized anxiety disorder, the child worries about performances, social situations, peer relations, and possible embarrassment, even in the absence of evaluation (Note: the absence of social evaluation distinguishes it from Social Phobia; *DSM-IV-TR*). Similarly, with agoraphobia and panic the fear and worry over embarrassment persist even into situations in which there is no evaluative component (*DSM-IV-TR*). While the *DSM-IV-TR* recommends examining the use of a safety companion in this diagnostic determination, this is likely to be of less value with children who frequently have parents or caregivers nearby anyway. Obsessive-compulsive disorder in children has been associated with increased loneliness and victimization by peers (Storch et al., 2006) and may interfere with social experiences and relationships (*DSM-IV-TR*). As is readily evident, across the anxiety disorders varying symptoms of social withdrawal, apprehension, avoidance, peer rejection, and concern over embarrassment impair children and frequently deny them access to social experiences which might otherwise be beneficial, possibly corrective, and maybe even enjoyable.

Etiology and Prevalence

Etiology

The etiology of anxiety disorders has long been attributed to four possible mechanisms acting either singly or in combination: classical conditioning, modeling, negative information transfer, and a non-associative mechanism (for more detailed reviews see Fisak & Grills-Taquechel, 2007; Muris, Merckelbach, de Jong, & Ollendick, 2002). Anxiety is thought to be transmitted through associative means by experiencing a negative event directly, by seeing someone else behave anxiously or being afraid, or by hearing or reading about being anxious or afraid. Non-associative accounts point to people having some innate, inborn biological or genetic predisposition to fear and anxiety. From these basic mechanisms, the etiology of anxiety has been broadly understood to be a consideration of how much association to a stimulus is necessary to bring

about a disorder given one's innate predisposition (Marks, 2002). Even so, the interaction of these four etiological mechanisms is poorly understood, and their description of coalescing into an anxiety disorder is greatly simplified.

A complete understanding of how anxiety disorders emerge may be that various etiological processes occasion the emergence of just one or more aspects of the emotional response instead of the entire emotion. These etiological risks then might accumulate over time. Such an occurrence might be supported by notions of desynchrony in which only partial emotional responses occur in response to an anxiety-provoking situation or stimulus (Rachman & Hodgson, 1974). Even so, etiological models of anxiety need to incorporate current progress in the understanding of developmental psychology and developmental psychopathology. It has long been observed that many children have similar experiences but develop differently and that children with differing experiences can arrive upon the same developmental trajectory. For example, two children have negative social experiences (e.g., getting teased and bullied), yet only one develops an anxiety disorder. These observations represent the constructs of multifinality (i.e., a single developmental event can have multiple outcomes) and equifinality (i.e., different developmental trajectories can lead to the same outcome; cf. Ollendick & Hirshfeld-Becker, 2002). As a result, the goal is to understand each child as an individual with his or her unique predispositions, learning histories, strengths, weaknesses, coping abilities, etc. at a particular point in time (Davis, in press).

Taken this way, developmental psychopathology seeks to understand the "developmental and psychological disturbances in children as the result of complex interactions over the course of development between the biology of brain maturation and the multidimensional nature of experience" (Mash & Dozois, 2003, p. 5). Increasingly, notions of multifinality and equifinality influence etiological models along with the recognition that psychopathology is influenced by both when a child is observed (e.g., developmental milestones negotiated, age, situation) and who is serving as observer (e.g., the observer's perspective, orientation, and biases; Mash & Dozois, 2003).

Child psychopathology is then a multifaceted construct which ties together factors both within and without the child as well as the impressions of those around him or her. Further, a child's behavior may or may not be pathological, but the caregivers' accommodation of disorder or intolerance of typical child behaviors may deny a child needed help or potentially contribute to the development of dysfunction.

As a result, adequate etiological models of anxiety disorders increasingly need to incorporate the negotiation of developmental milestones—in the case of this chapter, social development. Theorists have attempted to do just that, and integrated etiological theories have begun to emerge in which the previous mechanisms have been couched in developmental psychology. For example, etiological discussions of anxiety and social problems now commonly include the topics of genetics, temperament, childrearing and parenting, and negative social experiences as well as a variety of other factors (Elizabeth et al., 2006; Ollendick & Hirshfeld-Becker, 2002; Rapee & Spence, 2004). Social anxiety has been conceptualized as lying on a continuum with a child's risk for or resiliency to disorder being described as how developmental factors move a child up or down the continuum from a certain initial set point (Rapee & Spence, 2004). Several of these influential factors will be reviewed briefly below.

Genetics

Genetics has been tentatively linked to a variety of social developmental aspects, including emotionality, sociability, and broad internalizing tendencies. In particular, genetic research has pointed to the role of both broad vulnerabilities to internalizing disorders as well as specific vulnerabilities to social anxiety problems in particular (Ollendick & Hirshfeld-Becker, 2002; Rapee & Spence, 2004). For example, social phobia has been found to be more common among first degree relatives (e.g., Fyer, 1993; Fyer, Mannuzza, Chapman, Martin and Klein, 1995), and heritability estimates in twins of 0.48 have been found for broader social anxiety constructs like the fear of negative evaluation (Stein, Jang, & Livesley, 2002). In addition, the broader, generalized type of social phobia may be

more heritable than the specific type (Mannuzza et al., 1995; Stein, Chartier, Kozak, King and Kennedy, 1998). Unfortunately, research in this area has been hampered by polygenetic influences with limited impact, and, in the end, the genetic component may be more useful for determining psychopathological risk than response to treatment (Gregory & Eley, 2007). In addition, even genes must be understood as residing in cellular environments which can act to switch them "on" or "off" (e.g., Szyf, McGowan, & Meaney, 2008).

Temperament

For decades children have been understood to have different temperaments. A child's temperament is understood to involve several dimensions including his or her emotionality, activity, and sociability (Buss & Plomin, 1984). Children were classified into groups such as "easy" or "difficult" with difficult classifications (e.g., children with poor adaptability, withdrawal from novelty, intense reactivity) more strongly associated with anxiety and behavior problems (Thomas & Chess, 1977; Thomas, Chess, & Birch, 1968). Subsequent refinements have found the related concept of behavioral inhibition to be a particularly important temperamental construct for social anxiety and social withdrawal. Behavioral inhibition refers to a relatively stable pattern of behavioral and emotional responses in which a child is tentative, shy, and withdrawn in strange or novel situations (Kagan, Reznick, Clarke, Snidman, & Garcia Coll, 1984; Rapee & Spence, 2004). Behaviorally inhibited children have been theorized to have a low threshold and low tolerance for arousal in these novel situations (Kagan, Reznick, & Snidman, 1987). Given this, it is not surprising that social phobia has also been found to be more likely in behaviorally inhibited children compared to those who are not (Biederman et al., 2001).

Parent–Child Interaction

Investigations to date have failed to determine whether socially anxious children result from particular parenting styles or elicit them (Ollendick & Hirshfeld-Becker, 2002; Rapee & Spence, 2004). The likely answer is that child and parent impact each other reciprocally, with other variables such as temperament and genetics having long-standing contributions as well. Even so, in examining non-retrospective studies, Wood, McLeod, Sigman, Hwang, and Chu (2003) found anxious children had parents who were observed to be less accepting, more critical, overcontrolling, and overprotective. Moreover, parents who modeled anxiety tended to have children with increased anxiety. Importantly as well, parents are frequently influential in scheduling and monitoring play, with socially phobic parents potentially less proficient at these tasks (Masia & Morris, 1998; Ollendick & Hirshfeld-Becker, 2002). In other words, parents of anxious children have frequently been observed to have interactions in which they present the world as hostile, dangerous, and anxiety-provoking while also demanding compliance and being less accepting and more critical of deviation from their directives. Such interactions may be most impairing as risk factors for younger children who have other diatheses (Ollendick & Horsch, 2007); as a result, there is likely an unfortunate interaction of multiple familial factors which occasion social anxiety (e.g., inherited traits which affect parents and children alike, parenting styles, modeling, socioeconomic status, etc.).

Prevalence

Estimates of the prevalence of anxiety disorders in children have varied considerably, from roughly 3 to 24% of children based on the disorders included, sample, methodology, and time period (Cartwright-Hatton, McNicol, & Doubleday, 2006). According to one group of researchers, by the age of 16 years 36.7% of children will meet criteria for at least one *DSM-IV* disorder and 10% will have an anxiety disorder, with the 3-month prevalence of anxiety disorders being 2.4% (Costello, Mustillo, Erkanli, Keeler, & Angold, 2003). In addition, children reporting "childhood fears" had a diagnosable anxiety disorder in 22.8% of instances (Muris, Merckelbach, Mayer,

& Prins, 2000). High comorbidity with other disorders (including anxiety disorders) has also been found consistently (e.g., 41% comorbid, Beidel, Turner, & Morris, 2000; 54% comorbid, Spence, Donovan, & Brechman-Toussaint, 2000; 72% comorbid, Silverman et al., 1999).

Particularly relevant to this chapter, the 3-month prevalence of social phobia in the general population has been found to be 0.5% for a younger sample of children and adolescents (Costello et al., 2003; 9–13 years initially), while 1-year prevalence estimates of child and adolescent social phobia have been suggested to be 6.8% in primary care facilities (Chavira, Stein, Bailey, & Stein, 2004). Similarly, the adult 1-year prevalence in the population has been found to be 6.8%, the second most prevalent mental disorder (Kessler, Chiu, Demler, & Walters, 2005). Overall, lifetime prevalence rates for children and adolescents have been suggested to vary between 5 and 15% (Heimberg, Stein, Hiripi, & Kessler, 2000). Age of onset is usually in preadolescence to adolescence with more generalized social worries beginning earlier (Ollendick & Hirshfeld-Becker, 2002; Rapee & Spence, 2004). Further suggesting a later onset, a recent review of preadolescent children (defined to be under 12 years of age) found prevalence rates to be less than 1% (Cartwright-Hatton et al., 2006), similar to the slightly younger aged sample in Costello et al. (2003).

Social Skills Problems Unique to the Population

As alluded to above, children with anxiety disorders and phobias experience a variety of social problems that interact reciprocally with the psychopathology, further complicating aspects of both. Moreover, a threat-related attentional bias may exacerbate avoidance and the perception of situations as potentially anxiety provoking (Puliafico & Kendall, 2006). Anxiety in children has been associated with myriad risks including social withdrawal, social skills deficits, peer rejection and neglect, dysfunctional parent–child interactions, the use of maladaptive social strategies, and cognitive distortions (e.g., Elizabeth et al., 2006; Ollendick & Hirshfeld-Becker, 2002; Rapee & Spence, 2004; Sondaite & Zukauskiene, 2005; Spence et al., 1999; Strauss, Lease, Kazdin, Dulcan, & Last, 1989). As a result, anxious children have been somewhat consistently described as being socially maladjusted by parents, teachers, peers, and even the children themselves (e.g., Strauss et al., 1989; Verduin & Kendall, 2008). Overall, these factors may be associated with placing them upon a developmental trajectory toward further social withdrawal and dysfunction (Oh et al., 2008). In fact, social anxiety has been described as moderately stable across the lifespan (Rapee & Spence, 2004).

One of the larger areas of research in this area has been the impact of peer relationships. While shy children have been suggested to be as likely to have friends as other children, there are important differences in these relationships (Rubin, Wojslawowicz, Rose-Krasnor, Booth-LaForce, & Burgess, 2006), and examinations of adolescents with social anxiety have suggested that friendships may be impacted as well—particularly for girls (La Greca & Lopez, 1998). According to Rubin et al. (2006), withdrawn children's friends were more likely to be withdrawn and victimized by peers themselves; the quality of these friendships was also poorer than control children's relationships. La Greca and Lopez (1998) found that socially anxious adolescent boys and girls reported feeling less supported, accepted by, and attractive to peers; girls especially were found to report fewer friendships and less intimacy and support in existing relationships. Generally, it has been surmised that social anxiety in children is associated with long-standing social and peer problems which lead these boys and girls to experience peer rejection, neglect, and exclusion (Rapee & Spence, 2004).

Examinations of social functioning, relationships, and competence in children with other anxiety disorder diagnoses are more limited, but findings have been similar to those obtained with socially anxious children. For example, Strauss, Lahey, Frick, Frame, and Hynd (1988) used a peer nomination procedure (i.e., children wrote down the names of the three children they liked most and the three children they liked least) to determine peer social status among anxiety-disordered, conduct-disordered, and non-referred control children.

Broadly, they found the anxiety-disordered group and the conduct-disordered group were similarly disliked compared to the control group. Anxiety-disordered children were also more likely to be classified as socially neglected (i.e., few "like most" or "like least" nominations; Strauss et al., 1988). Additionally, Strauss et al. (1989) found that, compared to control children, anxiety-disordered children reported more loneliness and less social competence. Parents and teachers reported that the anxiety-disordered children were more withdrawn, maladjusted, socially deficient, and lacking in social skills (Strauss et al., 1989).

Examining the differences between two groups of anxiety-disordered children, Ginsburg, La Greca, and Silverman (1998) found that anxiety-disordered children with high social anxiety, compared to anxiety-disordered children with low social anxiety, had more negative peer interactions and lower self-esteem and social acceptance. Children diagnosed with social phobia in particular have also been found to have social skills deficits, poorer social competence, and more negative self-talk in socially evaluative situations when compared to a matched group of nonclinical children (Spence et al., 1999). Moreover, during direct observations of the children interacting with peers at school, children with social phobia were observed to experience similar percentages of interaction that were negative or in which the child was ignored, but fewer peer social interactions with positive outcomes (Spence et al., 1999).

More recently, Verduin and Kendall (2008) examined children's ratings of videotaped anxiety-disordered and non-anxiety-disordered children. Child raters were able to perceive anxiety in videotaped children, as indicated by positive correlations between raters' ratings of anxiety in the video-taped children and the video-taped children's ratings of themselves. Moreover, the effect was stronger for ratings of anxiety-disordered children than those children without an anxiety disorder. Correspondingly, children rated anxiety-disordered children as significantly less likeable; however, further analyses indicated that these differences were "wholly attributable to the presence of" social phobia and not diagnoses of generalized anxiety disorder or separation anxiety disorder (p. 465). Socially phobic children were even rated less likeable when the peer-raters' ratings of anxiety were controlled for—in other words, socially phobic children were disliked even if they were not perceived to be anxious (Verduin and Kendall, 2008). As a result, it would seem that the combination of anxiety and social problems causes peer difficulties for children even if they are able to keep their anxiety covert.

Anxiety-disordered children's problems with peer relations may even be stigmatizing and associated with victimization by peers. For example, Jorm and Wright (2008) surveyed 3746 children, adolescents, and young adults as well as 2005 parents in Australia by phone. Participants were interviewed after being read several vignettes of hypothetical clinically diagnosed 15-year-olds—one of which described the hypothetical teen as having symptoms of social phobia. Youth's ratings of the teen with social phobia were associated with higher scores on scales stigmatizing the teen as "weak not sick" and "stigma perceived in others" indicating perceptions that the hypothetical teen was weak-minded, stigmatized, and to be avoided (Jorm & Wright, 2008). Moreover, youth "weak not sick" beliefs were associated with parents' increased "weak not sick" beliefs and decreased "stigma perceived in others" beliefs. Overall, the authors concluded that "social phobia was more likely to be seen as a weakness rather than a sickness and was perceived as being more stigmatised [sic] by others in society" (p. 147).

Peer victimization is also a problem for children with anxiety. For example, Storch, Masia-Warner, Crisp, and Klein (2005) and Storch et al. (2006) examined the victimization of adolescents with social anxiety and children and adolescents with obsessive-compulsive disorder respectively. Victimization in these studies was defined to include both overt (e.g., hitting, yelling) and relational (e.g., spreading rumors and gossip, using relationships to isolate individuals) aggression by peers (Storch et al., 2005; 2006). A longitudinal investigation found that relational victimization predicted social phobia symptoms at 1 year, but not the reverse, and also did not predict more general symptoms of social anxiety (Storch et al., 2005). These results suggest a unidirectional influence of relational aggression; however, it may be that socially anxious children are already avoidant and excluded to the extent that little more relational aggression can occur. Additionally, it

may be that the 1-year follow-up was too brief to detect meaningful differences. Storch et al. (2006) found that children with obsessive-compulsive disorder were victimized more than control children or even the children with diabetes who were included. Victimization was associated with a number of factors, including depression and loneliness and fully or partially mediated the effects between obsessive-compulsive disorder severity and depression, externalizing behaviors, and loneliness. Taken together, it may be that socially anxious and awkward children are identified, disliked, and targeted for victimization by peers, even before they show significant overt anxiety symptoms (cf. Storch et al., 2005; Verduin & Kendall, 2008). Moreover, the social and anxiety problems these children experience may be viewed by peers and adults as abnormal and indicative of weakness instead of as symptoms of a treatable psychiatric condition (cf. Jorm & Wright, 2008; Storch et al., 2006).

From this brief review, one can discern that children with comorbid anxiety and social problems face a difficult developmental trajectory. Children experiencing loneliness, a lack of friends or stability in friendships, and peer exclusion have been found to be on a trajectory of increasing social withdrawal across the preadolescent to early adolescent years (Oh et al., 2008). Moreover, in significant percentages of adolescents, avoidant and helpless social strategies have been observed which may serve to maintain social problems and anxiety (Sondaite & Zukauskiene, 2005). Even so, the principles of developmental psychopathology should not be dismissed and trajectories should not be viewed as absolute. For example, high levels of familial stress have been associated with shyness, anxiety, and social skills deficits in urban youth; however, additional factors such as parental warmth and strong familial support have been suggested to be protective factors even in families experiencing high stress (McCabe, Clark, & Barnett, 1999). Overall, though, the social toll on children with anxiety is great—peer difficulties, stigma, parent–child interaction factors, deficits/distortions, and more—and these problems extend beyond the anxiety symptoms and varied diagnostic criteria. In addition, more research examining the extent to which social skills difficulties represent actual social skills deficits or production deficits (the child has the skill but does not implement it) would be ideal. As a result, a complex multi-method, multi-informant evidence-based assessment of both anxiety and comorbid disorders, as well as peer relations and social skills, is important when working with anxious children, especially when determining the best evidence-based treatment approach (2005; Silverman & Ollendick, 2005). Such an assessment needs to examine both the child's symptomatology and the possible presence of social skills deficits (both the lack of a particular skill and the possibility of just a lack of implementation).

Assessment

Given anxiety disorders do not seem to improve on their own over time (Beidel, Fink, & Turner, 1996), and they often lead to long-term problems for the child (Kendall, Safford, Flannery-Schroeder, & Webb, 2004), proper diagnosis is essential to ensure that the correct treatments are initiated. As a result, accurate assessment using evidence-based measures is crucial to ensuring that the correct diagnosis is made (2005; Silverman & Ollendick, 2005). Recently researchers have made incredible progress in the development and validation of evidence-based measures of anxiety (see Silverman & Ollendick, 2005 for a more complete review). It is now believed that the best strategy for assessment is a multi-method, multi-informant approach to provide the most comprehensive diagnostic picture possible and to be sure that important areas of emotional functioning or differing physical environments are not overlooked (Achenbach, McConaughy, & Howell, 1987).

Even so, the issue of multi-informant agreement and disagreement is a complex one (2005). There has commonly been a problem of multi-informant disagreement as to the presence and severity of child anxiety disorders (e.g., Grills & Ollendick, 2003; Jensen et al., 1999; Silverman & Ollendick, 2005). While discussion of this issue is beyond the space allotted here, it is important to note that disagreements should not be dismissed quickly or flippantly. For example, Muris and Merckelbach (2000) found that almost 20% of children with parent-reported

"childhood fears" met full criteria for specific phobia, while 23% of children reporting their own "childhood fears" met criteria for an anxiety disorder (Muris et al., 2000). Further, verification of diagnostic information from parents and children by trained clinicians has indicated that children were accurate in reporting existing anxiety disorders their parents did not and vice versa in roughly 59 and 65% of cases, respectively (Jensen et al., 1999). As a result, careful attention should be paid to discrepant information, and a thorough assessment is strongly recommended.

Common methods of assessment in anxiety include structured and semi-structured interviews, self-reports, parent and other reports, and analogue behavior observation methods (ABO). Assessments should also be constructed to probe the different components of the anxiety response (i.e., physiology, behavior, and cognition; 2005; Davis & Ollendick, 2005). The following brief review will include information on several commonly used measures from each of these categories. While several of the measures discussed include measures of social functioning, few actually measure social skills. Therefore, a separate discussion of measures of social skills commonly used in anxiety is also included. More information on the assessment of social skills is also included in Chapter 4 of this book.

Structured Diagnostic Interviews

The most commonly used method of assessment in the child anxiety literature is the clinical interview (Ollendick & Hersen, 1993; Silverman, 1994; Silverman & Ollendick, 2005); however, a variety of problems and limitations are associated with their use (e.g., reliability, validity, diagnostic specificity, and comprehensiveness). As a result, several structured and semi-structured interviews have been developed to address many of the difficulties associated with open clinical interviews. Table 11.1 describes some of the structured and semi-structured interviews that are most commonly used. Of these, the Anxiety Disorders Interview Schedule for Children DSM-IV: Child and Parent Versions (ADIS: C/P; Silverman & Albano, 1996) is

Table 11.1 Diagnostic interviews

Instrument	Description	Psychometric properties
Anxiety disorders interview schedule-child/parent schedules (ADIS-C/P; Silverman & Albano, 1996; Silverman, Saavedra, & Pina, 2001)	A semi-structured clinical interview designed for use with children aged 6–18 years used to diagnose a range of internalizing and externalizing disorders	Kappa coefficients for the anxiety disorders from parent/child combined assessment are as follows: GAD = 0.80, SAD = 0.84, SOP = 0.92, SP = 0.81. Kappa coefficients from the mood disorders and externalizing disorders range from 0.62 to 1.00
NIMH diagnostic interview schedule for children version IV (NIMH DISC-IV; Shaffer, Fisher, Lucas, Dulcan and Schwab-Stone, 2000)	A structured clinical interview designed for use with children aged 9–17 years used to diagnose a range of internalizing and externalizing disorders	Kappa coefficients for the anxiety disorders from parent/child combined assessment are as follows: GAD = 0.58, SAD = 0.51, SOP = 0.48, SP = 0.86. Kappa coefficients from the mood disorders and externalizing disorders range from 0.55 to 0.86
Schedule for affective disorders and schizophrenia for school-age children (K-SADS; Ambrosini, 2000)	A semi-structured clinical interview designed for use with children aged 6–18 years used to diagnose a range of internalizing and externalizing disorders	Kappa coefficients range from 0.55 to 0.80 for specific anxiety disorders from parent/child combined assessment

Note: GAD, generalized anxiety disorder; SAD, separation anxiety disorder; SOP, social phobia; SP, specific phobia.

the most popular in anxiety research (Silverman & Ollendick, 2005). The ADIS contains separate modules for each of the anxiety disorders (e.g., social phobia, specific phobia, generalized anxiety disorder) and other common psychological problems in children (e.g., attention-deficit/hyperactivity disorder, conduct disorder, major depressive disorder). Screening sections for many other problems are also included (e.g. eating disorders, pervasive developmental disorders, schizophrenia, enuresis). Modules may be administered individually or together. The modules ask questions that are closely modeled after the *DSM-IV* criteria and most also ask the children to rate their fear and avoidance of various situations that are commonly problems for those disorders on a scale from 0 (no problems or fear) to 8 (very severe or disturbing). They also rate the overall interference that each disorder is causing on the same 0–8 scale. A visual fear thermometer with numeric and qualitative descriptors helps younger children grasp the scale and allows for developmentally sensitive responses. At the end of the interview the clinician then assigns clinical severity ratings on the 0 (none) to 8 (very severely disturbing/impairing) scale to each of the disorders that were endorsed based on the information provided, with scores of 4 or higher being considered clinically significant.

While the ADIS does not include a scored assessment of social skills, there is a portion of the interview that inquires into the extent and quality of the interpersonal relationships of the child. This section includes questions such as "Compared to other kids, do you feel you have more friends, less friends, or about the same"; "Do you have a best friend"; and "Given the choice would you prefer to spend most of your time alone or with other kids." There are also questions in the social phobia and school refusal modules that ask the child to rate fear and avoidance of specific social situations, including starting or joining in on a conversation, working or playing in a group, and having difficulties with assertiveness. It is unclear, however, whether these problems are due to a lack of skill or just a general fear of negative evaluation.

Self-Report and Other-Report Questionnaires

Self-report questionnaires represent another method of assessment for the diagnosis of anxiety disorders. These measures are often collected from the children themselves, as well as from parents, teachers, and other reporters. Many of the commonly used questionnaires are described in Table 11.2. Questionnaires have the

Table 11.2 Self-report, parent-report, and other-report questionnaires in the assessment of anxiety

Measure	Description	Subscales	Psychometric properties
Behavior assessment system for children (BASC; Reynolds & Kamphaus, 1992)	A 148-item parent report measure of adaptive functioning and behavior problems in children aged 2–21	Broadband subscales (internalizing and externalizing symptoms) and narrowband subscales (aggression, anxiety, attention problems, atypicality, conduct problems, depression, hyperactivity, withdrawal, and somatization)	Internal consistency ranges from 0.70 to 0.99. Test–retest reliability ranges from 0.70 to 0.99
Child anxiety sensitivity index (CASI; Silverman, Fleisig, Rabian, & Peterson, 1991)	An 18-item questionnaire for children aged 6–17 that has the child rate how disturbing various anxiety symptoms are to them	Disease concerns, unsteady concerns, mental incapacitation concerns, and social concerns	Internal consistency for the total score = 0.87. Test–retest reliability for the total score = 0.76
Child behavior checklist (CBCL; Achenbach, 1991)	A 118-item measure that asks parents to rate the frequency of various problem behaviors that their child (aged 6–18) may experience	Two broad scales (internalizing and externalizing problems) and eight subscales (withdrawn, somatic complaints, anxious/ depressed, social problems, thought problems, attention problems, rule-breaking behavior, and aggressive behavior)	Internal consistency for the subscales ranges from 0.54 to 0.96. Test–retest reliability ranges from 0.86 to 0.89
Children's automatic thoughts scale (CATS; Schniering & Rapee, 2002)	A 40-item questionnaire for children aged 7–16 that asks the child to rate the frequency of each automatic thought about physical threat, personal failure, and hostility in the last week		Internal consistency = 0.94. Test–retest reliability = 0.79
Fear survey schedule for children-revised (FSS-R; Ollendick, 1983)	An 80-item measure for children aged 7–18 that has the children rate the amount of fear they experience for each object or situation	Fear of failure and criticism, fear of the unknown, fear of danger and death, medical fears, and small animals	Internal consistency for the subscales ranges from 0.92 to 0.95. Test–retest reliability for the total scale = 0.82. Has been shown to be able to discriminate between the different types of phobias (Weems, Silverman, Saavedra, Pina and Lumpkin, 1999)
Multidimensional anxiety scale for children (MASC; March, Parker, Sullivan, Stallings, & Conners, 1997)	A 39-item measure for children aged 8–18 that measures a range of anxiety symptoms	Physical symptoms (tense/ restlessness and somatic/ autonomic), harm avoidance (perfectionism and anxious coping), social anxiety (humiliation/ rejection and performance fears), separation/panic,	Internal consistency for the total score = 0.90. Test–retest for the total score and the subscales range from 0.34 to 0.93. Good convergent validity. Excellent discriminative validity

Table 11.2 (continued)

Measure	Description	Subscales	Psychometric properties
		and an overall anxiety disorder index	
Negative affect self-statement questionnaire (Ronan, Kendall, & Rowe, 1994)	A 31-item measure for children aged 7–15 that assesses how often the child experiences negative automatic thoughts		Internal consistency for the total score ranges from 0.89 to 0.96. Test–retest reliability ranges from 0.78 to 0.96
Penn state worry questionnaire for children (PSWQ; Chorpita, Tracey, Brown, Collica, & Barlow, 1997)	A 14-item questionnaire that has children aged 6–18 rate the frequency and controllability of worry		Internal consistency = 0.89. Test–retest reliability = 0.92
Revised children's manifest anxiety scale (RCMAS; Reynolds & Richmond, 1985)	A 37-item measure for children aged 6–18 that assesses anxiety symptoms in a yes/no format	Physiological anxiety, worry/oversensitivity, social concerns/concentration, and lie/social desirability	Good internal consistency. Test–retest reliability for subscales range from 0.64 to 0.76
Screen for child anxiety related emotional disorders (Birmaher et al., 1999, 1997)	A 38-item measure for children aged 9–18 that measures symptoms of separation anxiety disorder, generalized anxiety disorder, social phobia, and school phobia	Somatic/panic, generalized anxiety, separation anxiety, social phobia, and school phobia	Internal consistency range from 0.74 to 0.93. Test–retest reliability range from 0.70 to 0.90. Good discriminant validity
Screen for child anxiety related emotional disorders—revised (SCARED-R; Muris, Merckelbach, Schmidt, & Mayer, 1999; Muris & Steerneman, 2001)	A 66-item measure for children aged 6–18 that measures symptoms of anxiety disorders based on the DSM-IV	Separation anxiety disorder, generalized anxiety disorder, panic disorder, social phobia, obsessive-compulsive disorder, traumatic stress disorder, and specific phobias	Internal consistency = 0.94. Good convergent and discriminate validity
Social anxiety scale for children (SAS-C; La Greca, Dandes, Wick, Shaw, & Stone, 1988)	A 26-item measure that asks children aged 8–18 to rate how true each experience of social anxiety is for them	Fear of negative evaluation, social avoidance and distress in new situations, and general social avoidance and distress	Internal consistency for the subscales range from 0.69 to 0.86. Test–retest reliability ranges from 0.69 to 0.86
Social phobia and anxiety inventory for children (SPAI-C; Beidel, Turner, & Morris, 1995)	A 26-item measure for children aged 8–14 years that measures physiological, cognitive, and behavioral symptoms of social phobia on a 3-point Likert scale	Assertiveness/general conversation, traditional social encounters, and public performance	Good internal consistency, test–retest reliability
The social worries questionnaire (SWQ; Spence, 1995)	A measure of the degree of worry the child experiences in various social situations. A 10-item parent version and a 13-item pupil version are available		Internal consistency for the parent version = 0.82. Internal consistency for the pupil version = 0.85

Table 11.2 (continued)

Measure	Description	Subscales	Psychometric properties
State-trait anxiety inventory for children (STAI-C; Spielberger, 1973)	A 20-item measure for children aged 8–15 that measures chronic and transitory symptoms of anxiety	Anxiety-trait, anxiety-state	Internal consistency for the subscales range from 0.80 to 0.90. Test–retest reliability range from 0.31 to 0.71
Teacher report form (TRF; Achenbach, 1991)	A 120-item teacher report measure that is comparable to the CBCL described above	Two broad scales (internalizing and externalizing problems) and eight subscales (withdrawn, somatic complaints, anxious/ depressed, social problems, thought problems, attention problems, rule-breaking behavior, and aggressive behavior)	Internal consistency for the subscales ranges from 0.54 to 0.96. Test–retest reliability ranges from 0.86 to 0.89

advantage of being easier and cheaper to administer than interviews, as well as allowing a greater wealth of information to be obtained from multiple informants in an expedited fashion. The speed and efficiency of such instruments make them particularly valuable as screening tools and potentially add to the overall cost-effectiveness of services (Silverman & Ollendick, 2005). Parents and teachers may be particularly important informers for very young children or children with social skills deficits, as these children may be unable to fully express their symptoms (Choudhury, Pimentel, & Kendall, 2003).

Analogue Behavioral Observation (ABO)

ABO is another important method of assessment with children, as it provides an opportunity to objectively view how the child responds in various situations. Several assessment methods have been developed for this purpose and include myriad techniques such as role-plays, interaction tasks, think-aloud procedures, functional assessments, and behavioral avoidance tasks (BATs; S. N. Haynes, 2001). ABOs can also be conducted in a variety of settings from school classrooms to psychiatric facilities to research settings to the home. For example, the BAT involves asking the child to engage in some feared situation (e.g. touching a spider, giving a speech) and then measuring the extent to which the child complies, as well as the

amount of distress the child experiences during the task. This task is commonly used in phobia research (see Ollendick, Davis, & Muris, 2004) but has also been used in the assessment of obsessive-compulsive disorder (Barrett, Healy, & March, 2003) and social phobia (Coles & Heimberg, 2000). An adaptation of this task to a role-play format that has been used to measure social skills directly is the Revised Behavioral Assertiveness Test for Children (BAT-CR; Ollendick, 1981). The BAT-CR involves asking the child to participate in a series of role-plays of both positive and negative social situations. They can then be coded on things such as eye contact, latency of response, and length of response. This task has been used to evaluate the social skills of children with social phobia (Spence et al., 1999).

In addition to BATs, direct observations of behavior are also commonly used in the assessment of anxiety. These protocols allow the observer to view the anxious behaviors in the child's natural environment (i.e. home, classroom) and are coded based on the protocol being used (e.g. Glennon & Weisz, 1978). Other forms of ABO also provide valuable information. For example, interaction tasks in which families or children are observed interacting freely about a prescribed topic or situation can assist in determining the effects of parental influence or patterns of dysfunctional interaction (S. N. Haynes, 2001). Functional assessments are also useful in which the potential operant maintaining factors of anxiety are observed, codified, and recorded (2005; S. N. Haynes, 2001) or discussed through detailed interviewing with the child and/or parent (2005; Ollendick et al., 2004). Overall, ABO procedures provide a wealth of information and allow the clinician to directly observe how a child behaves in certain anxiety-provoking and/or social situations.

Measures Specific to Social Skills/Social Competence

There are also several measures designed specifically for the assessment of social skills or social competence that are commonly used in the assessment of child anxiety (see Table 11.3 for more detailed descriptions). The Matson Evaluation of Social Skills for Youngsters (MESSY; Matson, Rotatori, & Helsel, 1983) and the Social Skills Rating System Child and Parent Version (SSRS; Gresham & Elliot,

1990) are two of the most frequently used of these measures. Both are described in great detail in the broader social skills assessment chapter of this volume. Other less frequently used measures include the Social Skills Questionnaire—Parent (SSQ-P, Spence, 1995), the Social Competence Questionnaire—Parent (SCQ-P; Spence, 1995), the Friendship Questionnaire (Bierman & McCauley, 1987), and the Children's Assertive Behavior Scale (CABS; Michelson & Wood, 1982).

Summary and Recommendations for Assessment

In sum, for the assessment of anxiety disorders, we echo the recommendations of Davis and Ollendick

Table 11.3 Measures of social skills and social competence

Instrument	Description	Psychometric properties
The children's assertive behavior scale (CABS; Michelson & Wood, 1982)	A 27-item child report measure of social behavior. Each item represents a social situation and children indicate how they would respond on a 5-point scale from passive to aggressive	Internal consistency = 0.78. Test–retest reliability = 0.86. Good discriminant and convergent validity
The friendship questionnaire (Bierman & McCauley, 1987)	A 40-item child-report measure of peer interactions. Includes 3 subscales: positive interactions, negative interactions, and extensiveness of peer network	Internal consistency range from 0.72 to 0.82
The Matson evaluation of social skills for youngsters (MESSY; Matson, et al., 1983; Spence and Liddle, 1990)	A 62-item parent- and teacher-report measure of social skills in children aged 4–18. Various social behaviors are listed and respondents indicate how often the behavior is performed on a scale from 1 ("not at all") to 5 ("very much"). The scale yields six factors, appropriate social skills, inappropriate assertiveness, impulsive/recalcitrant, overconfident, jealousy/withdrawal, and miscellaneous	Internal consistency = 0.91 for the total score and ranges from 0.54 to 0.89 for the factors. Has been found to have good convergent and discriminant validity
The social competence questionnaire—parent (Spence, 1995)	Contains 9 items in which parents rate a child's social competence with peers from 0 (not true) to 2 (mostly true)	Guttman split-half reliability has been reported to be 0.87
The social skills questionnaire—parent (Spence, 1995)	Contains 30 items in which parents assess a child's perceived social skills	Split-half reliability has been reported to be 0.90
The social skills rating system child and parent version (SSRS; Gresham & Elliot, 1990)	Includes parent, teacher, and child (grade 3 and above) measures of social skills and problem behaviors. There are five social skills factors: cooperation, assertion, responsibility, empathy, and self-control	Internal consistency ranges from 0.65 to 0.95. Test–retest reliability ranges from 0.65 to 0.87. Has been shown to have good construct and criterion validity

(2005) and Silverman and Ollendick (2005) in that an evidence-based, multi-component (i.e., physiology, behavior, and cognition), and multi-method, multi-informant assessment is crucial. Given the numerous anxiety instruments and methods available (cf. Silverman & Ollendick, 2005), it is difficult to create a single, one-size-fits-all battery. However, current evidence suggests using the Multidimensional Anxiety Scale for Children (MASC) and Revised Children's Manifest Anxiety Scale (RCMAS) to screen for potential anxiety disorders, and using the Social Phobia and Anxiety Inventory for Children (SPAI-C) to screen specifically for social phobia (Silverman & Ollendick, 2005). These instruments not only capture the anxiety symptoms, but also other aspects of the emotional response (e.g., physiology). Further, the RCMAS has the benefit of including a "Lie" scale which may be beneficial in determining the extent to which a child may be engaging in impression management—potentially more important with a child with social-evaluative fears. A broadband measure of functioning is also recommended (e.g., the Child Behavior Checklist). Diagnostically, the semi-structured ADIS interviews are recommended for determining the presence or absence of diagnoses and for tracking treatment progress, and social skills can be assessed with the MESSY or the SSRS. If at all possible, clinicians should consider the use of an ABO method to further evaluate a child's functioning. Finally, clinicians should be aware that the social anxiety, deficits, and difficulties they are attempting to assess and treat may interfere with the actual assessment and treatment processes as well. As a result, clinicians should be mindful to allow more time to develop rapport and be especially mindful of the child's progress, anxiety, and frustration.

Treatment

Currently, a variety of efficacious treatment techniques have been examined for use with anxious children (2005; Davis & Ollendick, 2005). Over time, these various techniques, while therapeutic and researched in their own right, have been combined into increasingly efficacious behavioral

and cognitive-behavioral therapies (CBT). These treatment techniques include exposure, systematic desensitization, modeling, and contingency management. Each of these procedures is explained and evaluated below regarding its use in the treatment of symptoms of anxiety as well as the treatment of social skills problems in children with anxiety. Additionally, a particular focus will be the commonly used combination behavioral and cognitive-behavioral treatments for child social anxiety. Overall, however, it is important to remember that efficacious treatments for child anxiety have typically been designed to alleviate anxious symptomatology and not necessary social problems per se. In addition, and while progress has been made, many child treatments still need to account for child development and developmental psychopathology more thoroughly, and the field should be wary of overly simplistic downward extensions of adult therapies (Barrett, 2000). Given the implications of the review to this point, the treatment of both pathological emotion and social skills may be necessary and advisable, even in children having anxiety disorders other than social phobia.

Exposure

Exposure involves the anxious child encountering or experiencing the feared stimulus or situation either in vivo or imaginally and ideally remaining exposed until the anxiety or fear has had the opportunity to decrease. In vivo exposure involves the child being exposed to the actual feared stimulus, such as being around a dog or interacting with an unfamiliar person. For imaginal exposure the child is guided in imagining the feared stimulus or situation, such as imagining what it would be like to talk with a person at a restaurant and situations at school with peers. In vivo exposure is commonly included in treatments for children with a variety of anxiety disorders; for example, one review suggested that as many as 90–100% of anxiety treatments incorporate exposure (Chorpita & Southam-Gerow, 2006). Exposure can be administered all at once to the most feared situation, such as in flooding or implosive therapy; however, exposure is more commonly administered gradually by setting up a hierarchy of least to most fearful stimuli or situations for the client, then exposing the client starting with the least fearful stimulus or situation and working up to more and more fearful stimuli or situations as the client becomes comfortable with the previous steps. The latter is thought to be the more humane of the two doses of exposure and is preferred by most clients, parents, and professionals (King & Gullone, 1990). Overall, controlled exposure is thought to provide safe experiences with the feared stimulus or situation allowing for habituation and extinction of fear anxiety. New learning occurs as well which competes with previous fearful responding, and exposure sessions provide a structured environment in which to practice and develop coping skills and competency (Davis, in press).

Systematic Desensitization

One form of treatment which makes use of exposure is systematic desensitization. This treatment was developed by Wolpe (1958) and was initially based on the idea that a fear response could be counter-conditioned by pairing the feared stimulus with an activity that is reciprocal to and incongruent with anxiety. While such processes are now better understood as the development of competing, context-specific learning instead of new learning overwriting the old (Bouton, 2004), the procedure remains largely unchanged. The competing activity most often used is progressive muscle relaxation and diaphragmatic breathing; however, it can be any act in which the person will not be anxious at the same time (e.g., holding a favorite toy or eating). After relaxation skills are taught, a fear hierarchy is developed ranging from the least to the most feared stimulus or situation. The person then begins to engage in the competing activity (becomes relaxed) and is then gradually exposed to situations on the hierarchy. So long as the client remains relaxed and does not become anxious in the situation, the association between the stimulus and the fearful response is thought to decrease and the client's fear of the stimulus should decrease. Systematic desensitization can be administered either in vivo or imaginally. Typically, and particularly with

imaginal exposures, some sort of safety signal is utilized during progression along the hierarchy to designate when an individual begins to experience fear or anxiety and the exposure intensity needs to be halted or slightly decreased (e.g., raising a hand).

Modeling

Modeling involves the child observing another person engaging in appropriate behavior in the feared situation either on video or directly with that model demonstrating coping, competence, and skill. A model may engage in myriad behaviors to be learned, including appropriate conversation skills with peers, ordering at a restaurant, or asking questions in class. Models, further, can be other children, parents, or clinicians. Models can also be qualified as either mastery models, who demonstrate the mastery of interacting in the situation with ease, or coping models, in which the model is initially anxious in the situation but overcomes the anxiety (Chorpita & Southam-Gerow, 2006). In a different variation, Ritter (1965, 1968) developed participant modeling based on work grounded in social-learning theory. In participant modeling, the model demonstrates appropriate behavior for the child, and then the model interacts with the child to help him perform the skills. An example of this would be having a child watch a peer introduce himself on the playground, and then having the peer go with the child to introduce himself. Subsequently, the effectiveness of models during child treatment has been suggested to increase from using filmed models, to live models, to participant modeling (Ollendick, 1979).

Contingency Management

In contingency management, children are rewarded for appropriate behavior in anxiety-provoking situations. Rewards can be tangible items or verbal praise from therapists or caregivers. Silverman and colleagues (1999) examined the efficacy of a contingency management treatment in children with anxiety disorders. The children's parents awarded rewards for completing certain tasks on a fear hierarchy. Parents were also educated in basic behavioral principles such as positive rewards and extinction. Children with this treatment showed significant improvement on outcome measures assessing fear, anxiety, and depression, and 55% of children who received contingency management treatment no longer met criteria for an anxiety disorder according to diagnostic interviews (Silverman et al., 1999).

Behavioral and Cognitive-Behavioral Techniques

Behavioral treatments make use of a variety of techniques previously discussed and are based upon operant and classical conditioning. Cognitive-behavioral treatments (CBT) involve cognitive techniques such as cognitive restructuring and changing expectations about what will happen in a feared situation combined with the addition of behavioral techniques such as exposure, contingency management, or social skills training. In a meta-analysis, CBT was found to have strong effect sizes for reducing social anxiety and moderate effect sizes for increasing social competence (Segool & Carlson, 2008). Many of the more widely examined and relevant behavioral and cognitive-behavioral treatments are discussed below.

Coping Cat

The *Coping Cat* program is a manualized childhood anxiety treatment designed by Kendall, Kane, Howard, and Siqueland (1990). In addition to the therapist manual, there is also a *Coping Cat Workbook* that is given to children and used in each session (Kendall, 1990). The treatment consists of 16 individual sessions, two of which are parent meetings with the therapist. The first 8 sessions focus on psychoeducation, cognitive skills, and healthy coping skills; the last 8 sessions focus on working through an exposure hierarchy (Kendall et al., 1990). Kendall (1994) evaluated the effectiveness of this program in an RCT for children with

primary anxiety disorder diagnoses including overanxious disorder, separation anxiety disorder, and avoidant disorder. Children who received the *Coping Cat* treatment were compared with a waitlist control group. At post-treatment, 64% of children in the *Coping Cat* group no longer met criteria for an anxiety disorder, compared with 5% of children in the waitlist group (Kendall, 1994). The children who received the *Coping Cat* treatment also improved on a number of scales assessing anxiety; these results were maintained at 1-year follow-up (Kendall, 1994). Similar results for treatment outcome were found by Kendall (1997) in another RCT comparing the *Coping Cat* to waitlist control. Further, Kendall (1994) also included the social competency scale of the CBCL as an outcome measure. Children in the treatment group showed significant improvement in ratings on this scale compared to the waitlist group, and these effects were maintained at 1-year follow-up (Kendall, 1994).

Several authors have examined whether adding a family component increases efficacy of the treatment. Results from these studies indicate that there may be a marginal effect of adding parent training and parent education components to the *Coping Cat* and that these changes will have a greater efficacy with younger treatment clients than adolescents (Barrett, 1998; Barrett, Dadds, & Rapee, 1996). Nauta, Scholing, Emmelkamp, and Minderaa (2003), however, found no outcome differences between treatment groups with and without parent training components. The *Coping Cat* has also been implemented successfully in group formats, showing that it is superior to a psychological placebo procedure and waitlist control (Muris, Meesters, & van Melick, 2002). When compared with individual treatment, few differences were found and both treatments were superior to the waitlist control (Flannery-Schroeder & Kendall, 2000). Flannery-Schroeder and Kendall (2000) included several measures of social skills in a RCT comparing individual treatment, group treatment, and waitlist control. This study failed to show, however, that the treatment groups differed from the waitlist control at post-treatment on both child and parent measures of social skills (Flannery-Schroeder & Kendall, 2000). Although the *Coping Cat* is a well-received treatment and is effective in reducing symptoms of anxiety, it does not include a social skills component. Furthermore, few studies to date have examined the role it plays in helping anxious children with social skills deficits and those that do have produced mixed results.

FRIENDS

The FRIENDS program is a group format CBT procedure for children aged 6–16 years with anxiety disorders. Treatment consists of 10 child group sessions, 2 booster sessions, and 10 parent sessions. The treatment includes cognitive and coping skills similar to the *Coping Cat*, family management and communication skills training to facilitate practice of the skills children learn in session, and a peer component in which children are taught basic social skills including how to make friends (Shortt, Barrett, & Fox, 2001). FRIENDS is an acronym for the coping skills taught in session (i.e., F-Feeling worried? R-Relax and feel good; I-Inner thoughts; E-Explore plans; N-Nice work so reward yourself; D-Don't forget to practice; S-Stay calm, you know how to cope now). There is a therapist manual, children's workbook, and parent booklet that are used in the treatment. Shortt and colleagues (2001) examined the efficacy of FRIENDS treatment in an RCT compared to a waitlist control. Children included in the study met criteria for a primary anxiety disorder diagnosis including generalized anxiety disorder, separation anxiety disorder, or social phobia. At post-treatment, 69% of children in the FRIENDS group no longer met diagnosis criteria, compared with 6% of children in the waitlist control. These treatment effects were maintained at 1-year follow-up, with 68% of children who received treatment no longer meeting diagnosis criteria for a primary anxiety disorder (Shortt et al., 2001). Although the FRIENDS treatment contains a social skills component, there are no studies to date which include outcome measure of social skills or social competency.

Social Effectiveness Therapy for Children (SET-C)

SET-C is a behavioral group treatment for social anxiety disorder in children and adolescents. The treatment includes group sessions for education and social skills training focusing on conversation skills, skills for joining groups, assertiveness, and telephone skills. The treatment also includes peer generalization sessions in which anxious and non-anxious children engage in social activities, and individual in vivo exposure to feared social situations (Beidel et al., 2000). In an RCT, Beidel and colleagues (2000) compared SET-C to an attentional control called Testbusters. Children in the Testbusters group spent an equal amount of time in treatment, but were taught study skills and test-taking strategies. At post-treatment, 67% of children in the SET-C group no longer met criteria for social phobia, compared to 5% in the Testbusters group (Beidel et al., 2000). Children in the SET-C group were also rated as being more skilled during a role-play task and read-aloud task than children in the Testbusters group by independent observers post-treatment. At 6-month follow-up 80% of children who received SET-C no longer met criteria for social phobia (Beidel et al., 2000), and at 3-year follow-up, 72% of children who received SET-C no longer met criteria for social phobia. Ratings of children's skills during the role-play task decreased to pre-treatment levels following the post-treatment assessment, but effectiveness in performance during the read-aloud task was maintained (Beidel, Turner, Young, & Paulson, 2005).

Skills for Academic and Social Success (SASS)

Fisher, Masia-Warner, and Klein (2004) described a school-based social skills intervention to treat adolescents with social phobia. Skills for Academic and Social Success (SASS) is a cognitive-behavioral group treatment that includes psychoeducation, cognitive skills, social skills training (including conversation skills), listening skills and assertiveness, and gradual exposure and relapse prevention. It was developed from SET-C described above. Treatment consisted of 12 weekly group meetings that took place in school, two individual meetings, social events, including the use of peer assistants who were non-anxious adolescent classmates who assisted group members at school social events such as club meetings, two parent meetings which included education about social anxiety, and two teacher meetings which included education about anxiety and aided in setting up and working through the fear hierarchy for students (Fisher et al., 2004). Masia-Warner and colleagues (2007) examined the efficacy of SASS in a randomized clinical trial (RCT) comparing it to an attention control (Masia-Warner et al., 2007). Authors found that at post-treatment, 59% of the SASS treatment group no longer met criteria for social phobia, compared to 0% of the attention control group. These gains were maintained at 6-month follow-up (Masia-Warner et al., 2007). Measures of social skills or competency were not included in the study.

Cognitive-Behavioral Group Treatment for Adolescents (CBGT-A)

CBGT-A is a treatment for social anxiety disorder in adolescents. It was developed from an adult treatment for social phobia which followed a similar format (Albano & Barlow, 1996). The treatment is administered in 16 group sessions. The first 8 sessions focus on education, skill building including cognitive restructuring, social skills including those necessary for maintaining social relationships, and problem solving. The last 8 sessions focus on exposure to feared social situations. Parents are also educated about the disorder and help with exposure exercises (Albano & Barlow, 1996). Albano, Marten, Holt, Heimberg, and Barlow (1995) tested the efficacy of the protocol in 5 adolescents who met criteria for social phobia. At 3-month follow-up, 4 of the 5 participants no longer met criteria for social phobia, and at 12-month follow-up, none of the 5 participants met criteria for social phobia (Albano et al., 1995). Hayward and colleagues (2000) tested the efficacy of the treatment on a larger scale. These authors included 35 adolescent females who met criteria for social phobia. One half were assigned to CBGT-A, and the other half were assigned to a no-treatment control group. At post-treatment, 45% of girls in the CBGT-A group no longer met criteria for social phobia, compared with 4% of those in the no-treatment control group (Hayward et al., 2000). At 1-year follow-up, however, there was no statistical difference between the CBGT-A

group and the no-treatment control group. The treatment group continued to improve, and the control group improved as well. Authors suggested that this effect may have been due to children in the control group receiving treatment in the community (Hayward et al., 2000).

Cognitive-Behavioral Treatment with and Without Parent Involvement

Spence et al. (2000) used a social skills-based cognitive-behavioral treatment (CBT) to treat children aged 7–14 with social phobia. The children were divided into 3 treatment groups—CBT with parent involvement, CBT without parent involvement, and waitlist control. The treatment consisted of 12 group sessions, each of which was followed by a half-hour of games in which children could practice their skills with peers and be rewarded by the therapists for appropriate interactions. The treatment included social skills training covering conversation skills, listening skills, and identifying social cues in others. Children were also assigned weekly homework tasks. Parent involvement included parents observing children's group sessions and being taught about modeling and reinforcement. This treatment was successful in reducing symptoms of anxiety—87.5% of children in the CBT with parent involvement and 58% of children in the CBT without parent involvement no longer met criteria at post-treatment compared with 7% of children in the waitlist group. The authors also examined social skills, using the Social Skills Questionnaire-parent version (SSQ-P), Social Competence Questionnaire-parent version (SCQ-P), direct observation of social skills in the classroom and on the playground, and the Revised Behavioral Assertiveness Test for Children (BAT-CR). Improvement in children's social skills according to parent-report (SSQ-P) approached significance from pretreatment to posttreatment for both treatment groups but not the waitlist condition. Parent report of social competence (SCQ-P) and performance in role-play tasks for the BAT-CR improved for both treatment groups as well as the waitlist control group. Ratings of competence from direct observation by independent observers did not differ between the treatment groups and the waitlist control and did not improve over time (Spence et al., 2000). At 6- and 12-month follow-up assessments, treatment gains were maintained for the SSQ-P and the SCQ-P (Spence et al., 2000).

Brief Group Cognitive-Behavioral Treatment for Social Phobia

Similar to other CBT studies, Gallagher, Rabian, and McCloskey (2004) examined the effects of a small group CBT intervention composed of psychoeducation, cognitive strategies, and exposure in 23 children with social phobia. Children were either assigned to a wait-list or to small groups of 5–7 children for three 3-hour sessions of CBT. At 3-week follow-up, children treated with CBT generally showed improvement over those in the wait-list condition; however, no change in social competence was evident as measured by the CBCL (Gallagher et al., 2004).

Modular Treatment of Anxiety

Modular treatment of anxiety is an individual treatment for anxiety disorders in children developed by Chorpita, Taylor, Francis, Moffitt, and Austin (2004). The treatment consists of 13 modules which therapists can choose from and arrange to treat the individual needs of their clients. Four core modules which all children receive involve self-monitoring (fear ladder), psychoeducation, exposure, and maintenance/relapse prevention. These were thought by the authors to be essential principles in the treatment of childhood anxiety (Chorpita et al., 2004). Depending on the needs of the individual client, therapists can choose to include the other modules of cognitive restructuring, social skills training, rewards, differential reinforcement, and time-out as they pertain to individual client needs. The order of use for the modules is dictated by a flow chart in which modules for the basic skills of self-monitoring and psychoeducation are done first, then other optional modules are completed for behaviors that may interfere with exposure, then exposure and relapse prevention modules are completed. To the extent that parents or other adults are involved in the maintenance of the disorder, they are also involved in treatment such as the differential reinforcement and rewards modules (Chorpita et al., 2004). A pilot study examining the efficacy of this treatment was conducted with seven children suffering from primary diagnoses of anxiety disorders. Following their individual treatments none of the children met criteria for their primary anxiety diagnoses. These effects were maintained at 6-month follow-up (Chorpita et al., 2004). Although there has not been a large-scale RCT examining modular treatment, based on available evidence it does seem to hold promise for adding a protocol to the literature that is both efficacious and adaptable to both therapist and client needs (Chorpita, Daleiden, & Wisz, 2005). Modular treatment has also been suggested for disorders other than anxiety such as depression (Chorpita et al., 2005).

Conclusion

There are many available treatments for childhood anxiety in general and childhood social phobia in particular; however, these treatments often remain focused on reducing the symptoms of anxiety and arousal while ignoring social skills deficits common to children with this class of disorders. As a result, behavioral and cognitive-behavioral packages have been found to be particularly effective at treating anxiety disorder diagnoses and symptoms. Broadly, CBT has been found to meet well-established criteria for anxiety disorders and both behavioral and cognitive-behavioral programs have been found to be effective for social phobia in particular (i.e., probably efficacious status; 2005). However, even for treatments that do include social skills training as a component in treatment, few RCTs include outcome measures of social skills or social competency, and in those that do, it is unclear whether social skills improvements are evident (e.g., Flannery-Schroeder & Kendall, 2000; Gallagher et al., 2004) or maintained over time (Beidel et al., 2000, 2005; Spence et al., 2000). Because impairments in social skills often impact the lives of children with anxiety disorders, RCTs for childhood anxiety should include outcome measures of social skills. Social skills training should also be included in treatment of anxiety to the extent that it is relevant for individual cases.

Current Status and Future Directions

Children with anxiety suffer strained peer relationships, stigma, and victimization. Given the debilitating interaction of anxiety and social problems, it is surprising that as few as 10% of child anxiety treatment protocols include a social skills component (Chorpita & Southam-Gerow, 2006). Currently, many anxiety treatments seem geared toward alleviating anxious emotional responding, assessing and targeting behavioral symptoms in particular (cf. Davis, in press; Davis & Ollendick, 2005). While assessing avoidant and dysfunctional behavior is important, more research should be conducted using both a comprehensive assessment of anxiety (i.e., physiology, behavior, and cognition; Davis & Ollendick, 2005) as well as indicators of social functioning across a child's day-to-day environments (e.g., school, home, peers).

Specifically, beyond examinations of social anxiety, a great deal more needs to be done to target the interference and impairment in social relationships and functioning. Researchers should more frequently include measures of functioning in social and peer domains in child anxiety treatment studies. Findings from the extant literature on peer relations and social anxiety should increasingly be infused into broader treatment strategies to continue to develop comprehensive treatment packages, or, as is the case with the work by Chorpita, modular options which can be included as needed. Additional research needs to target the potential moderators and mediators of treatment as well. For example, incorporating parents into treatment may be important, but parental influence may be greatest for certain genders or ages (e.g., Ollendick & Horsch, 2007). Moreover, having greater knowledge of how treatments work could lead to better outcomes, treatment matching, and even more refined interventions. Given the rich data which can now be obtained through diagnostic, self/other-report questionnaires, and ABO methods,

continued research examining which treatments or techniques play to certain families' strengths or weaknesses would be beneficial. Finally, treatments should increasingly incorporate development and developmental psychopathology into assessment and treatment methods.

Future directions for those on the front lines of research and practice are as follows. Adapted from Davis, (in press), researchers developing and evaluating treatments should examine and address the weaknesses in the assessment and treatment literature, include more rigorous comparison groups (e.g., alternative treatments instead of only wait-lists), plan treatment evaluations around a comprehensive assessment of the anxiety response (including responses in social and peer contexts), include analysis of mediators and moderators of treatment outcome using a developmental psychopathological framework, and work harder to disseminate findings broadly to practitioners and the public. Front-line practitioners should continue the transition to evidence-based practice. Though the continual need to update practice standards to keep up with advances in research is daunting and potentially time consuming, inconvenience should not outweigh dated and possibly ineffectual and unethical practice. Realizing, however, that keeping up with the stream of new research is difficult, researchers have begun to organize their findings into more accessible formats and develop practitioner-friendly means of accessing evidence-based practices (cf. Ollendick & Davis, 2004). For example, Herschell, McNeil, and McNeil (2004) have suggested improvements in strategies which can lead practitioners to increased experience and expertise in evidence-based practice (e.g., graduate training, continuing education courses, practitioner-friendly manuals), while Ollendick and Davis (2004), building upon and integrating the suggestions of others, have suggested a web-based strategy geared toward sifting through the immense assessment and treatment literatures. Briefly, they recommend a five-step approach (cf. Sackett, Richardson, Rosenberg, & Haynes, 2000) common to many problem-solving strategies: Formulate the relevant assessment or treatment question, search for answers, evaluate the findings, implement the selected strategy, and evaluate the outcome. Further, they recommend melding these five steps with R. Haynes (2001) 4S strategy: Focus on systems, synopses, syntheses, and individual studies going from broad comprehensive resources to abstracts and reviews and finally down to individual research studies (Ollendick & Davis, 2004). Such an integrated search is likely necessary when attempting to determine current evidence-based practices with socially anxious and withdrawn children as much more work is needed for addressing social skills and social behaviors in the assessment, treatment, and relationships of these children.

Acknowledgments The participation of Thompson E. Davis III, Ph.D. was funded in part by an internal Louisiana State University grant. The terms "child" and "children" are used throughout and usually meant to include adolescents.

References

Achenbach, T. (1991). *Integrative guide for the 1991 CBCL/4-18, YSR, and TRF profiles*. Burlington: University of Vermont.

Achenbach, T. M., Mcconaughy, S. H., & Howell, C. T. (1987). Child/adolescent behavioural and emotional problems: Implications of cross-informant correlations for situational specificity. *Psychological Bulletin, 101,* 213–232.

Albano, A. M., & Barlow, D. H. (1996). Breaking the vicious cycle: Cognitive-behavioral group treatment for socially anxious youth. In E. D. Hibbs & P. S. Jensen (Eds.), *Psychosocial treatments for child and adolescent disorders: Empirically based strategies for clinical practice* (pp. 43–62). Washington, DC: American Psychological Association.

Albano, A. M., Marten, P. A., Holt, C. S., Heimberg, R. G., & Barlow, D. H. (1995). Cognitive-behavioral group treatment for social phobia in adolescents: A preliminary study. *The Journal of Nervous and Mental Disease, 183,* 649–656.

Ambrosini, P. J. (2000). Historical development and present status of the Schedule for affective Disorders and Schizophrenia for School-Age Children (K-SADS). *Journal of the American Academy of Child and Adolescent Psychiatry, 39,* 49–58.

American Psychiatric Association. (2000). *Diagnostic and statistical manual of mental disorders* (4th ed., text rev.). Washington, DC: Author.

Barrett, P. M. (1998). Evaluation of cognitive-behavioral group treatments for childhood anxiety disorders. *Journal of Clinical Child Psychology, 27,* 459–468.

Barrett, P. M. (2000). Treatment of childhood anxiety: Developmental aspects. *Clinical Psychology Review, 20,* 479–494.

Barrett, P. M., Dadds, M. R., & Rapee, R. M. (1996). Family treatment of childhood anxiety: A controlled trial. *Journal of Consulting and Clinical Psychology, 64,* 333–342.

Barrett, P., Healy, L., & March, J. S. (2003). Behavioral avoidance test for childhood obsessive-compulsive disorder: A home-based observation. *American Journal of Psychotherapy, 57,* 80–100.

Beidel, D. C., Fink, C. M., & Turner, S. M. (1996). Stability in anxious symptomatology in children. *Journal of Abnormal Child Psychology, 24,* 257–269.

Beidel, D. C., Turner, S. M., & Morris, T. L. (1995). A new inventory to assess childhood social anxiety and phobia: The social phobia and anxiety inventory for children. *Psychological Assessment, 7,* 73–79.

Beidel, D. C., Turner, S. M., & Morris, T. L. (2000). Behavioral treatment of childhood social phobia. *Journal of Consulting and Clinical Psychology, 68,* 1072–1080.

Beidel, D. C., Turner, S. M., Young, B., & Paulson, A. (2005). Social effectiveness therapy for children: Three-year follow-up. *Journal of Consulting and Clinical Psychology, 73,* 721–725.

Biederman, J., Hirshfeld-Becker, D., Rosenbaum, J., Herot, C., Friedman, D., Snidman, N., et al. (2001). Further evidence of association between behavioral inhibition and social anxiety in children. *American Journal of Psychiatry, 158,* 1673–1679.

Bierman, K. L., & Mccauley, E. (1987). Children's descriptions of their peer interactions: Useful information for clinical child assessment. *Journal of Clinical Child Psychology, 16,* 9–18.

Birmaher, B., Brent, D., Chiappetta, L., Bridge, j., Monga, S., & Baugher, M. (1999). Psychometric properties of the Screen for Child Anxiety Related Emotional Disorders (SCARED): A replication study. *Journal of the American Academy of Child and Adolescent Psychiatry, 38,* 1230–1236.

Birmaher, B., Khetarpal, S., Brent, D. A., Cully, M., Balach, L., Kauffman, J., et al. (1997). The Screen for Child Anxiety Related Emotional Disorders (SCARED): Scale construction and psychometric characteristics. *Journal of the American Academy of Child and Adolescent Psychiatry, 36,* 545–553.

Bouton, M. (2004). Context and behavioral processes in extinction. *Learning and Memory, 11,* 485–494.

Buss, A., & Plomin, R. (1984). *Temperament: Early developing personality traits*. Hillsdale, NJ: Erlbaum.

Cartwright-Hatton, S., Mcnicol, K., & Doubleday, E. (2006). Anxiety in a neglected population: Prevalence of anxiety disorders in pre-adolescent children. *Clinical Psychology Review, 26,* 817–833.

Chavira, D., Stein, M., Bailey, K., & Stein, M. (2004). Childhood anxiety disorders in primary care: Prevalent but untreated. *Depression and Anxiety, 20,* 155–164.

Chorpita, B. F., Daleiden, E. L., & Weisz, J. R. (2005). Modularity in the design and application of therapeutic interventions. *Applied and Preventive Psychology, 11,* 141–156.

Chorpita, B., & Southam-Gerow, M. (2006). Fears and anxieties. In E. J. Mash & R. A. Barkley (Eds.), *Treatment of child disorders* (3rd ed., pp. 271–335). New York: Guilford.

Chorpita, B. F., Taylor, A. A., Francis, S. E., Moffitt, C., & Austin, A. A. (2004). Efficacy of modular cognitive behavior therapy for childhood anxiety disorders. *Behavior Therapy, 35*, 263–287.

Chorpita, B. F., Tracey, S. A., Brown, T. A., Collica, T. J., & Barlow, D. H. (1997). Assessment of worry in children and adolescents: An adaptation of the Penn State Worry Questionnaire. *Behavior Research and Therapy, 35*, 569–581.

Choudhury, M. S., Pimentel, S. S., & Kendall, P. C. (2003). Childhood anxiety disorders: Parent–child (dis)agreement using a structured interview for the DSM-IV. *Journal of the American Academy of Child and Adolescent Psychiatry, 42*, 957–964.

Coles, M. E., & Heimberg, R. G. (2000). Patterns of anxious arousal during exposure to feared situations in individuals with social phobia. *Behaviour Research and Therapy, 38*, 405–424.

Costello, E. J., Mustillo, S., Erkanli, A., Keeler, G., & Angold, A. (2003). Prevalence and development of psychiatric disorders in childhood and adolescence. *Archives of General Psychiatry, 60*, 837–844.

Davis III, T. E. (2009). PTSD, anxiety, and phobias. In J. Matson, F. Andrasik, & M. Matson (Eds.), *Treating childhood psychopathology and developmental disorders* (pp. 183–220). New York: Springer Science and Business Media, LLC.

Davis, T. E., III, & Ollendick, T. H. (2005). A critical review of empirically supported treatments for specific phobia in children: Do efficacious treatments address the components of a phobic response? *Clinical Psychology: Science and Practice, 12*, 144–160.

Drobes, D. J., & Lang, P. J. (1995). Bioinformational theory and behavior therapy. In W. O'Donohue & L. Krasner (Eds.), *Theories of behavior therapy: Exploring behaviour change* (pp. 229–257). Washington, DC: American Psychological Association.

Elizabeth, J., King, N., Ollendick, T. H., Gullone, E., Tonge, B., Watson, S., et al. (2006). Social anxiety disorder in children and youth: A research update on aetiological factors. *Counselling Psychology Quarterly, 19*, 151–163.

Fisak, B., & Grills-Taquechel, A. E. (2007). Parental modeling, reinforcement, and information transfer: Risk factors in the development of child anxiety? *Clinical Child and Family Psychology Review, 10*, 213–231.

Fisher, P. H., Masia-Warner, C., & Klein, R. G. (2004). Skills for social and academic success: A school-based intervention for social anxiety disorder in adolescents. *Clinical Child and Family Psychology Review, 7*, 241–249.

Flannery-Schroeder, E. C., & Kendall, P. C. (2000). Group and individual cognitive-behavioral treatments for youth with anxiety disorders: A randomized clinical trial. *Cognitive Therapy and Research, 24*, 251–278.

Foa, E. B., & Kozak, M. J. (1986). Emotional processing of fear: Exposure to corrective information. *Psychological Bulletin, 99*, 20–35.

Foa, E. B., & Kozak, M. J. (1998). Clinical applications of bioinformational theory: Understanding anxiety and its treatment. *Behavior Therapy, 29*, 675–690.

Fyer, A. (1993). Heritability of social anxiety: A brief review. *Journal of Clinical Psychiatry, 54*, 10–12.

Fyer, A., Mannuzza, S., Chapman, T., Martin, L., & Klein, D. (1995). Specificity in familial aggregation of phobic disorders. *Archives of General Psychiatry, 52*, 564–573.

Gallagher, H., Rabian, B., & Mccloskey, M. (2004). A brief cognitive-behavioral intervention for social phobia in childhood. *Journal of Anxiety Disorders, 18*, 459–479.

Ginsburg, G., La Greca, A., & Silverman, W. (1998). Social anxiety in children with anxiety disorders: Relation with social and emotional functioning. *Journal of Abnormal Child Psychology, 26*, 175–185.

Glennon, B., & Weisz, J. R. (1978). An observational approach to the assessment of anxiety in young children. *Journal of Consulting and Clinical Psychology, 46*, 1246–1257.

Gregory, A., & Eley, T. (2007). Genetic influences on anxiety in children: What we've learned and where we're heading. *Clinical Child and Family Psychology Review, 10*, 199–212.

Gresham, F. M., & Elliot, S. N. (1990). *Social skill rating system.* Circle Pines, MN: American Guidance Service.

Grills, A. & Ollendick, T. H. (2003). Multiple informant agreement and the anxiety disorders interview schedule for parents and children. *Journal of the American Academy of Child and Adolescent Psychiatry, 42*, 30–40.

Haynes, R. (2001). Of studies, summaries, synopses, and systems: The "4S" evolution of services for finding current best evidence. *Evidence-Based Mental Health, 4*, 37–39.

Haynes, S. N. (2001). Introduction to the special section on clinical applications of analogue behavioral observation. *Psychological Assessment, 13*, 3–4.

Hayward, C., Varady, S., Albano, A. M., Thienemann, M., Henderson, L., & Schatzberg, A. F. (2000). Cognitive-behavioral group therapy for social phobia in female adolescents: Results of a pilot study. *Journal of the Academy of Child and Adolescent Psychiatry, 39*, 721–726.

Heimberg, R., Stein, M., Hiripi, E., & Kessler, R. (2000). Trends in the prevalence of social phobia in the United States: A synthetic cohort analysis of changes over four decades. *European Psychiatry, 15*, 29–37.

Herschell, A., Mcneil, C., & Mcneil, D. (2004). Clinical child psychology's progress in disseminating empirically supported treatments. *Clinical Psychology: Science and Practice, 11*, 267–288.

Jenson, P. S., Rubio-Stipec, M., Canino, G., Bird, H. R., Dulcan, M. K., Schwab-Stone, M. E., et al. (1999). Parent and child contributions to diagnosis of mental disorder: Are both informants always necessary? *Journal of the American Academy of Child and Adolescent Psychiatry, 38*, 1569–1579.

Jorm, A., & Wright, A. (2008). Influences on young people's stigmatising attitudes towards peers with mental disorders: National survey of young Australians and their parents. *The British Journal of Psychiatry, 192*, 144–149.

Kagan, J., Reznick, J., Clarke, C., Snidman, N., & Garcia Coll, C. (1984). Behavioral inhibition to the unfamiliar. *Child Development, 55*, 2212–2225.

Kagan, J., Reznick, J., & Snidman, N. (1987). The physiology and psychology of behavioural inhibition. *Child Development, 58*, 1459–1473.

Kendall, P. C. (1990). *The coping cat workbook.* Ardmore, PA: Workbook Publishing.

Kendall, P. C. (1994). Treating anxiety disorders in children: Results of a randomized clinical trial. *Journal of Consulting and Clinical Psychology*, *62*, 100–110.

Kendall, P. C. (1997). Therapy for youths with anxiety disorders: A second randomized clinical trial. *Journal of Consulting and Clinical Psychology*, *65*, 366–380.

Kendall, P. C., Kane, M., Howard, B., & Siqueland, L. (1990). *Cognitive-behavioral therapy for anxious children: Treatment manual*. Ardmore, PA: Workbook.

Kendall, P. C., Safford, S., Flannery-Schroeder, E. C., & Webb, A. (2004). Child anxiety treatment: Outcomes in adolescence and impact on substance use and depression at 7.4 year follow-up. *Journal of Consulting and Clinical Psychology*, *72*, 276–287.

Kessler, R., Chiu, W., Demler, O., & Walters, E. (2005). Prevalence, severity, and comorbidity of 12-months DSM-IV disorders in the national comorbidity survey replication. *Archives of General Psychiatry*, *62*, 617–627.

King, N. J., & Gullone, E. (1990). Acceptability of fear reduction procedures with children. *Journal of Behavioral Therapy and Experimental Psychiatry*, *21*, 1–8.

La Greca, A. M., Dandes, S. K., Wick, P., Shaw, K., & Stone, W. L. (1988). Development of the social anxiety scale for children: Reliability and concurrent validity. *Journal of Clinical Child Psychology*, *17*, 84–91.

La Greca, A., & Lopez, N. (1998). Social anxiety among adolescents: Linkages with peer relationships and friendships. *Journal of Abnormal Child Psychology*, *26*, 83–94.

Lang, P. J. (1979). A bio-informational theory of emotional imagery. *Psychophysiology*, *16*, 495–512.

Lang, P. J., Cuthbert, B. N., Bradley, M. M. (1998). Measuring emotion in therapy: Imagery, activation, and feeling. *Behavior Therapy*, *29*, 655–674.

Mannuzza, S., Schneier, F., Chapman, T., Liebowitz, M., Klein, D., & Fyer, A. (1995). Generalized social phobia: Reliability and validity. *Archives of General Psychiatry*, *52*, 230–237.

March, J. S., Parker, J. D. A., Sullivan, K., Stallings, P., & Conners, K. (1997). The Multidimensional Anxiety Scale for Children (MASC): Factor structure, reliability, and validity. *Journal of the American Academy of Child & Adolescent Psychiatry*, *36*, 554–565.

Marks, I. (2002). Innate and learned fears are at opposite ends of a continuum of associability. *Behaviour Research and Therapy*, *40*, 165–167.

Mash, E., & Dozois, D. (2003). Child psychopathology: A developmental-systems perspective. In E. Mash & R. Barkley (Eds.), *Child psychopathology* (2nd ed., pp. 3–71). New York: Guilford Press.

Masia, C., & Morris, T. (1998). Parental factors associated with social anxiety: Methodological limitations and suggestions for integrated behavioral research. *Clinical Psychology: Science and Practice*, *5*, 211–228.

Masia-Warner, C., Fisher, P. H., Shrout, P. E., Rathor, S., & Klein, R. G. (2007). Treating adolescent with social anxiety disorder in school: An attention control trial. *Journal of Child Psychology and Psychiatry*, *48*, 676–686.

Matson, J. L., Rotatori, A. F., & Helsel, W. J. (1983). Development of a rating scale to measure social skills in children: The Matson Evaluation of Social Skills with Youngsters (MESSY). *Behaviour Research and Therapy*, *21*, 335–340.

Mccabe, K., Clark, R., & Barnett, D. (1999). Family protective factors among urban African American youth. *Journal of Clinical Child Psychology*, *28*, 137–150.

Michelson, L., & Wood, R. (1982). Development and psychometric properties of the Children's Assertive Behavior Scale. *Journal of Behavioral Assessment*, *4*, 3–13.

Mineka, S., & Zinbarg, R. (2006). A contemporary learning theory perspective on the etiology of anxiety disorders. *American Psychologist*, *61*, 10–26.

Muris, P., Meesters, C., & van Melick, M. (2002). Treatment of childhood anxiety disorders: A preliminary comparison between cognitive-behavioral group therapy and a psychological placebo intervention. *Journal of Behavior Therapy and Experimental Psychiatry*, *33*, 143–158.

Muris, P., Merckelbach, H., De Jong, P., & Ollendick, T. H. (2002). The etiology of specific fears and phobias in children: A critique of the non-associative account. *Behaviour Research and Therapy*, *40*, 185–195.

Muris, P., Merckelbach, H., Schmidt, H., & Mayer, B. (1999). The revised version of the Screen for Child Anxiety Related Emotional Disorders (SCARED-R): Factor structure in normal children. *Personality and Individual Differences*, *26*, 99–112.

Muris, P., & Merkelbach, H. (2000). How serious are common childhood fears? II. The parent's point of view. *Behaviour Research and Therapy*, *38*, 813–818.

Muris, P., Merkelbach, H., Mayer, B., & Prins, E. (2000). How serious are common childhood fears? *Behaviour Research and Therapy*, *38*, 217–228.

Muris, P., & Steerneman, P. (2001). The revised version of the Screen for Child Anxiety Related Emotional Disorders (SCARED-R): First evidence for its reliability and validity in a clinical sample. *British Journal of Clinical Psychology*, *40*, 35–44.

Nauta, M. H., Scholing, A., Emmelkamp, P. M. G., & Minderaa, R. B. (2003). Cognitive-behavioral therapy for children with anxiety disorders in a clinical setting: No additional effect of a cognitive parent training. *Journal of the American Academy of Child and Adolescent Psychiatry*, *42*, 1270–1278.

Oh, W., Rubin, K., Bowker, J., Booth-Laforce, C., Rose-Krasnor, L., & Laursen, B. (2008). Trajectories of social withdrawal from middle childhood to early adolescence. *Journal of Abnormal Child Psychology*, *36*, 553–566.

Ollendick, T. H. (1979). Fear reduction techniques with children. In M. Hersen, R. M. Eisler, & P. M. Miller (Eds.), *Progress in behavior modification* (Vol. 8, pp. 127–168). New York: Academic.

Ollendick, T. H. (1981). Assessment of social interaction skills in school children. *Behavioral Counseling Quarterly*, *1*, 227–243.

Ollendick, T. H. (1983). Reliability and validity of the Revised Fear Survey Schedule for Children (FSSC-R). *Behaviour Research and Therapy*, *21*, 395–399.

Ollendick, T. H., & Davis, T. E., III (2004). Empirically supported treatments for children and adolescents: Where to from here? *Clinical Psychology: Science and Practice*, *11*, 289–294.

Ollendick, T. H., Davis, T. E., & Muris, P. (2004). Treatment of specific phobia in children and adolescents. In P. Barrett & T. H. Ollendick (Eds.), *The handbook of interventions that work with children and adolescents: From prevention to treatment* (pp. 273–299). West Sussex, England: John Wiley and Sons.

Ollendick, T. H., & Hersen, M. (1993). Child and adolescent behavioral assessment. In T. H. Ollendick & M. Hersen (Eds.), *Handbook of child and adolescent assessment* (pp. 3–14). New York: Pergamon.

Ollendick, T. H., & Hirshfeld-Becker, D. (2002). The developmental psychopathology of social anxiety disorder. *Biological Psychiatry, 51*, 44–58.

Ollendick, T. H., & Horsch, L. (2007). Fears in clinic-referred children: Relations with child anxiety sensitivity, maternal overcontrol, and maternal phobic anxiety. *Behavior Therapy, 38*, 402–411.

Puliafico, A., & Kendall, P. C. (2006). Threat-related attentional bias in anxious youth: A review. *Clinical Child and Family Psychology Review, 9*, 162–180.

Rachman, S., & Hodgson, R. (1974). Desynchrony in measures of fear. *Behaviour Research and Therapy, 12*, 319–326.

Rapee, R., & Spence, S. (2004). The etiology of social phobia: Empirical evidence and an initial model. *Clinical Psychology Review, 24*, 737–767.

Reynolds, C. R., & Kamphus, R. W. (1992). *Behavioral assessment scale for children*. Circle Pines, MN: American Guidance Service.

Reynolds, C. R., & Richmond, B. O. (1985). *Revised children's manifest anxiety scale: Manual*. Los Angeles: Western Psychological Services.

Ritter, B. (1965). *The treatment of a dissection phobia*. Unpublished manuscript, Queens College.

Ritter, B. (1968). The group desensitization of children's snake phobias using vicarious and contact desensitization procedures. *Behaviour Research and Therapy, 6*, 1–6.

Ronan, K. R., Kendall, P. C., & Rowe, M. (1994). Negative affectivity in children: Development and validation of a self-statement questionnaire. *Cognitive Therapy and Research, 18*, 509–528.

Rubin, K., Wojslawowicz, J., Rose-Krasnor, L., Booth-Laforce, C., & Burgess, K. (2006). The best friendships of shy/withdrawn children: Prevalence, stability, and relationship quality. *Journal of Abnormal Child Psychology, 34*, 143–157.

Sackett, D., Richardson, W., Rosenberg, W., & Haynes, B. (2000). *Evidence-based medicine* (2nd ed.). London: Churchill Livingston.

Schniering, C. A., & Rapee, R. M. (2002). Development and validation of a measure of children's automatic thoughts: The Children's Automatic Thoughts Scale. *Behaviour Research and Therapy, 40*, 1091–1109.

Segool, N. K., & Carlson, J. S. (2008). Efficacy of cognitive-behavioral and pharmacological treatments for children with social anxiety. *Depression and Anxiety, 25*, 620–631.

Shaffer, D., Fisher, P., Lucas, C., Dulcan, M. K., & Schwab-Stone, M. E. (2000). NIMH Diagnostic Interview Schedule for Children Version IV (NIMH DISC-IV): Description, differences from previous versions, and reliability of some common diagnoses. *Journal of the American Academy of Child and Adolescent Psychiatry, 39*, 28–38.

Shortt, A. L., Barrett, P. M., & Fox, T. L. (2001). Evaluating the FRIENDS program: A cognitive-behavioral group treatment for anxious children and their parents. *Journal of Clinical Child Psychology, 30*, 525–535.

Silverman, W. K. (1994). Structured diagnostic interviews. In T. H. Ollendick, N. J. King, & W. Yule (Eds.), *International handbook of phobic and anxiety disorders in children and adolescents* (pp. 293–315). New York: Plenum.

Silverman, W. K., & Albano, A. M. (1996). *Anxiety disorders interview schedule for DSM-IV (child and parent versions)*. San Antonio, TX: Psychological Corporation.

Silverman, W. K., Fleisig, W., Rabian, B., & Peterson, R. A. (1991). Childhood anxiety sensitivity index. *Journal of Clinical Child Psychology, 20*, 162–168.

Silverman, W. K., Kurtines, W. M., Ginsburg, G. S., Weems, C. F., Rabian, B., & Serafini, L. T. (1999). Contingency management, self-control, and education support in the treatment of childhood phobic disorders: A randomized clinical trial. *Journal of Consulting and Clinical Psychology, 67*, 675–687.

Silverman, W., & Ollendick, T. H. (2005). Evidence-based assessment of anxiety and its disorders in children and adolescents. *Journal of Clinical Child and Adolescent Psychology, 34*, 380–411.

Silverman, W. K., Saavedra, L. M., & Pina, A. A. (2001). Test–retest reliability of anxiety symptoms and diagnoses using the anxiety disorders interview schedule for DSM-IV: Child and Parent Versions (ADIS for DSM-IV: C/P). *Journal of the American Academy of Child & Adolescent Psychiatry, 40*, 937–944.

Sondaite, J., & Zukauskiene, R. (2005). Adolescents' social strategies: Patterns and correlates. *Scandinavian Journal of Psychology, 46*, 367–374.

Spence, S. H. (1995). *Social skills training: Enhancing social competence with children and adolescents*. Windsor, Berkshire, England: NFER-NELSON.

Spence, S., Donovan, C., & Brechman-Toussaint, M. (1999). Social skills, social outcomes, and cognitive features of childhood social phobia. *Journal of Abnormal Psychology, 108*, 211–221.

Spence, S. H., Donovan, C., & Brechman-Toussaint, M. (2000). The treatment of childhood social phobia: The effectiveness of a social skills training-based, cognitive-behavioural intervention, with and without parent involvement. *Journal of Child Psychology and Psychiatry, 41*, 713–726.

Spence, S. H., & Liddle, B. (1990). Self-report measures of social competence for children: An evaluation of Social Skills for Youngsters and the List of Social Situation Problems. *Behavioral Assessment, 12*, 317–336.

Spielberger, C. D. (1973). *Manual for the state-trait anxiety inventory for children*. Palo Alto, CA: Consulting Psychologists Press.

Stein, M., Chartier, M., Kozak, M., King, N., & Kennedy, J. (1998). Genetic linkage to the serotonin transporter protein and 5HT2A receptor genes excluded in generalized social phobia. *Psychiatry Research, 81*, 283–291.

Stein, M., Jang, K., & Livesley, W. (2002). Heritability of social anxiety-related concerns and personality characteristics: A twin study. *Journal of Nervous and Mental Disease*, *190*, 219–224.

Storch, E. A., Ledley, D., Lewin, A., Murphy, T., Johns, N., Goodman, W., et al. (2006). Peer victimization in children with obsessive-compulsive disorder: Relations with symptoms of psychopathology. *Journal of Clinical Child and Adolescent Psychology*, *35*, 446–455.

Storch, E. A., Masia-Warner, C., Crisp, H., & Klein, R. G. (2005). Peer victimization and social anxiety in adolescence: A prospective study. *Aggressive Behavior*, *31*, 437–452.

Strauss, C., Lahey, B., Frick, P., Frame, C., & Hynd, G. (1988). Peer social status of children with anxiety disorders. *Journal of Consulting and Clinical Psychology*, *56*, 137–141.

Strauss, C., Lease, C., Kazdin, A., Dulcan, M., & Last, C. (1989). Multimethod assessment of the social competence of children with anxiety disorders. *Journal of Clinical Child Psychology*, *18*, 184–189.

Szyf, M., Mcgowan, P., & Meaney, M. (2008). The social environment and the epigenome. *Environmental and Molecular Mutagenesis*, *49*, 46–60.

Thomas, A., & Chess, S. (1977). *Temperament and development*. New York: Brunner/Mazel.

Thomas, A., Chess, S., & Birch, H. (1968). *Temperament and behavior disorders in children*. New York: New York University Press.

Verduin, T. L., & Kendall, P. C. (2008). Peer perceptions and liking of children with anxiety disorders. *Journal of Abnormal Child Psychology*, *36*, 459–469.

Weems, C. F., Silverman, W. K., Saavedra, L. M., Pina, A. A., & Lumpkin, P. W. (1999). The discrimination of children's phobias using the Revised Fear Survey Schedule for Children. *Journal of Child Psychology and Psychiatry*, *40*, 941–952.

Wolpe, J. (1958). *Psychotherapy by reciprocal inhibition*. Stanford, CA: Stanford University Press.

Wood, J. J., Mcleod, B. D., Sigman, M., Hwang, W. C., & Chu, B. C. (2003). Parenting and childhood anxiety: Theory, empirical findings, and future directions. *Journal of Child Psychology and Psychiatry*, *44*, 134–151.

Chapter 12
Major Depression

Jill C. Fodstad and Johnny L. Matson

Definition of the Population

For years, debate existed concerning whether it was possible for preadolescent children to experience depression. Thought to be primarily a mood dysfunction that manifested in late adolescence to adulthood, children were viewed by experts to be incapable of experiencing many of the phenomena associated with clinical depression. Symptomatic markers, such as mood disturbance, were viewed as being part of the normal progression of childhood development and, therefore, were attributed to "childhood moodiness" or "adolescent turmoil" (Baker, 2006; Rochlin, 1959). In the 1980s, enough substantial evidence had accumulated to suggest that young children can indeed suffer from this problem. It was also determined that children who evince depression exhibit symptoms paralleling those experienced in adolescence and adulthood. Thus, the myth that depression is "masked" in the juvenile population was refuted (Milling, 2001). Since then, research in the area of childhood depression has flourished; however, questions about its nature, causes, and treatment remain.

Childhood depression is a complex disorder. Its presentation is influenced by developmental factors, the degree to which it is associated with other disorders, and the negative long-lasting impact it has on all areas of psychosocial functioning. While other psychopathologies, such as schizophrenia,

adversely affect thought, the principal symptoms of Major Depressive Disorder (MDD) are mood and affect. According to Kazdin and Marciano (1998), depression should be viewed as a disorder which encompasses a whole myriad of characteristics and domains of functioning "well beyond mood-related symptoms." Children who experience depression have impairments in many areas of daily life, but unfortunately, these children may not come to the attention of mental health professionals until later adolescence or adulthood when their symptoms become pervasive and debilitating (Wu et al., 1999).

Potentially the most difficult problem in the area of childhood depression lies in its definition. Depression, in lay terminology, is most synonymously associated with sadness or unhappiness. While sadness may be a single symptom, individuals with depression can experience a wide range of socio-emotional deficits including diminished interest in activities, feelings of worthlessness or guilt, sleep disturbances, changes in appetite, and excessive fatigue. In mental health, however, depression refers to a cluster of symptoms (i.e., behaviors and emotions, including a depressed mood) that are interrelated and reflect several clinical disorders described in the *Diagnostic and Statistical Manual of Mental Disorders* [DSM-IV-TR; American Psychiatric Association (APA), 2000]. Therefore, the manner in which depression is defined determines the nature of research as well as how the nature, etiology, and course of the disorder are perceived.

The current classification system of the DSM-IV-TR does not describe depression in the disorders of childhood. Instead, it is encompassed in the section

J.C. Fodstad (✉)
Department of Psychology, Louisiana State University,
Baton Rouge, LA 70803, USA
e-mail: jcwill482@gmail.com

J.L. Matson (ed.), *Social Behavior and Skills in Children*, DOI 10.1007/978-1-4419-0234-4_12,
© Springer Science+Business Media, LLC 2009

on adult mood disorders. While experts suggest that encapsulating childhood depression within the adult psychopathologies is adequate given the overlap of the essential features of depression, this fails to account for developmental differences in symptom expression (Lewinsohn, Pettit, Joiner, & Seeley, 2003; Kazdin & Marciano, 1998). The only exceptions currently stated in the DSM-IV-TR in regard to childhood depression include irritable mood as a proxy for depressed mood and a failure to make expected weight gains as a proxy for weight loss.

Despite the overlap in core symptoms of depression, there is evidence that age differences exist. Researchers have noted that irritability is more likely to be seen among children than depressed mood and that somatic complaints, extreme fatigue, separation anxiety, difficulty with schoolwork, phobias, increased guilt, low self-esteem, and behavior problems are more likely to be the presenting concerns (Birmaher et al., 1996). On the other hand, adolescence is the period where somatic complaints begin to decrease and hypersomnia, reduced appetite (for girls), depressed mood, irritability, hopelessness, anhedonia, social withdrawal, and psychomotor retardation increases (Kashani, Rosenberg, & Reid, 1989). Additionally, suicidal behavior (ideation and attempts) starts to become problematic for depressed girls (middle adolescence) and boys (late adolescence) during this period of development (Kovacs, Obrosky, & Sherill, 2003).

The depressive disorder that is most often seen in children and adolescence is MDD or a subclinical variation of MDD. According to the DSM-IV-TR (2000), a diagnosis of MDD is made when, during the span of at least 2 weeks, one or more episodes occur where a marked change in the child's functioning is noted. This change in functioning can include a depressed mood and/or irritability or a loss of interest or pleasure in most activities. In some cases, both of these symptoms occur. Additionally, the child must experience at least four of the following symptoms nearly every day and must evince significant impairment in functioning: (1) a significant loss of weight or failure to gain weight; (2) sleep disturbance (hypersomnia or insomnia); (3) psychomotor retardation or agitation; (4) fatigue or a decrease in energy; (5) worthlessness or guilt; (6) concentration problems or indecisiveness; and (7) recurrent thoughts about death or suicide (APA, 2000).

One final issue in regard to defining childhood depression is comorbidity with other psychiatric disorders. In community studies, 40–50% of depressed adolescents meet criteria for at least one other diagnosis; however, some researchers suggest that these rates can be as high as 80–90% (Kazdin & Marciano, 1998). In one of the few studies to look at comorbidty separately in children and adolescents, Birmaher et al. (1996) noted that childhood depression was most commonly associated with anxiety disorders (30–80%), with conduct disorder, oppositional defiant disorder, and ADHD (10–80%). These high percentages are a reflection of the overlap that exists between symptoms of depression, anxiety disorders, conduct disorders, and ADHD. However, given that depressed children experience widespread dysfunction, whether the child meets or does not meet criteria for another disorder is a restrictive way of conceptualizing the nature of depression. Dysfunction in other domains such as cognitive processes (e.g., negative beliefs, attributions of failure), social relationships (e.g., isolation, communication deficits), interpersonal problem solving, academic skills (e.g., failing to complete homework, tardiness or absence, repetition of a grade, school dissatisfaction), and poor peer relations (e.g., lower popularity, greater rejection) have also been identified as being associated features that are well outside of the diagnostic criteria of childhood depression (Kazdin & Marciano, 1998; Schroeder & Gordon, 2002). Given development, it would seem to be a natural phenomenon that clinically depressed children are likely to show multiple symptoms that extend to other disorders, whether or not they meet criteria for those other disorders. It is up to clinicians, then, to assess for a broad range of symptoms and to determine how this wide range of dysfunction will contribute to overall functioning, treatment strategy, and long-term prognosis.

Etiology and Prevalence

Prevalence

Current research and epidemiological data suggest that children and adolescents are experiencing depression at an unprecedented rate. In Western cultures, prevalence rates of depression have escalated to epidemic proportions and, as a result, the average age of onset has vastly decreased. Only in recent years, how-ever, have methodologically sound surveys of child-hood disorders been conducted. This is largely due to the lack of a firmly agreed-upon conceptualization of childhood depression and the varying methods of assessment (Kessler, Avenevoli, & Merikangas, 2001). With the advent of more appropriate modes of diagnosis and assessment and an increase in what is known about its course and development, better esti-mates of the prevalence rates of childhood depression can be made.

Recent research suggests that the prevalence of depression in community settings ranges from 0.4 to 2.5% in children and 0.4 to 8.3% in adolescents (Bir-maher et al., 1996; Ford, Goodman, & Meltzer, 2003). In addition, it is estimated that in the community more than 7% of boys and almost 12% of girls will develop a depressive disorder by the age of 16 years (Costello, Mustillo, Erkanli, Keeler, & Angold, 2003). To further extrapolate the seriousness of this issue from a mental health perspective, knowing at what ages depression can be identified is necessary.

Preschoolers

Researchers suggest that a clinically significant depressive disorder can arise in children as young as 3 years of age (Luby, Belden, Pautsch, Si, & Spitznagel, 2008). This is contrary to historical developmental theory that stated preschool children were incapable of evincing "true" psychopathology because of the belief that young children were cog-nitively, socially, and emotionally immature (Egger & Angold, 2006). Kashani and colleagues were the first to systematically investigate the probability of depression in young children and found that "con-cerning symptoms" such as extreme feelings of guilt, fatigue, crying, low self-esteem, anhedonia, and play themes involving death do occur (Kashani & Ray, 1983; Kashani & Carlson, 1985; Kashani, Hol-comb, & Orvaschel, 1986). Since then, large-scale studies investigating the preschool population (e.g., American Preschool Age Psychiatric Assessment Test–Retest Study) have reported rates of depres-sive disorders in nonclinical samples of preschoolers being 1.4% for MDD, 0.6% for dysthymic disorder, and 0.7% for depression NOS/minor depression (Egger & Angold, 2006). Furthermore, Egger and

Angold (2006) found that MDD was more common in older preschoolers (3%) than in toddlers (0.3%).

Children

In children approximately 6–12 years of age, pre-valence rates of depression have been reported to be generally less than 3% (Cohen et al., 1993). In the largest U.S. study of children (ages, 9, 11, and 13), Costello et al. (1996) reported a 3-month prevalence rate of 0.03% for MDD, 0.13% for dysthymia, and 1.45% for depression NOS, for a total of 1.52% depressive disorders. Furthermore, 6- to 12-month prevalence estimates are somewhat higher, with ranges from less than 1% (Costello et al., 1988) to almost 3% (Velez, Johnson, & Cohen, 1989).

Adolescents

Rates of diagnosed depression among adolescents are comparable to those of adults. In adolescents (ages 13–18 years), point prevalence estimates of MDD range from about 1 to 7% (Fergusson, Hor-wood, & Lynskey, 1993; Garrison et al., 1997). As would be expected, 6- to 12-month prevalence esti-mates are somewhat higher, with a range from 2 to 13% (McGee et al., 1990; Feehan, McGee, Raja, & Williams, 1994). Lifetime prevalence of MDD has been estimated to occur in 14% of adolescents, with an additional 11% reporting minor depression symptoms (Kessler & Walters, 1998; Lewinson, Hops, Roberts, Seeley, & Andrews, 1993). It is important to note that prior to adolescence girls and boys have similar rates of depression; however, during adolescence, rates of depression onset is gen-erally reported to be higher for girls. This prepon-derance of MDD in females continues into adult-hood with females evincing MDD symptomatology two-fold that of males. This gender difference is stated to emerge between 13 and 15 years of age (Cohen et al., 1993).

Etiology

Depression is a multi-factorial syndrome with many causal agents. Risk factors for developing MDD can be divided into those that predispose (i.e., increase vulnerability) and those that precipitate (i.e., lead to the development of depression at a specific point in time). It is unlikely that there is any one risk factor that can fully explain the development of MDD; therefore, reducing the chances of occurrences of a single risk factor is not sufficient to prevent depression. It is more likely that the accumulation and interaction of these concomitant risk factors increase the likelihood that an individual will express diagnosable MDD or a lesser clinical depressive disorder. Once established, depressive episodes may be prolonged by maintenance factors including persistent depressive symptoms, high levels of anxiety, low self-esteem, social deficits, and family dysfunction. These maintenance factors are generally the target of alleviation in therapeutic treatment.

Formulations of the precipitants of childhood depression are important in helping professionals understand how depression develops and knowing how to treat, prevent, and diagnose individuals who are symptomatic. Originated as adaptations of adult models, current views on the etiology, concomitants, and consequences of childhood depression have been restructured to underscore the development of psychopathology as it relates to the interplay between vulnerability, ontogeny, and the phenomenology of depression. As such, there are a number of factors which contribute to depression. Some of the more general, evidenced-based models of depression will be highlighted. Existing theories can be broadly classified into two areas: biological and environmental/psychological.

Biological Factors

Genetics

Depression is a familial syndrome. It has been well established that having a parent with MDD is one of the strongest predictors of childhood or adolescent depression (Beardslee, Versage, & Gladstone, 1998). Furthermore, longitudinal studies have determined that children of depressed parents have persistent and recurrent depressive disorders that are associated with considerable impairment (Hammen, Burge, Burney, & Adrian, 1990).

Twin, family, and adoption studies all strongly suggest that genetic factors are significant determinants of depression (Sullivan, Neale, & Kendler, 2000). Children raised by depressed parents are noted to be approximately four times more likely to have an episode of MDD than children of normal controls (Rice, Harold, & Thapar, 2002). Additionally, offspring of depressed parents are two times more likely to develop a depressive disorder than children of parents with other psychiatric disorders or medical conditions. This incidence continues to increase with age (Beardslee et al., 1998; Weissman, Warner, Wickramaratne, Moreau, & Olfson, 1997). By late adolescence, cumulative probability of MDD at some point during the lifespan for offspring of depressed parents is estimated to be almost 70% (Hammen et al., 1990).

Although genetic heritability of MDD may be one substantiated risk factor, the influence of adverse psychosocial factors associated with having a depressed parent (e.g., disordered parent–child relationships, stressful life events and conditions, and marital discord) cannot be overlooked (Goodman & Gotlib, 1999). Most twin studies suggest that there is only a moderate genetic influence for childhood depressive symptoms with heritability estimates ranging from 30 to 80% (Eley & Plomin, 1997; Scourfield et al., 2003; Sullivan et al., 2000). Additionally, researchers note that in child/adolescent samples, there appear to be different origins of childhood-onset and adolescent-onset depression. Thapar and McGuffin (1994) studied the heritability of depressive symptoms in 411 British child and adolescent twins. Results from this and subsequent investigations revealed that there is stronger evidence of heritability in adolescents, whereas depressive symptoms in children tend to be more strongly associated with environmental factors (Thapar & McGuffin, 1994; Scourfield et al., 2003). Furthermore, the shared environment between monozygotic twins is believed to only have a negligible influence on the etiology of depression, except in very severe cases (Eley, 1999). Non-shared environmental factors, therefore, seem to have a substantial contribution to the variance of depression seen in children. Offspring of depressed parents who would have a higher genetic risk may be more vulnerable to environmental influence than those with low genetic risk (Birmaher et al., 1996). However, without a clearly defined genetic marker of depression, it can be deduced that, at best, what is inherited may simply be a vulnerability or predisposition to depressive symptomatology that must be exacerbated by stressors in the environment to develop into clinically significant depression.

Neurobiology

There have been a number of neurobiological factors implicated in childhood depression. Perhaps the most researched of these potential variants of depression in children are based on the dysregulation of the human stress system through the activation of the hypothalamic-pituitary-adrenal (HPA) axis (Nestler et al., 2002). One area that the HPA axis has been implicated is in the gender bias that arises in mid-adolescence. A significant number of researchers have suggested that it is the increase in female sex steroids (i.e., progesterone and estrogen) coupled with a significant suppression along the HPA axis that increases their vulnerability to depression (Young & Altemus, 2004). This research is still in its infancy and, therefore, conclusive evidence at this point is not available. Aside from stress reactivity, other biological systems that have been implicated include sleep dysregulation, circadian rhythm disturbances, and impaired reward and motivational pathways (Birmaher & Heydl, 2001; Davidson et al., 2003; Heim & Nemerolf, 2001; Shaffery, Hoffmann, & Armitage, 2003). Alteration in hormonal systems has also been implicated as being potential trait markers for MDD. Mainly an outgrowth of pharmacological research, studies of growth hormone, prolactin, and cortisol levels in currently depressed, remitted, and at-risk children have shown that, in all three groups, abnormalities in the secretion of these hormones exist (Birmaher & Heydl, 2001).

Preliminary evidence in imaging studies suggests that there are functional and anatomical brain differences in depressed and at-risk children when compared to normal controls. It is well-known that the frontal lobe plays a primary role in the regulation of mood and affect. Researchers studying brain asymmetry have pinpointed left frontal hypoactivation in infant, child, and adolescent offspring of depressed versus nondepressed mothers (Dawson, Frey, Panagiotides, Osterling, & Hessl,

1997; Field, Fox, Pickens, & Nawrocki, 1995; Tomarken, Dichter, Garber, & Simien, 2004). In a study by Nolan et al. (2002), children diagnosed with MDD who had no history of familial MDD had significantly larger left-sided prefrontal cortical volumes and greater levels of activation when compared to children with familial MDD and a control group. This decreased activation in the left front cortex suggests that there is an underactivation of the approach system in the brain and a reduced positive emotionality (Davidson, Pizzagalli, Nitschke, & Putnam, 2002). Evidence for anomalies in brain regions other than the frontal cortex (e.g., temporal and limbic systems) has been somewhat inconsistent, and results vary in regard to age, gender, maturation, psychiatric family history, severity, and exposure to stress. More research appears warranted to determine the extent to which neurobiological risk factors predict the onset of MDD either in isolation or in combination with other vulnerability markers.

Environmental and Psychosocial Factors

Learned Helplessness

Learned helplessness, as a theory, developed from primarily animal models to account for depressive behavior. The original model, proposed by Seligman (1975), stated that depression occurs in response to uncontrollable, noncontingent events. Furthermore, when individuals experience these events, they believe that control will never be attained and, as a result, deficits in motivation, cognition, and emotions occur (Seligman, 1975). Depression, therefore, is only alleviated when the individual begins to regain his/her sense of control over the environment. Based on subsequent research, a number of problems were identified in Seligman's seminal formulation and, therefore, the learned helplessness model has been reformulated. In the most recent version referred to as the helplessness/hopelessness model, Abramson, Metalsky, and Alloy (1989) suggest that it is the interaction between negative life events and depressogenic attributions (i.e., pessimistic expectations about the future) that exacerbates and maintains depressive symptoms. Central to this theory are three general premises, including (1) the expectation that negative outcomes are probable or that highly desirable outcomes are improbable; (2) the belief that there is no response that will change the likelihood of the events from occurring; and (3) failure or negative outcomes are attributed to internal events, but success occurs due to external factors. Due to these beliefs, when a negative event occurs, the depressed individual is likely to make negative inferences, which leads them to give up and not try in similar situations in the future (Matson, 1989). Once this state of helplessness develops, hopelessness is unavoidable.

The applicability of the hopelessness/helplessness model to childhood depression is currently under debate. In adolescence, the ability to determine the causality of behavior is established; however, developmental psychologists suggest that young children do not have the cognitive capacity to develop hopelessness because the child is not yet able to sequence events, determine probabilities, or have a full understanding of time (Kaslow, Adamson, & Collins, 2000). Recent examinations including a wider range of cognitive vulnerability factors (e.g., rumination, dysfunctional attitudes, self-criticism, etc.) and developmentally sensitive measures of attributional style have determined that children are able to attribute negative connotations to life events and develop an age-appropriate variant of hopelessness (Conley, Haines, Hilt, & Metalsky, 2001). Furthermore, the cognitive distortions are externally derived from the environment or another individual (Nolen-Hoeksema, Mumme, Wolfson, & Guskin, 1995; Gibb et al., 2006). For example, a child is told that he/she did not get picked for the kick-ball team because he/she is "stupid." As a result, the child is given an internal, stable, and global attribution for his/her lack of social success. Because social messages (e.g., peer rejection, teasing, humiliation, criticism, negative feedback, etc.) are salient cues, this results in a greater likelihood that depressive symptoms will be elicited and maintained.

There are additional etiological perspectives related to the helplessness model. In general, these theories pertain to the role of self-regulation and cognitive competency. This states that depressive behavior and negative emotions are related to the individual's expectations of the outcomes of events (e.g., control, competence, potential short-term and long-term consequences) and their personal investment in those outcomes (e.g., goals, standards, values) (Rehm, 1977; Weisz, Sweeney, Proffitt, & Carr, 1994). Depressed individuals are more likely to dwell on and accentuate the negative versus positive aspects of the environment. Therefore, depressed individuals set unrealistic standards for themselves or believe that there is nothing they can physically do to achieve that perceived standard.

Social Learning Theory

Traditional behavioral models conceptualize depression as a consequence of skill deficits and an inability to derive positive feedback. Lewinsohn (1974) hypothesized that depression is a result of low rates of response-contingent positive reinforcement. This low rate of positive reinforcement is a consequence of competency deficits that interfere with the attainment of success, the formation of stable relationships, and the ability to derive positive affect from experiences. According to social learning theory, these sources of reduced reinforcement can then lead to depressive symptoms such as withdrawal, fatigue, lack of interest, and somatic complaints (Lewinsohn, 1974). Therefore, the environment acts as the primary maintaining factor for depressive behavior.

Traditional behavioral theories of depression, such as Lewinsohn's, have received little empirical attention, but have formed the basis for more elaborate models of depression. For example, in their competency-based model of depression, Cole, Martin, and Powers (1997) propose that negative feedback from others is internalized by children in the form of negative self-perception. Furthermore, it is this internalization that increases the probability of future depression (Cole et al., 1997). According to interpersonal theorists, it is the child's interaction with his/her social world that induces depressive symptomatology. Thus, depressive symptoms and associated behaviors elicit aversive social experiences that maintain and exacerbate depressed affect. Consistent with interpersonal models, researchers have found that social difficulties and deficits exist in depressed children. Social impairments including difficulties making and maintaining friends and maladaptive problem solving, coping, and emotion regulation can cause pervasive negative effects on multiple areas of functioning.

Social Skills Problems Unique to the Population

Though not a diagnostic criterion, children with depression are often described as having extensive social skill deficits. Many experts believe that these deficits in socio-behavioral competency are a primary factor in the maintenance of depressive symptoms throughout the lifespan (Lewinsohn, 1974). The characteristics associated with depression often disrupt peer relationships by evoking negative responses from others and generating interpersonal stress and conflict (Joiner, Coyne, & Blalock, 1999; Rudolph et al., 2000). Given the consequences that social dysfunction can cause in interacting with one's social world, being familiar with what the most common skill deficits are for depressed children is beneficial for evaluation, diagnostic issues, treatment planning, and symptom monitoring.

Empirical investigations of social skill deficits in children with depression resemble those conducted on adults. For example, depressed children rate themselves as less socially competent (e.g., less able to resolve conflict or provide emotional support to peers, less able to make friends, etc.) than their nondepressed peers (Kupersmidt & Patterson, 1991; Hammen, Shih, & Brennan, 2004). In addition, these children are more likely to be rejected by their peers, are perceived as less likable, and have more negative social behaviors (Milling, 2001). Children with depression are often described as having deficits in prosocial behavior such as direct eye gaze, negative statements regarding self and peers, poor problem-solving and coping skills, etc. and, in addition, have higher level of aggression and withdrawal (Rudolph & Clark, 2001). While a lack of appropriate social behaviors are evinced by children with depression, Ollenburg and Kerns (1997) suggest that children who are predisposed (either genetically or biochemically) to depression may already possess poor social skills which can prompt the onset of depression. Furthermore, the results of longitudinal studies have shown that children may experience poor peer relations (e.g., withdrawal, no

best friend, and peer rejection) prior to the onset of depression (Kupersmidt & Patterson, 1991).

Through observations and parent interviews, researchers have been able to pinpoint a wide range of specific social deficits that characterize MDD in children. Altmann and Gotlib (1988) observed children playing during two 6-min periods. During their observation, depressed children were noted to be alone more often, initiate fewer interactions, and engage in more aversive and aggressive behaviors than nondepressed children (Altmann & Gotlib, 1988). Focusing on interpersonal behaviors, Rudolph, Hammen, and Burge (1994) found that children with depressive symptoms had more difficulty resolving peer conflict (e.g., problem solving, positive thinking, less assertiveness) and more emotional dysregulation (e.g., hostility, aggression) during stressful peer encounters. The findings from Rudolph et al. (1994) give further support to researchers who suggest that childhood depression may be linked to lower levels of active or problem-focused coping, decreased assertiveness, and elevated levels of passive or ruminative coping, avoidance, and helpless responses to negative affect or social conflict (Rudolph, Kurlakowsky, & Conley, 2001; Zahn-Waxler, Klimes-Dougan, & Slattery, 2000). Other overt social behaviors that have been noted to be indicative of children who are depressed include a restricted range of facial expressions, less communicative gesturing, and more speech latency and negative self-evaluation than nondepressed peers (Segrin, 2000).

Assessment

With the vast array of etiological models, the assessment of childhood depression can be a rather difficult process. There is, to date, no single measure that can account for the multiple facets of dysfunction that depression evokes. Therefore, the clinician must adopt a broad-based method to assessing depression that includes multiple measures that embody different methods of assessment (e.g., checklists, behavioral observations, diagnostic interviews, etc.), perspectives (e.g., child, parent, teacher), and domains (e.g., affect, cognitions, behavior).

Not only is it suggested that numerous approaches be utilized, but specific findings within the area of childhood depression make such strategies essential. Renouf and Kovacs (1994) suggest that practitioners must consider the child's age and sex, parent psychopathology, parental cognizance of the child's actual symptom severity, and agreement across raters. In addition, the clinician must consider maintaining the child's attention, motivation, and rapport. For younger children and those with special problems (e.g., hyperactivity) who may have short attention spans, using fewer and shorter measures should be regarded relative to other childhood problems. To ensure the child understands what is being asked, the clinician may need to read and repeat questions to the child, paraphrase, give examples, and have the child repeat what was said. Taking breaks and incorporating play periods into the assessment or providing other means of reinforcement may also be necessary to sustain motivation. Adaptive devices such as pictorial representations of topics, drawings, or puppets can be useful aids in conveying various ideas. These strategies may be necessary to ensure understanding of sensitive topics by young children. Another issue that must be addressed by the clinician is the competency of the parent. Because childhood depression has a familial link, it is possible that one or both parents may have a diagnosable psychopathology and, as such, it is up to the clinician to determine whether the parent is competent and has enough insight to be a valid information source for the child's problems. For example, mothers who are clinically depressed are more likely to over-report the child's depressive symptoms regardless of the child's age (Renouf & Kovacs, 1994).

Therefore, to properly diagnose depression in "at risk" children, an assessment battery should, at minimum, include different sources of information (e.g., the child, parent, teacher), performance in different settings (e.g., home, academic, and social), prior course of the depression (e.g., previous episodes, chronicity), diverse symptom domains (e.g., depression, comorbid psychiatric symptoms, general medical conditions, developmental delays, etc.), family history and environment, and impairment in everyday functioning. Utilizing such an approach will help to not only increase diagnostic accuracy but will inform appropriate treatment procedures and general prognosis of the child.

A familiarity with the most up-to-date and systematic ways of evaluating childhood psychopathology is essential to the diagnosis of depression in children. Therefore, a general description of the various modes of assessing depression in "at risk" children will be given. Traditional measurement topics such as checklists and rating scales, behavioral observations, and structured and semistructured interviews will be briefly covered and a few examples of appropriate measures for the childhood population will be given. Due to space limitations, this discussion will only be limited to general measures. There are a variety of measures that target specific components of the depressive syndrome, such as self-esteem, hopelessness, depressive cognitions, and suicidality that may be useful for particular cases (refer to Winters, Myers, & Proud, 2002, for a review); however, they are not reviewed here. In addition, interpersonal and social assessment methods will be discussed. Given the significant social deficits evinced by depressed children, including such measures would be valuable additions to the evaluation and diagnostic process (Segrin, 2000).

Interviews

Discussing symptomatology with a client or parent in an open-ended format continues to be the oldest form of assessment and is still the most widely used in applied, non-university-based settings. The unstructured interview, however, falters in that because there is no standardization, the format may vary from clinician to clinician with respect to duration and breadth of coverage. These differences attributed to the open-endedness of the questions have the potential to significantly alter the amount, quality, and type of information elicited with respect to depressive symptoms. Likewise, when clinicians use unstructured interviews, it has been noted that they often fail to inquire about key aspects of psychopathology presentation (especially if it is inconsistent with their initial diagnostic impression) and make fewer diagnoses than clinicians who use structured interviews (Zimmerman, 2003).

Despite the continued use of unstructured interviews, the current trend in clinical practice is to provide more structured means of obtaining information from children, parents, and other important individuals (e.g., teachers). Structured interviews can be divided into two main categories: semistructured and fully structured. Semistructured interviews are referred to as being "interview based" assessments due to the interviewer being responsible for criteria rating and for providing questions to garner additional information. In contrast, fully structured interviews are referred to as "respondent based" because the interviewer's role is limited to reading the questions verbatim and recording the respondent's answers. Both are appropriate for assessing childhood depression. The structured interview involves a prearranged set of questions that are asked in a sequential order that usually gather information about a specific DSM disorder. In addition, they employ specific rules for assessing syndromes in terms of frequency of specific characteristic symptoms, duration, and impairment. This emphasis on more overt, objective behaviors (e.g., inability to gain weight, irritability, emotionality) lends itself to producing material that is more reliably indicative of childhood depression. Since childhood depression is more prevalent than previously thought, there have been structured interviews developed that can be utilized in a standard assessment battery.

There are several structured and semistructured interviews available for assessing psychopathology in children. These typically include interviews that require the administration and interpretation of responses by a trained clinician. The most widely used interviews include the Schedule for Affective Disorders and Schizophrenia for School Aged Children (K-SADS; Puig-Antich & Chambers, 1978) and the Child and Adolescent Psychiatric Assessment (CAPA; Angold et al., 1995) The K-SADS and CAPA are not specific for diagnosing major depression but assesses the criteria for most of the major child psychiatric disorders. In addition, there are parallel versions for parents and children. These measures have been shown to have acceptable test–retest and inter-rater reliability (Angold & Costello, 1995; Kaufman et al., 1997). Other interviews, such as the Diagnostic Interview for Children and Adolescents (DICA-IV; Reich, 2000) and the Diagnostic Interview Schedule for Children (DISC-IV; Shaffer, Fisher, Lucas, Dulcan, & Schwab-Stone, 2000) are respondent-based measures that do not require extensive training by the interviewer. Both the DISC and DICA have acceptable test–retest reliability for major depression in children and have shown to be correlated with other measures of child psychopathy (Reich, 2000; Shaffer et al., 2000).

Checklist/Rating Scales

Checklists include clinician-administered, self-report, and parent and teacher measures. For good reasons, these types of measures are the most extensively studied and used methods to diagnose depression in children. First, checklists can be administered easily and in a timely manner. Second, assessments of this type usually give a standardized list of items which allows for a uniform comparison across children. Third, normative data are often available with cutoff scores for depression, thereby making checklists less subjective. Fourth, it is easy to obtain data from caregivers of the child and mental health professionals who are best acquainted with the client. Fifth, depression scales, unlike interviews or direct behavioral observations, are based on the last 2 or 3 weeks of the child's behavior rather than on a prolonged period of time or past occurrences of symptoms. Finally, the cost of the evaluation is not as prohibitive as other assessment methods because they can be filled out by parents, teachers, caregivers, or the child. Therefore, for practical reasons these are instruments that may be used in settings (e.g., mental health center) as a screening instrument where the need for more directive assessment is needed due to time and cost constraints.

Several measures can be used as a direct evaluation of the child via self-report, clinician, and multi-informant rating scales for depression. The discussion will begin with the most popular of the child depression checklists, the Child Depression Inventory (CDI; Kovacs, 1992). This will then be followed by a discussion of the Children's Depression Rating Scale-Revised (CDRS; Poznanski & Mokros, 1999), the Children's Depression Scale (CDS; Tisher & Lang, 1983), and the Reynolds Child Depression Scale (RCDS; Reynolds, 1989).

Child Depression Inventory (CDI)

The CDI (Kovacs, 1992) is the most widely used depression rating scale for children and adolescents. Developed based on an adult measure, the Beck

Depression Inventory (Kovacs & Beck, 1977), the CDI assesses severity of depression during the previous 2 weeks in children ranging in age from 7 to 17 years. Normative data on the CDI was initially collected based on the responses of randomly selected school-age children, but it has also been shown to be useful for children who are diagnosed as functioning in the range of intellectual disabilities (Matson, Helsel, & Barrett, 1988). It is comprised of 27 items covering a broad range of depression symptoms and associated features, with emphasis on cognitive symptoms. Each item consists of 3 Likert-type responses scored as 0, 1, or 2, based on the response chosen by the rater and can easily be completed in 10–20 min.

There has been a good deal of research to support the efficacy of the CDI. Researchers have reported that the CDI has acceptable internal consistency and good short-term test–retest reliability (Brooks & Kutcher, 2001; Kovacs, 1992). The CDI has been factor analyzed and, as such, is composed of five subdomains (negative mood, interpersonal problems, ineffectiveness, anhedonia, and negative self-esteem) and a total composite score. The factor structure of the CDI has been shown to vary by age; however, this is not surprising given that symptom expression also varies in regard to the child's age and developmental level (Cole, Hoffman, Tram, & Maxwell, 2000; Weiss & Garber, 2003). In addition, the CDI is moderately to highly correlated with the CDRS as well as with other self-rated depression scales and other measures of associated symptoms (e.g., negative cognitions, self-esteem), thereby providing evidence of its convergent validity (Brooks & Kutcher, 2001). The discriminant validity, however, has been found to be questionable, as it is almost as highly correlated with anxiety measures as it is with depression measures (Reynolds, 1998). Since anxiety disorders and depression are highly comorbid in the childhood population, an overlap between symptomatology is to be expected. Therefore in cases where being able to distinguish between depression or an anxiety-related disorder is needed, the clinician may need to follow up with more discernable measures.

Children's Depression Rating Scale-Revised (CDRS-R)

The CDRS-R is a clinician administered scale for rating the severity depression in children 6–12 years of age (Poznanski & Mokros, 1999). The measure contains 17 items assessing somatic, cognitive, affective, and psychomotor symptoms and draws on the respondent's responses and the interviewer's behavioral observations. The CDRS-R takes approximately 15–20 min to administer. It is administered separately to the child and, if necessary, an adult informant. The clinician integrates the data to rate the child using a Likert-type scale of 1–7 for the child's response on 14 items and from 1 to 5 for sleep, appetite, and tempo of speech. Cutoff scores are provided to aid in interpreting the level of depression severity. A rating of 5 or higher indicates definite abnormal symptoms and a total of 40 is a reliable indicator of depression. The items rated cover schoolwork, social withdrawal, capacity to have fun, appetite, sleep, irritability, physical complaints, guilt, self-esteem, depressed feelings, suicidal ideation, morbid thoughts, weeping, and nonverbal items such as tempo of speech, depressed affect, and hypoactivity.

In regard to psychometric properties of the CDRS-R, it has moderate internal consistency and good interrater reliability (Poznanski et al., 1984). In addition, the measure is moderately to highly correlated with the Hamilton Rating for Depression and other self-rated depression scales (Jain et al., 2007; Shain, Naylor, & Alessi, 1990). Potential drawbacks of the CDRS-R center around the subjectivity of the clinician ratings, lack of clarity as to how data are weighted, and the potential "halo effect" in determining correlation with the global rating (Strober & Werry, 1986). In addition, the CDRS-R has been found to have difficulty distinguishing between depression and anxiety and overestimates the severity of depression in children who have general medical conditions. This is largely due to the measures emphasis on somatic symptoms of depression (Brooks & Kutcher, 2001).

Children's Depression Scale (CDS)

The CDS was developed by Tisher and Lang (1983). The CDS consists of 66 items, 44 of which focus on depressive symptoms and 18 on positive experiences. Primarily used as a self-report rating scale for children aged 9–16, there is also an adult form to use with parents, teachers, and caregivers. To administer, the child (or adult) is asked to sort statements printed on cards into one of five boxes, labeled *very wrong, don't know, not sure, right*, and *very right*. The subscales of the CDS were derived from the literature on depressive symptomatology. There are a variety of symptom categories such as affective symptoms (e.g., sadness and unhappiness, weeping, low self-esteem, worthlessness), decreases in mental productivity and drive (e.g., boredom, withdrawal, lack of energy, discontent, low capacity for pleasure, motor retardation, inability to accept help or comfort), and psychosomatic complaints (e.g., headaches, abdominal pains, insomnia or other sleep disturbances). Other items such as preoccupation with death and aggressive tendencies are also included. Responses are tallied on a scale from 1 to 5, with low scores being indicative of depression. Factor analysis has found one general factor so there are no separate symptom subscales (Bath & Middleton, 1985).

Psychometric properties of the CDS have been found to be adequate. Internal consistency coefficients range from 0.90 for total depression to 0.79 for positive affect (Bath & Middleton, 1985; Kazdin, 1987). Test–retest reliability has been tested and was found to be 0.74 (Tisher, Lang-Takac, & Lang, 1992). Additionally, the CDS has been found to be moderately correlated to other measures of depression, such as the CDS and CDI ($r = 0.48$–0.84; Kazdin, 1987; Knight, Hensley, & Waters, 1988; Rotundo & Hensley, 1985). The correlation between parent and child ratings is very poor ($r = 0.04$; Kazdin, 1987). The CDS is able to discriminate between depressed and nondepressed children using the child form but not the adult form (Fine, Moretti, Haley, & Marriage, 1984).

The CDS is an acceptable addition as a self-report measure to an assessment battery for childhood depression. It would be best to use this measure in instances where a child has had prior difficulty with paper-and-pencil formats or needs additional encouraging and enhancing interactions from the clinician to maintain attention and motivation. The main drawback to the CDS is that, given its format, it can be quite cumbersome to administer.

Reynolds Child Depression Scale (RCDS)

The RCDS is a 30-item self-report measure designed to use with children aged 8–13 years (Reynolds, 1989).

The first 29 items use a 4-point Likert-type response scale (*almost never, hardly ever, sometimes*, and *most of the time*) to assess depressive symptomatology. The last item consists of a gradient of facial expressions ranging from sad to happy and the child is instructed to place an "X" over the face that demonstrates how he or she feels that particular day. The test takes approximately 10 min to complete, although some children may require additional time.

The measure was normed on 1600 children of varying economic and ethnic backgrounds and has been found to have acceptable psychometric properties. Internal consistency coefficients are reported to be 0.90 with a test–retest reliability of 0.85 (Reynolds & Graves, 1989). The correlation between the RCDS and other measures of childhood depression, such as the CDI and CDRS, range from 0.7 to 0.79 (Stark, Reynolds, & Kaslow, 1987) and with structured clinical interviews, such as the SADS, at 0.76 (Reynolds, 1989). The RCDS is, in addition, sensitive to treatment outcomes and, based on a few investigations, can discriminate between depressed and nondepressed children (Stark et al., 1987).

Behavioral Observations

In addition to rating scales and interviews, including a direct observation of the child's behavior in multiple settings and domains is a crucial addition to any standard assessment battery. Observational techniques can acquire beneficial information on overt behaviors characteristic of depression as well as provide an objective view on the nature, antecedents, and consequences of the child. Often disregarded in the assessment process, a direct observation of behavior may be necessary to help the clinician understand and delineate the underlying problem(s), as well as monitor the progress the treatment.

Before beginning the observation, there are a few essential steps the clinician must take to maximize the amount and quality of data collected. First, the clinician must operationally define the target behaviors to be observed. This involves breaking the behavior down into discrete observable behaviors that are described in simple, directed words that can be observed by multiple observers. Selecting responses that are overt and observable would be ideal so as to decrease the amount of subjective interpretation by the clinician or multiple observers. Second, the clinician must select the most appropriate setting in which to observe the behavior. Observations can be conducted either in the child's natural environment (e.g., home, school, etc.), or in the clinic, a laboratory, or an analogue setting. Third, the clinician must establish a way to conduct independent reliability assessments of the targeted behavior(s) and include a way to capture the nature of the behavior. The way in which the behavior is recorded is dependent on the manner in which the behavior is evinced (e.g., tics, sleep, on-task behavior). Methods that should be considered include counting the number of times the behavior occurs (i.e., event recording), noting the length of time from the beginning to end of the behavior (i.e., duration recording), and indicating whether or not the behavior occurred during a preset time interval (i.e., time sampling). For example, Robinson and Lewinsohn (1973) conducted an observation for the target behavior of slowed rate of speech in a chronically depressed psychiatric patient. To accurately capture this behavior, the observer counted the number of words per 30-s intervals.

Kazdin (1990) developed an observational system for use in depressed children. Based on the findings from previous observations with adult and diagnostic criteria, Kazdin (1990) selected three broad categories of behavior characteristic of the responses of children diagnosed with MDD (Kazdin, Esveldt-Dawson, Sherick, & Colbus, 1985). Although this behavioral code was developed initially for use during the free-play of inpatient children, it could easily be adapted for use in a clinic or school-based setting. The responses and categories are listed below so that the clinician is given a systematic, objective example of how an observation should be structured. In addition, the target behaviors are given to serve as a model for clinicians who choose to include this type of approach in the evaluation and treatment of depressed children.

1. *Social activity.* This category was composed of the following four behaviors: (1) *Talking* was operationally defined as a verbal exchange of comments or ongoing dialogue with another child. (2) *Playing a game* was operationally defined as the participation in a social game (e.g., Checkers) with one or more individuals.

(3) *Participating in a group activity* was operationally defined as either interacting with peers via taking turns, looking at materials together, or working together on a special task. (4) *Interacting with staff* included contacting staff members through conversation or a play activity.

2. *Solitary behavior.* This category was composed of the following five behaviors: (1) *Playing a game alone* was operationally defined as engaging in a game activity (i.e., board game, cards, or tasks with play materials) by oneself. (2) *Working on an academic task* was operationally defined as reading, studying, or writing by oneself. (3) *Listening and watching* was operationally defined as looking, listening, and reacting to a TV program, radio, or music by oneself. (4) *Straightening one's room* was defined as placing personal belongings in their proper place or cleaning one's room. (5) *Grooming* was defined as engaging in self-care behaviors including getting dressed, changing clothes, personal hygiene routines, and bathing.

3. *Affect-related expression.* This category was composed of the following four behaviors: (1) *Smiling* was defined as using facial muscles to upturn the corners of the mouth and/or facial expressions of joy or pleasure. (2) *Frowning* was the lowering of eyebrows or downward turning of the mouth and/or facial expressions of displeasure. (3) *Arguing* included tense, emotional, verbal interactions such as using a loud voice, shouting, losing one's temper, or engaging in an outburst of anger. (4) *Complaining* was defined as a verbal expression indicative of unhappiness, dissatisfaction, or pain.

If a more standardized approach to direct observation is needed, there are a few noteworthy observational systems that have been shown to be acceptable for recording childhood behavior. The Behavior Assessment System for Children-Student Observation System (BASC-SOS; Reynolds & Kamphaus, 1992) and the Child Behavior Checklist-Direct Observation Form (CBCL-DOF; Achenbach, 1986) are two examples of standardized approaches to observation used primarily for classroom behaviors. Both of these measures are companion measures to broad-based social skills questionnaires. The BASC-SOS is structured as a 15-min observation of 65 target classroom behaviors grouped into one of 13 categories (response to teacher/lesson, peer interaction, work on school subjects, transition movement, inappropriate movement, inattention, inappropriate vocalization, somatization, repetitive motor movements, aggression, self-injurious behavior, inappropriate sexual behavior, and bowel/bladder problems). To conduct the observation, a momentary time-sampling recording procedure is utilized in which the clinician denotes (via a checklist) whether any of the 13 categories of behaviors occurred after a 3-s observation every 30 s. The CBCL-DOF is a 10-min systematic observation that consists of the observer (1) writing a narrative description of the child's behavior noting the occurrence, duration, and intensity of specific problems; (2) coding the child's behavior as on or off task; and (3) rating the child on 96 behaviors using a Likert-type 4-point scale (0 = behavior was not observed to 3 = definite occurrence of behavior at a severe intensity or behavior occurred for greater than 3-min).

In addition to the aforementioned observational assessments there are a few that can be used to aid the clinician in observing parent–child interactions. The Dyadic Parent–Child Interaction Coding System-II (DPICS-II; Eyberg, Bessmer, Newcomb, Edwards, & Robinson, 1994) is one such highly structured coding system that can be used in the clinic to assess the current level of parenting skills, the child's responsiveness to the parent, and qualitative aspects of the parent–child interaction in three 5-min standardized situations: (1) Child-Directed Interaction where the parents play with the child in an activity of the child's choice using the child's rules; (2) Parent-Directed Interaction where the parents select the activity, determines the rules, and guides the play; and (3) Cleanup where the parents instruct the child to clean up the toys.

Interpersonal and Social

Evidence suggests that children who are diagnosed with MDD have deficits in socially appropriate behavior. Researchers investigating certain social behavior problems (e.g., slow speech rate, excessively long pauses and silences, diminished vocal pitches, diminished gestures, sad facial expressions,

and reduced eye contact) note that social skills (or the lack thereof) is highly correlated to the presence of childhood depression and also to the severity and long-term prognosis of symptoms (Segrin, 2000). As such, including an assessment component of the child's social skills and deficits would be essential to a depression evaluation.

To assess social skills and social competence in children, a multi-method approach should be utilized. Unfortunately for the typical clinician, limited resources and time constraints, oftentimes, makes conducting a thorough evaluation of social skills in addition to assessing depressive symptomatology difficult. It is advised that necessary steps are taken to include a valid measure of social behavior and an in-clinic observation. In addition, the clinician should attempt to gain information about the nature of the child's social behaviors or deficits, the amount and quality of friendships/relationships the child has with others (e.g., peers, adults), type and frequency of social activities, situations which may be aversive or difficult for the child, and the child's behavior in social settings.

Several behavior ratings scales exist to aid the clinician in assessing the social competence and social behaviors of children. The Matson Evaluation of Social Skills for Youngsters (MESSY; Matson, Rotatori, & Helsel, 1983) is one measure that is useful in the assessment of social behaviors for children aged 4–18 years. Found to be psychometrically acceptable, the MESSY has child and teacher/parent versions that rate social behaviors in terms of frequency of occurrence (1 = not at all; 2 = a little; 3 = some; 4 = much of the time; and, 5 = very much) and cover both appropriate and inappropriate behaviors that influence the quality of relationships with others. Furthermore, the scale can be reliably used with children who are typically developing and those who are diagnosed with hearing and visual impairment, developmental disabilities, intellectual disabilities, and psychopathology (Matson, Macklin, & Helsel, 1985; Matson, Heinze, Helsel, Kapperman, & Rotatori, 1986; Matson, LoVullo, Boisjoli, & Gonzales, 2008). Scores on the MESSY have been found to have a strong relationship between scores on other measures of childhood depression, such as the CDI; therefore, this measure could be an additional tool to assist in the evaluation, treatment planning, and monitoring of social behaviors of depressed children (Matson, 1988; Roberts, Kane, Thomson, Bishop, & Hart, 2003). Other useful measures of childhood social functioning include the Social Skills Rating System (Greshman & Elliot, 1990) and the School Social Behaviour Scales (Merrell, 1993).

Treatment

Depression is a serious psychological disturbance that affects a large number of children. Therefore, effectively treating this phenomenon in children is an extremely important issue to clinicians, mental health workers, and parents. Determining the most effective mode of intervention is not something to be taken lightly but should, instead, be given much consideration and time. Furthermore, given the complex nature of childhood depression, selecting the treatment approach is not a "one-size fit all" phenomena. The clinician must take into account etiological variables attributing to depressive symptoms in addition to the skill set, competence, developmental level, and needs of their client to ensure maximum results. Despite significant growth and interest in the occurrence of childhood depression, literature pertaining to ameliorating or preventing depression in youngsters is, unfortunately, still considered to be sparse. The need for more research is significant.

Adapted from primarily adult outcome studies and clinical observations, there are many intervention strategies that have been used for depressed children. The majority of interventions that are suggested to be effective choices for decreasing depressive symptoms include cognitive, emotional, and social components. A thorough review of the different types of treatment modalities is beyond the scope of this chapter; however, we will focus our discussion specifically on social skills training.

Given the connection between depressive symptomatology and social behavioral deficits in children, specifically targeting these skills would appear to be an appropriate target for intervention. Researchers and clinicians assert that social skills training is one method that can be used to increase necessary prosocial skills in depressive children. Furthermore, social skills training for children who are depressed has been shown to be as effective

as other interventions and can easily be incorporated into a comprehensive treatment package. The purpose of training prosocial behaviors is to enable the child to be able to recognize and utilize a complex set of appropriate behavioral responses. As a result, this will allow the child to adapt to various problems he/she might encounter in social situations. For the clinician, teaching social skills requires implementing several standard procedures that target to increase more appropriate social behaviors and decrease negative social behaviors including providing explicit instructions, modeling, corrective feedback, social reinforcement, role-playing, rehearsal or practice, and tangible reinforcement of discrete behaviors. Typically, these procedures occur in one-to-one training sessions between the client and therapist. However, small groups of four to six children may be trained simultaneously as long as they have similar skill level and type of problem.

Matson and colleagues (1980) provide a good example of evidence-based social skills direct training for children with depression who have deficits in rudimentary prosocial behaviors. Each of the four participants, two males and two females from 9 to 11 years of age, were receiving short-term inpatient treatment for emotional disturbance and challenging behaviors concomitant with diagnosable depression. All the children were noted to have difficulty adapting both at school and home and were noted to evince antisocial behaviors including fighting, provoking, and being noncompliant. In addition, these children were socially withdrawn and had many psychosomatic complaints.

The behaviors targeted for intervention were appropriate verbal content (e.g., giving a compliment, giving help, or making appropriate requests), appropriate affect (e.g., smiles when complimented, facial expression matches situation), makes eye contact, and body posture (e.g., faces the clinician, maintains appropriate stance). Intervention involved instructions, performance feedback, role-playing, and social reinforcement for appropriate responding (i.e., verbal behavior, affect, eye contact, and body posture). The children were trained individually through the use of vignettes. Using index cards with social scenarios written on them, the clinician read the information aloud and then attempted to elicit a response from the child who was participating in the role-play. The therapist provided feedback and, based on the quality of the child's response, would either re-present the same scene and model appropriate responding or present and narrate the next scene. Via a multiple-baseline research design, the children improved in their targeted behavioral responses and also showed gains in vignettes for which they had not received the specialized training. In addition, these gains were maintained at a 15-week follow-up in an outpatient therapy session.

Marchant and colleagues (2007) describe a somewhat different variation of this type of direct behavioral instruction that utilizes modeling, feedback, rehearsal, self-monitoring, goal setting, and reinforcement. They treated three children aged 7, 11, and 11 years old. All of the participants had been previously identified as being "at risk" for developing depression due to internalizing behavior problems. In addition, the children engaged in socially withdrawn playground behavior such as hiding in the bushes during recess, playing by himself/herself, not interacting with other children, complaining of somatic problems (e.g., headache), staying inside to finish class assignments, and engaging in aggressive behavior just prior to recess.

The behavioral targets for intervention were effective communication (i.e., engaging a peer by looking at him/her and initiating verbal communication) and appropriate peer-play (i.e., follow the rules of the game, use equipment in a safe way, how to invite others to play, how to ask to play with others, let everyone play, keep your hands and feet to yourself, and use kind words). For each social skill, the clinician explained the steps of each social skill, modeled the skill steps, practiced the skill with the child, provided verbal praise, gave feedback and correction on performance, and discussed playground situations where the skill could be used appropriately. Next, each participant was required to verbally recite all the steps of the social skill with 100% accuracy. Then, the child practiced implementing the behavior via role-playing various scenarios on a vacant playground while receiving feedback from the clinician. Once the skill was mastered, the child was instructed in how to self-monitor his/her behavior by recording how many times they engaged in a specific behavior with a peer during normal recess time. If the child's predetermined goal was met for the day, he/she received reinforcement in the form of special privileges (e.g., five extra minutes of recess) as well as tangible or edible reinforcers (e.g., candy bars, soda, bouncy balls).

Using a multiple baseline design, the authors were able to demonstrate immediate increases in effective peer communication and appropriate play on the playground. These gains continued to increase throughout treatment. Social gains were maintained at post-study observations conducted 4 months following the intervention. In addition, reports from the participants' parents and teachers indicated that the intervention positively influenced behavior in other settings, such as at home and in the classroom.

Including same-age peers in the therapeutic process may be another strategy that the clinician considers to increase social skills in children with depression. Most researchers who utilize peer-mediated learning focus on the use of a more socially-competent peer to provide an example of appropriate prosocial behaviors. Fantuzzo, Manz, Atkins, and Meyers (2005) used this type of approach to improve the social skills of withdrawn preschool children who evinced low levels of interactive play. These children, in addition, had experienced maltreatment or physical abuse by their parents. In their study, peers/classmates were selected who were rated as having a high level of compliance and prosocial play interaction. Each of the 15 sessions took place in a designated corner of the classroom that contained an array of the target child's preferred toys. The items were provided to help facilitate interaction between the child and the peer. The clinician began each session by, first, providing the buddy instructions, modeling, and assistance on the different activities that may be used to promote play behaviors from the withdrawn child. Then, the peer was prompted to invite the target child to "come play." During the play session, the two children engaged in play and were rated on their levels of solitary play, social attention, associative play, and collaborative play interactions by the clinician. At the end of the session, the clinician gave feedback (e.g., reinforcement, corrective feedback, and modeling) to the target child and the play buddy about their interactive play behaviors. The treatment resulted in significant gains in the level of collaborative play interactions for the withdrawn children. At follow-up, teacher ratings of play interactions and classroom behavior indicated that the target children continued to show overall higher levels of interactive play and self- control and lower levels of disconnected and disruptive play behavior than when compared to pre-treatment data and to the data of withdrawn children whose play partner was of average social competence and did not receive instruction from the clinician.

Social problem solving (i.e., anger management, conflict resolution, relaxation, self-monitoring, etc.) is another area that children with depression have difficulty engaging in and provides another target for social skill intervention. Given that depressed children have a poor ability to handle stressful social situations effectively, ensuring that the child has the tools to help manage a challenging social situation is necessary. There are many methods to train problem-solving skills in children. In brief, these methods teach children a wide range of strategies that allow them to develop and maintain positive relationships with peer and adults through coping with difficult social situations, problem solving, and resolving conflict. To ensure success, the child must, at minimum, be able to identify the occurrence of a social problem, generate alternative responses rather than respond impulsively, predict the consequences of each alternative, and select and perform the strategy most likely to lead to a successful outcome (Amish, Gesten, Smith, Clark, & Stark, 1988; Spivack, Platt, & Shure, 1976). These steps are generally taught as a combination of modeling, rehearsal, exercises, and games that illustrates the steps in real-world situations. In addition, many of these programs utilize a mnemonic device to make the steps easier for young children to recall (Vaughn & Lancelotta, 1990).

Webster-Stratton, Reid, and Hammond (2001) incorporated a problem-solving paradigm into a curriculum-based treatment package for 51 children 4–8 years of age. These children evinced poor social coping skills, emotional disturbances, and had a variety of conduct problems (aggression, noncompliance, oppositional behavior). The intervention used, *The Incredible Years Dinosaur Social Skills and Problem-solving Child Training Program*, consisted of 18–22 structured lessons that occurred for approximately 40 min once a week. Six broad social-emotional behaviors (social and conflict-resolution skills, loneliness and negative attributions, inability to emphasize or understand others' perspective, limited use of feeling language, and poor problem solving at school) were

the intervention targets. Techniques including group discussion and practice, videotape modeling, role-play, social stories, activity scheduling, and homework assignments were utilized to allow the children to practice a varied repertoire of acceptable solutions and coping skills for social situations frequently encountered. To ensure that the children remained motivated and focused, a variety of developmentally-appropriate strategies (cue cards, coloring books, cartoons, books, tokens, stickers, prizes, child-sized puppets) were use to reinforce key concepts and newly acquired skills. When compared to a control group, the children in the treatment group showed significant reductions in aggressive and disruptive behavior and had increases in prosocial behaviors and positive conflict management skills. These treatment gains were maintained 1 and 2 years later.

The procedures we have reviewed here constitute the primary intervention strategies for teaching appropriate social skills to children with depression. Unfortunately, there has not been a great number of empirically-based investigations conducted using these training strategies. This is consistent with other treatment modalities (e.g., cognitive behavioral therapy, interpersonal therapy, etc.) used with children diagnosed with depression. To ensure effective treatment planning, then, the clinician is advised to conduct a thorough assessment of the skills and deficits of the client and tailor the intervention to the individual needs of the child. Given the dearth of information on treatment efficacy in children, being able to provide an individualized treatment plan will better equip the child with the skills necessary to handle their depressive tendencies and be able to make and maintain friendships with peers. The child with depression who is able to achieve success in his/her social world will have more confidence and self-esteem, thereby, translating into better outcomes.

Current Status and Future Directions

Once believed incapable of occurring, childhood depression is experienced by a significant proportion of children. Developmentally distinct from adolescent or adult depressive symptoms, early onset depression in the young can have detrimental and deleterious effects which can translate into a whole host of problems that are long-lasting. Perhaps because of recognition of the seriousness of the disorder, and the growing number of children affected by it, research in the area has increased. The knowledge-base that has been amassed regarding this is still regarded to be meager when compared to that of the adolescent or adult population. Questions still exist regarding the nature of the disorder, the impact of depressive symptoms on the child and his/her family, its course, and common co-occurring disturbances. Given that there is much yet to be determined about the basic etiology and presentation of depression in children, this has resulted in a dearth of empirically based assessment and treatment models.

In this chapter, we have highlighted the current state of what is known in regard to the best way to assess and define childhood depression. There is no single method to assess and diagnose depression in the very young; therefore, it is suggested that the clinician utilize a broad-based multi-method approach to gather information about the frequency and severity of the mood-related problems typically seen (i.e., aggression, social withdrawal, irritability, low self-esteem, extreme fatigue, etc.) in children. By doing so, the clinician will be better able to formulate and implement an intervention which will be effective at ameliorating the targeted symptoms. In regard to treatment, there is no standard as to the most effective way to decrease depression in the young child. Therefore, the clinician must be able to glean information from depression assessments, behavioral observations, and their clinical knowledge to be able to know what is the best intervention for their client.

Social skills training is one such method that has demonstrated viability for treating depression in children. Given that deficits in positive social behaviors and excesses in negative social skills are a hallmark of depressive symptomatology in children, targeting these types of behaviors for treatment purposes would seem to be an intuitive choice. Through the use of evidenced-based approaches, increasing a child's ability to interact with his/her social world in a more appropriate manner will not only allow for greater success with peers but will also, as a result, increase self-concept, enable better problem-solving strategies, and provide a more effective way to handle stressful social situations.

Obviously, as with other treatment research in the very young, there have not been a great number of studies utilizing a social skills model. Those studies that have appeared show the utility of this training method with a variety of target behaviors of clients from mild to very severe depressive disorders. Regardless, given that research is only just beginning to investigate the child population, more work is needed to develop a comprehensive and effective approach to treating children.

References

Abramson, L. Y., Metalsky, F. I., & Alloy, L. B. (1989). Hopelessness depression: A theory based subtype of depression. *Psychological Review, 96*, 358–372.

Achenbach, T. M. (1986). *Child behavior checklist: Direct observation form* (rev. ed.). Burlington: University of Vermont, Department of Psychiatry.

Altmann, E. O., & Gotlib, I. H. (1988). The social behavior of depressed children: An observational study. *Journal of Abnormal Child Psychology, 16*, 29–44.

American Psychiatric Association. (2000). *Diagnostic and statistical manual of mental disorders-text revision* (4th ed.). Washington, DC: Author.

Amish, P. L, Gesten, E. L., Smith, J. K., Clark, H. B., & Stark, C. (1988). Social problem-solving training for severely emotionally and behaviorally disturbed children. *Behavioral Disorders, 13*, 175–186.

Angold, A., & Costello, E. J. (1995). A test–retest reliability study of child-reported psychiatric symptoms and diagnoses using the child and adolescent psychiatric assessment (CAPA-C). *Psychological Medicine, 25*, 755–762.

Angold, A., Prendergast, M., Cox, A., Harrington, R., Simonoff, E., & Rutter, M. (1995). The child and adolescent psychiatric assessment (CAPA). *Psychological Medicine, 25*, 739–753.

Baker, K. (2006). Treatment and management of depression in children. *Current Paediatrics, 16*, 478–483.

Bath, H. I., & Middleton, M. R. (1985). The children's depression scale: Psychometric properties and factor structure. *Australian Journal of Psychology, 37*, 81–88.

Beardslee, W. R., Versage, E. M., & Gladstone, T. R. (1998). Children of affectively ill parents: A review of the past 10 years. *Journal of the American Academy of Child and Adolescent Psychiatry, 37*, 1134–1141.

Birmaher, B. & Heydl, P. (2001). Biological studies in depressed children and adolescents. *International Journal of Neuropsychopharmacology, 4*, 149–157.

Birmaher, B., Ryan, N. D., Williamson, D. E., Brent, D. A., Kaufman, J., Dahl, R. E., et al. (1996). Childhood and adolescent depression: A review of the past 10 years. Part I. *Journal of the American Academy of Child and Adolescent Psychiatry, 35*, 1427–1439.

Brooks, S. J., & Kutcher, S. (2001). Diagnosis and measurement of adolescent depression: A review of commonly utilized instruments. *Journal of Child and Adolescent Psychopharmacology, 11*, 341–376.

Cohen, P., Cohen, J., Kasen, S., Velez, C. N., Hartmark, C., Johnson, J., et al. (1993). An epidemiological study of disorders in late childhood and adolescence: I. Age-and gender-specific prevalence. *Journal of Child Psychology and Psychiatry, 34*, 851–867.

Cole, D. A., Hoffman, K., Tram, J. M., & Maxwell, S. E. (2000). Structural differences in parent and child reports of children's symptoms of depression and anxiety. *Psychological Assessment, 12*, 174–185.

Cole, D. A., Martin, J. M., & Powers, B. (1997). A competency-based model of child depression: A longitudinal study of peer, parent, teacher, and self-evaluations. *Journal of Child Psychology an Psychiatry, 38*, 505–514.

Conley, C. S., Haines, B. A., Hilt, L. M., & Metalsky, G. I. (2001). The children's attributional style interview: Developmental tests of cognitive diathesis-stress theories of depression. *Journal of Abnormal Child Psychology, 29*, 445–463.

Costello, E. J., Angold, A., Burns, B. J., Stangl, D. K., Tweed, D. L., Erkanli, A., et al. (1996). The Great Smoky Mountains Study of Youths: Goals, design, methods, and the prevalence of DSM-III-R disorders. *Archives of General Psychiatry, 53*, 1129–1136.

Costello, E. J., Costello, A. J., Edelbrock, C., Burns, B. J., Dulcan, M. K., Brent, D. A., et al. (1988). Psychiatric disorders in pediatric primary care: Prevalence and risk factors. *Archives of General Psychiatry, 45*, 1107–1116.

Costello, E. J., Mustillo, S., Erkanli, A., Keeler, G., & Angold, A. (2003). Prevalence and development of psychiatric disorders in childhood and adolescence. *Archives of General Psychiatry, 60*, 837–844.

Davidson, R. J., Kabat-Zinn, J., Schumacher, J., Rosenkranz, M., Muller, D., Santorelli, S. F., et al. (2003). Alterations in brain and immune function produced by mindfulness meditation. *Psychosomatic Medicine, 65*, 564–570.

Davidson, R. J., Pizzagalli, D., Nitschke, J. B., & Putnam, K. (2002). Depression: Perspectives from affective neuroscience. *Annual Review of Psychology, 53*, 545–574.

Dawson, G., Frey, K., Panagiotides, H., Osterling, J., & Hessl, D. (1997). Infants of depressed mothers exhibit atypical frontal brain activity: A replication and extension of previous findings. *Journal of child Psychology and Psychiatry, 38*, 179–186.

Egger, H. L., & Angold, A. (2006). Common emotional and behavioral disorders in preschool children: Presentation, nosology, and epidemiology. *Journal of Child Psychology and Psychiatry, 47*, 313–337.

Eley, T. C. (1999). Behavioral genetics as a tool for developing psychology: Anxiety and depression in children and adolescents. *Clinical Child and Family Psychology Review, 2*, 21–36.

Eley, T. C., & Plomin, R. (1997). Genetic analyses of emotionality. *Current Opinion in Neurobiology, 7*, 279–284.

Eyberg, S. M., Bessmer, J., Newcomb, K., Edwards, D., & Robinson, E. (1994). Manual for the dyadic parent–child interaction coding system-II. *Social and behavioral sciences documents* (MS. No. 2897). San Rafel, CA: Select Press.

Fantuzzo, J., Manz, P., Atkins, M., & Meyers, R. (2005). Peer-mediated treatment of socially withdrawn maltreated preschool children: Cultivating natural community resources. *Journal of Clinical Child and Adolescent Psychology, 34*, 320–235.

Feehan, M., Mcgee, R., Raja, S. N., & Williams, S. M. (1994). DSM-III-R disorders in New Zealand 18-year-olds. *Australian and New Zealand Journal of Psychiatry, 28*, 87–99.

Field, T., Fox, N. A., Pickens, J., & Nawrocki, T. (1995). Relative frontal EEG activation in 30 to 6-month-old infants of depressed mothers. *Developmental Psychology, 31*, 358–363.

Fergusson, D. M., Horwood, L. J., & Lynskey, M. T. (1993). Prevalence and comorbidity of DSM-III-R diagnoses in a birth cohort of 15-year-olds. *Journal of the American Academy of Child and Adolescent Psychiatry, 32*, 1127–1134.

Fine, S., Moretti, M., Haley, G., & Marriage, K. (1984). Depressive disorder in children an adolescents: Dysthymic disorder and the use of self-rating scales in assessment. *Child Psychiatry and Human Development, 14*, 223–229.

Ford, T., Goodman, R., & Meltzer, H. (2003). The British child and adolescent mental health survey, 1999: The prevalence of DSM-IV disorders. *Journal of the American Academy of Child and Adolescent Psychiatry, 42*, 1203–1211.

Garrison, C. Z., Waller, J. L., Cuffee, S. P., Mckeown, R. E., Addy, C. L., & Jacson, K. L. (1997). Incidence of major depressive disorder and dysthymia in young adolescents. *Journal of the American Academy of child and Adolescent Psychiatry, 36*, 458–465.

Gibb, B. E., Alloy, L. B., Walshaw, P. D., Comer, P. D., Comer, J. S., Shen, G. H. C., et al. (2006). Predictors of attributional style change in children. *Journal of Abnormal Child Psychology, 34*, 1573–2835.

Goodman, S. H., & Gotlib, I. H. (1999). Risk for psychopathology in the children of depressed mothers: A developmental model for understanding mechanisms of transmission. *Psychological Review, 106*, 458–490.

Gresham, F. M., & Elliot, S. N. (1990). *Social skills rating system.* Circle Pines, MN: American Guidance Service.

Hammen, C., Burge, D., Burney, E., & Adrian, C. (1990). Longitudinal study of diagnoses in children of women with unipolar and bipolar affective disorder. *Archives of General Psychiatry, 47*, 1112–1117.

Hammen, C., Shih, J. H., & Brennan, P. A. (2004). Intergenerational transmission of depression: Test of an interpersonal stress model in a community sample. *Journal of Consulting and Clinical Psychology, 72*, 511–522.

Heim, C. & Nemerolf, C. B. (2001). The role of childhood trauma in the neurobiology of mood and anxiety disorders: Preclinical and clinical studies. *Biological Psychiatry, 57*, 867–872.

Jain, S., Carmody, T. J., Trivedi, M., Hughes, C., Bernstein, I. H., Morrism, D. W., et al. (2007). A psychometric evaluation of the CDRS and MADRS in assessing depressive symptoms in children. *Journal of the American*

Academy of Child and Adolescent Psychiatry, 46, 1204–1212.

Joiner, Jr., T. E., Coyne, J. C., & Blalock, J. (1999). Overview and synthesis. In T. E. Joiner & J. C. Coyne (Eds.), *The interactional nature of depression* (pp. 3–19). Washington, DC: American Psychological Association.

Kaufman, J., Birmaher, B., Brent, D., Rao, U., Flynn, C., Moreci, P., et al. (1997). Schedule for affective disorders and schizophrenia for school-age children-present and lifetime version (K-SADS-PL): Initial reliability and validity data. *Journal of the American Academy of Child & Adolescent Psychiatry, 36,* 980–988.

Kashani, J. H. & Carlson, G. A. (1985). Major depressive disorder in a preschooler. *Journal of the American Academy of Child Psychiatry, 24,* 490–494.

Kashani, J. H., Holcomb, W. R., & Orvaschel, H. (1986). Depression and depressive symptoms in preschool children from the general population. *American Journal of Psychiatry, 143,* 138–1143.

Kashani, J. H. & Ray, J. S. (1983). Depressive related symptoms among preschool-age children. *Child Psychiatry and Human Development, 13,* 233–238.

Kashani, J. H., Rosenberg, T. K., & Reid, J. C. (1989). Developmental perspectives in child and adolescent depressive symptoms in a community sample. *American Journal of Psychiatry, 146,* 871–875.

Kaslow, N. J., Adamson, L. B., & Collins, M. H. (2000). A developmental psychopathology perspective on the cognitive components of child and adolescent depression. In A. J. Sameroff, M. Lewis, & S. M. Miller (Eds.), *Handbook of developmental psychopathology* (2nd ed., pp. 491–510). New York: Plenum Press.

Kazdin, A. E. (1987). Children's depression scale: Validation with child psychiatric inpatients. *Journal of Child Psychology and Psychiatry, 28,* 29–41.

Kazdin, A. E. (1990). Childhood depression. *Journal of Child Psychology and Psychiatry, 13,* 121–160.

Kazdin, A. E., Esveldt-Dawson, K., Sherick, R. B., & Colbus, D. (1985). Assessment of overt behavior and childhood depression among psychiatrically disturbed children. *Journal of Consulting and Clinical Psychology, 53,* 201–210.

Kazdin, A. E., & Marciano, P. L. (1998). Childhood and adolescent depression. In E. J. Mash & R. A. Barkley (Eds.), *Treatment of childhood disorders* (2nd ed., pp. 211–248). New York: Guilford Press.

Kessler, R. C., Avenevoli, S., & Merikangas, K. R. (2001). Mood disorders in children and adolescents: An epidemiologic perspective. *Biological Psychiatry, 49,* 1002–1014.

Kessler, R. C., & Walters, E. E. (1998). Epidemiology of DSM-III-R major depression and minor depression among adolescents and young adults in the National Comorbidity Survey. *Depression and Anxiety, 7,* 3–14.

Knight, D., Hensley, V. R., Waters, B. (1988). Validation of the children's depression scale and the children's depression inventory in a prepubertal sample. *Journal of Child Psychology and Psychiatry, 29,* 853–863.

Kovacs, M. (1992). *Children's depression inventory manual.* North Tonawanda, NY: Multi-Health Systems.

Kovacs, M., & Beck, A. T. (1977). An empirical-clinical approach toward a definition of childhood depression. In J. G. Schulterbrandt & A. Raskin (Eds.), *Depression in childhood: Diagnosis, treatment, and conceptual models* (pp. 1–25). New York: Raven Press.

Kovacs, M., Obrosky, D. S., & Sherill, J. (2003). Developmental changes in the phenomenology of depression in girls compared to boys from childhood onward. *Journal of Affective Disorders, 74,* 33–48.

Kupersmidt, J. B., & Patterson, C. J. (1991). Childhood peer rejection, aggression, withdrawal, and perceived competence as predictors of self-reported behaviors in preadolescence. *Journal of Abnormal Child Psychology, 19,* 427–449.

Lewinsohn, P. M. (1974). A behavioral approach to depression. In R. Friedman & M. Katz (Eds.), *The psychology of depression: Contemporary theory and research* (pp. 157–185). Washington, DC: Winston-Wiley.

Lewinson, P. M., Hops, H., Roberts, R. E., Seeley, J. R., & Andrews, J. A. (1993). Adolescent psychopathology: I. Prevalence and incidence of depression and other DSM-II-R disorders in high school students. *Journal of Abnormal Psychology, 102,* 133–144.

Lewinsohn, P. M., Pettit, J. W., Joiner, T. E., & Seeley, J. R. (2003). The symptomatic expression of major depressive disorder in adolescents and young adults. *Journal of Abnormal Psychology, 112,* 244–252.

Luby, J. L., Belden, A. C., Pautsch, J., Si, X., & Spitznagel, E. (2008). The clinical significance of preschool depression: Impairment in functioning and clinical markers of the disorder. *Journal of Affective Disorders,* doi:10.1016/j.jad.2008.03.026.

Marchant, M. R., Solano, B. R., Fisher, A. D., Caldarella, P., Young, K. R., & Renshaw, T. L. (2007). Modifying socially withdrawn behavior: A playground intervention for students with internalizing behaviors. *Psychology in the Schools, 44,* 779–794.

Matson, J. L. (1988). The Maston Evaluation of Social Skills in Youngsters (MESSY). Woshington, Ohio: International Diagnostic Systems. Translated into Spanish, Norweigan, Dutch, Swedish, and Italian.

Matson, J. L. (1989). *Treating depression in children and adolescents.* New York: Pergamon Press.

Matson, J. L., Esveldt-Dawson, K., Andrasik, F., Ollendick, T., Petti, T. H., & Hernsen, M. (1980). Direct, observational, and generalization effects of social skills training with emotionally disturbed children. *Behavior Therapy, 11,* 522–531.

Matson, J. L., Heinze, A., Helsel, W. J., Kapperman, G., & Rotatori, A. F. (1986). Assessing social behaviors in the visually handicapped: The Matson evaluation of social skills with youngsters (MESSY). *Journal of Clinical Child Psychology, 15,* 78–87.

Matson, J. L., Helsel, W. J., & Barrett, R. P. (1988). Depression in mentally retarded children. *Research in Developmental Disabilities, 9,* 39–46.

Matson, J. L., Lovullo, S. V., Boisjoli, J. A., & Gonzales, M. L. (2008). The behavioural treatment of an 11-year-old girl with autism and aggressive behaviors. *Clinical Case Studies, 7,* 313–326.

Matson, J. L., Macklin, G. F., & Helsel, W. J. (1985). Psychometric properties of the Matson evaluation of social skills with youngsters (MESSY) with emotional problems an self-concept in deaf children. *Journal of Behavior Therapy and Experimental Psychiatry, 14,* 117–123.

Matson, J. L., Rotatori, A. F., & Helsel, W. J. (1983). Development of a rating scale to measure social skills in children: The Matson evaluation of social skills in youngsters (MESSY). *Behaviour Research and Therapy, 21,* 335–340.

Mcgee, R., Feehan, M., Williams, S., Partridge, F., Silva, P. A., & Kelly, J. (1990). DSM-III disorders in a large sample of adolescents. *Journal of the American Academy of Child and Adolescent Psychiatry, 29,* 611–619.

Merrell, K. W. (1993). Using behavioral rating scales to assess social skills and antisocial behavior in school settings: Development of the School Social Behavior Scales. *School Psychology Review, 22,* 115–133.

Milling, L. S. (2001). Depression in preadolescents. In C. E. Walker & M. Roberts (Eds.), *Handbook of clinical child psychology* (3rd ed., pp. 373–392). New York: Wiley.

Nestler, E. J., Barrot, N., Dileone, R. J., Eisch, A. J., Gold, S. J., & Monteggia, L. M. (2002). Neurobiology of depression. *Neuron, 34,* 13–25.

Nolan, C. L., Moore, G. J., Madden, R., Farchione, T., Bortoi, M., Lorch, E., et al. (2002). Prefrontal cortical volume in childhood-onset major depression: Preliminary findings. *Archives of General Psychiatry, 59,* 173–179.

Nolen-Hoeksema, S., Mumme, D., Wolfson, A., & Guskin, K. (1995). Helplessness in children of depressed and nondepressed mothers: Special section: Parental depression and distress: Implications for development in infancy, childhood, and adolescence. *Developmental Psychology, 31,* 337–387.

Ollenburg, C. M., & Kerns, K. A. (1997). Associations between peer relationships and depressive symptoms: Testing moderator effects of gender and age. *Journal of Early Adolescence, 17,* 319–337.

Poznanski, E. O., Cook, S. C., & Carroll, B. J. (1979). A depression rating scale for children. *Pediatrics, 64,* 442–450.

Poznanski, E., Grossman, J., Buchsbaum, Y., Banegas, M., Freeman, L., & Gibbons, R. (1984). Preliminary studies of the reliability and validity of the Children's Depression Rating Scale. *Journal of the American Academy of Child Psychiatry 23,* 191–197.

Poznanski, E. O., & Mokros, H. B. (1999). *Children depression rating scale-revised (CDRS-R).* Los Angeles: Western Psychological Services.

Puig-Antich, J., & Chambers, W. (1978). *The schedule for affective disorders and schizophrenia for school-age children (Kiddie-SADS).* New York: New York State Psychiatric Institute.

Rehm, L. P. (1977). A self-control model of depression. *Behavior Therapy, 8,* 787–804.

Reich, W. (2000). Diagnostic interview for children and adolescents (DICA). *Journal of the American Academy of Child & Adolescent Psychiatry, 39,* 59–66.

Renouf, A., & Kovacs, M. (1994). Concordance between mothers' reports and children's self-reports of depressive symptoms: A longitudinal study. *Journal of the American Academy of Child and Adolescent Psychiatry, 33,* 208–216.

Reynolds, W. M. (1989). *Reynolds child depression scale: Professional manual.* Odessa, FL: Psychological Assessment Resources.

Reynolds, W. M. (1998). Depression in children and adolescents. In T. H. Ollenick (Ed.), *Comprehensive clinical psychology: Vol. 4. Children and adolescents: Clinical formulations and treatment* (pp. 419–461). New York: Pergamon Press.

Reynolds, W. M., & Graves, A. (1989). Reliability of children's reports of depressive symptomatology. *Journal of Consulting an Clinical Psychology, 54,* 653–660.

Reynolds, C. R., & Kamphans, R. W. (1992). Behavior Assessment System for Children. Circle Pines, MN: American Guidance Service.

Rice, F., Harold, G., & Thapar, A. (2002). The genetic aetiology of childhood depression: A review. *Journal of Child Psychology and Psychiatry, 43,* 65–79.

Rochlin, G. (1959). The loss complex. *Journal of the American Psychoanalytic Association, 7,* 299–316.

Roberts, C., Kane, R., Thomson, H., Bishop, B., & Hart, B. (2003). The prevention of depressive symptoms in rural school children: A randomized controlled trial. *Journal of Consulting and Clinical Psychology, 71,* 622–628.

Robinson, J. C., & Lewinsohn, P. M. (1973). Behavior modification of speech characteristics in a chronically depressed man. *Behavior Therapy, 4,* 150–155.

Rotundo, N., & Hensley, V. R. (1985). The children's depression scale. A study of its validity. *Journal of Child Psychology and Psychiatry, 26,* 917–927.

Rudolph, K. D., & Clark, A. G. (2001). Conceptions of relationships in children with depressive and aggressive symptoms: Social-cognitive distortion or reality? *Journal of Abnormal Child Psychology, 29,* 41–56.

Rudolph, K. D., Hammen, C., & Burge, D. (1994). Interpersonal functioning and depressive symptoms in childhood: Addressing the issues of specificity and comorbidity. *Journal of Abnormal Child Psychology, 22,* 355–371.

Rudolph, K. D., Hammen, C., Burge, D., Lindberg, N., Herzberg, D., & Daley, S. E. (2000). Toward an interpersonal life-stress model of depression: The developmental context of stress generation. *Development and Psychopathology, 12,* 215–234.

Rudolph, K. D., Kurlakowsky, K. D., & Conley, C. S. (2001). Developmental and social-contextual origins of depressive control-related beliefs and behaviors. *Cognitive Therapy and Research, 25,* 447–475.

Schroeder, C. S., & Gordon, B. N. (2002). *Assessment and treatment of childhood problems: A clinician's guide* (2nd ed.). New York: Guilford Press.

Scourfield, J., Rice, F., Thapar, A., Harold, G. T., Martin, N., & Mcguffin, P. (2003). Depressive symptoms in children and adolescents: Changing aetiological influences with development. *Journal of Child Psychology and Psychiatry, 44,* 968–976.

Segrin, C. (2000). Social skills deficits associated with depression. *Clinical Review, 20,* 379–403.

Seligman, M. E. P. (1975). *Helplessness: On depression, development, and death.* San Francisco: W. H. Freeman.

Shaffer, D., Fisher, P., Lucas, C. P., Dulcan, M. K., Schwab-Stone, M. E. (2000). NIMH diagnostic interview schedule for children version IV (NIMH DISC-IV): Description, differences from previous versions, an reliability of some common diagnoses. *Journal of the American Academy of Child and Adolescent Psychiatry, 39,* 28–38.

Shain, B. N., Naylor, M., & Alessi, N. (1990). Comparison of self-rated and clinician-rated measures of depression in adolescents. *The American Journal of Psychiatry, 147*, 793–795.

Spivack, G., Platt, J. J., Shure, M. B. (1976). *The problem solving approach to adjustment: A guide to research and intervention.* San Francisco: Jossey-Bass.

Strober, M., & Werry, J. S. (1986). The assessment of depression in children and adolescents. In N. Sartorius & T. A. Ban (Eds.), *Assessment of depression* (pp. 324–342). Berlin: Springer-Verlag.

Sullivan, P. F., Neale, M. C., & Kendler, K. S. (2000). Genetic epidemiology of major depression: Review and meta-analysis. *American Journal of Psychiatry, 157*, 1552–1562.

Shaffery, J., Hoffmann, R., & Armitage, R. (2003). The neurobiology of depression: Perspectives from animal and human sleep studies. *Neuroscientist, 9*, 82–98.

Stark, K., Reynolds, W. M., & Kaslow, N. J. (1987). A comparison of the relative efficacy of self-control therapy and behavioral problem-solving therapy for depression in children. *Journal of Abnormal Child Psychology, 15*, 91–113.

Thapar, A., & Mcguffin, P. (1994). A twin study of depressive symptoms in childhood. *British Journal of Psychiatry, 165*, 259–265.

Tisher, M., Lang, M. (1983). The children's depression scale: Review and further developments. In D. P. Cantwell & G. A. Carlson (Eds.), *Affective disorders in childhood and adolescents—An update* (pp. 181–203). Jamaica, NY: Spectrum Publications.

Tisher, M., Lang-Takac, E., & Lang, M. (1992). The children's depression scale: Review of Australian and overseas experience. Australian Journal of Psychology, 44, 27–35.

Tomarken, A. J., Dichter, G. S., Garber, J., & Simien, C. (2004). Relative left frontal hypoactivation in adolescents at risk for depression. *Biological Psychology, 67*, 77–102.

Vaughn, S., & Lancelotta, G. X. (1990). Teaching interpersonal skills to poorly accepted students: Peer-paring versus non-peer-pairing. *Journal of School Psychology, 28*, 181–188.

Velez, C., Johnson, J., & Cohen, P. (1989). A longitudinal analysis of selected risk factors for childhood psycho-pathology. *Journal of the American Academy of Child and Adolescent Psychiatry, 28*, 861–864.

Webster-Stratton, C., Reid, J., & Hammond, M. (2001). Social skills and problem-solving training for children with early-onset conduct problems: Who benefits? *Journal of Child Psychology an Psychiatry, 42*, 943–952.

Weiss, B., & Garber, G. (2003). Developmental differences in the phenomenology of depression. *Development and Psychopathology, 15*, 403–430.

Weissman, M. M., Warner, V., Wickramaratne, P., Moreau, D., & Olfson, M. (1997). Offspring of depressed parents: Ten years later. *Archives of General Psychiatry, 54*, 932–940.

Weisz, J. R., Sweeney, L., Proffitt, V., & Carr, T. (1994). Control-related beliefs and self-reported depressive symptoms in late childhood. *Journal of Abnormal Psychology, 102*, 411–418.

Winters, N. C., Myers, K., & Proud, L. (2002). Ten-year review of rating scales. III: Scales assessing suicidality, cognitive style, and self-esteem. *Journal of the American Academy of Child and Adolescent Psychiatry, 41*, 1150–1181.

Wu, P., Hoven, C. W., Bird, H. R., Moore, R. E., Cohen, P., Alegria, M., et al. (1999). Depressive and disruptive disorders and mental health service utilization in children and adolescents. *Journal of the American Academy of Child and Adolescent Psychiatry, 38*, 1081–1090.

Young, E. A., & Altemus, M. (2004). Puberty, ovarian steroids, and stress. *Annals of the New York Academy of Science, 1021*, 124–133.

Zahn-Waxler, C., Klimes-Dougan, B., & Slattery, M. J. (2000). Internalizing problems of childhood and adolescence: Prospects, pitfalls, and progress in understanding the development of anxiety and depression. *Development and Psychopathology, 12*, 443–446.

Zimmerman, M. (2003). What should the standard of care for psychiatric diagnostic evaluations be? *Journal of Nervous and Mental Disease, 191*, 281–286.

Chapter 13
Medical and Physical Impairments and Chronic Illness

Tessa T. Rivet and Johnny L. Matson

Children with chronic conditions face a number of challenges which place them at risk for difficulties in psychosocial functioning. Aspects related to the condition itself or the treatment of the condition may serve as significant stressors. These include hospitalizations, excessive school absences, pain, fatigue, changes in physical appearance, teasing, restrictions on physical activity, extensive monitoring and treatment regimens, lifestyle modifications, and mobility, sensory, or neurocognitive impairments (La Greca, 1990; Schuman & La Greca, 1999). Multiple aspects of social functioning have important implications in several areas for children with chronic conditions, including adjustment to and management of the condition. For example, peers may be a significant source of social support, influence treatment adherence, and impact health-promoting and health-risk behaviors (La Greca, Bearman, & Moore, 2002). Therefore, for the child with chronic medical conditions, the ability to make and maintain lasting bonds with same-age peers is important, if not a necessity.

The following is an overview of the definition and prevalence of chronic childhood conditions; presentation of theoretical frameworks as applied to psychosocial adjustment; review of the literature on psychosocial adjustment, social functioning, related risk and resilience factors, assessment, and treatment; and implications for further research regarding the social functioning of children with chronic conditions. By understanding the information regarding these factors, the clinician will be better prepared to serve and treat their young clients with medical, physical, or chronic illness difficulties which are impacting their ability to effectively function in their social environment.

Definition of the Population

Two different approaches have been used to define chronic pediatric conditions: categorical and noncategorical. Traditionally, a categorical approach has been employed via the use of lists of diseases and conditions by which children are grouped (Gortmaker & Sappenfield, 1984). Numerous potential problems with this diagnostic approach exist (Stein, Bauman, Westbrook, Coupey, & Ireys, 1993). These lists are non-exhaustive and, thus, exclude children with conditions that are not included. Exclusion may also occur due to the lag between symptom onset and diagnosis of a condition. Furthermore, the use of a categorical approach causes a selection bias to occur toward children with access to medical care and those who have more apparent or less rare conditions. Additionally, diagnoses are not applied consistently across clinicians and settings. Finally, information on the extent of morbidity from the condition was not obtained when solely using a present or absent distinction.

Rather than focusing on the type or diagnosis a child has, a noncategorical approach focuses on the

T.T. Rivet (✉)
Department of Psychology, Louisiana State University,
Baton Rouge, LA 70803, USA
e-mail: tessatr@gmail.com

J.L. Matson (ed.), *Social Behavior and Skills in Children*, DOI 10.1007/978-1-4419-0234-4_13,
© Springer Science+Business Media, LLC 2009

consequences of having pediatric conditions (Pless & Pinkerton, 1975; Stein & Jessop, 1982). This approach recognizes that children experience common consequences from different conditions and may, in addition, experience different consequences from the same types of conditions (Stein et al., 1993). Chronic conditions can be described via a range of common dimensions, including duration (brief to lengthy), age of onset (congenital or acquired), limitation of age-appropriate activities, visibility, expected survival, course (progressive, constant, relapsing), uncertainty (episodic or predictable), and degree of impairment in the areas of mobility, physiologic functioning, cognition, emotional/social, sensory functioning, and communication (Perrin, Newacheck et al., 1993).

A wide variety of definitions have been employed to study chronic conditions in children for various purposes. In a systematic review, van der Lee, Mokkink, Grootenhuis, Heymans, and Offringa (2007) identified the four commonly used definitions of chronic health conditions (also referred to as chronic illness or special health care needs) in children (McPherson et al., 1998; Perrin, Newacheck et al., 1993; Pless & Douglas, 1971; Stein et al., 1993). These definitions take into account factors such as the impact of the condition in multiple domains of functioning (e.g., physical, cognitive, behavioral, etc.) and the need for medical care and assistance. For example, McPherson and colleagues (1998) defined children with special health care needs as those who have or are at increased risk of a chronic physical, developmental, behavioral, or emotional condition and who also require health and related services of a type or amount beyond that generally required by children. This chapter is organized according to a noncategorical approach rather than by specific conditions or illnesses. This conceptualization lends itself well to examining factors relevant to psychosocial outcomes, assessment, and treatment in children with chronic conditions.

Etiology and Prevalence

Advances in medical technology have resulted in improved early diagnosis and treatment and an increase in survival during the early years of life for children with serious conditions; however, this is coupled with an increase in the number of children living with disabilities, as well as complex, demanding treatments (Perrin, Bloom, & Gortmaker, 2007; Perrin & Hicks, 2008; van der Veen, 2003). Other factors related to the increase in children with chronic health conditions include increased survival of premature infants, emergence of new conditions such as human immunodeficiency virus (HIV) and prenatal drug exposure, deinstitutionalization of children with disabilities, and inclusion of conditions not accounted for by prior methods of categorical lists of diagnoses (Newacheck, Budetti, & Halfon, 1986; Thompson & Gustafson, 1996a). Prevalence has risen due to increased survival rates, especially for conditions such as cystic fibrosis, sickle cell disease, and cancer, while conditions such as asthma, type 2 diabetes, and HIV have increased in their occurrence (Thompson & Gustafson, 1996a).

Prevalence rates for chronic childhood conditions vary widely from 0.22% (children with very serious health problems who must often depend on technology for vital functions) to 44% (children visiting an urban health center identified by diagnosis list; van der Lee et al., 2007). Multiple factors may contribute to this variability, including the definitions used, characteristics of the sample (e.g., age, access to medical services), source and method of information (e.g., physical exam, interview, medical or claims records), and study characteristics (setting, year, purpose; van der Lee et al., 2007). Using the 1992–1994 National Health Interview Survey on Disability, Newacheck and colleagues (1998) found that 12% of noninstitutionalized children in the United States had special health care needs, and an additional 6% experience limitations in social role activities (e.g., school, play) because of chronic physical or mental conditions.

Regarding specific conditions, asthma is the most common chronic health condition in children (Bloom & Tonthat, 2002) and is a leading cause of school absences, hospitalizations, and activity restrictions for children with chronic conditions (Newacheck & Taylor, 1992). The most common pediatric genetic illnesses include cystic fibrosis and sickle cell disease (Barakat & Boyer, 2008). Cystic fibrosis is more common among Caucasians and is characterized by progressive pulmonary disease and pancreatic insufficiency. It is associated with delayed puberty, small physical stature, school absences, and extensive treatment demands (Cystic Fibrosis Foundation, 2008; DiGirolamo, Quittner, Ackerman, & Stevens, 1997). Sickle cell disease is more common among African Americans and is characterized by red blood cells restricting blood flow. It is associated with pain, stroke, delayed physical maturation, activity restrictions, school absences, fatigue, and extensive treatment demands (Barakat, Lash, Lutz, & Nicolaou, 2006). Conditions with mixed genetic and environmental causes include diabetes and cancer (Barakat & Boyer, 2008). Diabetes requires extensive lifestyle modifications (e.g., diet) and complex monitoring and treatment (Wysocki, 2006). Cognitive functioning may be impacted by the cancer itself (e.g., brain tumors) or the treatment (e.g., radiation). Cancer also causes school absences, changes in physical appearance (e.g., hair loss), and physical symptoms from treatment (e.g., nausea, fatigue). Epilepsy, cerebral palsy, and spina bifida are among the most common central nervous system (CNS) conditions in children (Nassau & Drotar, 1997) and can involve cognitive and mobility impairments. Additionally, for children with epilepsy, side effects from antiepileptic medications may impact functioning. Numerous other chronic pediatric conditions have been examined in relation to psychosocial functioning including neurofibromatosis, HIV, hemophilia, juvenile rheumatic diseases, cardiac conditions, craniofacial conditions, diabetes, liver disease, hearing loss, and visual impairments. Each of these conditions has different aspects that vary in the extent of impact these aspects may have on social functioning.

Social Skills Problems Unique to the Population

Theoretical Models of Psychosocial Adjustment

A number of theoretical models have been proposed to explain children's adaptation to chronic conditions (see Drotar, 2006b). The models vary with

regard to extent of focus on child, condition, or social-ecological influences. For example, Pless and Pinkerton's (1975) model views adaptation to illness as resulting from reciprocal interactions between the child and his or her environment. The child's self-concept and coping style (influenced by biological and social processes) determines how he or she reacts to stress. The social ecological model (Bronfenbrenner, 1979; Kazak, 1989), outlines proximal and distal influences on adaptation, including microsystems (the child, illness, family), mesosystems (neighborhood, peers, school, hospital/medical team), and exosystems (culture, social class, religion, social policy). Rolland's family systems-illness model (Rolland, 1984, 1987) provides a framework for examining illness characteristics and phases, as well as the interaction between child, illness, and family development. The model incorporates three dimensions: (1) a psychosocial typology of the illness and disability, including the onset (acute or gradual), course (progressive, constant, relapsing), outcome (nonfatal, shortened life span or sudden death, fatal), degree of incapacitation (none, mild, moderate, severe), and level of uncertainty; (2) the time phase of the illness (crisis, chronic, and terminal); and (3) family systems variables. These three models provide examples of varying degrees of focus on child (Pless & Pinkerton, 1975), social-ecological (Bronfenbrenner, 1979; Kazak, 1989), and condition (Rolland, 1984, 1987) influences.

Two common integrative theoretical models, or risk-and-resistance models, include the disability-stress-coping model (Wallander & Varni, 1992; Wallander, Varni, Babani, Banis, & Wilcox, 1989) and the transactional stress and coping model (Thompson, Gustafson, Hamlett, & Spock, 1992). In the disability-stress-coping model, risk factors include condition parameters (diagnosis, visibility, brain involvement, severity); functional independence; and psychosocial stressors (disability-related problems, major life events, daily hassles). Resistance or protective factors include intrapersonal factors (e.g., temperament, competencies, effectance motivation, problem-solving skills); stress processing (cognitive appraisal, coping strategies); and social-ecological factors (e.g., family environment, social support, parental adjustment, utilitarian resources). In the transactional stress and coping model, adjustment is the cumulative result of interactions of biomedical, developmental, and psychosocial processes, with the focus on psychosocial contributions. The type and severity of the illness, as well as demographic parameters such as child gender, child age, and socio-economic status are incorporated. Psychosocial processes are included in terms of maternal and child adaptational processes. Maternal adaptational processes include cognitive processes (appraisal stress including daily hassles and illness tasks; expectations including efficacy and health locus of control); methods of coping (palliative, adaptive); and family functioning (supportive, conflicted, controlling). Child adaptational processes include cognitive processes (expectations, self-esteem, health locus of control) and coping methods.

More recently, two additional models have been proposed. In view of data suggesting "hardiness" in children with chronic conditions, Noll and Kupst (2007) proposed the Human EvolutionAry Response to Trauma/Stress (HEART) model. The model posits that random and traumatic pediatric events do not result in dysfunction unless they impact the central nervous system (e.g., brain tumors, closed head injury, neurofibromatosis) or are directly related to the child's family (e.g., death of a parent, abuse, neglect). As an integration of the categorical and risk-resistance models, Boyer (2008) presented the Model for Integrating Medicine and Psychology (MI-MAP). The MI-MAP incorporates disease factors (onset, progression, types of symptoms); treatment regimen factors (complexity, intrusiveness, accessibility, cost, side-effects); individual factors (intelligence, information, literacy, culture, trust, health beliefs, coping, family and social support); and comorbid psychopathology (depression, anxiety, substance abuse/addiction, dementia, psychosis, personality disorders). The model was proposed for utility in guiding comprehensive assessment and treatment planning.

Theoretical models of psychosocial adjustment have important implications in guiding research and clinical practice in children with chronic conditions. These models can pinpoint what the mediating and moderating factors are in relation to psychosocial adjustment, assessment, and response to treatment. Conversely, further research findings can inform model revision and testing. Further research

and development is warranted in the refinement and application of these models.

Psychosocial Adjustment

Overall, children with chronic conditions have an increased risk for difficulties in psychosocial adjustment; however, the majority of these children do not experience clinically significant symptomatology (for reviews see Barlow & Ellard, 2006; Lavigne & Faier-Routman, 1992; Noll & Kupst, 2007; Wallander, Thompson, & Alriksson-Schmidt, 2003). In general, rates of significant psychopathology or social dysfunction in children with chronic conditions are not significantly different from those found in appropriate comparison groups of children. This is not to say that chronic conditions do not impact psychosocial adjustment. Rather, for children with chronic conditions, a subclinical impact can be found in multiple domains of functioning (Noll & Kupst, 2007). Thus, chronic conditions should be characterized as significant stressors which produce significant challenges for the child, resulting in an increased risk for adjustment problems.

Due to the fact that most children with chronic conditions do not differ significantly from healthy comparison peers in terms of clinically significant psychosocial dysfunction, researchers have moved from between group comparisons to within group comparisons (La Greca et al., 2002). This research has examined psychosocial functioning within conditions and across various chronic conditions. These comparisons have, at times, produced conflicting results (Barlow & Ellard, 2006). Thus, a wide range of heterogeneity within and between conditions exists with regard to psychosocial outcome. Several issues have been discussed as contributing to this disparity. These include methodological issues and research into the correlates or risk and resilience factors involved in psychosocial adjustment.

Several methodological issues have been pointed out as contributing to the heterogeneity of findings in the literature on psychosocial adjustment in children with chronic conditions. Adjustment has been defined inconsistently across multiple domains such as behavior problems, social functioning, and self-esteem (Perrin, Ayoub, & Willett, 1993). Approaches to assessment have varied by method types, instruments, and informants (Perrin, Ayoub et al., 1993). Therefore, the various approaches to assessment have been questioned regarding their sensitivity to illness-related aspects of functioning, as well as validity related to several concerns (e.g., items reflecting somatic complaints; assessment of social participation rather than capacity). These concerns will be discussed further in the "Assessment" section. In terms of informants, parents consistently provide the most negative ratings of children's psychosocial functioning compared to self and teacher reports (Barlow & Ellard, 2006). Discrepant results have also been found depending on whether control group or normative comparisons were used. For example, Lavigne and Faier-Routman (1992) found risk to be highest when using norms, while Bennett (1994) found risk of depression lowest when using norms. McQuaid, Kopel, and Nassau (2001) found that in children with asthma, risk was the same when using normative and control group comparisons. Regarding participants, small sample sizes and single site recruitment have consistently been noted as a problem in the literature (Barlow & Ellard, 2006).

Several research syntheses have examined the psychosocial well-being of children with chronic conditions. Lavigne and Fraier-Routman (1992) conducted a meta-analysis which included children aged 3–19 years who were diagnosed as having chronic conditions, including sensory and physical impairments. Examples of commonly used instruments included the Child Behavior Checklist and Piers-Harris Self Concept Scale. Children with chronic conditions were found to be at increased risk for adjustment problems such as internalizing (i.e., withdrawal, depression, anxiety) and externalizing (i.e., aggression, hyperactivity) disorders. Additionally, rates of adjustment problems varied according to variables such as condition type, informant, and comparison group characteristics. Children with sensory and neurological disorders and those with conditions having unpredictable courses showed the greatest risk, though there were only a small number of studies within individual conditions. Children with chronic conditions had lower self-concepts than healthy children; however, when careful matching or normative comparisons were used, self-concept differences were not significant. Lavigne and Fraier-Routman (1992) note that communalities across conditions which tend to impact psychosocial functioning (e.g., the visibility of the condition, is it life-threatening, does the condition require demanding or intrusive treatment, and does it causes learning impairments) should be considered.

Additional research syntheses have been conducted examining specific areas of adjustment or in specific conditions. In a meta-analysis, Bennett (1994) examined depressive symptoms in children aged 4–18 years with chronic conditions, including sensory and physical impairments. Most children with chronic conditions did not have clinical depression but did have a slightly elevated risk for depressive symptoms. Some of the researchers included in Bennett's meta-analysis found that children with conditions such as asthma, recurrent abdominal pain, and sickle cell anemia had a greater risk for depressive symptoms than those with conditions such as cancer, cystic fibrosis, and diabetes (Bennett, 1994). However, considerable heterogeneity in depressive symptoms was found in within conditions as well. Specifically, the relationship between depressive symptoms and condition severity was found to be inconsistent, and condition duration, gender, and age were unrelated. In children with rheumatic diseases, Miller (1993), in a traditional review, did not find evidence of psychological or social dysfunction. Contrary to Miller's findings, LeBovidge, Lavigne, Donenberg, and Miller (2003) conducted a meta-analysis and found that there was an increased risk of overall adjustment problems and internalizing symptoms for children with chronic conditions but not externalizing symptoms or poor self-concept. In a meta-analysis comparing children with sickle cell disease to a control group, Midence, Mcmanus, Fuggle, and Davies (1996) found no significant differences on depression or self-concept. However, teachers rated children with a milder form of sickle cell disease as having more behavioral problems, and this was associated with maternal mental health (Midence et al., 1996). Finally, McQuaid and colleagues (2001) conducted a meta-analysis and found that children with asthma had significantly more internalizing and externalizing problems, which increased with asthma severity.

Correlates of Psychosocial Adjustment

Research has also expanded to examine the mediating and moderating factors that are involved in the psychosocial adjustment of children with chronic illnesses. Correlates of psychosocial adjustment can be framed into child parameters (e.g., gender, age/age of onset, temperament, coping methods, cognitive processes), condition parameters (e.g., type, severity, functional status, duration), and social-ecological parameters (e.g., family functioning, parental stress and adjustment, peer relationships). In a review of this literature, Wallander and colleagues (2003) note that most factors have only been examined in one study. Furthermore, inconsistencies exist in the findings of multiple studies which investigate psychosocial correlates. Relatively stronger support does, however, exist for the associations between poor adjustment and factors such as brain involvement, child-reported stress and low self-esteem, low family cohesion and supportiveness, high family conflict, and maternal distress (Wallander et al., 2003).

Using the framework of child, illness, and social-ecological influences, research has examined supporting evidence for specific correlates of psychosocial functioning. In a meta-analysis, Lavigne and Faier-Routman (1993) examined correlates of psychosocial adjustment in children aged 3–19 years. These researchers found that child characteristics showed the strongest relationship to psychosocial adjustment, including self-concept, poor coping, and low cognitive ability (Lavigne & Faier-Routman, 1993). In terms of condition parameters, Lavigne and Faier-Routman (1993) found relationships between psychosocial adjustment and severity, prognosis, and functional status. In Wallander and colleagues' (2003) review of the literature, consistent findings suggest that condition parameters including brain involvement, increased asthma severity, and decreased functional abilities have been associated with poorer social functioning. Regarding socio-ecological parameters, Lavigne and Faier-Routman (1993) found that maternal adjustment, marital/family adjustment/conflict, and family support/cohesion were associated with adjustment; however, socio-economic status was not. Family psychological functioning and cohesion has been found to significantly impact social

functioning in children with chronic conditions (Wallander et al., 1989). High levels of social support from family and peers have been shown to be associated with better adjustment in children with chronic conditions (Wallander & Varni, 1989) and important for adolescents with diabetes (La Greca & Thompson, 1998).

Social Functioning

Though social functioning has been incorporated into broader studies of psychosocial adjustment in children with chronic conditions, it is often not the primary focus (La Greca, 1990, 1992; Spirito, DeLawyer, & Stark, 1991). When social functioning has been examined as the primary focus, similar methodological issues to those in the psychosocial adjustment literature hamper available conclusions. For example, early studies primarily used methods such as interviews (Spirito et al., 1991) and, even currently, much of the literature is founded on social competence as measured by the Achenbach System of Empirically Based Assessment (ASEBA) measures (see "Assessment" section).

Several authors have reviewed the available literature specific to social functioning in children with chronic conditions (see La Greca et al., 2002; La Greca, Bearman, & Moore, 2004; Reiter-Purtill, Noll, & Roberts, 2003; Schuman & La Greca, 1999; Thomas & Warschausky, 2006; Thompson & Gustafson, 1996b). Overall, children with chronic conditions do not seem to have significantly more social difficulties in comparison to peers; however, they are at increased risk. Additionally, significant heterogeneity exists with regard to social outcomes, both between and within chronic conditions. This may be in part due to the multifaceted nature of the construct of social functioning. Research has varied in terms of which aspects of social functioning are studied, as well as which outcome variables are assessed.

Social functioning in children with chronic conditions has been examined in regards to a number of aspects, including peer acceptance/status, friendships, social skills, and social support. Peer acceptance/status involves whether the child is liked or accepted by the peer group. Categories of peer acceptance/status include popular, rejected, neglected, controversial, and average children (Coie, Dodge, & Coppotelli, 1982). Peer friendships involve close ties with peers which vary in number, features, and quality (Furman & Robbins, 1985; Parker & Asher, 1993). In adolescence, peer acceptance/status and friendships become more complex primarily due to the emergence of peer crowds (e.g., jocks, brains, druggies, etc.), cliques, and dyads (Brown, 1989). Another aspect of social functioning involves social skills, which include specific abilities that enable an individual to perform competently at specific social tasks (McFall, 1982). Social skills deficits may be due to acquisition ("can't do"), performance ("won't do), or fluency deficits, and competing problem behaviors may also be present (Gresham, 1981). Social support encompasses four main functional types (House, 1981): emotional support (e.g., caring empathy, trust); instrumental support (e.g., tangible assistance, money, time); informational support (e.g., suggestions, advice); and appraisal support (e.g., affirmation, feedback, social comparison). Social support can be provided by different people (e.g., parent, sibling, peer, teacher). Finally, research examining different aspects of social information processing in children with chronic conditions hase emerged (e.g., Boni, Brown, Davis, Hsu, & Hopkins, 2001; Bonner et al., 2008; Yeates et al., 2007). Steps in social information processing include encoding social cues, representation and interpretation, clarification, response construction, response selection, and behavioral enactment (Crick & Dodge, 1994). Thus, the research on the social functioning of children with chronic conditions has varied considerably in the aspects of social functioning examined and the assessment methods utilized.

More recent studies have incorporated measures to tap various aspects (e.g., behavioral, cognitive, and emotional) of social functioning using a noncategorical approach. For example, Meijer, Sinnema, Bijstra, Mellenbergh, and Wolters (2000a, 2000b) examined social functioning separately in children and adolescents with chronic illnesses, including cystic fibrosis, diabetes, arthritis, osteogenesis imperfect, eczema, and asthma in a normative comparison. Children with chronic illness reported significantly less aggressive social behavior and gave significantly more socially

desirable responses. No significant differences were found in social self-esteem. Parents reported more submissive social behavior, and in male children, less aggressive social behavior. Male children reported less social anxiety (Meijer et al., 2000b). Regarding adolescents, female adolescents with chronic illnesses reported participation in fewer social activities, but more assertive social skills. Male adolescents reported less inappropriate social behaviors, such as teasing (Meijer et al., 2000a).

Just as the conceptualization and measurement of social functioning has varied, so have the outcome variables and focus. Some researchers have examined the differences in various aspects of social functioning in children with chronic conditions, using normative comparisons, comparisons to healthy control groups, or comparisons between and within types of conditions. Rather than examining the impact of the chronic condition on social functioning, another approach has been to examine the influence of social functioning variables on illness adaptation, illness management and treatment adherence, and health-promoting and health-risk behaviors (La Greca et al., 2002). Finally, as with the literature on psychosocial adaptation in general, research has moved toward examining condition, child, and social-ecological risk and resilience factors related to social functioning in children with chronic conditions.

Correlates of Social Functioning

Aspects of either the chronic condition itself or the management of the condition may impact social functioning. Conditions that impact normal daily activities, physical activity, appearance, or cognitive functioning or involve management requirements causing school absences, physical activity restrictions, physical appearance alterations, or lifestyle modifications may impact social functioning (La Greca, 1990; Schuman & La Greca, 1999). In addition, conditions involving the central nervous system (CNS) have been shown to have more impact on social functioning than non-CNS-related conditions (Nassau & Drotar, 1997).

Cognitive Impairment

Chronic CNS conditions pose an increased risk for problems in social functioning (Nassau & Drotar, 1997). Chronic conditions associated with cognitive impairments include cerebral palsy, spina bifida, epilepsy, congenital heart disease, sickle cell disease, and HIV infection (La Greca et al., 2004). Nassau and Drotar (1997) reviewed the literature base of social competence in children with cerebral palsy, epilepsy, and spina bifida, which are among the most prevalent chronic CNS conditions. The authors described several factors which contribute to the social difficulties of children with CNS conditions. The cognitive impairments (e.g., intelligence, memory, attention, problem solving) which sometimes present in CNS conditions may result in deficits in social understanding. Peer stigmatization resulting from the visible manifestations of CNS conditions (e.g., use of assistive devices, seizure activity) may reduce opportunities to participate in age-appropriate peer activities. Furthermore, children with CNS conditions may be faced with unique social stressors (e.g., teasing, disclosure regarding the condition, difficulty finding social outlets and activities due to condition constraints). Finally, many children with CNS conditions are placed in special education settings. Placement in special education may result in stigma and social isolation. For example, special education has been associated with more problem behaviors and decreased social competence in children with leukemia (Shelby, Nagle, Barnett-Queen, Quattlebaum, & Wuori, 1998).

Based on Nassau and Drotar's (1997) review, children with CNS conditions were found to have lower social adjustment in comparison to normative data, healthy controls, or children with non-CNS conditions. However, the strength of the results varied based on how social adjustment was operationalized and measured (Nassau & Drotar, 1997). Only four studies (compared to 18 for social adjustment) examined social performance and social skills. Children with CNS conditions were less competent in social performance compared to healthy children or children with non-CNS conditions (Howe, Feinstein, Reiss, Molock, & Berger, 1993; Tin & Teasdale, 1985); however, no differences in social skills via role-play tests were found

between children with and without spina bifida (Ammerman, Van Hasselt, Hersen, & Moore, 1989; Van Hasselt, Ammerman, Hersen, Reigel, & Rowley, 1991). Six out of seven studies found that increased condition severity (e.g., functional impairments in cognition, mobility, etc.) was associated with decreased social competence. Nassau and Drotar (1997) point out several problematic issues in the literature, including the operationalization and measurement of social competence, methods of comparison, lack of attention to age and cognitive functioning, and use of single sites limiting generalizability.

More recent studies continue to support a relationship between cognitive impairments and multiple domains of social functioning. In children with neurofibromatosis type 1, severity of neurological impairment was associated with decreased peer acceptance and friendships, decreased ratings of popularity and leadership behavior, and increased ratings of socially sensitive-isolated characteristics (e.g., often left out, trouble making friends; Noll et al., 2007). In comparing children with sickle cell disease, those who had cerebrovascular accidents had more errors on facial and vocal emotional decoding task compared to those without CNS pathology (Boni et al., 2001). Children with encephalopathic HIV displayed less social and emotional responsivity than children with nonencephalopathic HIV (Moss, Wolters, Brouwers, Hendricks, & Pizzo, 1996). In children with neurofibromatosis type 1, Barton and North (2004) found lower intelligence and achievement scores, as well as lower social competence and skills, particularly in those with comorbid attention-deficit/hyperactivity disorder. Neurological variables in children with epilepsy such as learning disability, intractability, and use of antiepileptic medications, as well as abnormal family functioning, have been shown to be related to lower assertive and overall social skills as reported by parents (Tse, Hamiwka, Sherman, & Wirrell, 2007). Lower intelligence quotients (but not seizure related variables) have been found to be associated with lower parent reported social competence in children with epilepsy (Caplan et al., 2005).

In children with cancer, it is not clear whether social skills impairments and decreased academic functioning is related to cognitive side-effects from treatment, frequent absences from school, or other variables (Newby, Brown, Pawletko, Gold, & Whitt, 2000). Newby and colleagues (2000) found that academic functioning was associated with parent and teacher rated impairments in social skills. In children with non-CNS cancer, intensity of CNS-directed treatment has been found to predict peer-rated acceptance and friendships, decreased leadership/popularity, and increased sensitive-isolated social behavior (Vannatta, Gerhardt, Wells, & Noll, 2007). Multiple medical treatments in children with brain tumors has been shown to predict social competence (Kullgren, Morris, Morris, & Krawiecki, 2003). Some researchers have found differences in social functioning related to cranial irradiation (Bonner et al., 2008; Vannatta, Zeller, Noll, & Koontz, 1998), while some have not (Noll, Bukowski, Rogosch, LeRoy, & Kulkarni, 1990; Noll et al., 1991; Shelby et al., 1998).

Physical Restrictions and Interruptions in Daily Activity

Children with chronic conditions may participate in fewer social activities due to pain (e.g., sickle cell disease), fatigue (e.g., rheumatic disease), mobility impairments (e.g., spina bifida, cerebral palsy), and physical activity restrictions that limit participation in certain activities (e.g., risk of bleeding in hemophilia; La Greca, 1990; Spirito et al., 1991). Eiser, Havermans, Pancer, and Eiser (1992) found that as illness restrictions increased, children with chronic conditions were reported to have more difficulties with peer relations. In children with chronic illnesses, decreased participation in social activities has been found to be associated with frequency of hospitalizations, physical restrictions, and pain, though not with social skills or self-esteem (Meijer et al., 2000b). Pain has also been found to be associated with social anxiety, especially in participation in physical activities (Meijer et al., 2000b). In adolescents with chronic illnesses, functional limitations were not found to be associated with social functioning, and, in boys, pain was associated with reduced social activities (Meijer et al., 2000a).

Interruptions in daily activities, such as frequent school absences, may occur due to hospitalizations, illness exacerbations, physician visits, or treatment and management demands (e.g., diabetes). As a result, these periods of absence may influence the child's ability to effectively interact with his/her social and academic environment. Children with asthma who had more hospitalizations have been found to be less popular, more lonely, and exhibit more sensitive-isolated behavior (Graetz & Shute, 1995). In boys with hemophilia (56% also had HIV), absences from school were associated with lower teacher ratings of scholastic, social, and athletic competence, physical attractiveness, and social activities (Colegrove & Huntzinger, 1994). Decreased participation in activities and reduced peer contact may result in fewer opportunities to develop social skills needed to make and keep friends (Reiter-Purtill, Noll et al., 2003). Thus, lack of participation in activities may be associated with increased risk for a wide range of social difficulties (King et al., 2007).

King and colleagues (2006) examined factors contributing to participation in activities for children with chronic conditions. They found that children's functional ability (i.e., intelligence, communication skills, physical functioning), activity preferences, and family participation in social and recreational activities were significant predictors of participation in both formal and informal activities. Other contributing factors included family cohesion, parental perceptions of environments as unsupportive (i.e., inaccessible, less facilitative regarding policies, attitudes, etc.), and child's social support and relationships (King et al., 2006).

Physical Appearance

Physical appearance is a contributing factor to peer acceptance and friendships. Thus, chronic conditions that impact a child's physical appearance (e.g., craniofacial anomalies, small stature in cystic fibrosis, tumors and skin alterations in neurofibromatosis) pose a risk for difficulties in social functioning (La Greca, 1990; Spirito et al., 1991). Children with visible differences in physical appearance may experience more peer victimization and teasing (e.g., Carroll & Shute, 2005). They may also exhibit symptoms consistent with social anxiety. Social anxiety may result in decreased initiation of and responsiveness to interactions with peers

(Kapp-Simon & McGuire, 1997). Self-perceived facial appearance in adolescents with craniofacial anomalies has been found to be associated with peer relationship difficulties and low self-esteem (Pope & Ward, 1997b). In adolescents with craniofacial anomalies, Shute, Mccarthy, and Roberts (2007) found that decreased self-worth was associated with fear of negative evaluation, which predicted social competence with perceived parental social support as a mediator. Additionally, social avoidance and distress predicted social competence, with perceived peer social support as a mediator (Shute et al., 2007). In contrast, some researchers have not found a relationship between physical appearance and social functioning (e.g., in neurofibromatosis; Noll et al., 2007).

Treatments for chronic conditions can also result in changes in physical appearance, such as hair loss from chemotherapy or weight gain and puffy facial features from corticosteroids (La Greca, 1990). Physical appearance changes due to treatments can impact social functioning via a range of pathways. In adolescents with cancer, negative body image has been correlated with social anxiety, loneliness, and low self-worth, though not with peer network or activities (Pendley, Dahlquist, & Dryer, 1997). In children who had received a bone marrow transplant, social difficulties (i.e., active isolation and peer acceptance) were mediated by physical appearance, athletic ability, and whether cranial irradiation was received (Vannatta et al., 1998). Further research into the impact of various aspects of physical appearance on domains of social functioning in children with chronic conditions is needed.

Mediators and Moderators

Recently, researchers have begun to investigate the mediating and moderating factors of social functioning in children with chronic conditions. For example, King and colleagues (2005) examined influences on the prosocial behavior and academic functioning of children with chronic conditions. Children with activity-limiting conditions were found to be at increased risk for academic problems, and this relationship was mediated by cognitive functioning deficits (e.g., memory, problem solving). Lower levels of recreational participation and poorer behavioral functioning resulted in increased risk for poorer prosocial behavior. In addition, cognitive functioning was found to influence recreational participation and hyperactivity/inattention. Furthermore, greater social support to parents and neighborhood cohesion resulted in improved family functioning and greater recreational participation (King et al., 2005). Regarding family functioning, in children with liver disease, parent-reported family functioning (i.e., family cohesion and adaptability, parenting stress, and parenting esteem) was found to be associated with parent-reported social competence (Hoffman, Rodrigue, Andres, & Novak, 1995). In contrast to findings in typically developing children, Thomas, Warschausky, Golin, and Meiners (2008) did not find a relationship between direct parenting strategies (e.g., facilitating play activities or involvement in extracurricular activities) and social outcomes in children with cerebral palsy.

Alderfer, Wiebe, and Hartmann (2002) examined illness characteristics and social behavior in relation to peer acceptance in diabetes. Overall, peer acceptance was enhanced by prosocial behavior and hampered by aggressive behavior. However, children with more observable disease symptoms and management (e.g., blood testing, taking medications, food intake or refusal, symptoms) experienced higher levels of peer acceptance regardless of social behavior, while those with less obvious disease characteristics who exhibited aggressive behavior were significantly less accepted by peers. Impact of disease in multiple domains (e.g., appearance, athletic ability, school performance, self-esteem, family relationships, independence, conduct), but not poor medical control, also predicted peer acceptance.

Meijer, Sinnema, Bijstra, Mellenbergh, and Wolters (2002) examined coping styles and locus of control in relation to psychosocial functioning in adolescents with chronic conditions (i.e., asthma, cystic fibrosis, eczema, and arthritis). Coping styles were associated with social adjustment, global self-esteem, and externalizing behavior problems. Confrontation coping (i.e., active and purposeful problem solving) predicted social self-esteem, adequate social skills, decreased social anxiety, and assertive behavior (Meijer et al., 2002). Coping through seeking social support predicted adequate social skills and assertive behavior. A depressive coping style predicted decreased self-esteem and increased social anxiety and internalizing problems, and avoidant coping was related to behavior problems. Locus of control (expectations of control over one's environment) was related to externalizing and total behavior problems.

Social Functioning in Children with Hearing Loss

Due to the significant heterogeneity in children with hearing loss, a number of factors must be considered. Some of these factors that may cause social challenges in the child with hearing loss include degree, onset, and cause of hearing loss; amplification; communication mode; and language fluency (Hauser, Wills, & Isquith, 2006). Language ability may influence communication with peers, resulting in decreased frequency and duration of peer interactions (Antia & Kriemeyer, 2003). Nunes, Pretzlik, and Olsson (2001) found that while, on average, students who were deaf were not disliked by peers, they were more neglected and less likely to have a friend in the classroom, and communication was noted to be an obstacle to friendship.

For the child with hearing loss, his/her social functioning may also vary with the degree of inclusiveness of the school setting. For example, in adolescents attending public versus residential schools, no differences were found in teacher-rated social skills (Cartledge, Paul, Jackson, & Cochran, 1991). However, self-reported social skills were higher for adolescents in public school settings (Cartledge & Cochran, 1996). In their review of the literature concerning social functioning in children who are deaf in mainstreamed settings, Kluwin, Stinson, and Colarossi (2002) drew several conclusions, though cautioned that methodological issues pose limitations to the findings. First, students who were deaf were rated by teachers as less socially mature (i.e., based on behaviors associated with performing competently, functioning independently, relating well to others, and acting responsibly). Second, observational studies as well as self-report data have indicated that children who were deaf interacted more frequently with children who were deaf

rather than hearing classmates. Third, studies of peer-rated acceptance and perceived social acceptance have yielded mixed results. Finally, no differences were found in self-image, self-esteem, perceived social competence, or loneliness.

More recently, Wauters and Knoors (2008) examined multiple domains of social functioning as well as correlates in children in inclusive settings. No differences were found between peers and children who were deaf, in peer acceptance, social status, mutual friendships, or mutual antipathies, though children who were deaf were often involved in a network without friendships. Children who were deaf were nominated less on prosocial behavior (e.g., cooperating and helping) and more on socially withdrawn behavior (e.g., seeking help and being bullied). Contrary to previous studies, no relationship was found between peer acceptance and social competence and other variables (i.e., use of a cochlear implant, inclusive setting, grade level, and gender). Regarding academics, children with a high social impact (i.e., received many like and/or dislike nominations) scored lower on mathematics.

Social Functioning in Children with Visual Impairments

Numerous aspects involved with having visual impairments may impact children's social functioning. Visual impairments may impact children's ability to learn social behavior through modeling and imitation. Likewise, these impairments may hinder their ability to receive and comprehend feedback pertaining to their social performance through visual cues, such as facial expression and body language (Ammerman, Van Hasselt, & Hersen, 1998). Children with visual impairments may have fewer social experiences due to inability to participate in activities such as sports or games, or inability to obtain a driver's license (Rosenblum, 2000). Additionally, they may experience stigma due to physical appearance (e.g., ocular deformities) or use of adaptive equipment (Hunter, Griffin-Shirley, & Noll, 2006). Adolescents with visual impairments have been found to have more difficulties in relationships with friends, have fewer friends and dating experiences, and spend less time engaging in leisure time with friends compared to adolescents with other chronic conditions and adolescents with no disabilities (Huurre & Aro, 2000).

Researchers have identified certain social skills particularly difficult for children with visual impairments. Verdugo and Caballo (1996) found that children with visual impairments participated in less social activities and had deficits in verbal and non-verbal social skills (i.e., one to one interaction, appearance, body language, play skills, verbal skills, assertion skills). Specific social skills such as verbal skills, body language, play skills, cooperation skills, and expression and recognition of emotions skills have been found to predict the quality of participation in one-to-one and larger group social interactions for children with visual impairments (Caballo & Verdugo, 2007). Buhrow, Hartshorne, and Bradley-Johnson (1998) found that while there were no significant differences in overall social behavior, children who were blind had lower parent-rated assertive social skills (e.g., difficulty making friends) and teacher-rated cooperative social skills (e.g., using time appropriately while waiting for help, attending to instructions) and academic competence, as well as higher teacher-rated problem behaviors.

Assessment

Assessment of social functioning in children with chronic conditions is fundamental to treatment planning and service provision. As discussed earlier, social functioning encompasses multiple domains such as social skills, social support, peer relationships, and social-cognitive skills. In order to obtain comprehensive data, these areas should be assessed using multiple methods, informants, and settings because results may vary significantly depending on these factors. Once specific areas of need are identified, treatment target areas can be derived based on assessment results. Finally, the assessment of targeted intervention outcomes should be done before, during, and after treatment. Thus, assessment is critical to selection of treatment targets, progress monitoring, treatment revisions, and evaluation of outcomes.

A wide variety of measures have been employed to assess a broad range of psychosocial aspects relevant to pediatric populations. Measures have been developed to assess important areas such as health status and quality of life, adherence, pain, behavior, development, stress/coping, cognitions/attributions/attitudes, family communication/conflict/responsibility, and consumer satisfaction (for reviews see Naar-King, Ellis, & Frey, 2004; Streisand & Michaelidis, 2007). Assessment specific to social functioning in children with chronic conditions has been approached in various ways including using measures designed for children without chronic conditions, using subscales of quality of life measures, modifying adult measures pertaining to adjustment to illness, or developing new measures for use in particular studies with specific populations (Adams, Streisand, Zawacki, & Joseph, 2002). Each of these approaches is not without its limitations. Concerns with modifying adult measures for use in assessing social functioning in children with a chronic condition include readability, pertinence of areas of functioning (e.g., work or employment-related items), and inclusion of areas other than those specific to social functioning (Adams et al., 2002). Furthermore, developing measures individually for specific studies may be inefficient, costly, and time consuming, and also cause inconsistency across studies making it difficult to contrast and interpret findings (Adams et al., 2002).

Scale development efforts have been initiated in an attempt to address the limitations of current methods of assessing social functioning in children with chronic conditions. Specifically, Adams and colleagues (2002) developed the Living with a Chronic Illness (LCI) scale and examined its initial psychometric properties in 115 children aged 9–18 years with a broad range of conditions (i.e., asthma, seizure disorder, cancer, arthritis/lupus, sickle cell disease, cystic fibrosis, and other conditions such as organ transplant, headaches, etc.). Parent and youth versions of the LCI have been developed as well. Adams and colleagues used a noncategorical approach when developing the LCI and its accompanying measures. In doing so, variables which are shared by multiple dimensions were considered, and therefore Adams and colleagues incorporated aspects found to impact peer relationships (e.g., physical activity restrictions, interruption of daily activities, physical appearance changes, lifestyle modifications). This was done to aid the clinician to gain an accurate picture of the child's ability to socially function amidst having a medical condition. Items of the LCI cover three areas of social functioning, including home, school, and extracurricular activities, in addition to whether the difficulties are illness related or non-illness related (e.g., lack of opportunity, socioeconomic status) and the child's level of satisfaction in each area or how much the child is upset by the difficulties.

Adams and colleagues (2002) found that internal consistency reliability was satisfactory for the parent (KR-20 = 0.86) and youth (KR-20 = 0.82) versions of the LCI. Pearson correlations between parent and youth LCI scores were 0.34 for illness-related, and 0.45 for non-illness-related social difficulties. Convergent and divergent validity was established with The Achenbach System of Empirically Based Assessment (ASEBA) measures (including parent, teacher, and self-report measures) and the Harter self-perception profiles for children and adolescents (see below for detailed descriptions of the ASEBA and Harter measures). Scores on the ASEBA and Harter measures were within the average range. Overall, children reported less psychosocial and behavioral symptoms than did parents. Children with seizure disorders were more likely to receive special education services and reported significantly more non-illness related social difficulties than children with other conditions. Additional analyses were conducted using information from the School Information Form (SIF; e.g., school absences, grades) and Medical Chart Review Form (e.g., frequency of clinic visits, hospitalizations, etc.). Higher health-care utilization was associated with more psychosocial and illness-related difficulties. Further examination of the psychometric properties of the LCI is needed, such as test-retest reliability and factor analysis.

Though efforts have been initiated to improve assessment methods of social functioning in children with chronic conditions, currently the most common approach appears to be the use of general measures and subscales of quality of life measures, either alone or in combination with each other or additional measures. General measures developed for the general population of children and adolescents (including both broadband and social functioning specific measures) and quality of life measures will be reviewed in detail. A discussion of the strengths and weaknesses of each of these approaches will be incorporated into the following discussion.

General Measures Developed for the General Population of Children and Adolescents

The ASEBA instruments such as the Child Behavior Checklist (CBCL), Teacher Report Form (TRF), and Youth Self Report (YSR) have been commonly used in assessing psychosocial adjustment in children with chronic conditions (Achenbach & Rescorla, 2000, 2001). These measures provide broadband, syndrome, DSM-oriented, and competence scales. Specific to social functioning, all three measures contain a Social Problems syndrome scale and competence scales in areas of activities (CBCL and YSR); social (CBCL and YSR); school (CBCL); and academic performance, working hard, behaving appropriately, learning, and happiness (TRF). The ASEBA measures have been used in examining social functioning in studies of children with a wide range of chronic conditions. The Behavior Assessment System for Children (BASC; Reynolds & Kamphaus, 2002), a broadband measure similar to the ABEBA measures, has also been used to examine psychosocial functioning in children with leukemia (Shelby et al., 1998).

Despite their widespread use, multiple concerns have been raised pertaining to the applicability of using measures such as the ASEBA with children who have chronic conditions. First, unique aspects of illness (e.g., illness-related discomfort, worry about medical procedures, parenting stressors in care-giving or financial issues) which affect psychosocial functioning are not assessed (Streisand & Michaelidis, 2007). Second, the validity of these measures is an area of concern due to various factors. For example, because the ASEBA assessment instruments were designed to distinguish between psychopathology and normal functioning rather than a continuum of functioning within chronic conditions, they may be limited in their ability to identify less serious adjustment problems (Adams et al., 2002; Perrin, Stein, & Drotar, 1991; Streisand & Michaelidis, 2007; Wallander et al., 2003). In addition, these measures were not designed to solely assess social functioning and, as such, their assessment of social competence may be misleading for this population (Perrin et al., 1991; Thompson & Gustafson, 1996a; Wallander et al., 2003). The competence scales of the ASEBA measures assess time spent in activities with peers, structured activities outside of school, and number of friends rather than social skills. Furthermore, the competence scales may also be affected by other condition-related variables (e.g., neurological factors such as clumsiness; Tse et al., 2007). Thus, they may measure social participation rather than social capacity (Perrin et al., 1991; Streisand & Michaelidis, 2007). Finally, the ASEBA instrument items which reflect somatic complaints could either overestimate internalizing symptoms or fail to reflect true internalizing symptoms if wrongly attributed to the illness (Drotar, Stein, & Perrin, 1995; Perrin et al., 1991). For example, items which address issues pertaining to fatigue or stomach aches (intended to measure anxiety or depression) or attention, disobedience, or peer interactions may be endorsed due to physical discomfort, treatment nonadherence, or treatment side effects (Streisand & Michaelidis, 2007).

Some efforts have been made to examine the validity of the ASEBA measures, specifically the somatic items. Holmes, Respess, Greer, and Frentz (1998) found that when somatic items rated by medical personnel as being related to diabetes were eliminated, children with diabetes still had higher CBCL internalizing scores than healthy controls. Thus, Holmes and colleagues concluded that these findings suggest that use of the CBCL was not confounded for use in this population. In contrast, Friedman, Bryant, and Holmbeck (2007) found that maternal ratings of somatic complaints on the CBCL did not measure internalizing problems in children with spina bifida and a comparison group in the same manner. This suggests that this scale should be interpreted with caution regarding internalizing problems when used with children with chronic illness. The authors of two recent studies examining the validity of the CBCL in children with epilepsy concluded that it has clinical utility in this population (Bender, Auciello, Morrison, MacAllister, & Zaroff, 2008; Gleissner et al., 2008).

Though there are a number of concerns and limitations involved with using measures developed for the general population in children with chronic conditions, there are several advantages as well. Many of these measures have sound psychometric properties and well-established norms. In addition, they have the ability to assess multiple domains of functioning, provide forms for the use of multiple informants across a broad age range, and can be administered repeatedly to measure change over time (Streisand & Michaelidis, 2007).

Social Functioning Measures Developed for the General Population of Children and Adolescents

Regarding instruments designed specifically to assess social skills, the Matson Evaluation of Social Skills with Youngsters (MESSY; Matson, Rotarori, & Helsel, 1983) and Social Skills Rating System (SSRS; Gresham & Elliott, 1990) have been the most researched instruments in the child population (Matson & Wilkins, 2008). In children with chronic conditions, these scales, as well as direct measures (e.g., observation, role-play), sociometric methods, and rating scales of self-esteem have been employed. Table 13.1 provides references for studies of social functioning in children with chronic conditions by condition type and the assessment method employed.

The MESSY is a Likert-type rating scale (from 1-*not at all* to 5-*very much*) for ages 4–18 years. The MESSY has both a self-report and a teacher report version (which can be used for all caregivers, including parents). The teacher report form has two factors: Inappropriate Assertiveness/Impulsiveness and Appropriate Social Skills. The self-rating form has five factors: Appropriate Social Skills, Inappropriate Assertiveness, Impulsive/Recalcitrant, Overconfident, and Jealousy/Withdrawal. Norms are provided by age and gender. Scores that fall one standard deviation below the normative mean are considered "problematic," while scores that fall two standard deviations below the mean are

Table 13.1 References for studies of social functioning in children with chronic conditions by condition type and assessment method

	ASEBA measures	MESSY	SSRS	Harter scales	Observation/role-play	Sociometric methods
Asthma	Zbikowski and Cohen (1998)			Asthma and diabetes (Nassau & Drotar, 1995; Pelletier & LePage, 1999)		Graetz and Shute (1995), Zbikowski and Cohen (1998)
Cancer	Bonner et al. (2008), Fossen, Abrahamsen, and Storm-Mathisen (1998), Kullgren et al. (2003), Mulhern, Carpentieri, Shema, Stone, and Fairclough (1993), Mulhern, Wasserman, Friedman, and Fairclough (1989), Newby et al. (2000), Noll et al. (1999), Shelby et al. (1998), Spirito et al. (1990)		Bonner et al. (2008), Newby et al. (2000)	Eapen, Revesz, Mpofu, and Daradkeh (1999), Katz, Rubinstein, Hubert, and Blew (1988), Noll et al. (1999), Noll et al. (2000), Noll et al. (1991), Pendley et al. (1997), Spirito et al. (1990)		Noll, Bukowski, Davies, Koontz, and Kulakrni (1993), Noll et al. (1990), Noll et al. (1999), Noll et al. (1991), Vannatta et al. (2007)
Cardiac conditions	Casey, Sykes, Craig, Power, and Mulholland (1996), Oates, Turnbull, Simpson, and Cartmill (1994)			Russo et al. (2008 a,b)		
Cerebral palsy						Center and Ward (1984)
Craniofacial conditions	Heneman-De Boer, De Haan, and Beemer (1999), Pope and Ward			Kapp-Simon, Simon, and Kristovich (1992), Pope and Ward	Kapp-Simon and McGuire (1997), Kapp-Simon et al. (2005)	

Table 13.1 (continued)

	ASEBA measures	MESSY	SSRS	Harter scales	Observation/role-play	Sociometric methods
Epilepsy	(1997a, 1997b), Shute et al. (2007) Apter et al. (1991), Caplan et al. (2005), Cunningham, Johnson, Austin, and Dunn (2006), Elliott, Lach, Kadis, and Smith (2008), Jakovljevic and Martinovic (2006), Tse et al. (2007)		Tse et al. (2007)	(1997a, 1997b), Shute et al. (2007)		
Hearing loss	Vostanis, Hayes, Feu, and Warren (1997)	Burley (1996), Macklin and Matson (1985), Matson, Macklin, and Helsel (1985), Raymond and Matson (1989)	Cartledge and Cochran (1996), Cartledge et al. (1991)		Antia and Kreimeyer (1996), Ducharme and Holborn (1997)	Broesterhuizen, Van Lieshout, and Riksen-Walraven (1991) Cappelli, Daniels, Durieux-Smith, McGrath, and Neuss (1995), Coyner (1993), Craig (1965), Hagborg (1987), Kennedy and Bruininks (1974), Kurkjian and Evans (1988), Nunes et al. (2001), Ridsdale and Thompson (2002), Suárez (2000), Wauters and Knoors (2008)
Hemophilia/HIV	Colegrove and Huntzinger (1994), Moss, Bose, Wolters, and Brouwers (1998)		Colegrove and Huntzinger (1994)	Colegrove and Huntzinger (1994), Moss et al. (1998)	Moss et al. (1996)	
Liver disease	Hoffman et al. (1995), Schwering et al. (1997), Tornqvist et al. (1999)			Hoffman et al. (1995), Tornqvist et al. (1999)		
Neuro-fibromatosis	Barton and North (2004), Johnson, Saal, Lovell, and		Barton and North (2004)	Noll et al. (2007)		Noll et al. (2007)

Table 13.1 (continued)

	ASEBA measures	MESSY	SSRS	Harter scales	Observation/role-play	Sociometric methods
Rheumatic diseases	Schorry (1999), Noll et al. (2007), Daltroy et al. (1992), Noll et al. (2000)			Noll et al. (2000)	Harris, Newcomb, and Gewanter (1991)	Noll et al. (2000), Reiter-Purtill, Gerhardt, Vannatta, Passo, and Noll (2003)
Sickle cell disease	Rodrigue, Streisand, Banko, Kedar, and Pitel (1996)		Boni et al. (2001)			Noll et al. (1996)
Spina bifida	Hommeyer, Holmbeck, Wills, and Coers (1999), Van Hasselt et al. (1991), Wallander, Feldman, and Varni (1989)		Lemanek, Jones, and Lieberman (2000)	Aksnes, Diseth, Helseth, Aafos, and Emblem (2002), Buran, Sawin, Brei, and Fastenau (2004), Edwards, Borzyskowski, Cox, and Badcock (2004), Thill et al. (2003)	Tin and Teasdale (1985), Van Hasselt et al. (1991)	
Visual impairments		Matson, Heinze, Helsel, Kapperman, and Rotatori (1986), Sharma, Sigafoos, and Carroll (2000), Verdugo and Caballo (1996)	Buhrow et al. (1998)	Visual impairments and other chronic conditions (Huurre & Aro, 2000)	Ammerman et al. (1989), Markovits, Gariépy, Huet, and Strayer (1982), Van Hasselt, Hersen, and Kazdin (1985), Verdugo and Caballo (1996)	Verdugo and Caballo (1996)
Various chronic conditions	Meijer et al. (2000a, 2000b), Wallander, Varni, Babani, Banis, and Wilcox (1988)	Meijer et al. (2000a, 2000b, 2002)		Armstrong, Rosenbaum, and King (1992), Meijer et al. (2000a, 2000b)		Armstrong et al. (1992), Spina bifida or other paralysis, cerebral palsy, or muscular dystrophy (de Apodaca, Watson, Mueller, & Isaacson-Kailes, 1985)

considered "very problematic." Validity has been established with direct observation and teacher nominations of social competence (Matson, Esveldt-Dawson, & Kazdin, 1983). Additionally, the MESSY has been translated into nine languages and studied in the UK and Australia (Matson & Wilkins, 2008).

The SSRS consists of rating scales for ages 3–18. Teacher, parent, and student rating forms are available according to age: preschool, elementary, and secondary. Items are rated on perceived frequency and importance on a scale from 0 to 2. It consists of a Social Skills Scale (Cooperation, Empathy, Assertion, Self-Control, and Responsibility), a Problem Behaviors Scale (Externalizing Problems, Internalizing Problems, and Hyperactivity), and an Academic Competence Scale (reading and mathematics performance, general cognitive functioning, motivation, and parental support). Separate norms are provided by gender and for students with and without disabilities. The SSRS has been translated into four languages (Matson & Wilkins, 2008).

The Self-Perception Profile for Children (SPPC; Harter, 1985a) is a revision of the Perceived Competence Scale for Children (PCSC; Harter, 1982). The SPPC is for children aged 8–15 and is designed to evaluate specific judgments of children's perceived competence in the domains of Scholastic Competence, Athletic Competence, Peer Likability, Physical Appearance, and Behavioral Conduct, as well as a subscale of Global Self-Worth. Respondents first rate whether they are more like kids described in one of two statements. Then, ratings are made regarding whether the statement is "really true for me" or "sort of true for me." There is also a parallel teacher-rating scale of the child's actual behavior which can be modified into a parent-rating scale (Cole, Gondoli, & Peeke, 1998; Harter, 1985a; Thill et al., 2003). The parent- and teacher-rating scales exclude the Global Self-Worth scale of the SPPC. The Pictorial Scale of Perceived Competence and Social Acceptance for Young Children (Harter & Pike, 1984) was designed for children up to age 7. There are two versions: one for children in preschool and kindergarten and one for children in first and second grade. Items evaluate self-perception in four domains: Cognitive Competence, Physical Competence, Peer Acceptance, and Maternal Acceptance. Factor analysis revealed a 2-factor solution: General

Competence (Cognitive and Physical Competence) and Social Acceptance (Peer and Maternal Acceptance). There is also a parallel teacher rating scale of the child's actual behavior which can be modified into a parent rating scale (Harter & Pike, 1984). The parent and teacher rating scales exclude the Maternal Acceptance domain. The Self-Perception Profile for Adolescents (SPPA; Harter, 1988) is for adolescents aged 15–18. The SPPA includes 3 additional subscales (Romantic Appeal, Job Competence, and Close Friendship) in addition to those measured in the SPPC.

Many studies using the Harter scales (e.g., SPPC, SPPA) in children with chronic conditions failed to find differences in the measures (Harter & Fischer, 1999). Therefore, their use in this population has been questioned (Aasland & Diseth, 1999). Harter and Fischer (1999) propose five possible reasons for the lack of differences in self-concept and competence in children with chronic conditions compared to normative or control groups. First, children with chronic conditions may be basing their judgments on a similar social reference group. Also, child respondents may be providing socially desirable responses. Denial or confusion between their actual and desired competency may be present. Finally, children with chronic conditions may have made a healthy adjustment of their self-standards to the actual limitations imposed by their condition.

In addition to behavior rating scales, other approaches, alone or in combination with rating scales, have been utilized to examine social functioning in children with chronic conditions. Observational methods, including role-play and naturalistic observation, have been utilized in children with chronic conditions. Sociometric methods may be used and can include peer (or teacher) nominations, ratings, and rankings. Sociometric methods such as the Revised Class Play (Masten, Morison, & Pellegrini, 1985), Three Best Friends (Gottman, Gonso, & Rasmussen, 1975), and Like Rating Scale (Asher, Singleton, Tinsley, & Hymel, 1979) have been used to assess social functioning in children with a wide variety of chronic conditions. In the Revised Class Play, the student (or teacher) assigns students to roles in an imaginary play. The Revised Class Play has four factors (Zeller, Vannatta, Schafer, & Noll, 2003): popular-leader (e.g., someone everybody likes, someone who has many friends); prosocial (e.g., polite, helps others); aggressive-disruptive (e.g., bossy, picks on others, gets into fights); and sensitive-isolated (e.g., sad, often left out, shy, plays alone).

Quality of Life Measures

Quality of life has been defined in numerous ways and can be generic or health related. In Wallander, Schmitt, and Koot (2001, p. 6) it was defined as "the combination of objectively and subjectively indicated well-being in multiple domains of life considered salient in one's culture and time, while adhering to universal standards of human rights." The social domain of quality of life includes the child's perceptions and satisfaction with social relationships (e.g., friends, family, school) and may be related to culture and socioeconomic variables (Kuyken, Orley, Hudelson, & Sartorius, 1994). Coping is also related to family and social contexts which may be more influential than characteristics of the child or illness (Koot & Wallander, 2001). In a recent review of quality of life measures for children and adolescents, Solans and colleagues (2008) identified 30 generic and 64 condition-specific instruments. Numerous measures include domains related to social functioning such as self-esteem, social functioning (social life, getting along with others, social support, role function, communication, relationship), friends, and bullying/peer rejection (Solans et al., 2008). A commonly used instrument, the Pediatric Quality of Life Inventory[TM] (PedsQL; Varni, Seid, & Kurtin, 2001), contains generic core scales (i.e., physical, emotional, social, and school functioning) and disease-specific modules for conditions such as asthma, arthritis, cancer, cardiac disease, cerebral palsy, diabetes, rheumatology, fatigue, and pain. For example, Storch and colleagues (2008) found that parents and children reported lower social functioning on the PedsQL in children with glycogen storage disease type 1 compared to healthy controls. In children with cerebral palsy, lower child and parent reported social functioning on the PedsQL has been found the reported level of social functioning was related to pain (Russo, Goodwin, Miller, Haan, Connel, & Crotty, 2008a; Russo, Miller, Haan, Cameron, & Crotty, 2008b).

A strength of quality of life measures is that many assess a variety of additional domains which are linked to social functioning such as physical activity, daily activities, cognitive functioning, self-esteem, pain, family functioning, and environmental factors (Solans et al., 2008). While quality of life measures incorporate a broad range of domains, they are not designed solely to assess social functioning and may not include sufficient items for this purpose (Adams et al., 2002). Thus, quality of life measures should be supplemented with measures that adequately assess social functioning.

Treatment

Psychological Interventions

Psychological interventions for children with chronic conditions vary on several parameters such as the primary target of the intervention, the intervention techniques and target areas, and the outcome variables assessed. Targets for interventions have included the primary caregiver, family, school environment, peer relationships, and the child with the chronic condition (Drotar, 2006a). Interventions typically have included both information and skills training components (Beale, 2006). Skills training components have targeted areas such as self-management, coping skills, problem solving, and stress management. Interventions employed have included cognitive behavior therapy (CBT), biofeedback, interactive computer games or educational tutorials, and social support. Psychological interventions have been conducted both in group and individual formats Outcome variables have included physical and symptom variables, illness knowledge, psychological adjustment, self-care and coping behaviors, and attitudinal variables (Beale, 2006), though more attention has been paid to disease management than psychosocial factors (Barlow & Ellard, 2004).

Psychological interventions in children with chronic conditions have been shown to be effective; however, most interventions have multiple components which are difficult to categorize. Thus, it remains unclear which specific types of interventions are more effective for which subgroups of children (Beale, 2006; Kibby, Tyc, & Mulhern, 1998). When designing and implementing psychological interventions, individual differences must be taken into account. Drotar (2006a) describes three main areas of relevant individual differences in psychological interventions with childhood chronic illness. The first is the type, severity, and stage of the psychological issues. As the severity and time course of the problem progresses, interventions progress from primary, secondary, and tertiary prevention approaches. Primary prevention focuses on those at high risk, secondary prevention focuses on reducing the impact of identified problems on functioning, while tertiary prevention focuses on the impact of serious mental health conditions or health-related morbidity on child and family functioning (Drotar, 2006a). Second, the nature and stage of the illness (onset, long-term adaptational phase, exacerbation/ complications, deterioration/terminal phase) must be incorporated. Substantial heterogeneity exists between conditions in factors such as age of onset, course, impact, treatment demands, and so forth (Rolland, 1984, 1987). Finally, the child's age/developmental stage (infancy/early childhood, school age, adolescence, transition to adulthood, young adulthood) is relevant to intervention design and implementation. Factors such as cognitive and physical maturity as well as periods of developmental transitions (e.g., transition into adolescence or beginning school) substantially impact design and implementation of interventions (Drotar, 2006).

Numerous authors have reviewed a broad range of psychological interventions for children with chronic illness (see Barakat, Gonzalez, & Weinberger, 2007; Barlow & Ellard, 2004; Bauman, Drotar, Leventhal, Perrin, & Pless, 1997; Beale, 2006; Drotar, 2006a; Elkin & Stoppelbein, 2008; Kibby et al., 1998; Plante, Lobato, & Engel, 2001). Overall, effect sizes of psychological interventions in children with chronic conditions have been large (Beale, 2006; Kibby et al., 1998). Evaluating results of various psychological intervention studies proves difficult due to wide variations in the approach and implementation of the intervention, research design, assessment type and timeline, and analysis/interpretation of the results (Beale, 2006). Furthermore, many studies do not provide an adequate description of the details of the intervention procedures (Barlow & Ellard, 2004; Bauman et al., 1997). In reviewing psychological interventions specific to psychosocial functioning, Bauman and colleagues (1997) describe several areas in need of further development in psychosocial interventions for children with chronic conditions including the need for power analyses to ensure sufficient sample sizes, inclusion of comparison groups, employing adequate assessment measures, conducting process evaluations prior to outcome evaluations of new programs, prioritizing outcome measures used to judge intervention effectiveness, increased attention to clinical significance, incorporating theory to guide interventions, evaluating whether interventions are better for certain subgroups or are uniformly effective, and maximizing contributions from multiple professional backgrounds through the use of interdisciplinary teams.

Social Skills Interventions

In comparison to the large number of studies examining multi-component psychological interventions for children with chronic illness, much less attention has been afforded to psychosocial interventions. Likewise, even fewer researchers have focused specifically on social skills intervention. Most social skills interventions for children with chronic conditions have been conducted in a group format. Populations have included children with cancer, craniofacial conditions, cerebral palsy, and spina bifida. Studies of interventions specific to social skills for children with chronic conditions will be reviewed in further detail.

Varni, Katz, Colegrove, and Dolgin (1993) compared a standard school reintegration program alone to the program in addition to a manualized individual social skills training in 5- to 13-year-olds with cancer ($N = 64$). Participants were randomized into experimental conditions. Training was conducted in three 1-h sessions and two booster sessions and involved multiple components such as didactic discussions, modeling, role-play, video vignettes, and cue-controlled relaxation. Targeted skills included social cognitive problem solving (i.e., promoting optimism in ability to improve things, identifying specific problems, considering antecedents and associated factors, brainstorming alternative solutions, planning, implementation, and outcome evaluation), assertiveness (i.e., identifying thoughts, wishes, and concerns, and how to express them effectively to others), and handling teasing and name calling (i.e., coping, extinguishing through withdrawing attention, giving age-appropriate explanations for physical changes, and using authoritative adults for support and assistance). The standard intervention involved education emphasizing the importance of an early return to school, school conferences and classroom presentations to demystify cancer, and regular follow-ups with patients, parents, teachers, classmates, and medical staff. Nine months post-intervention, the social skills training group, compared to the control group, had higher degrees of child-perceived social support from classmates and teachers (as measured by the Social Support Scale; Harter, 1985b), as well as parent-reported decreases in behavior problems and increases in school competence (as measured by the CBCL).

Barakat and colleagues (2003) evaluated a manualized group social skills training intervention for 13 children with brain tumors using role-play and homework assignments. In 6 weekly sessions, skills were targeted with the goal of reducing social isolation (starting, maintaining, and ending conversations; giving and receiving compliments) and improving friendships (nonverbal social skills, empathy, cooperation, conflict resolution). A parent component and homework assignments were included to improve generalization. The SSRS, ASEBA measures, and the Miami Pediatric Quality of Life Questionnaire (MPQLQ) were administered at baseline and follow-up (9 months). Child-rated MPQLQ social competence and parent-rated CBCL total competence were significantly improved, and child-rated internalizing behavior problems were significantly reduced. Non-significant reductions in child- and teacher-reported externalizing behavior problems and teacher-reported SSRS problem behaviors were found. A number of children moved from the clinical to the nonclinical range in behavior problems and social competence. Effect sizes ranged from small to medium. Parents and children reported that the intervention met their goals and that they were highly or extremely satisfied with the intervention.

Kapp-Simon, Mcguire, and Simon (2005) evaluated an outpatient social skills training group compared to a waitlist control group in 12 to 14-year-olds with craniofacial conditions ($N = 20$). The waitlist control group was unable to participate in the social skills group primarily due to transportation/scheduling difficulties. Training was conducted in 12 weekly group sessions lasting 90 min each. Teaching methods included modeling, role playing, didactic teaching, coaching, and behavioral practice. Skills targeted included attending skills (nonverbal communication such as using eye contact and posture to communicate interest); self-awareness (awareness of the interplay between feelings, thoughts, experiences, and behavior); social initiation and conversations skills (entering a conversation and maintaining conversations); responding to uncomfortable questions, negative comments, and stares; empathy (focusing on another's feelings/experiences and communicating interest through active listening to decrease self-consciousness); immediacy (skills for handling difficult issues in a relationship); anxiety management; and conflict resolution and problem-solving skills. In addition, 45-min observations were conducted pre- and post-intervention for each child during his/her school lunch break. Observational data was coded for type, frequency, and duration of social contact. Data categories included participant or peer: initiation, response, conversation, and nondirected comments. Initiation and response events included vocal/verbal behaviors (e.g., questions, statements, greetings or insults) and were coded as positive or negative based on facial expressions and tone of voice. Conversations were coded for interactions that progressed beyond a three-chain exchange (target initiation, peer response, target response). Nondirected comments were vocal/verbal behaviors which were not directed toward a specific peer and were discordant with the group process. Significant improvements in total communication, participant initiated conversations, peer responses, and nondirected communication were found for the group who received the social skills training compared to the waitlist control group.

King and colleagues (1997) examined a group social skills training intervention called "Joining In" for children aged 8–14 years with cerebral palsy or spina bifida ($N = 11$). Participants were selected for participation if they exhibited social withdrawal based on teacher ratings on the School

Social Skills scale (Brown, Black, & Downs, 1984) and were unpopular based on sociometric measures of popularity. Training was conducted in biweekly 90-min sessions for 10 weeks. Five skills were targeted: interpersonal problem solving, verbal and nonverbal communication, initiating interactions with peers, conversational skills, and coping with difficult peers. Training was based on a cognitive-social learning model and used verbal and visual instruction; symbolic videotaped modeling; rehearsal through role-play, feedback, and re-rehearsal; reality check (coping strategies and appropriate attributions in situations where performance is not successful); and homework assignments. Participants were evaluated before and after the intervention and at a 6-month follow-up. Outcome measures included the Global Self-Worth and Social Acceptance subscales of the SPPC (Harter, 1985a), the Close Friend Support and Classmate Support subscales of the Social Support Scale for Children (Harter, 1985b), and the Loneliness Scale (Asher, Hymel, & Renshaw, 1984). Perceived social acceptance initially improved but was not maintained at follow-up. However, a clinically significant reduction in loneliness was noted to have occurred at follow-up (King et al., 1997).

Die-Trill, Bromberg, Lavally, and Portales (1996) conducted a group social skills intervention with eight boys (10–14 years of age) with brain tumors. The first 8 sessions focused on specific social skills (e.g., assertiveness, making new friends, handling teasing), while the final 8 sessions focused on skill reinforcement, medical education, and social support. A parallel parent group included social support. Parent and child visual-analog ratings suggested that sessions were helpful in skill acquisition and social support; however, no standardized measures were used.

In summary, the literature base for social skills interventions in children with chronic conditions is small. Only Varni and colleagues (1993) randomly assigned participants to conditions and compared treatment to an alternative program. Furthermore, three of the five studies reviewed here did not include a comparison group. Sample sizes were notably small (< 20), with the exception of Varni and colleagues (1993). Systematic methods for target skill selection were not employed, although King and colleagues (1997) used teacher ratings of

social withdrawal and sociometric unpopular ratings to select participants. Interventions have included components targeting social skills and social information processing variables, as well as some illness-related skills (e.g., giving explanations for physical changes, responding to uncomfortable questions, handling teasing and stares). All intervention studies used role-play in combination with various other procedures. A wide range of outcome methods and measures were used, including quality of life, social skills, social competence, psychopathology, social support, peer interaction (observation), peer acceptance, self-esteem, and loneliness. Barakat and colleagues (2003) incorporated generalization as well as conducted program evaluations for the intervention meeting parent and child goals and satisfaction with the intervention. Three studies conducted follow-up assessments (one study at 6 months and two studies at 9 months). In conclusion, as with the research in general for psychological interventions in children with chronic conditions, much more methodologically sound research is needed in the area of social skills interventions.

Peer Interventions Targeting Illness Factors

Throughout this chapter, the impact of illness or condition factors on social functioning and peer relationships has been described. The reverse of the relationship has also received attention in the intervention literature. Peer relationships can significantly influence illness adaptation and management. Friendships can serve as a significant source of social support, influence treatment adherence, and impact health-promoting and health-risk behaviors such as diet, exercise, smoking, drug/alcohol use, and risky sexual behavior (La Greca et al., 2002). For example, in a group of teenagers with diabetes, Kaplan, Chadwick, and Schimmel (1985) found improved metabolic control through participation in daily social-learning exercises to improve social skills and ability to resist peer influence. Group social skills training has also been shown to improve adherence in diabetes (Citrin, La Greca, & Skyler, 1985).

Social interventions have also been examined in the context of improving medical outcome variables via skills such as assertiveness. For example, Gross, Heimann, Shapiro, and Schultz (1983) evaluated group social skills training for children aged 9–12 years who were diagnosed with diabetes. Eleven children were randomly assigned to the social skills intervention group ($N = 6$) or a control group ($N = 5$). The social skills group met biweekly in 45-min sessions for 5 weeks. Techniques used included modeling, coaching, role-play, feedback, and praise. Target skills included verbal responses (e.g., explaining what diabetes is, refusing inappropriate foods) and affect (e.g., eye contact, posture, voice volume) in stressful illness-related social situations (e.g., peer pressure to violate diabetic regimen, teasing, parent–child conflicts about diabetes management). Assessment was conducted at baseline, post-training, and 1 and 6 week follow-ups. As a measure of metabolic control, hemoglobin A1c levels were taken at baseline and posttest (spanning 12 weeks). Compared to controls, children who received social skills training showed large improvements in target variables which were maintained and generalized across role-play scenes and experimenters. In contrast, no differences in metabolic control were observed.

Social Skills Interventions in Children with Hearing Loss

Social interventions programs in children with hearing loss have taken two main approaches (Suárez, 2000). One approach aims to improve social skills, using strategies such as instructions, modeling, prompting, role-play, group discussion, feedback, home activities, and positive reinforcement (Antia & Kreimeyer, 1996, 1997; Antia, Kreimeyer, & Eldredge, 1994; Ducharme & Holborn, 1997; Lemanek, Williamson, Gresham, & Jensen, 1986; Rasing & Duker, 1992, 1993; Schloss, Selinger, Goldsmith, & Morrow, 1983; Schloss, Smith, & Schloss, 1984; Smith, Schloss, & Schloss, 1984). Target skills have included smiling, body posture, eye contact, communication responses, turn waiting, greeting, cooperating, sharing, assisting, initiating and maintaining conversations, complimenting, and praising. A second

approach has been to incorporate cognitive skills, such as social information processing (Dyck & Denver, 2003; Greenberg & Kusché, 1993, 1998; Lytle, Johnson, & Smith, 1987; Suárez, 2000). Overall, short-term interventions have shown improvements primarily in the nonlinguistic interactions of children with hearing loss, but increases in interactions between children with and without hearing loss have not been noted to occur. This is possibly due to communication barriers (Antia & Kriemeyer, 2003). Long-term, intensive interventions may show more success due to increased familiarity (Antia & Kriemeyer, 2003).

The PATHS (Promoting Alternative Thinking Strategies) program is a school-based curriculum based on the affective-behavioral-cognitive-dynamic (ABCD) model of development and change (Greenberg & Kusché, 1993). Target areas include self-control, awareness and communication of feelings, and problem-solving skills. The PATHS program has been shown to increase social problem solving, emotion recognition, and teacher- and parent-rated social competence in children with hearing loss compared to controls, with gains maintained at 2 years post-intervention (Calderon & Greenberg, 2003; Greenberg & Kusché, 1998).

Social Skills Interventions in Children with Visual Impairments

Several researchers have investigated outcomes of a variety of social skills interventions for children with visual impairments. Positive reinforcement procedures, including praise and tangible reinforcement have been employed to increase appropriate social behaviors (Farkas, Sherick, Matson, & Loebig, 1981; Yarnall, 1979). Van Hasselt, Hersen, Kazdin, Simon, and Mastantuono (1983) used direct instructions, performance feedback, behavior rehearsal, modeling, and manual guidance to increase assertive behavior in four female adolescents who were blind. Peer-mediated interventions have been shown to have improved generalization and maintenance outcomes in comparison to teacher-mediated interventions (Sacks & Gaylord-Ross, 1989). Through a peer-mediated intervention, Sisson, Van Hasselt, Hersen, and Strain (1985) found increases in appropriate play and the number and quality of social interactions. D'Allura (2002) found increased social interaction in preschool students through cooperative learning strategies and integration of sighted peers into special education classes. Finally, Jindal-Snape and colleagues have used self-evaluation and peer feedback interventions to increase social interaction skills in children with visual impairments (Jindal-Snape, 2004, 2005a, 2005b; Jindal-Snape, Kato, & Maekawa, 1998).

The Social Skills Training Program (SSTP) is one of the first comprehensive efforts specifically targeting interpersonal effectiveness in children with visual impairments (Ammerman et al., 1998). In the SSTP, assessment includes role-play tests, standardized interviews, self-report questionnaires, and parent- and teacher-ratings. Instruments used include the MESSY, ASEBA measures, and the Children's Assertive Behavior Scale. Specific target skills include expressive verbal skills (e.g., speech duration, speech latency, speech disturbances, speech intonation, hostility of tone, voice volume), verbal content skills (e.g., compliance, requests for new behavior, giving compliments, showing appreciation, offering help), nonverbal behaviors (e.g., direction of gaze, smiling, gestures, posture, social distance, reducing stereotypies), and interactive balance (e.g., coordinated delivery of social skills components, "give and take" in interaction). Skill repertoire areas targeted include positive assertion (e.g., giving compliments, communicating affection, apologizing, offering approval or praise), negative assertion (e.g., refusing unreasonable requests, expressing disapproval and annoyance, and asking others to behave differently in the future, compromise), and conversational skills (e.g., initiating and maintaining interactions, displaying appropriate verbal and nonverbal responses, giving reinforcement, terminating conversations). Social perception training is also included, defined as "the ability to understand social mores, recognize and identify expressed emotions in others, and predict the social consequence of one's interpersonal behavior" (Ammerman et al., 1998, pg. 513). Training methods include direct instructions, performance feedback, modeling, behavior rehearsal, and manual guidance. Booster sessions and follow-up are incorporated. Future research should investigate the effectiveness of the SSTP, as well as generalization and maintenance of outcomes.

Current Status and Future Directions

Overall, the majority of children with chronic conditions do not experience significant psychosocial dysfunction; however, they are at an increased risk. Research has moved from categorical approaches and between group designs to examining risk and resilience factors related to psychosocial outcomes. Risk and resilience factors can include aspects related to the child, the condition, and social-ecological parameters. Specific to social functioning, cognitive impairment, activity restrictions or interruptions, and physical appearance have been associated with increased risk for poorer social outcomes.

Social functioning is multifaceted and has been operationalized and assessed in various ways, including peer acceptance/status, friendships, social skills, social support, and social information processing. Peer relationships should be assessed comprehensively by examining both positive (e.g., social support, quality of friendships) and negative (e.g., teasing, social anxiety, exclusion) aspects (La Greca et al., 2002). Influences of both general peer-crowds and close friendships should be considered (La Greca et al., 2002). Assessment of social functioning has included general broadband measures, social skills rating scales, measures of self-esteem, observational and role-play methods, and sociometric assessments. Some research has moved toward new approaches in examining social functioning, such as social information processing and brain imaging (e.g., Boni et al., 2001; Bonner et al., 2008; Yeates et al., 2007).

Future research should use a multi-trait, multi-method framework. This should include the multiple aspects of social functioning, multiple measurement methods (e.g., interviews, psychometrically sound instruments, observations, sociometric measures), and multiple informants (e.g., self, parent, teacher, and peers). In addition, for children with chronic conditions, various child, condition, and social-ecological parameters should be assessed, including developmental level, emotional and behavioral functioning, illness-related characteristics (i.e., pain, quality of life, stress/coping, knowledge and expectations, adherence, family communication/conflict/responsibility), cognitive functioning, and family functioning (Streisand & Michaelidis, 2007). The reciprocal interactions between these factors and multiple domains of social functioning should be examined.

Regarding treatment, most interventions for children with chronic conditions have focused on disease-related outcomes and knowledge, with few focusing on health promotion/prevention or psychosocial outcomes, and fewer still focusing on social functioning. Numerous methodological issues have been discussed, including the need for larger sample sizes from multiple sites, adequate comparison groups, attention to attrition, control for demand characteristics, attention to treatment integrity, psychometrically sound assessment and outcome measures, and longer follow-ups. Skills to be targeted for intervention should be selected systematically. Additionally, mediating and moderating variables need to be examined. Problem severity, developmental considerations, and illness stage and progression should be taken into account. As reviewed in the social skills training literature for other child populations, treatment should target socially significant behaviors that will improve peer status/acceptance and friendships inclusive of number as well as quality (i.e., support, reciprocity, conflict, intimacy; Foster & Bussman, 2008). Programming for generalization and maintenance, as well as treatment integrity, should be incorporated (Foster & Bussman, 2008).

In general, most children with chronic conditions do not experience clinically significant psychosocial dysfunction. However, they face significant stressors which place them at increased risk for difficulties with social functioning. In comparison to the literature base concerning areas such as disease factors and treatment adherence, much less attention has been afforded to social aspects. Further work investigating the risk and resilience factors which impact psychosocial outcomes is needed. Methodologically sound research involving assessment techniques and interventions in children with chronic conditions is sorely needed. Social functioning has been shown to have an important influence on both adjustment to and management of childhood conditions, and research efforts should continue in this important area of functioning.

References

Aasland, A., & Diseth, T. H. (1999). Can the Harter self-perception profile for adolescents (SPPA) be used as an indicator of psychosocial outcome in adolescents with chronic physical disorders? *European Child and Adolescent Psychiatry, 8*(2), 78–85.

Achenbach, T. M., & Rescorla, L. A. (2000). *Manual for ASEBA preschool forms & profiles.* Burlington, VT: University of Vermont, Research Center for Children, Youth, & Families.

Achenbach, T. M., & Rescorla, L. A. (2001). *Manual for ASEBA school-age forms & profiles.* Burlington, VT: University of Vermont, Research Center for Children, Youth, & Families.

Adams, C. D., Streisand, R. M., Zawacki, T., & Joseph, K. E. (2002). Living with a chronic illness: A measure of social functioning for children and adolescents. *Journal of Pediatric Psychology, 27*(7), 593–605.

Aksnes, G., Diseth, T. H., Helseth, A., Aafos, G., & Emblem, R. (2002). Appendicostomy for antegrade enema: effects on somatic and psychosocial functioning in children with myelomeningocele. *Pediatrics, 109*(3), 484–489.

Alderfer, M. A., Wiebe, D. J., & Hartmann, D. P. (2002). Predictors of the peer acceptance of children with diabetes: Social behavior and disease severity. *Journal of Clinical Psychology in Medical Settings, 9*(2), 121–130.

Ammerman, R. T., Van Hasselt, V. B., & Hersen, M. (1998). Social skills training for children and youth with visual disabilities. In *Handbook of psychological treatment protocols for children and adolescents* (pp. 501–517). Mahwah, NJ: Lawrence Erlbaum Associates Publishers.

Ammerman, R. T., Van Hasselt, V. B., Hersen, M., & Moore, L. E. (1989). Assessment of social skills in visually impaired adolescents and their parents. *Behavioral Assessment, 11*(3), 327–351.

Antia, S. D., & Kreimeyer, K. H. (1996). Social interaction and acceptance of deaf or hard-of-hearing children and their peers: A comparison of social-skills and familiarity-based interventions. *Volta Review, 98*(4), 157–180.

Antia, S. D., & Kreimeyer, K. H. (1997). The generalization and maintenance of the peer social behaviors of young children who are deaf or hard of hearing. *Language, Speech, and Hearing Services in Schools, 28*(1), 59–69.

Antia, S. D., Kreimeyer, K. H., & Eldredge, N. (1994). Promoting social interaction between young children with hearing impairments and their peers. *Exceptional Children, 60*(3), 262–275.

Antia, S. D., & Kriemeyer, K. H. (2003). Peer interactions of deaf and hard-of-hearing children. In M. Marschark & P. E. Spencer (Eds.), *Oxford handbook of deaf studies, language, and education* (pp. 164–176). New York: Oxford University Press.

Apter, A., Aviv, A., Kaminer, Y., Weizman, A., Lerman, P., & Tyano, S. (1991). Behavioral profile and social competence in temporal lobe epilepsy of adolescence. *Journal of the American Academy of Child & Adolescent Psychiatry*, 30, 887–892.

Armstrong, R. W., Rosenbaum, P. L., & King, S. (1992). Self-perceived social function among disabled children in regular classrooms. *Journal of Developmental & Behavioral Pediatrics*, 13(1), 11–16.

Asher, S. R., Hymel, S., & Renshaw, P. D. (1984). Loneliness in children. *Child Development*, 55(4), 1456–1464.

Asher, S. R., Singleton, L. C., Tinsley, B. R., & Hymel, S. (1979). A reliable sociometric measure for preschool children. *Developmental Psychology*, 15(4), 443–444.

Barakat, L. P., & Boyer, B. A. (2008). Pediatric psychology. In B. A. Boyer & M. I. Paharia (Eds.), *Comprehensive handbook of clinical health psychology* (pp. 371–394). Hoboken, NJ: John Wiley & Sons Inc.

Barakat, L. P., Gonzalez, E. R., & Weinberger, B. S. (2007). Using cognitive-behavior group therapy with chronic medical illness. In R. W. Christner, J. L. Stewart, & A. Freeman (Eds.), *Handbook of cognitive-behavior group therapy with children and adolescents: Specific settings and presenting problems* (pp. 427–446). New York: Routledge/Taylor & Francis Group.

Barakat, L. P., Hetzke, J. D., Foley, B., Carey, M. E., Gyato, K., & Phillips, P. C. (2003). Evaluation of a social-skills training group intervention with children treated for brain tumors: A pilot study. *Journal of Pediatric Psychology*, 28(5), 299–307.

Barakat, L. P., Lash, L. A., Lutz, M. J., & Nicolaou, D. C. (2006). Psychosocial adaptation of children and adolescents with sickle cell disease. In R. T. Brown (Ed.), *Comprehensive handbook of childhood cancer and sickle cell disease: a biopsychosocial approach* (pp. 471–495). New York: Oxford University Press.

Barlow, J. H., & Ellard, D. R. (2004). Psycho-educational interventions for children with chronic disease, parents and siblings: An overview of the research evidence base. *Child: Care, Health and Development*, 30(6), 637–645.

Barlow, J. H., & Ellard, D. R. (2006). The psychosocial well-being of children with chronic disease, their parents and siblings: An overview of the research evidence base. *Child: Care, Health and Development*, 32(1), 19–31.

Barton, B., & North, K. (2004). Social skills of children with neurofibromatosis type 1. *Developmental Medicine & Child Neurology*, 46(8), 553–563.

Bauman, L. J., Drotar, D., Leventhal, J. M., Perrin, E. C., & Pless, I. B. (1997). A review of psychosocial interventions for children with chronic health conditions. *Pediatrics*, 100(2), 244–251.

Beale, I. L. (2006). Scholarly literature review: Efficacy of psychological interventions for pediatric chronic illnesses. *Journal of Pediatric Psychology*, 31(5), 437–451.

Bender, H. A., Auciello, D., Morrison, C. E., Macallister, W. S., & Zaroff, C. M. (2008). Comparing the convergent validity and clinical utility of the behavior assessment system for children-parent rating scales and child behavior checklist in children with epilepsy. *Epilepsy & Behavior*, 13(1), 237–242.

Bennett, D. S. (1994). Depression among children with chronic medical problems: A meta-analysis. *Journal of Pediatric Psychology*, 19(2), 149–169.

Bloom, B., & Tonthat, L. (2002). Summary health statistics for U.S. children: National Health Interview Survey, 1997. *Vital and Health Statistics. Series 10, Data from the National Health Survey* (203), 1–46.

Boni, L. C., Brown, R. T., Davis, P. C., Hsu, L., & Hopkins, K. (2001). Social information processing and magnetic resonance imaging in children with sickle cell disease. *Journal of Pediatric Psychology*, 26(5), 309–319.

Bonner, M. J., Hardy, K. K., Willard, V. W., Anthony, K. K., Hood, M., & Gururangan, S. (2008). Social functioning and facial expression recognition in survivors of pediatric brain tumors. *Journal of Pediatric Psychology*, 33(10), 1142–1152.

Boyer, B. A. (2008). Theoretical models of health psychology and the model for integrating medicine and psychology. In B. A. Boyer & M. I. Paharia (Eds.), *Comprehensive handbook of clinical health psychology* (pp. 3–30). Hoboken, NJ: John Wiley & Sons Inc.

Broesterhuizen, M., Van Lieshout, C. F., & Riksen-Walraven, J. M. (1991). Sociometrie door nominatie bij prelinguaal dove adolescenten [Sociometric nominations in prelingually deaf adolescents]. *Pedagogische Studiën*, 68(2), 78–85.

Bronfenbrenner, U. (1979). *The ecology of human development: Experiments by nature and design*. Cambridge, MA: Harvard University Press.

Brown, B. B. (1989). The role of peer groups in adolescents' adjustment to secondary school. In T. J. Berndt & G. W. Ladd (Eds.), *Peer relationships in child development* (pp. 188–215). New York: Jhon Wiley and Sons.

Brown, L. J., Black, D. D., & Downs, J. C. (1984). *School social skills (S³) manual*. New York: Slosson Educational Publications, Inc.

Buhrow, M. M., Hartshorne, T. S., & Bradley-Johnson, S. (1998). Parents' and teachers' ratings of the social skills of elementary-age students who are blind. *Journal of Visual Impairment & Blindness*, 92(7), 503.

Buran, C. F., Sawin, K. J., Brei, T. J., & Fastenau, P. S. (2004). Adolescents with myelomeningocele: activities, beliefs, expectations, and perceptions. *Developmental Medicine & Child Neurology*, 46(4), 244–252.

Burley, S. K. (1996). *Factors influencing the development of social competence in deaf and hard-of-hearing adolescents: An ecological approach*. Lincoln: University of Nebraska.

Caballo, C., & Verdugo, M. Ã. (2007). Social skills assessment of children and adolescents with visual impairment: Identifying relevant skills to improve quality of social relationships. *Psychological Reports*, 100(3), 1101–1106.

Calderon, R., & Greenberg, M. T. (2003). Social and emotional development of deaf children: Family, school, and program effects. In M. Marschark & P. E. Spencer (Eds.), *Oxford handbook of deaf studies, language, and education* (pp. 177–189). New York: Oxford University Press.

Caplan, R., Sagun, J., Siddarth, P., Gurbani, S., Koh, S., Gowrinathan, R., et al. (2005). Social competence in pediatric epilepsy: insights into underlying mechanisms. *Epilepsy & Behavior*, 6(2), 218–228.

Cappelli, M., Daniels, T., Durieux-Smith, A., Mcgrath, P. J., & Neuss, D. (1995). Social development of children with hearing impairments who are integrated into general education classrooms. *Volta Review, 97*(3), 197–208.

Carroll, P., & Shute, R. (2005). School peer victimization of young people with craniofacial conditions: A comparative study. *Psychology, Health & Medicine, 10*(3), 291–304.

Cartledge, G., & Cochran, L. (1996). Social skill self-assessments by adolescents with hearing impairment in residential and public schools. *Remedial & Special Education, 17*(1), 30.

Cartledge, G., Paul, P. V., Jackson, D., & Cochran, L. L. (1991). Teachers' perceptions of the social skills of adolescents with hearing impairment in residential and public school settings. *RASE: Remedial & Special Education, 12*(2), 34.

Casey, F. A., Sykes, D. H., Craig, B. G., Power, R., & Mulholland, H. C. (1996). Behavioral adjustment of children with surgically palliated complex congenital heart disease. *Journal of Pediatric Psychology, 21*, 335–352.

Center, Y., & Ward, J. (1984). Integration of mildly handicapped cerebral palsied children into regular schools. *Exceptional Child, 31*(2), 104–113.

Citrin, W., La Greca, A. M., & Skyler, J. S. (1985). Group intervention in type 1 diabetes mellitus. *Coping with Juvenile Diabetes, 181*–204.

Coie, J. D., Dodge, K. A., & Coppotelli, H. (1982). Dimensions and types of social status: A cross-age perspective. *Developmental Psychology, 18*(4), 557–570.

Cole, D. A., Gondoli, D. M., & Peeke, L. G. (1998). Structure and validity of parent and teacher perceptions of children's competence: A multitrait-multimethod-multigroup investigation. *Psychological Assessment, 10*(3), 241–249.

Colegrove, R., & Huntzinger, R. M. (1994). Academic, behavioral, and social adaptation of boys with hemophilia/HIV disease. *Journal of Pediatric Psychology, 19*, 457–473.

Coyner, L. (1993). Academic success, self-concept, social acceptance and perceived social acceptance for hearing, hard of hearing and deaf students in a mainstream setting. *Journal of the American Deafness and Rehabilitation Association, 27*(2), 13–20.

Craig, H. B. (1965). A sociometric investigation of the self-concept of the deaf child. *American Annals of the Deaf, 110*(4), 456–478.

Crick, N. R., & Dodge, K. A. (1994). A review and reformulation of social information-processing mechanisms in children's social adjustment. *Psychological Bulletin, 115*(1), 74–101.

Cunningham, N. C., Johnson, C. S., Austin, J. K., & Dunn, D. W. (2006). The relationship between seizure variables, demographics, IQ and social competence in adolescents with epilepsy. *Journal of Adolescent Health, 38*(2), 115–115.

Cystic Fibrosis Foundation. (2008). *Patient registry 2006 annual report.* Bethesda, MD: Cystic Fibrosis Foundation.

D'Allura, T. (2002). Enhancing the social interaction skills of preschoolers with visual impairments. *Journal of Visual Impairment & Blindness, 96*(8), 576.

Daltroy, L. H., Larson, M. G., Eaton, H. M., Partridge, A. J., Pless, I. B., & Rogers, M. P. (1992). Psychosocial adjustment in juvenile arthritis. *Journal of Pediatric Psychology, 17*, 277.

de Apodaca, R. F., Watson, J. D., Mueller, J., & Isaacson-Kailes, J. (1985). A sociometric comparison of mainstreamed, orthopedically handicapped high school students and nonhandicapped classmates. *Psychology in the Schools, 22*(1), 95–101.

Die-Trill, M., Bromberg, J., Lavally, B., & Portales, L. A. (1996). Development of social skills in boys with brain tumors: A group approach. *Journal of Psychosocial Oncology, 14*(2), 23–41.

Digirolamo, A. M., Quittner, A. L., Ackerman, V., & Stevens, J. (1997). Identification and assessment of ongoing stressors in adolescents with a chronic illness: an application of the behavior-analytic model. *Journal of Clinical Child Psychology, 26*(1), 53–66.

Drotar, D. (2006a). *Psychological interventions in childhood chronic illness.* Washington, DC: American Psychological Association.

Drotar, D. (2006b). Theoretical models and frameworks for psychological intervention. In *Psychological interventions in childhood chronic illness* (pp. 33–55). Washington, DC: American Psychological Association.

Drotar, D., Stein, R. E. K., & Perrin, E. C. (1995). Methodological issues in using the child behavior checklist and its related instruments in clinical child psychology research. *Journal of Clinical Child & Adolescent Psychology, 24*(2), 184–192.

Ducharme, D. E., & Holborn, S. W. (1997). Programming generalization of social skills in preschool children with hearing impairments. *Journal of Applied Behavior Analysis, 30*(4), 639–651.

Dyck, M. J., & Denver, E. (2003). Can the emotion recognition ability of deaf children be enhanced? A pilot study. *Journal of Deaf Studies and Deaf Education, 8*(3), 348–356.

Eapen, V., Revesz, T., Mpofu, C., & Daradkeh, T. (1999). Self-perception profile in children with cancer: Self vs parent report. *Psychological Reports, 84*(2), 427–432.

Edwards, M., Borzyskowski, M., Cox, A., & Badcock, J. (2004). Neuropathic bladder and intermittent catheterization: social and psychological impact on children and adolescents. *Developmental Medicine & Child Neurology, 46*(3), 168–177.

Eiser, C., Havermans, T., Pancer, M., & Eiser, J. R. (1992). Adjustment to chronic disease in relation to age and gender: Mothers' and fathers' reports of their children's behavior. *Journal of Pediatric Psychology, 17*, 261–275.

Elkin, T. D., & Stoppelbein, L. (2008). Evidence-based treatments for children with chronic illnesses. In R. G. Steele, T. D. Elkin & M. C. Roberts (Eds.), *Handbook of evidence-based therapies for children and adolescents: Bridging science and practice* (pp. 297–309). New York: Springer Science + Business Media.

Elliott, I. M., Lach, L., Kadis, D. S., & Smith, M. L. (2008). Psychosocial outcomes in children two years after epilepsy surgery: Has anything changed? *Epilepsia, 49*(4), 634–641.

Farkas, G. M., Sherick, R. B., Matson, J. L., & Loebig, M. (1981). Social skills training of a blind child through differential reinforcement. *the Behavior Therapist, 4*(2), 24–26.

Fossen, A., Abrahamsen, T. G., & Storm-Mathisen, I. (1998). Psychological outcome in children treated for brain tumor. *Pediatric Hematology and Oncology, 15*(6), 479–488.

Foster, S. L., & Bussman, J. R. (2008). Evidence-based approaches to social skills training with children and adolescents. In R. G. Steele, T. D. Elkin & M. C. Roberts (Eds.), *Handbook of evidence-based therapies for children and adolescents: Bridging science and practice* (pp. 409–427). New York: Springer Science + Business Media.

Friedman, D., Bryant, F. B., & Holmbeck, G. N. (2007). Brief report: Testing the factorial invariance of the CBCL Somatic Complaints scale as a measure of internalizing symptoms for children with and without chronic illness. *Journal of Pediatric Psychology, 32*(5), 512–516.

Furman, W., & Robbins, P. (1985). What's the point: Issues in the selection of treatment objectives. In B. H. Schneider, K. H. Rubin, & J. E. Ledingham (Eds.), *Children's peer relations: Issues in assessment and intervention* (pp. 41–56). New York: Springer-Verlag.

Gleissner, U., Fritz, N. E., Von Lehe, M., Sassen, R., Elger, C. E., & Helmstaedter, C. (2008). The validity of the Child Behavior Checklist for children with epilepsy. *Epilepsy & Behavior, 12*(2), 276–280.

Gortmaker, S. L., & Sappenfield, W. (1984). Chronic childhood disorders: prevalence and impact. *Pediatric Clinics of North America, 31*(1), 3–18.

Gottman, J., Gonso, J., & Rasmussen, B. (1975). Social interaction, social competence, and friendship in children. *Child Development, 46*(3), 709–718.

Graetz, B., & Shute, R. (1995). Assessment of peer relationships in children with asthma. *Journal of Pediatric Psychology, 20*(2), 205–216.

Greenberg, M. T., & Kusché, C. A. (1993). *Promoting social and emotional development in deaf children: The PATHS project.* Seattle, WA: University of Washington Press.

Greenberg, M. T., & Kusché, C. A. (1998). Preventive interventions for school-age deaf children: The PATHS curriculum. *Journal of Deaf Studies and Deaf Education, 3*(1), 49–63.

Gresham, F. M. (1981). Assessment of children's social skills. *Journal of School Psychology, 19*(2), 120–133.

Gresham, F. M., & Elliott, S. N. (1990). *Social skills rating system.* Circle Pines, MN: American Guidance Service.

Gross, A. M., Heimann, L., Shapiro, R., & Schultz, R. M. (1983). Children with diabetes: Social skills training and hemoglobin A-sub-1c levels. *Behavior Modification, 7*(2), 151–164.

Hagborg, W. (1987). Hearing-impaired students and sociometric ratings: An exploratory study. *Volta Review, 89*(4), 221–228.

Harris, J. A., Newcomb, A. F., & Gewanter, H. L. (1991). Psychosocial effects of juvenile rheumatic disease: The family and peer systems as a context for coping. *Arthritis Care and Research, 4*, 123–130.

Harter, S. (1982). The Perceived Competence Scale for Children. *Child Development, 53*(1), 87–97.

Harter, S. (1985a). *Manual for the self-perception profile for children.* Denver, CO: University of Denver.

Harter, S. (1985b). *Manual for the social support scale for children.* Denver, CO: University of Denver.

Harter, S. (1988). *Manual for the self-perception profile for adolescents.* Denver, CO: University of Denver.

Harter, S., & Fischer, K. W. (1999). *The construction of self: A developmental perspective.* New York: Guilford Press.

Harter, S., & Pike, R. (1984). The pictorial scale of perceived competence and social acceptance for young children. *Child Development, 55*(6), 1969.

Hauser, P. C., Wills, K. E., & Isquith, P. K. (2006). Hard-of-hearing, deafness, and being deaf. In J. E. Farmer, J. Donders, & S. Warschausky (Eds.), *Treating neurodevelopmental disabilities: Clinical research and practice* (pp. 119–131). New York: Guilford Press.

Heneman-De Boer, J. A., De Haan, M., & Beemer, F. A. (1999). Behavioural and personality aspects of 37 VCFS children. *Genetic Counseling, 10*(1), 110.

Hoffman, R. G., Rodrigue, J. R., Andres, J., & Novak, D. A. (1995). Moderating effects of family functioning on the social adjustment of children with liver disease. *Children's Health Care, 24*, 107–117.

Holmes, C. S., Respess, D., Greer, T., & Frentz, J. (1998). Behavior problems in children with diabetes: Disentangling possible scoring confounds on the child behavior checklist. *Journal of Pediatric Psychology, 23*(3), 179–185.

Hommeyer, J. S., Holmbeck, G. N., Wills, K. E., & Coers, S. (1999). Condition severity and psychosocial functioning in pre-adolescents with spina bifida: Disentangling proximal functional status and distal adjustment outcomes. *Journal of Pediatric Psychology, 24*(6), 499–509.

House, J. S. (1981). *Work stress and social support.* Reading, MA: Addison-Wesley Publishing Company.

Howe, G. W., Feinstein, C., Reiss, D., Molock, S., & Berger, K. (1993). Adolescent adjustment to chronic physical disorders—I. Comparing neurological and non-neurological conditions. *Journal of Child Psychology & Psychiatry & Allied Disciplines, 34*(7), 1153–1171.

Hunter, S. J., Griffin-Shirley, N., & Noll, L. (2006). Visual impairments. In J. E. Farmer, J. Donders, & S. Warschausky (Eds.), *Treating neurodevelopmental disabilities: Clinical research and practice* (pp. 132–146). New York: Guilford Press.

Huurre, T., & Aro, H. (2000). The psychosocial well-being of Finnish adolescents with visual impairments versus those with chronic conditions and those with no disabilities. *Journal of Visual Impairment & Blindness, 94*(10), 625–637.

Jakovljevic, V., & Martinovic, Z. (2006). Social competence of children and adolescents with epilepsy. *Seizure, 15*(7), 528–532.

Jindal-Snape, D. (2004). Generalization and maintenance of social skills of children with visual impairments: Self-evaluation and the role of feedback. *Journal of Visual Impairment & Blindness, 98*(8), 470–483.

Jindal-Snape, D. (2005a). Self-evaluation and recruitment of feedback for enhanced social interaction by a student with visual impairment. *Journal of Visual Impairment & Blindness, 99*(8), 486–498.

Jindal-Snape, D. (2005b). Use of feedback from sighted peers in promoting social interaction skills. *Journal of Visual Impairment & Blindness, 99*(7), 403–412.

Jindal-Snape, D., Kato, M., & Maekawa, H. (1998). Using self-evaluation procedures to maintain social skills in a child who is blind. *Journal of Visual Impairment & Blindness, 92*(5), 362–366.

Johnson, N. S., Saal, H. M., Lovell, A. M., & Schorry, E. K. (1999). Social and emotional problems in children with neurofibromatosis type 1: Evidence and proposed interventions. *Journal of Pediatrics, 134,* 767.

Kaplan, R. M., Chadwick, M. W., & Schimmel, L. E. (1985). Social learning intervention to promote metabolic control in type I diabetes mellitus: pilot experiment results. *Diabetes Care, 8*(2), 152.

Kapp-Simon, K. A., & Mcguire, D. E. (1997). Observed social interaction patterns in adolescents with and without craniofacial conditions. *Cleft Palate-Craniofacial Journal, 34,* 380–384.

Kapp-Simon, K. A., Mcguire, D. E., & Simon, D. J. (2005). Addressing quality of life issues in adolescents: Social skills interventions. *Cleft Palate-Craniofacial Journal, 42*(1), 45–50.

Kapp-Simon, K. A., Simon, D., & Kristovich, S. (1992). Self-perception, social skills, adjustment, and inhibition in young adolescents with craniofacial anomalies. *Cleft Palate-Craniofacial Journal, 29,* 352–356.

Katz, E. R., Rubinstein, C. L., Hubert, N. C., & Blew, A. (1988). School and social reintegration of children with cancer. *Journal of Psychosocial Oncology, 6*(3), 123–140.

Kazak, A. E. (1989). Families of chronically ill children: A systems and social-ecological model of adaptation and challenge. *Journal of Consulting and Clinical Psychology, 57*(1), 25–30.

Kennedy, P., & Bruininks, R. H. (1974). Social status of hearing impaired children in regular classrooms. *Exceptional Children, 40*(5), 336–342.

Kibby, M. Y., Tyc, V. L., & Mulhern, R. K. (1998). Effectiveness of psychological intervention for children and adolescents with chronic medical illness: A meta-analysis. *Clinical Psychology Review, 18*(1), 105–117.

King, G., Law, M., Hanna, S., King, S., Hurley, P., Rosenbaum, P., et al. (2006). Predictors of the leisure and recreation participation of children with physical disabilities: A structural equation modeling analysis. *Children's Health Care, 35*(3), 209–234.

King, G., Mcdougall, J., Dewit, D., Hong, S., Miller, L., Offord, D., et al. (2005). Pathways to children's academic performance and prosocial behaviour: Roles of physical health status, environmental, family, and child factors. *International Journal of Disability, Development and Education, 52*(4), 313–344.

King, G. A., Law, M., King, S., Hurley, P., Hanna, S., Kertoy, M., et al. (2007). Measuring children's participation in recreation and leisure activities: Construct validation of the CAPE and PAC. *Child: Care, Health and Development, 33*(1), 28–39.

King, G. A., Specht, J. A., Schultz, I., Warr-Leeper, G., Redekop, W., & Risebrough, N. (1997). Social skills training for withdrawn unpopular children with physical disabilities: A preliminary evaluation. *Rehabilitation Psychology, 42*(1), 47–60.

Kluwin, T. N., Stinson, M. S., & Colarossi, G. M. (2002). Social processes and outcomes of in-school contact between deaf and hearing peers. *Journal of Deaf Studies and Deaf Education, 7*(3), 200–213.

Koot, H. M., & Wallander, J. L. (2001). *Quality of life in child and adolescent illness: Concepts, methods, and findings.* Philadelphia, PA: Brunner-Routledge.

Kullgren, K. A., Morris, R. D., Morris, M. K., & Krawiecki, N. (2003). Risk factors associated with long-term social and behavioral problems among children with brain tumors. *Journal of Psychosocial Oncology, 21*(1), 1–15.

Kurkjian, J. A., & Evans, I. M. (1988). Effects of sign language instruction on social interaction between hearing-impaired and normal-hearing children. *Child & Family Behavior Therapy, 10*(2), 121–134.

Kuyken, W., Orley, J., Hudelson, P., & Sartorius, N. (1994). Quality of life assessment across cultures. *International Journal of Mental Health, 23*(2), 5–27.

La Greca, A. M. (1990). Social consequences of pediatric conditions: Fertile area for future investigation and intervention. *Journal of Pediatric Psychology, 15*(3), 285.

La Greca, A. M. (1992). Peer influences in pediatric chronic illness: An update. *Journal of Pediatric Psychology, 17*(6), 775–784.

La Greca, A. M., Bearman, K. J., & Moore, H. (2002). Peer relations of youth with pediatric conditions and health risks: Promoting social support and healthy lifestyles. *Journal of Developmental & Behavioral Pediatrics, 23*(4), 271–280.

La Greca, A. M., Bearman, K. J., & Moore, H. (2004). Peer relations. In R. T. Brown (Ed.), *Handbook of pediatric psychology in school settings* (pp. 657–678). Mahwah, NJ: Lawrence Erlbaum Associates.

La Greca, A. M., & Thompson, K. M. (1998). Family and friend support for adolescents with diabetes. *Análise Psicológica, 1*(16), 101–113.

Lavigne, J. V., & Faier-Routman, J. F. (1992). Psychological adjustment to pediatric physical disorders: A meta-analytic review. *Journal of Pediatric Psychology, 17,* 133–157.

Lavigne, J. V., & Faier-Routman, J. F. (1993). Correlates of psychological adjustment to pediatric physical disorders: A meta-analytic review and comparison with existing models. *Journal of Developmental & Behavioral Pediatrics, 14*(2), 117–123.

LeBovidge, J. S., Lavigne, J. V., Donenberg, G. R., & Miller, M. L. (2003). Psychological adjustment of children and adolescents with chronic arthritis: a meta-analytic review. *Journal of Pediatric Psychology, 28*(1), 29–39.

Lemanek, K. L., Jones, M. L., & Lieberman, B. (2000). Mothers of children with spina bifida: Adaptational and stress processing. *Children's Health Care, 29*(1), 19–35.

Lemanek, K. L., Williamson, D. A., Gresham, F. M., & Jensen, B. J. (1986). Social skills training with hearing-impaired children and adolescents. *Behavior Modification, 10*(1), 55–71.

Lytle, R. R., Johnson, R. C., & Smith, D. (1987). A social skills training program for deaf adolescents. *Perspectives for Teachers of the Hearing Impaired, 6,* 19–22.

Macklin, G. F., & Matson, J. L. (1985). A comparison of social behaviors among nonhandicapped and hearing impaired children. *Behavioral Disorders, 11*(1), 60–65.

Markovits, H., Gariépy, L., Huet, D., & Strayer, F. F. (1982). Une étude comparée du fonctionnement social des jeunes enfants handicapés de la vue [A comparative study of social functioning of young children with disabilities of sight]. *Apprentissage et Socialisation, 5*(2), 87–97.

Masten, A. S., Morison, P., & Pellegrini, D. S. (1985). A revised class play method of peer assessment. *Developmental Psychology, 21*(3), 523–533.

Matson, J. L., Esveldt-Dawson, K., & Kazdin, A. E. (1983). Validation of methods for assessing social skills in children. *Journal of Clinical Child Psychology, 12*(2), 174.

Matson, J. L., Heinze, A., Helsel, W. J., Kapperman, G., & Rotatori, A. F. (1986). Assessing social behaviors in the visually handicapped: The Matson evaluation of social skills with youngsters (MESSY). *Journal of Clinical Child & Adolescent Psychology, 15*(1), 78–87.

Matson, J. L., Macklin, G. F., & Helsel, W. J. (1985). Psychometric properties of the Matson evaluation of social skills with youngsters (MESSY) with emotional problems and self concept in deaf children. *Journal of Behavior Therapy and Experimental Psychiatry, 16*(2), 117–123.

Matson, J. L., Rotarori, A. F., & Helsel, W. J. (1983). Development of a rating scale to measure social skills in children: The Matson evaluation of social skills with youngsters (MESSY). *Behaviour Research and Therapy, 21*(4), 335–340.

Matson, J. L., & Wilkins, J. (2008). Psychometric testing methods for children's social skills. *Research in Developmental Disabilities*, doi:10.1016/j.ridd.2008.04.002.

Mcfall, R. M. (1982). A review and reformulation of the concept of social skills. *Behavioral Assessment, 4*(1), 1–33.

McPherson, M., Arango, P., Fox, H., Lauver, C., Mcmanus, M., Newacheck, P. W., et al. (1998). A new definition of children with special health care needs. *Pediatrics, 102*(1), 137–140.

McQuaid, E. L., Kopel, S. J., & Nassau, J. H. (2001). Behavioral adjustment in children with asthma: A meta-analysis. *Journal of Developmental and Behavioral Pediatrics, 22*(6), 430–439.

Meijer, S. A., Sinnema, G., Bijstra, J. O., Mellenbergh, G. J., & Wolters, W. H. G. (2000a). Peer interaction in adolescents with a chronic illness. *Personality and Individual Differences, 29*(5), 799–813.

Meijer, S. A., Sinnema, G., Bijstra, J. O., Mellenbergh, G. J., & Wolters, W. H. G. (2000b). Social functioning in children with a chronic illness. *Journal of Child Psychology and Psychiatry (formerly Journal of Child Psychology and Psychiatry and Allied Disciplines), 41*(3), 309–317.

Meijer, S. A., Sinnema, G., Bijstra, J. O., Mellenbergh, G. J., & Wolters, W. H. G. (2002). Coping styles and locus of control as predictors for psychological adjustment of adolescents with a chronic illness. *Social Science & Medicine, 54*(9), 1453–1461.

Midence, K., Mcmanus, C., Fuggle, P., & Davies, S. (1996). Psychological adjustment and family functioning in a group of British children with sickle cell disease: Preliminary empirical findings and a meta-analysis. *British Journal of Clinical Psychology, 35*(3), 439–450.

Miller, J. J., III (1993). Psychosocial factors related to rheumatic diseases in childhood. *Journal Of Rheumatology, 20*(Suppl. 38), 1–11.

Moss, H. A., Bose, S., Wolters, P. L., & Brouwers, P. (1998). A preliminary study of factors associated with psychological adjustment and disease course in school-age children infected with the human immunodeficiency virus. *Journal of Developmental & Behavioral Pediatrics, 19*(1), 18–25.

Moss, H. A., Wolters, P. L., Brouwers, P., Hendricks, M. L., & Pizzo, P. A. (1996). Impaired of expressive behavior in pediatric HIV-infected patients with evidence of CNS disease. *Journal of Pediatric Psychology, 21*(3), 379–400.

Mulhern, R. K., Carpentieri, S., Shema, S., Stone, P., & Fairclough, D. (1993). Factors associated with social and behavioral problems among children recently diagnosed with brain tumor. *Journal of Pediatric Psychology, 18*(3), 339–350.

Mulhern, R. K., Wasserman, A. L., Friedman, A. G., & Fairclough, D. (1989). Social competence and behavioral adjustment of children who are long-term survivors of cancer. *Pediatrics, 83*(1), 18.

Naar-King, S., Ellis, D. A., & Frey, M. A. (2004). *Assessing children's well-being: A handbook of measures.* Mahwah, NJ: Lawrence Erlbaum Associates Publishers.

Nassau, J. H., & Drotar, D. (1995). Social competence in children with IDDM and asthma: Child, teacher, and parent reports of children's social adjustment, social performance, and social skills. *Journal of Pediatric Psychology, 20*, 187.

Nassau, J. H., & Drotar, D. (1997). Social competence among children with central nervous system-related chronic health conditions: A review. *Journal of Pediatric Psychology, 22*(6), 771–793.

Newacheck, P. W., Budetti, P. P., & Halfon, N. (1986). Trends in activity-limiting chronic conditions among children. *American Journal of Public Health, 76*(2), 178–184.

Newacheck, P. W., Strickland, B., Shonkoff, J. P., Perrin, J. M., Mcpherson, M., Mcmanus, M., et al. (1998). An epidemiologic profile of children with special health care needs. *Pediatrics, 102*(1), 117–123.

Newacheck, P. W., & Taylor, W. R. (1992). Childhood chronic illness: prevalence, severity, and impact. *American Journal of Public Health, 82*(3), 364–371.

Newby, W. L., Brown, R. T., Pawletko, T. M., Gold, S. H., & Whitt, K. (2000). Social skills and psychological adjustment of child and adolescent cancer survivors. *Psycho-Oncology, 9*, 113.

Noll, R. B., Bukowski, W., Davies, W., Koontz, K., & Kulakrni, R. (1993). Adjustment in the peer system of children with cancer: A two-year follow-up study. *Journal of Pediatric Psychology, 18*, 351–364.

Noll, R. B., Bukowski, W., Rogosch, F., Leroy, S., & Kulkarni, R. (1990). Social interactions between children with cancer and their peers: Teacher ratings. *Journal of Pediatric Psychology, 15*, 43–56.

Noll, R. B., Gartstein, M. A., Vannatta, K., Correll, J., Bukowski, W. M., & Davies, W. H. (1999). Social, emotional, and behavioral functioning of children with cancer. *Pediatrics, 103*, 71–78.

Noll, R. B., Kozloqski, K., Gerhardt, C., Vannatta, K., Taylor, J., & Passo, M. (2000). Social, emotional, and behavioral functioning in children with juvenile rheumatoid arthritis. *Arthritis and Rheumatism, 43*, 1387.

Noll, R. B., & Kupst, M. J. (2007). Commentary: The psychological impact of pediatric cancer hardiness, the exception or the rule? *Journal of Pediatric Psychology, 32*(9), 1089–1098.

Noll, R. B., Leroy, W. M., Bukowski, W. M., Rogosh, F. A., Davies, W. H., & Rogosch, F. A. (1991). Peer relationships and adjustment in children with cancer. *Journal of Pediatric Psychology, 16*, 307–326.

Noll, R. B., Nannatta, K., Koontz, K., Kalinyak, K., Bukowski, W. M., & Davies, W. H. (1996). Peer relationships and emotional well-being of youngsters with sickle cell disease. *Child Development, 67*, 423–436.

Noll, R. B., Reiter-Purtill, J., Moore, B. D., Schorry, E. K., Lovell, A. M., Vannatta, K., et al. (2007). Social, emotional, and behavioral functioning of children with NF1. *American Journal of Medical Genetics, Part A, 143*(19), 2261–2273.

Nunes, T., Pretzlik, U., & Olsson, J. (2001). Deaf children's social relationships in mainstream schools. *Deafness & Education International, 3*(3), 123–136.

Oates, R. K., Turnbull, J. A. B., Simpson, J. M., & Cartmill, T. B. (1994). Parent and teacher perceptions of child behaviour following cardiac surgery. *Acta Paediatrica, International Journal of Paediatrics, 83*(12), 1303–1307.

Parker, J. G., & Asher, S. R. (1993). Beyond group acceptance: Friendship and friendship quality as distinct dimensions of peer adjustment. In W. H. Jones & D. Perlman (Eds.), *Advances in personal relationships* (Vol. 4, pp. 261–294). London: Kinglsey.

Pelletier, L., & Lepage, L. (1999). L'ajustement psychosocial à l'asthme et au diabète juvénile chez des enfants d'age scolaire [Psychological adjustment to asthma and juvenile diabetes in school age children]. *Canadian Journal of Community Mental Health, 18*(1), 123–144.

Pendley, J. S., Dahlquist, L. M., & Dryer, Z. (1997). Body image and psychosocial adjustment in adolescent cancer survivors. *Journal of Pediatric Psychology, 22*, 29–43.

Perrin, E. C., Ayoub, C. C., & Willett, J. B. (1993). In the eyes of the beholder: Family and maternal influences on perceptions of adjustment of children with a chronic illness. *Journal of Developmental and Behavioral Pediatrics, 14*(2), 94.

Perrin, E. C., Newacheck, P. W., Pless, I. B., Drotar, D., Gortmaker, S. L., Leventhal, J., et al. (1993). Issues involved in the definition and classification of chronic health conditions. *Pediatrics, 91*(4), 787–793.

Perrin, E. C., Stein, R. E. K., & Drotar, D. (1991). Cautions in using the Child Behavior Checklist: Observations based on research about children with chronic illness. *Journal of Pediatric Psychology, 16*, 411.

Perrin, J. M., Bloom, S. R., & Gortmaker, S. L. (2007). The increase of childhood chronic conditions in the United States. *Journal of the American Medical Association, 297*(24), 2755–2759.

Perrin, J. M., & Hicks, P. J. (2008). The future of disability in America: Review of the institute of medicine report. *Ambulatory Pediatrics, 8*(2), 71–72.

Plante, W. A., Lobato, D., & Engel, R. (2001). Review of group interventions for pediatric chronic conditions. *Journal of Pediatric Psychology, 26*(7), 435–453.

Pless, I. B., & Douglas, J. W. (1971). Chronic illness in childhood. I. Epidemiological and clinical characteristics. *Pediatrics, 47*(2), 405–414.

Pless, I. B., & Pinkerton, P. (1975). *Chronic childhood disorders: Promoting patterns of adjustment*. St. Louis, MO: Mosby-Year Book.

Pope, A., & Ward, J. (1997a). Factors associated with peer social competence in preadolescents with craniofacial anomalies. *Journal of Pediatric Psychology, 22*, 455–469.

Pope, A., & Ward, J. (1997b). Self-perceived facial appearance and psychosocial adjustment in preadolescents with craniofacial anomalies. *Cleft Palate-Craniofacial Journal, 34*, 396–401.

Rasing, E. J., & Duker, P. C. (1992). Effects of a multifaceted training procedure on the acquisition and generalization of social behaviors in language-disabled deaf children. *Journal of Applied Behavior Analysis, 25*(3), 723–734.

Rasing, E. J., & Duker, P. C. (1993). Acquisition and generalization of social behaviors in language-disabled deaf children. *American Annals of the Deaf, 138*(4), 362–369.

Raymond, K. L., & Matson, J. L. (1989). Social skills in the hearing impaired. *Journal of Clinical Child Psychology, 18*(3), 247–258.

Reiter-Purtill, J., Gerhardt, C. A., Vannatta, K., Passo, M. H., & Noll, R. B. (2003). A controlled longitudinal study of the social functioning of children with juvenile rheumatoid arthritis. *Journal of Pediatric Psychology, 28*, 17.

Reiter-Purtill, J., Noll, R. B., & Roberts, M. C. (2003). Peer relationships of children with chronic illness. In *Handbook of pediatric psychology* (3rd ed., pp. 176–197). New York: Guilford Press.

Reynolds, C. R., & Kamphaus, R. W. (2002). *The clinician's guide to the behavior assessment system for children (BASC)*. New York: Guilford Press.

Ridsdale, J., & Thompson, D. (2002). Perceptions of social adjustment of hearing-impaired pupils in an integrated secondary school unit. *Educational Psychology in Practice, 18*(1), 21–34.

Rodrigue, J. R., Streisand, R., Banko, C. G., Kedar, A., & Pitel, P. A. (1996). Social functioning, peer relations, and internalizing and externalizing problems among youths with sickle cell disease. *Children's Health Care, 25*, 37–52.

Rolland, J. S. (1984). Toward a psychosocial typology of chronic and life-threatening illness. *Family Systems Medicine, 2*(3), 245–262.

Rolland, J. S. (1987). Chronic illness and the life cycle: A conceptual framework. *Family Process, 26*(2), 203–221.

Rosenblum, L. P. (2000). Perceptions of the impact of visual impairment on the lives of adolescents. *Journal of Visual Impairment & Blindness, 94*(7), 434.

Russo, R. N., Goodwin, E. J., Miller, M. D., Haan, E. A., Connell, T. M., & Crotty, M. (2008a). Self-esteem, self-concept, and quality of life in children with hemiplegic cerebral palsy. *The Journal of Pediatrics, 153*(4), 473–477. e 2.

Russo, R. N., Miller, M. D., Haan, E., Cameron, I. D., & Crotty, M. (2008b). Pain characteristics and their association with quality of life and self-concept in children with hemiplegic cerebral palsy identified from a population register. *Clinical Journal of Pain, 24*(4), 335–342.

Sacks, S., & Gaylord-Ross, R. (1989). Peer-mediated and teacher-directed social skills training for visually impaired students. *Behavior Therapy*, 20(4), 619–640.

Schloss, P. J., Selinger, J., Goldsmith, L., & Morrow, L. (1983). Classroom-based approaches to developing social competence among hearing-impaired youth. *American Annals of the Deaf*, 128(6), 842–850.

Schloss, P. J., Smith, M. A., & Schloss, C. N. (1984). Empirical analysis of a card game designed to promote consumer-related social competence among hearing-impaired youth. *American Annals of the Deaf*, 129(5), 417–423.

Schuman, W. B., & La Greca, A. M. (1999). Social correlates of chronic illness. In R. T. Brown (Ed.), *Cognitive aspects of chronic illness in children* (pp. 289–311).

Schwering, K. L., Febo-Mandl, F., Finkenauer, C., Rime, B., Hayez, J. Y., & Otte, J. B. (1997). Psychological and social adjustment after pediatric liver transplantation as a function of age at surgery and of time elapsed since transplantation. *Pediatric Transplantation*, 1(2), 138–145.

Sharma, S., Sigafoos, J., & Carroll, A. (2000). Social skills assessment of Indian children with visual impairments. *Journal of Visual Impairment & Blindness*, 94(3), 172–176.

Shelby, M. D., Nagle, R. J., Barnett-Queen, L. L., Quattlebaum, P. D., & Wuori, D. F. (1998). Parental reports of psychosocial adjustment and social competence in child survivors of acute lymphocytic leukemia. *Children's Health Care*, 27(2), 113–129.

Shute, R., Mccarthy, K. R., & Roberts, R. (2007). Predictors of social competence in young adolescents with craniofacial anomalies. *International Journal of Clinical and Health Psychology*, 7(3), 595–613.

Sisson, L. A., Van Hasselt, V. B., Hersen, M., & Strain, P. S. (1985). Peer interventions: Increasing social behaviors in multihandicapped children. *Behavior Modification*, 9(3), 293–321.

Smith, M. A., Schloss, P. J., & Schloss, C. N. (1984). An empirical analysis of a social skills training program used with hearing impaired youths. *Journal of the American Deafness and Rehabilitation Association*, 18(2), 7–14.

Solans, M., Pane, S., Estrada, M. D., Serra-Sutton, V., Berra, S., Herdman, M., et al. (2008). Health-related quality of life measurement in children and adolescents: A systematic review of generic and disease-specific instruments. *Value in Health*, 11(4), 742–764.

Spirito, A., Delawyer, D. D., & Stark, L. J. (1991). Peer relations and social adjustment of chronically ill children and adolescents. *Clinical Psychology Review*, 11, 539.

Spirito, A., Stark, L. J., Cobiella, C., Drigan, R., Androkites, A., & Hewett, K. (1990). Social adjustment of children successfully treated for cancer. *Journal of Pediatric Psychology*, 15(3), 359–371.

Stein, R. E. K., Bauman, L. J., Westbrook, L. E., Coupey, S. M., & Ireys, H. T. (1993). Framework for identifying children who have chronic conditions: The case for a new definition. *Journal of Pediatrics*, 122(3), 342–347.

Stein, R. E. K., & Jessop, D. J. (1982). A noncategorical approach to chronic childhood illness. *Public Health Reports*, 97(4), 354–362.

Storch, E., Keeley, M., Merlo, L., Jacob, M., Correia, C., & Weinstein, D. (2008). Psychosocial functioning in youth with glycogen storage disease type I. *Journal of Pediatric Psychology*, 33(7), 728.

Streisand, R., & Michaelidis, T. (2007). Assessment in pediatric health. In S. R. Smith & L. Handler (Eds.), *The clinical assessment of children and adolescents: A practitioner's handbook* (pp. 507–525). Mahwah, NJ: Lawrence Erlbaum Associates Publishers.

Suárez, M. (2000). Promoting social competence in deaf students: The effect of an intervention program. *Journal of Deaf Studies and Deaf Education*, 5(4), 323–333.

Thill, A. D. W., Holmbeck, G., Bryant, F., Nelson, C., Skocic, A., & Uli, N. (2003). Assessing the factorial invariance of Harter's self-concept measures: Comparing preadolescents with and without spina bifida using child, parent, and teacher report. *Journal of Personality Assessment*, 81(2), 111–122.

Thomas, P. D., Warschausky, S., Golin, R., & Meiners, K. (2008). Direct parenting methods to facilitate the social functioning of children with cerebral palsy. *Journal of Developmental and Physical Disabilities*, 20(2), 167–174.

Thomas, P. J., & Warschausky, S. (2006). Social integration of children with physical disabilities. In J. E. Farmer, J. Donders & S. Warschausky (Eds.), *Treating neurodevelopmental disabilities: Clinical research and practice* (pp. 234–248). New York: Guilford Press.

Thompson, R. J., Jr., & Gustafson, K. E. (1996a). *Adaptation to chronic childhood illness*. Washington, DC: American Psychological Association.

Thompson, R. J., Jr., & Gustafson, K. E. (1996b). Social adjustment, peer relationships, and school performance. In R. J. Thompson Jr. & K. E. Gustafson (Eds.), *Adaptation to chronic childhood illness*. Washington, DC: American Psychological Association.

Thompson, R. J., Jr., Gustafson, K. E., Hamlett, K. W., & Spock, A. (1992). Stress, coping, and family functioning in the psychological adjustment of mothers of children and adolescents with cystic fibrosis. *Journal of Pediatric Psychology*, 17(5), 573–585.

Tin, L. G., & Teasdale, G. R. (1985). An observational study of the social adjustment of spina bifida children in integrated settings. *The British Journal of Educational Psychology*, 55(Pt 1), 81–83.

Tornqvist, J., Van Broeck, N., Finkenauer, C., Rosati, R., Schwering, K. L., Hayez, J. Y., et al. (1999). Long-term psychosocial adjustment following pediatric liver transplantation. *Pediatric Transplantation*, 3(2), 115–125.

Tse, E., Hamiwka, L., Sherman, E. M. S., & Wirrell, E. (2007). Social skills problems in children with epilepsy: Prevalence, nature and predictors. *Epilepsy & Behavior*, 11(4), 499–505.

van der Lee, J. H., Mokkink, L. B., Grootenhuis, M. A., Heymans, H. S., & Offringa, M. (2007). Definitions and measurement of chronic health conditions in childhood. *Journal of the American Medical Association*, 297(24), 2741–2751.

van der Veen, W. J. (2003). De kleine epidemiologische transitie: Verdere daling van de zuigelingensterfte door medische interventie rond zwangerschap en bevalling, maar geen daling van handicaps op de kinderleeftijd [The small epidemiologic transition: further decrease in infant mortality due to medical intervention during pregnancy and childbirth, yet no decrease in childhood disabilities]. *Nederlands tijdschrift voor geneeskunde*, 147(9), 378–381.

Van Hasselt, V. B., Ammerman, R. T., Hersen, M., Reigel, D. H., & Rowley, F. L. (1991). Assessment of social skills and problem behaviors in young children with spina bifida. *Journal of Developmental & Physical Disabilities, 3*, 69–80.

Van Hasselt, V. B., Hersen, M., & Kazdin, A. E. (1985). Assessment of social skills in visually-handicapped adolescents. *Behaviour Research and Therapy, 23*(1), 53–63.

Van Hasselt, V. B., Hersen, M., Kazdin, A. E., Simon, J., & Mastantuono, A. K. (1983). Training blind adolescents in social skills. *Journal of Visual Impairment & Blindness, 77*(5), 199–203.

Vannatta, K., Gerhardt, C. A., Wells, R. J., & Noll, R. B. (2007). Intensity of CNS treatment for pediatric cancer: Prediction of social outcomes in survivors *Pediatric Blood and Cancer, 49*(5), 716–722.

Vannatta, K., Zeller, M., Noll, R. B., & Koontz, K. (1998). Social functioning of children surviving bone marrow transplantation. *Journal of Pediatric Psychology, 23*, 169–178.

Varni, J. W., Katz, E. R., Colegrove, R., & Dolgin, M. (1993). The impact of social skills training on the adjustment of children with newly diagnosed cancer. *Journal of Pediatric Psychology, 18*(6), 751–767.

Varni, J. W., Seid, M., & Kurtin, P. S. (2001). PedsQL™ 4.0: Reliability and Validity of the Pediatric Quality of Life Inventory™ Version 4.0 Generic Core Scales in Healthy and Patient Populations. *Medical Care, 39*(8), 800–812.

Verdugo, M. A., & Caballo, C. (1996). Evaluación de las habilidades sociales de alumnos con deficiencias visuales. Un estudio de investigación [Evaluation of the social skills of students with visual deficiencies: An investigation]. *Análise Psicológica, 14*(2), 313–323.

Vostanis, P., Hayes, M., Feu, M., & Warren, J. (1997). Detection of behavioural and emotional problems in deaf children and adolescents: comparison of two rating scales. *Child: Care, Health and Development, 23*(3), 233–246.

Wallander, J. L., Feldman, W. S., & Varni, J. W. (1989). Physical status and psychosocial adjustment in children with spina bifida. *Journal of Pediatric Psychology, 14*(1), 89–102.

Wallander, J. L., Schmitt, M., & Koot, H. M. (2001). Quality of life measurement in children and adolescents: Issues, instruments, and applications. *Journal of Clinical Psychology, 57*(4), 571–585.

Wallander, J. L., Thompson, R. J., Jr., & Alriksson-Schmidt, A. (2003). Psychosocial adjustment of children with chronic physical conditions. In M. C. Roberts (Ed.), *Handbook of pediatric psychology* (3rd ed., pp. 141–158). New York: Guilford Press.

Wallander, J. L., & Varni, J. W. (1989). Social support and adjustment in chronically ill and handicapped children. *American Journal of Community Psychology, 17*(2), 185–201.

Wallander, J. L., & Varni, J. W. (1992). Adjustment in children with chronic physical disorders: Programmatic research on a disability-stress-coping model. In A. M. La Greca, L. J. Siegel, J. L. Wallander, & C. E. Walker (Eds.), *Stress and coping in child health* (pp. 279–298). New York: Guilford Press.

Wallander, J. L., Varni, J. W., Babani, L., Banis, H., & Wilcox, K. (1989). Family resources as resistant factors for psychological development in chronically ill and handicapped children. *Journal of Pediatric Psychology, 14*, 157–173.

Wallander, J. L., Varni, J. W., Babani, L., Banis, H. T., & Wilcox, K. T. (1988). Children with chronic physical disorders: Maternal reports of their psychological adjustment. *Journal of Pediatric Psychology, 13*(2), 197–212.

Wauters, L. N., & Knoors, H. (2008). Social integration of deaf children in inclusive settings. *Journal of Deaf Studies and Deaf Education, 13*(1), 21–36.

Wysocki, T. (2006). Behavioral assessment and intervention in pediatric diabetes. *Behavior Modification, 30*(1), 72–92.

Yarnall, G. D. (1979). Developing eye contact in a visually impaired, deaf child. *Education of the Visually Handicapped, 11*(2), 56–59.

Yeates, K. O., Bigler, E. D., Dennis, M., Gerhardt, C. A., Rubin, K. H., Stancin, T., et al. (2007). Social outcomes in childhood brain disorder: A heuristic integration of social neuroscience and developmental psychology. *Psychological Bulletin, 133*(3), 535–556.

Zbikowski, S., & Cohen, R. (1998). Parent and peer evaluations of the social competence of children with mild asthma. *Journal of Applied Developmental Psychology, 19*, 249–265.

Zeller, M., Vannatta, K., Schafer, J., & Noll, R. B. (2003). Behavioral reputation: A cross-age perspective. *Developmental Psychology, 39*(1), 129–139.

Index